BIOPSY INTERPRETATION

OF THE LIVER

BIOPSY INTERPRETATION SERIES

BIOPSY INTERPRETATION
OF THE LIVER

Michael S. Torbenson, MD
Professor
Department of Laboratory Medicine and Pathology
Mayo Clinic
Rochester, Minnesota

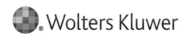
Wolters Kluwer

Philadelphia • Baltimore • New York • London
Buenos Aires • Hong Kong • Sydney • Tokyo

Acquisitions Editor: Nicole Dernosky
Development Editor: Ariel S. Winter
Editorial Coordinator: Remington Fernando
Editorial Assistant: Maribeth Wood
Marketing Manager: Kirsten Watrud
Production Project Manager: Justin Wright
Design Coordinator: Stephen Druding
Manufacturing Coordinator: Beth Welsh
Prepress Vendor: TNQ Technologies

4th edition

Copyright © 2022 Wolters Kluwer.

9 8 7 6 5 4 3 2 1

Printed in Mexico

Library of Congress Cataloging-in-Publication Data

ISBN-13: 978-1-975157-29-6

Cataloging in Publication data available on request from publisher.

LWW.com

PREFACE

I hope this book will become a well-used resource for you. I like liver pathology very much and have a fine collection of liver pathology books, a collection that has become quite extensive after so many years. All have strengths and some books are truly excellent. I can easily tell which books I have found most useful—it's the few books that sit permanently on my desk, near at hand. They have dog-eared pages, well-creased spines, and occasional stains from spilled diet coke. It is my hope that this book will appear similar, after some time in your office.

Many liver biopsies benefit from being shared with colleagues and trainees, shared because they are hard, shared because they are interesting, or shared because they have teaching points. Opportunities for sharing, when taken, strengthen both parties and improve patient care. I am grateful for the many cases shared with me by outstanding colleagues in places where I have worked. I am also very grateful to the pathologists who have sent consults over the years; it has been a privilege to review them, and I have learned much from interacting with pathology and clinical colleagues around the world.

I am also indebted through my association with the many outstanding liver pathologists who are members of the Laennec Society and the Gnomes, powerful intellects and great company, from which I have greatly benefitted.

A special thank you to Drs. Jason Daniels and Matt Sebenik, who both read the prior edition very carefully and provided invaluable feedback, feedback that I believe has greatly improved the book and that I hope will make it even more useful to you.

Regards,
Michael Torbenson, MD

CONTENTS

1

GENERAL APPROACH TO BIOPSY SPECIMENS

There are many ways to approach interpretation of a liver biopsy, all of which have some value. The approach outlined here has worked successfully for many pathologists for many years and may be helpful as a starting point for those of you who do not have an established routine. Careful attention to these core general elements of evaluating a liver biopsy specimen will improve your diagnostic liver pathology skills.

ROUTINE STAINS FOR LIVER BIOPSY SPECIMEN EVALUATION

In most centers, a liver biopsy is processed up front to produce at least two hematoxylin-eosin (H&E) stains, an iron stain, and a trichrome stain. Some centers may prefer a Sirius red stain over the trichrome stain for evaluating fibrosis. H&E stains and a stain for fibrosis should be performed on all medical liver biopsy specimens. There are no additional mandatory stains needed to evaluate a liver biopsy specimen, but many centers include an upfront Perls iron stain and an upfront periodic acid-Schiff (PAS) stain with digest (PASD) to screen for iron overload disease and for $\alpha 1$-antitrypsin deficiency. Less commonly, some centers also perform up front reticulin stain and PAS stains on all medical liver biopsy specimens; reticulin stains in medical biopsies are used to screen for nodular regenerative hyperplasia, while some pathologists like how PAS stains help bring out foci of lobular hepatitis in negative relief. Outside the H&E and trichrome (or Sirius red) stains, the up-front staining panel to choose should reflect what you believe is best for patient care, that is, the panel that best helps you make excellent diagnoses and avoid missing things.

CLINICAL AND LABORATORY INFORMATION

An important step in evaluating liver biopsy specimens is taking the time to understand the clinical history as thoroughly as possible. The clinical history may be scant in many situations, ranging from a consult biopsy

1

sent from another hospital with little or no information to an acutely ill patient who has just presented to the emergency room in your hospital. Nonetheless, it is important to review and understand as much of the clinical history as you can reasonably obtain. The available laboratory results should also be reviewed. At times, the actual laboratory results will not be available, but you may be told verbally that certain laboratory test results are positive or negative. These verbal results can be very helpful but should be confirmed by your reviewing the actual laboratory results whenever possible, as laboratory results can be sometimes misunderstood or conveyed to you inaccurately. If verbal information is all that is available, a useful approach is to use terminology in the surgical pathology note such as "By report, laboratory testing showed…"

After the liver biopsy specimen has been fully reviewed, the findings may prompt you to ask for additional information. For example, if you find granulomas, you may inquire about a history of sarcoidosis or other granulomatous diseases, even if that history was not initially provided. This second, focused request for clinical information or laboratory results is driven by the biopsy findings and can provide critical information that, in many cases, fully establishes the diagnosis. In fact, treating physicians may be unaware of the potential importance of specific clinical information, so did not provide it until asked, even though it was available.

Some pathologists prefer to have no clinical information when they first look at the biopsy, as they are concerned that clinical information and laboratory findings may bias their review of the biopsy. Clinicians sometimes share this same perspective and so may not provide relevant information that is available. In many ways, however, this is like a patient refusing to tell the doctor why they came to the doctor's office out of fear that their medical history and current symptoms will bias the physical examination. Nonetheless, the approach of reviewing the biopsy prior to examining relevant information is also fine if you prefer it, and the basic philosophy of wanting to do a thorough, systematic review is sound; however, at some point the pathologist should review and incorporate all reasonably available clinical information and laboratory results into the overall interpretation of the liver biopsy.

As part of your first review of the clinical history, it is very important to understand why the biopsy was performed. In some cases, the disease process is well known clinically and the biopsy is performed to assess the amount of inflammation and fibrosis. In fact, not that many years ago, this was one of the more common indications for liver biopsies, as treatment decisions for chronic hepatitis C and B took into account the grade and stage of the disease. With improvements in noninvasive testing for fibrosis, this indication has diminished considerably but will still be occasionally encountered. In other cases, the underlying liver disease may be known, such as with fatty liver disease or chronic biliary tract disease, but the biopsy is performed to investigate other unusual clinical or laboratory findings. In this setting, you will still want to comment on the amount of active injury and fibrosis but will also need to address the specific clinical question that prompted the biopsy. As an example, an individual with long-standing chronic hepatitis C with mildly active disease presents with a sudden spike in liver enzyme levels, fivefold above the usual baseline. In this case, the clinician already knows the patient has hepatitis C and the indication for biopsy is not staging and grading the known liver disease. Instead, their reason for performing the biopsy, and thus your report, should focus on diagnosing, or providing a differential for, the cause of the sudden spike in liver enzyme levels. The hepatitis C grade and stage should be included, of course, but are not the focus of the report in this example.

BIOPSY ADEQUACY

Specimen adequacy for clinical care cannot be determined solely by length. While length does matter, adequacy is an interpretation for the pathologist to make. For example, a biopsy of a tumor that samples only a small portion of histologically typical hepatocellular carcinoma may be entirely adequate to make clinical decisions. However, a biopsy with a similarly small amount of tissue on a diagnostically challenging tumor may not be adequate to make a complete diagnosis.

Specimen adequacy for staging and grading chronic liver diseases is an important issue for clinical trials and for similar research studies, and, in this setting, adequacy is formally defined by the specific study to meet its specific needs. Adequacy is usually assessed in the research setting by either measuring the length of the biopsy core or counting portal tracts. When counting portal tracts, any identifiable portal tract is usually counted, even if it is incomplete.

In the clinical setting, determining the adequacy of a liver biopsy specimen for diagnosing, grading, and staging of medical liver disease is a decision best made by the pathologist after reviewing the specimen and taking into consideration the specimen size, the findings on the biopsy, the underlying liver disease, and the clinical indication for the biopsy. For example, a relatively small biopsy specimen that shows unequivocal cirrhosis is adequate for fibrosis staging, while a larger biopsy specimen may by chance include few portal tracts and be inadequate. As a rule of thumb, an adequate medical liver biopsy specimen for clinical care will typically have at least 10 portal tracts and be at least 1 cm in length.[1] Smaller biopsy specimens tend to understage the degree of inflammation and fibrosis.[2] If the biopsy specimen size limits your interpretation in a specific case, it is important to state that in the report. It is just as important to state what information you can with confidence, given the material on hand. For example, fibrosis evaluation on a small biopsy specimen with just a few portal tracts that shows moderate portal fibrosis might say in the pathology report: "The biopsy specimen is too small to confidently stage the fibrosis, but there is at least moderate portal fibrosis in this biopsy specimen."

Sampling Error

The literature often notes that a biopsy specimen represents only about 1/50,000 of the entire liver. This is reasonably true, but of course a small sample size per se is not the best explanation for sampling error. After all, scientists make good use of much smaller samples when they measure, for example, wind speeds, air temperature, and precipitation. The small samples in these examples work very well because of the relative homogeneity of the sampled material. One can quickly think of dozens of other examples, all making the same point that a sample size of 1/50,000 is not unreasonable or invalid in and of itself. Thus, sampling error in liver pathology is a function of sample size *relative* to the heterogeneity of the disease process. If a disease process is patchy, then a small biopsy specimen is less likely to be representative. Early changes in chronic biliary tract disease, for example, are often quite patchy. Inflammatory changes and fibrosis in chronic hepatitis can also be patchy, especially with milder disease, leading to some of the sampling errors noted in the literature. Another well-recognized area of disease heterogeneity is older inactive cirrhotic livers that have undergone some degree of fibrosis regression. These cases often have a large macronodular pattern of cirrhosis with relative thin fibrous bands. Thus, small biopsy specimens can underestimate the amount of fibrosis, if by chance most of the sample comes from the center of a large macronodule.

PREDOMINANT PATTERN OF INJURY

As your first step in assessing a liver biopsy, low-power examination (such as 4× or 10×) is very helpful to understand the basic pattern of injury (Table 1.1). Is the injury predominately hepatitic (inflammatory)? Or predominately fatty change? Or that of biliary tract disease? There are many other disease patterns listed in Table 1.1 and their recognition will aide in making an accurate diagnosis.

One of the keys to excellence in liver pathology is understanding that you will often observe a large number of abnormalities in liver biopsy specimens but that not all changes are of equal significance. Your goal is not to list all the abnormal findings in the pathology report but instead to recognize when the various abnormalities coalesce together to form a predominant pattern of injury. For example, a liver biopsy specimen with primary biliary cirrhosis/cholangitis (PBC) may have mild fatty change, mild cholestasis, minimal lobular chronic inflammation, and mild nodular regenerative hyperplasia, in addition to the predominant findings of chronically inflamed, medium-sized bile ducts (septal bile ducts) with active duct injury. Recognizing the predominant injury pattern leads to an accurate diagnosis of PBC; listing all abnormal findings without further interpretation leads to confusion.

A further example illustrates a second important point: histological injury patterns can have very different meanings depending on the context

TABLE 1.1   **Patterns of Injury in Liver Biopsies**
Predominant Injury Pattern
Lobular hepatitis
Portal based chronic inflammation
Fatty change
Biliary tract obstruction
Biliary tract inflammation and injury
Bland lobular cholestasis (with little or no inflammation and no changes of obstruction)
Necrosis
Abnormal inclusions or pigment
Granulomas
Vascular disease
Infiltrates in the sinusoids
Tumors

This table is not comprehensive but lists the most common patterns of liver injury.

of other findings in the biopsy. Bile ductular proliferation is a key pattern of injury that often indicates downstream biliary tract obstructive disease from stones, strictures, tumors, etc. However, bile ductular proliferation in severe acute viral hepatitis can reach levels seen in obstructive disease.[3] In addition, bile ductular proliferation in some cases of vascular outflow disease, such as Budd-Chiari syndrome, can reach levels seen in obstructive disease.[4] Thus, one can see that patterns of injury, such as bile ductular proliferation in this example, should bring to your mind a differential and not a single diagnosis. The pathologist can then help prioritize the differential from most to least likely. In this example, the pattern of bile ductular proliferation as a sole dominant pattern would suggest biliary tract obstruction, but in the setting of other dominant patterns (marked cholestatic lobular hepatitis or venous outflow disease) the ductular proliferation is most likely a secondary change in response to the dominant form of injury.

Be Systematic

After the major pattern of disease has been identified, systematically go through the biopsy specimen, examining the architecture and each compartment carefully. While any systematic approach will work fine, one reasonable method is to start in the portal tracts and work toward the central veins. In the portal tracts examine the hepatic artery, portal vein, and bile ducts. Examine the inflammatory cells in the portal tracts. In the lobules look for inflammation, fatty change, cholestasis, and glycogenosis and examine the hepatocytes for abnormal inclusions or pigmented material.

Examine the sinusoids for dilatation, for abnormal cells, and for extracellular material such as amyloid and fibrosis. Finally examine the central veins for inflammation or other pathologies.

EVALUATING FIBROSIS

Fibrosis is most commonly evaluated by either a trichrome stain or a Sirius red stain. In cases of chronic hepatitis, fibrosis progresses through several well-defined steps: no fibrosis, portal fibrosis, bridging fibrosis, and cirrhosis. There are many different formal staging systems available, but each share these common fibrosis categories and the systems vary only in how the various categories are subdivided. Fatty liver disease is similar but has a pericellular fibrosis pattern that precedes and/or co-occurs with the portal fibrosis. Fibrosis evaluation is considered in greater detail in Chapter 2.

BIOPSIES OF TUMORS

Biopsies directed at mass lesions are commonly performed to establish a tissue-based diagnosis. In these situations, immunostains can often be very helpful in making a diagnosis (please see Chapters 19-23 for specific details by tumor type). However, biopsy material is often limited and it is important to use the tissue wisely. In this regard, the single most important question to consider is the following:

- Does the biopsy clearly show liver tissue, but I am not sure if the tissue is benign liver, a benign liver tumor, or a malignant liver tumor?
- Or, in contrast, is there clearly cancerous tissue, and I am not sure if this is hepatocellular carcinoma or some other type of carcinoma?

Based on reviewing consult material for many years, it seems that pathologists do not consistently consider this point carefully, as many times stains are performed that are useful to answer a question they did not intend to ask. For example, if you have a biopsy of a well-differentiated hepatic tumor and your differential is hepatocellular carcinoma versus a hepatic adenoma, then a Hep-Par stain or arginase stain or other stains that identify hepatic differentiation will not be helpful. In fact, the best panel of histochemical and immunostain markers is quite different for these two fundamental questions and recognizing what question you are asking will allow you to choose the most appropriate set of ancillary stains.

GENERAL APPROACH TO BIOPSY REPORTS

Structure of pathology reports. Surgical pathology reports for liver biopsies typically have a section for relevant clinical history (sometimes this is included in the note or comment section), a diagnosis section, and a note or comment section. Some institutions also have a microscopic description. As a general guideline, an excellent pathology report includes a clear diagnosis as well as a concise note or comment that expands or refines the diagnosis when necessary. An excellent pathology report also directly addresses the clinical indication for the liver biopsy. As an illustration, a biopsy was performed for low-titer antinuclear antibody (ANA) elevations and mild aspartate aminotransferase (AST) and alanine aminotransferase (ALT) elevations and the clinical question is to rule out autoimmune hepatitis. The biopsy shows mildly active fatty liver disease. The diagnosis of fatty liver disease will be conveyed in the diagnosis section, but the note or comment section should also indicate whether or not there is any evidence for autoimmune hepatitis, as that was the original clinical question.

Microscopic descriptions are included in the pathology report by some pathologists, and they can add value to the report when used wisely. They are not necessary, however, and it is best to include all key pathologic findings in the diagnosis or note/comment section.

Don't write long boring reports. There can be a tendency to write very long notes or comments for medical liver biopsy specimens. Occasionally, pathologists will detail every single thought they had while examining the specimen, even ones that turned out to be not important ("I considered this, then I considered that, but then I wasn't sure so I thought about that and this, but the biopsy is challenging so other this's and thats can't be completely excluded, and there you have it"). Sometimes these reports further include exhaustive and jumbled lists of all histological changes that could be identified, including those that are trivial, and then, still not content, go on to include detailed lists of things that were not seen but diligently looked for.

Such reports have good intentions of not missing anything and documenting all things that were considered, but they become a burden for clinicians to process and it is often hard for even fellow pathologists to finish reading them, let alone have a good mental picture of what the biopsy showed after reading the report. Certainly, writing pathology reports is as much art as science, and there are many reasonable styles. The best styles manage to clearly indicate the main pattern(s) of injury, provide a histological differential, indicate the amount of fibrosis, and directly address any clinical question that was posed at the time of the biopsy. Only pertinent negatives need to included, and pertinence is in reference to the current histological findings/clinical questions. For example, if there is a known history of sarcoidosis, or if there is clinical concern for sarcoidosis, then not finding granulomas is relevant and their absence should be in the pathology report. On the other hand, if the biopsy is to grade and stage fatty liver disease, then there is no need to mention the lack of granulomas or the many other things you did not see and are not relevant to that specific case.

Should I use a formal grading or staging system? It is important to accurately convey the amount of inflammation and fibrosis in a biopsy. The amount of fibrosis in chronic hepatitis C, for example, predicts liver-related morbidity and mortality.[5,6] There are many grading and staging systems for chronic liver diseases, the most common in use being for chronic hepatitis C, chronic hepatitis B, and nonalcoholic fatty liver disease. Other non-disease-specific systems exist for grading the results of iron stains in liver biopsies. These systems are discussed in more detail under their specific chapters. But here we consider the more general question of whether you should be using a formal numerical system, instead of traditional pathology descriptions, to convey the amount of inflammation and fibrosis. The answer is "no," if you and/or the clinicians at your hospital do not find them useful and the answer is "yes," as long as you and/or the clinicians find them useful.

Of note, numerical systems are most useful for research studies that analyze composite data from large groups of patients; there is no evidence that they provide benefit for routine clinical care over that of words that actually describe the pathologic findings. In fact, it is likely self-evident to readers that the numbers in grading and staging schemas are in most cases the direct equivalents of the pathology words. For example, if a biopsy shows focal bridging fibrosis and you convey that accurately in the report, either by stating "focal bridging fibrosis" or by stating "fibrosis stage METAVIR 2," it is exactly the same for clinical care and there is no advantage for the numerical staging system.

It is also a common misconception that using a numerical system creates a "universal" fibrosis stage that is not otherwise present and allows more accurate comparison of fibrosis stage between reports and institutions. This is not necessarily true for any well-written pathology report, as again it is words that define the numbers and not the other way around. Is there any harm in using the numbers? No. However, one potential downside risk is that a pathologist can become so focused on filling out the scoring sheet that they forget to carefully examine the overall biopsy. This seems to be more of an issue for pathologists who have seen relatively few liver biopsies and for whom the numerical staging and grading itself becomes the focus of the evaluation. Another subtle downside to using a numerical system is that it implies greater precision than the words that describe the pathology: to many, the words "METAVIR fibrosis stage 2" have a greater ring of authority than the words "focal bridging fibrosis." Yet the numbers are, again, used as synonyms for the words. Thus, they are in no way more accurate or authoritative.

If numerical systems are used, it is best practice to include the name of the system in the pathology report. This is important because there are some differences in the meaning of the numbers between the different systems. It is also best practice to follow the system faithfully. Even if you feel strongly that you have a terrific improvement to a published numerical grading or staging system, please do not use your "improvements" when using the published system, as the end result is one of confusion.

Also, it is important to be aware that not all pathologists interpret published systems the same. As one example, the Ishak score[7] (or modified Hepatic Activity Index grade) includes a score for confluent necrosis. Some pathologists, including academically active pathologists who are contributing to the literature in this area, do not score actual hepatocyte necrosis for this category but instead score central lobular inflammation regardless of whether there is any necrosis. Thus, biopsies may receive very different scores by different pathologists, even when using the exact same scoring system because of the difference in interpretation of what was meant by "necrosis." As a second example, when using the Ishak system to score portal chronic inflammation, the official scoring system is 1 for "mild, some or all portal areas" and 2 for "moderate, some or all portal areas." However, a subset of pathologists interprets the published system to require two or more portal tracts to show moderate levels of chronic portal inflammation in order to be scored as a 2. In this case, the same biopsy could again receive somewhat different scores by different pathologists using the exact same scoring system because of the difference in interpretation of the meaning of the word "some." These examples should not dissuade you from using a formal numerical grading and staging system if you or your clinical colleagues find it useful, but hopefully these examples and the overall discussion in this section will make you a wiser user of these tools.

Should I use a cancer synoptic report? Synoptic reports for cancer resections are mandated by most institutions and provide value by making sure that every report covers the critical information needed for clinical care. Remember that synoptic reports are focused on the most common types of cancer and are not intended to be limiting. When reporting a rare variant of carcinoma, or when there are other unusual findings, make sure the relevant information gets into the pathology report. Synoptic cancer reports are generally not used for biopsy specimens.

USE OF OUTSIDE CONSULTANTS

The use of both internal and external consultants is an important part of being an excellent pathologist; it is impossible to know all things about liver pathology in this life, so sometimes we all need help. When using external consultants, in most cases, it is best to have access to a "panel" of experts with different areas of expertise. To illustrate, if you are in general practice and have a difficult liver case, then it is best to show the case to a liver pathology expert and not a breast pathology expert, and vice versa when you have a difficult breast case. The sun has largely set on those days when a single pathologist can be an expert consultant in all areas of pathology.

Another consideration is the reputation of the institution versus the pathologist who sees the case. If you focus only on the name of the institution, you may, for example, send your very difficult case to a top-notch institution only to have it reviewed by a junior faculty member with just a year or two of actual experience or by a basic scientist who has been around for many years, but spends most of his or her time with rats and mice. They may be an excellent pathologist, but it is still up to you to make wise choices and make sure you are happy with the qualification of the person seeing your case. If you are uncomfortable with the diagnosis you get back from a consultant pathologist, it is entirely appropriate to discuss the case with them and explain your reservations about the diagnosis. Perhaps they overlooked an important part of the history or missed seeing an important histological finding. At times, it can be appropriate to ask them to share the case with other experts at their center, especially if they express uncertainty about the diagnosis in their report or phone conversation.

An important part of using consultants is that you should learn from the experience. Read the diagnosis and note portion of the report so that you understand how the case was approached and how a diagnosis was made. If it is not clear or if you still have questions, then do not be hesitant to call and discuss the case. This can be a very rewarding part of the experience and a key source of continuing education for your own personal growth. As a caveat, however, there is little value in calling to perseverate or complain over minor differences. For example, if you thought the background liver in a tumor case showed mild fatty change but the consultant pathologist signs out the background liver as having moderate fatty change, well that is a difference that in most cases is not worthy of further discussion.

If you have a difficult case that you have worked up and the diagnosis is not clear, then it is best to send the slides **and** the blocks to the consulting pathologist in order to get back a diagnosis as soon as possible. The block may not be needed, but sending the block up-front can help improve the overall turnaround time.

If you obtain follow-up information on difficult cases, consultant pathologists appreciate a quick phone call or email. So please take the time to provide that follow-up information on cases when it becomes available. Most consultant pathologists will welcome the feedback, even if their diagnosis was not entirely correct. Consultant pathologists do not always get the diagnosis right, and given a long-enough time line, every consultant pathologist will get it wrong at some point. So if new information develops that indicates a prior consult diagnosis should be revised, please share that information too.

Studies have examined the accuracy of consultant diagnoses by correlating them with clinical follow-up and outcomes and found that the consultant diagnosis is correct in 65% of fine-needle aspiration (FNA) specimens[8] and 90% of surgical biopsy specimens.[9-11] Incomplete or incorrect information submitted with the consult material is one of the most important reasons for an inaccurate diagnosis,[10] underscoring the importance of taking the extra step to submit with the consult material, as best as possible, the relevant clinical, imaging, and laboratory findings. To this point, a multicenter study of gastrointestinal (GI) and liver consults found that 30% of cases were lacking relevant laboratory information and 20%, relevant clinical information.[12]

EVALUATING THE LITERATURE

When you want to review the literature on both general topics and specific entities, review articles are an excellent resource. When you are reading primary articles, there are a few general guidelines that are helpful to remember. First, many reported findings in the literature are either not reproduced or only partially reproduced. Thus, observations that have been confirmed by several different groups are significantly more robust and should influence your thoughts and your pathology approach more strongly than those that are single articles. This is particularly true regarding the sensitivity and specificity of various antibodies used in diagnostic pathology. The sensitivity and specificity of a given antibody will strongly depend on the composition of the study population. For example, the diagnostic utility of a given antibody for diagnosing hepatocellular carcinoma may be excellent in a given study, but when the same or similar studies are repeated in a different hospital, the overall results may be less impressive because of the different underlying liver diseases, different proportions of tumor grades, and different laboratory staining methods.

Also be aware that sometimes authors have potential conflicts of interest. For example, a proportion of the literature that argues that blood tests should replace liver biopsies is written by authors who have financial interests in the company selling the blood tests. These conflicts are dutifully disclosed in the manuscripts and lectures, but those small blips of disclosures are easily lost once you start reading the article or listening to the lecture. A good clue that an article likely has a strong bias is when straw man arguments are used. A common trope, for example, is liver histology being portrayed as the "inaccurate/flawed gold stand," followed by heroic performances of the testing advocated by the authors. This is a straw man argument because no one ever claimed that tissue-based diagnoses are perfect or that they are always the best way to diagnose liver disease in every patient. Every test has limitations, including histology evaluation, and "gold standards" in science are really the "currently best standard approach in certain situations." This is fully understood by most physicians and scientists, who understand that no test is perfect in every situation and that testing improves over time, with new technology replacing old technology. Papers that rely on straw man arguments usually do so because of weak scientific understandings, sloppy writing, or conflicts of interest; in any case, these papers should be read with a grain of salt.

PERSONAL IMAGE/SLIDE LIBRARIES

An excellent tool in diagnostic pathology is to create over time a set of slides or images that will be of help in challenging cases. Of course, images in books and online are very helpful and are sufficient for most purposes, but they can be supplemented in those areas that you find particularly challenging or particularly interesting. For example, over many years, I have collected and curated a large collection of slides/images representing unusual morphological findings/immunostain findings in primary liver tumors. Then, when I encounter an unusual finding in active clinical cases, I have essentially a focused, deep library I can go through as an aide in both making the diagnosis and understanding what the unusual finding may mean. As a second example, early in my career, I created a reference set of images that I could use when grading hepatocellular carcinomas, with many examples of each of the different Edmondson-Steiner grades, which proved to be very useful over the years.

REFERENCES

1. Schiano TD, Azeem S, Bodian CA, et al. Importance of specimen size in accurate needle liver biopsy evaluation of patients with chronic hepatitis C. *Clin Gastroenterol Hepatol.* 2005;3:930-935.
2. Colloredo G, Guido M, Sonzogni A, et al. Impact of liver biopsy size on histological evaluation of chronic viral hepatitis: the smaller the sample, the milder the disease. *J Hepatol.* 2003;39:239-244.
3. Johnson K, Kotiesh A, Boitnott JK, et al. Histology of symptomatic acute hepatitis C infection in immunocompetent adults. *Am J Surg Pathol.* 2007;31:1754-1758.
4. Kakar S, Batts KP, Poterucha JJ, et al. Histologic changes mimicking biliary disease in liver biopsies with venous outflow impairment. *Mod Pathol.* 2004;17:874-878.
5. Limketkai BN, Mehta SH, Sutcliffe CG, et al. Relationship of liver disease stage and antiviral therapy with liver-related events and death in adults coinfected with HIV/HCV. *J Am Med Assoc.* 2012;308:370-378.
6. Everhart JE, Wright EC, Goodman ZD, et al. Prognostic value of Ishak fibrosis stage: findings from the hepatitis C antiviral long-term treatment against cirrhosis trial. *Hepatology.* 2010;51:585-594.
7. Ishak K, Baptista A, Bianchi L, et al. Histological grading and staging of chronic hepatitis. *J Hepatol.* 1995;22:696-699.
8. Bomeisl PE Jr, Alam S, Wakely PE Jr. Interinstitutional consultation in fine-needle aspiration cytopathology: a study of 742 cases. *Cancer.* 2009;117:237-246.
9. Swapp RE, Aubry MC, Salomao DR, et al. Outside case review of surgical pathology for referred patients: the impact on patient care. *Arch Pathol Lab Med.* 2013;137:233-240.
10. Coffin CS, Burak KW, Hart J, et al. The impact of pathologist experience on liver transplant biopsy interpretation. *Mod Pathol.* 2006;19:832-838.
11. Manion E, Cohen MB, Weydert J. Mandatory second opinion in surgical pathology referral material: clinical consequences of major disagreements. *Am J Surg Pathol.* 2008;32:732-737.
12. Torbenson MS, Arnold CA, Graham RP, et al. Identification of key challenges in liver pathology: data from a multicenter study of extramural consults. *Hum Pathol.* 2019;87:75-82.

2

LIVER INJURY PATTERNS

The discipline of liver pathology is built on recognizing key patterns of liver injury. Master these key patterns and their differentials and you will comfortably handle most medical liver biopsies. If you do not, medical liver biopsy interpretation will never quite lose an aura of mystery and uncertainty.

Sometimes it helps to remember that you do not need to be all-knowing and that the diagnosis/management of the patient does not rest solely on your diagnostic shoulders. Instead, you are part of a team and the biopsy findings will be fully integrated by the clinical team into a composite picture created by the histologic findings plus the clinical history, physical examination, laboratory results, and imaging findings, many of which may not be available to you when you examine the biopsy specimen; clinical decisions are then based on the integrated, composite findings. Your role is very important, as patients and clinicians depend on you to make three principle determinations: (1) establish the major pattern of injury and provide a reasonable differential, a diagnosis and differential that incorporates whatever clinical, imaging, or laboratory findings that are available to you; (2) determine the degree of active injury (grade); and (3) determine the amount of fibrosis (stage).

The first step, correctly recognizing the basic histologic pattern of liver injury, is almost always accomplished using your low-power lenses. Do not skip this first step and go straight to grading and staging; although the latter two determinations are important, their primary importance is that they indicate how bad the main pattern of injury is and if it has led to liver scarring. To aid in step one, this chapter focuses on succinct descriptions of the most common patterns of liver injury; more detailed descriptions for specific causes are found in their respective chapters.

We begin with a brief review of normal live histology. The next section discusses acute liver failure from a clinical perspective. While this information is not histologic, it can be helpful when you are providing a differential for the biopsy findings in a patient with acute liver failure. In the subsequent sections, key patterns of liver injury are reviewed and illustrated. Some patterns are seen only in acute liver injury and some only in chronic liver disease, but many injury patterns can be seen in both.

NORMAL LIVER

Portal Tracts

Most portal tracts contain a hepatic artery, portal vein, and bile duct. Occasionally, normal portal tracts can have several bile duct profiles or several hepatic artery profiles.[1] In general, the hepatic artery is approximately the same size as the bile duct (ie, has a similar diameter) and the two are usually found close together, often within a distance that is about the same as the bile duct's diameter. The portal veins are considerably larger, typically with a diameter that is fivefold or greater than the diameter of the bile ducts and arteries, at least in a well-oriented portal tract.

About 10% of the smallest branches of the portal tracts may not have a bile duct evident on hematoxylin-eosin (H&E) stains and yet still be normal.[1] Medium-sized and larger portal tracts, however, should always have bile ducts, if the complete portal tract is present on the slide. If they do not, this provides evidence for ductopenia. Portal dyads, where only two of the normal three structures are seen, are more common in the periphery of the liver, in the smallest sized portal tracts.[1]

All portal tracts will have collagen, with the amount of collagen correlating with the overall size of the portal tract. Normal portal tracts generally have a smooth border where the collagen interfaces with the hepatocytes. This collagen is normal and is not the same as fibrosis, which is always an abnormal finding. Because of this, statements such as "no abnormal fibrosis" have an element of redundancy, as all fibrosis is abnormal.

Lobules

The hepatic lobules contain cords or plates of hepatocytes that are typically two to three cells in thickness. The thickness of the hepatic plates is often best appreciated on a reticulin stain. The sinusoids are lined by endothelial cells, Kupffer cells, and stellate cells. You cannot reliably tell these sinusoidal cells apart in a normal liver without special stains. The hepatic lobules are divided into three roughly equal-sized zones based on their association with normal structures. The hepatocytes around the portal tracts are defined as zone 1, the hepatocytes around the central vein as zone 3, and those that are not clearly in either zone 1 or 3 are called zone 2 hepatocytes. These three zones have a gradient of blood flow, with hepatocytes in zone 1 having richer oxygen and nutrient supplies compared with zone 3 hepatocytes, and takes the lead in protein synthesis, β-oxidation of fatty acids, cholesterol synthesis, and gluconeogenesis. Hepatocytes in zones 2 and 3, on the other hand, play key roles in chemical detoxification and bile production.[2]

Connecting the Lobules and the Biliary Tree

The biliary system drains bile created by hepatocytes, moving it from the lobules into the bile ducts and then out of the liver. To do this, hepatocytes secrete bile into bile canaliculi, small structures that are formed where two hepatocytes come together, each hepatocyte forming half of the bile canaliculi. The bile then moves from the bile canaliculi into the canals of Hering, which are structures lined on one side by cholangiocytes and another side by hepatocytes. The canals of Hering extend from about mid-zone of the lobules into the portal tracts, where they connect directly to the bile ducts themselves. The bile canaliculi are not evident on H&E unless there is cholestasis, while the canals of Hering are not seen without special stains.

Central Veins

The central veins vary in size, being smallest in the periphery of the liver and gradually getting larger until they leave the liver via the hepatic veins. The thickness of the vein wall varies accordingly, and larger vein walls can have smooth muscle. The central vein and the surrounding hepatocytes are used to define zone 3 of the liver.

Normal Age-Related Changes in the Liver

With increasing age, there is an overall decline in liver volume of between 20% and 40%.[3] This decreased volume results from both fewer total hepatocytes and a reduction in the size of individual hepatocytes. This age-related liver atrophy is also associated with a decline in blood flow to the liver. These changes are subtle at the histologic level, not readily evident by routine histology. At the individual cell level, hepatocytes often show increased lipofuscin with age, as well as a decline in the smooth endoplasmic reticulum compartment. Age also leads to a decline in hepatocyte proliferative capacity.[3]

ACUTE LIVER FAILURE

Acute liver failure is a clinical term used when patients present with abrupt onset, severe liver disease. While a wide range of specific clinical definitions are used in the literature for acute liver failure, shared key elements are a short time interval from first clinical presentation to the development of hepatic encephalopathy and coagulopathy, as well as a lack of preexisting liver disease.[4] Coagulopathy is typically defined as a prothrombin time greater than 15 seconds or an international nationalized ratio (INR) greater than or equal to 1.5. Acute liver failure can be further divided into hyperacute liver failure (less than 1 week from initial presentation to encephalopathy or coagulopathy), acute liver failure (8-28 days), and subacute liver failure (4-13 weeks).[5] Of note, the term "acute hepatitis" is often used clinically to describe any sudden increase in hepatic enzyme levels, and this term should not be misinterpreted as "acute liver failure."

The most common causes of acute liver failure are acetaminophen (approximately 40% of cases in the United States and Europe); idiosyncratic drug reactions (10%-15%); acute hepatitis, most commonly hepatitis

A or B (15%-20%); and idiopathic (20%-30%). Other well-known but less common causes include alcoholic liver disease, fatty liver of pregnancy, autoimmune hepatitis, Wilson disease, Budd-Chiari syndrome, and uncommon viral infections.

The histologic findings in acute liver failure will depend to some degree on the cause of the liver injury, but biopsies typically show some combination of inflammation and/or necrosis. With toxic or ischemic injury, the liver can show massive necrosis with relatively little inflammation. With idiosyncratic drug-induced liver injury and with acute viral hepatitis, the specimens typically show marked inflammation and cholestasis, along with necrosis. With fatty liver of pregnancy and other mitochondrial pathologies, there will be diffuse microvesicular steatosis.

If sufficient time has elapsed between the onset of injury and the time of the biopsy, there may be significant bile ductular proliferation adjacent to the areas of parenchymal collapse; in time, the bile ductular proliferation can extend throughout the areas of parenchymal collapse. Survival prognostic information can be provided by the percentage of hepatocyte necrosis on transjugular liver biopsy. In general, death is rare with less than 25% necrosis. In contrast, with approximately 75% or more necrosis, death or the need for liver transplantation is the most likely outcome.[6-8]

ACUTE HEPATITIS, CHRONIC HEPATITIS, AND ACUTE ON CHRONIC HEPATITIS

The terms *acute hepatitis* and *chronic hepatitis* are largely defined by clinical findings, typically using a definition of at least 6 months of elevated liver enzyme levels. In most cases, the clinical findings provide sufficient information about whether the hepatitis is acute or chronic and the pathologist does not need to specifically classify the histologic findings as acute, chronic, or acute on chronic. For cases where the histologic distinction is relevant to clinical management, however, histologic findings can provide insights, although many biopsy specimens will show changes compatible with either acute or chronic liver disease.

The only histologic findings that provide strong evidence for an acute hepatitis is the presence of moderate diffuse or marked lobular hepatitis, and/or confluent or greater lobular necrosis, as these injury patterns are too severe to be chronic; the liver cannot survive long with such severe injury. Patterns with lesser degrees of active injury can be either acute or chronic.

If there is definite fibrosis, then the liver disease is classified as chronic. On the other hand, there are many cases of chronic hepatitis that lack fibrosis, including all the most common causes of chronic liver disease, such as chronic viral hepatitis, autoimmune hepatitis, fatty liver disease, and some examples of drug-induced liver injury. Thus, the lack of fibrosis should not be interpreted as indicating a lack of chronicity. Other structural abnormalities such as bile duct duplication, ductopenia, periductal fibrosis, or portal vein loss can also suggest chronicity.

Acute on chronic injury is defined as an underlying chronic hepatitis that either has an acute flair of disease activity—which is seen almost exclusively in autoimmune hepatitis and chronic hepatitis B—or in cases of chronic hepatitis with a superimposed but unrelated injury, for example, steatohepatitis from ethanol (ETOH) use with superimposed acute hepatitis C. Acute on chronic injury patterns may not have fibrosis but they typically have too much active injury for the underlying chronic injury pattern, or an additional disease pattern that does not fit for the underlying disease.

There are two recurring misperceptions concerning the histologic distinction of acute versus chronic hepatitis. First, sometimes the presence of interface activity is used as evidence for chronic hepatitis, but it is not. Instead, interface activity is common in both acute and chronic hepatitis from many different causes. The more common second misperception is that finding more portal inflammation than lobular inflammation is sometimes thought to be evidence for a chronic hepatitis. This also is not true; this notion seems to have arisen during the heydays of liver biopsies for chronic hepatitis C, as these cases did indeed have a known chronic hepatitis (hepatitis C) and almost always had more portal than lobular inflammation. Because this indication for liver biopsy dwarfed all others for more than decades—before the modern era of highly active antiviral agents—it appears to have led to or fed into this wrong notion. In truth, acute hepatitis can at times have predominately portal inflammation, in particular with some examples of drug-induced liver injury. Likewise, there are many examples of both acute and chronic hepatitis where the inflammation is similar in intensity between the portal tracts and the lobules, a pattern that also does not distinguish between acute and chronic hepatitis.

MOST COMMON LIVER INJURY PATTERNS
Hepatitic Pattern

Main Features

Inflammation can be portal based or lobular based; usually a combination of both.
Plasma-cell-rich inflammation suggests autoimmune hepatitis, but infection and drug-induced liver injury still need to be excluded.

Key Supporting Stains

Epstein-Barr virus (EBV) with acute hepatitis pattern
Trichrome

The hepatitic pattern of injury is very common and shows lobular and portal inflammation that is composed predominately of T lymphocytes and can range from mild to marked (Figure 2.1). There may be scattered apoptotic hepatocytes, ballooned hepatocytes, and areas of zone 3 confluent necrosis (Figure 2.2). The normal lobular organization is often

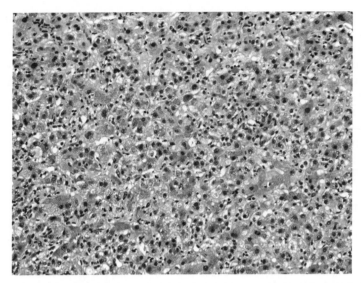

FIGURE 2.1 **Lobular hepatitis pattern.** The lobules show marked lymphocytic inflammation with occasional acidophil bodies.

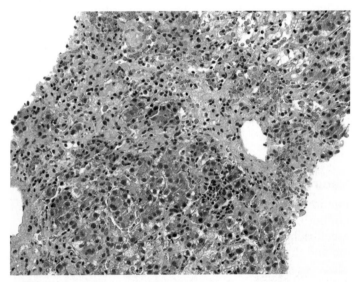

FIGURE 2.2 **Hepatitis with zone 3 necrosis.** This case of markedly active autoimmune hepatitis also has zone 3 necrosis.

disrupted; the usual neat rows or cords of hepatocytes are replaced by a more haphazard arrangement of hepatocytes, a finding called lobular disarray. Cholestasis may be present, particularly in cases with moderate to severe hepatitis. In some cases of severe hepatitis, there can be central necrosis or bridging necrosis.

The portal tracts show predominately lymphocytic inflammation in most cases, often with smaller numbers of plasma cells, histiocytes, and occasional eosinophils. The lymphocytes will be mostly T cells, with fewer admixed B cells and occasionally small lymphoid aggregates of B cells. In cases of severe acute hepatitis, the portal tracts also may show mild bile ductular proliferation (Figure 2.3). This finding can be an important diagnostic pitfall, as the ductular reaction can sometimes be sufficiently prominent to suggest an additional component of downstream biliary tract disease.[9] The presence of moderate to marked lobular hepatitis, however, is usually sufficient to indicate the proper diagnosis.

Possible Histological Clues to the Etiology

As noted previously, the specific cause of an acute hepatitis will not be apparent by histologic examination in most cases and the differential in 99% of cases is that of acute viral hepatitis, idiopathic drug-induced liver injury, or autoimmune hepatitis. One finding that may push the differential in one direction is prominent plasma cells (Figure 2.4), which suggests autoimmune hepatitis. Be aware, however, that some cases of drug-induced liver injury and some cases of acute viral hepatitis, particularly hepatitis A or B, can have prominent plasma cells. Plasma cells in the lobules also favor autoimmune hepatitis (Figure 2.5). Prominent eosinophils would suggest an allergic type drug reaction, but remember that most cases of drug-induced liver injury are idiosyncratic and do not have prominent eosinophils and are, instead, predominately lymphocytic in nature.

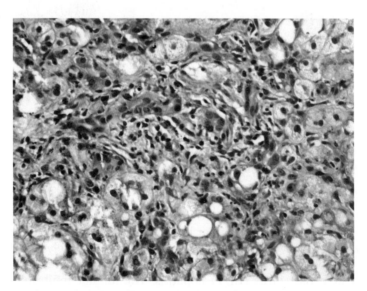

FIGURE 2.3 **Ductular proliferation with marked hepatitis.** In this idiosyncratic drug reaction, the hepatitis was associated with patchy bile ductular proliferation.

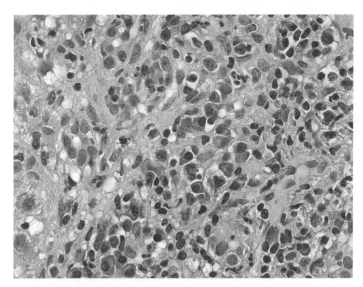

FIGURE 2.4 **Plasma-cell-rich hepatitis.** The portal tract shows marked inflammation with numerous plasma cells in this case of autoimmune hepatitis.

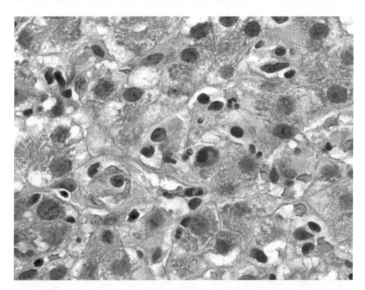

FIGURE 2.5 **Plasma cells in lobules.** This case of autoimmune hepatitis has plasma cells in the lobular inflammation.

A cholestatic hepatitis with neutrophils in the lobule suggests the possibility of acute hepatitis E; the lobular hepatitis is usually mild. Sinusoids that are densely packed with lymphocytes, often with relatively mild hepatocyte injury for the amount of lymphocytosis, suggests the possibility of acute Epstein-Barr virus (EBV) hepatitis. The lobular infiltrates in EBV infection can be patchy and vary in density. Sometimes, the lymphocytes will be lined up or "beaded" within the sinusoids (Figure 2.6). Of course,

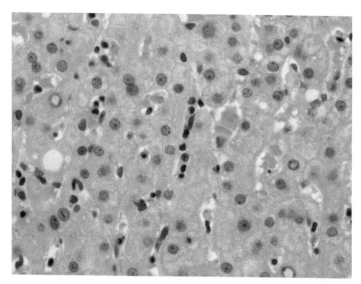

FIGURE 2.6 **Epstein-Barr virus (EBV) hepatitis.** The lobules show a mild hepatitis with no significant hepatocyte injury. The lymphocytes are lined up in a single file in this image, a finding sometimes called *beading*.

the presence of specific viral inclusions, such as those seen in cytomegalovirus (CMV) infection, are useful in identify a cause. There are relatively few other useful findings that will aid in suggesting a specific diagnosis. A zone 3 predominant pattern of hepatitis, often with a mild lymphocytic venulitis, can be seen in autoimmune hepatitis, as well as in acute drug-induced liver injury and acute viral hepatitis.

RESOLVING HEPATITIS PATTERN

Main Features

Minimal lobular and/or portal inflammation
Scattered clusters of pigmented macrophages in the lobules and portal tracts

Key Supporting Stains

Periodic acid-Schiff with diastase (PASD) (highlights pigmented macrophages)
Ki-67 (typically shows mildly increased proliferation in hepatocytes)

The resolving hepatitis pattern of injury is encountered most often in patients who presented with an acute hepatitis, but one that essentially resolved by the time the biopsy was performed. The most common causes for this pattern are acute self-limited viral infection and cases of idiosyncratic drug-induced liver injury, where the medication use was stopped before the biopsy was taken. The histologic findings tend to be very mild, with absent or minimal inflammation in the lobules and portal tracts. The lobules contain occasional, scattered clusters of pigmented macrophages that represent "cleanup" in a site of prior mild hepatitis; the clusters of macrophages often stand out on periodic acid-Schiff with diastase (PASD) stain (Figure 2.7). A Ki-67 often shows a mildly increased hepatocellular proliferative rate (Figure 2.8).

FATTY LIVER DISEASE

Main Features

Steatosis is classified as microvesicular versus macrovesicular. Macrovesicular pattern is divided into steatosis versus steatohepatitis. Steatohepatitis has fat plus active injury (balloon cells, lobular hepatitis, acidophil bodies).

Key Supporting Stains

Trichrome

Fat in the liver can be predominately macrovesicular or predominately microvesicular. The macrovesicular pattern of fat is more common by far, so much so that most pathologists will go their entire career without seeing a case of microvesicular steatosis.

Macrovesicular steatosis (Figure 2.9) is further divided into steatosis versus steatohepatitis, as discussed in detail in Chapter 9. The primary

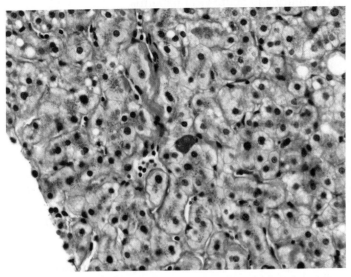

FIGURE 2.7 **Resolving hepatitis pattern, periodic acid-Schiff with diastase (PASD) stain.** In this biopsy, the lobules showed occasional pigmented macrophages but was otherwise essentially normal.

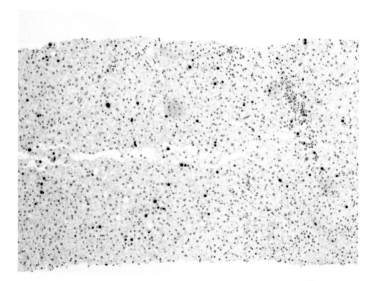

FIGURE 2.8 **Resolving hepatitis pattern, Ki-67.** This biopsy looked almost normal, with only a few scattered periodic acid-Schiff with diastase (PASD)-positive macrophage clusters in the lobules. A Ki-67, however, shows a clearly increased proliferative rate.

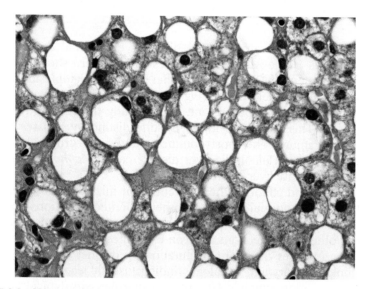

FIGURE 2.9 **Macrovesicular steatosis.** Large droplets of fat are evident.

differential for this pattern of injury is alcohol-related liver disease, the metabolic syndrome–related liver disease (central obesity, diabetes mellitus, hypertension, dyslipidemia), and drug effects. Fatty liver can also be caused by inherited diseases that affect metabolism in infants and children. Malnutrition is another cause, but one rarely seen on liver biopsy. Other causes are listed in Table 2.1.

TABLE 2.1	Differential for Macrovesicular Steatosis
Cause	Comment or Examples
Alcoholic liver disease	
Metabolic syndrome associated fatty liver disease	
Other metabolic conditions	Diabetes mellitus (even in patients without the full metabolic syndrome), hypothyroid disease, growth hormone deficiency
Various genetic diseases	Cystic fibrosis, Wilson disease, porphyria cutanea tarda, Prader-Willi syndrome, Turner syndrome
Malnutrition	More commonly reported with protein malnutrition
Small bowel disease	Crohn disease, celiac disease, small bowel bypass surgery or extensive small bowel resection
Drug effect	Many different drugs, please see drug chapter
Miscellaneous	Volatile petrochemical products

Microvesicular steatosis has a different differential than macrovesicular steatosis (Table 2.2). The microvesicular pattern shows (1) diffuse liver involvement with (2) hepatocytes that have their cytoplasm filled with numerous small droplets of fat (Figure 2.10). Modest amounts of macrovesicular fat may also be present, but typically there is relatively little inflammation. This pattern of injury is quite distinctive and results from mitochondrial injury. The most common causes are drug-induced liver injury, a rare form of alcoholic liver disease called *alcoholic foamy liver degeneration*, or fatty liver of pregnancy.

In infants and children, the differential for microvesicular steatosis is focused on mitochondrial defects or other inherited mutations that affect the urea cycle or fatty acid oxidation. Finally, the differential also includes a number of other rare infections or toxin exposures (Table 2.2). The clinical setting in most cases of inherited mutations is distinct and the combination of clinical history and histologic findings usually leads to a clear diagnosis. Of note, approximately 10% of liver biopsies with typical fatty liver disease resulting from the metabolic syndrome will have small discrete foci of microvesicular steatosis,[12] but this finding does not have the same significance as a diffuse microvesicular pattern of steatosis. Also, of note, after a massive liver necrosis from many different causes, ranging from ischemia to acetaminophen injury, the surviving hepatocytes may show mild microvesicular steatosis. In this setting, the finding of microvesicular steatosis is nonspecific and does not necessarily engender the differential listed in Table 2.2.

TABLE 2.2	**Differential for Microvesicular Steatosis**
Cause	Comment/Representative Reference
Acute fatty liver of pregnancy	10
Alcoholic foamy degeneration	11
Typical metabolic syndrome–related fatty liver disease	Usually seen as small discrete patches, present in about 10% of cases[12]
Genetic mitochondrial disease	
Alpers syndrome	13
Mitochondrial DNA depletion syndrome	14
Navajo neuropathy	15
Pearson syndrome	16
Oxidative phosphorylation deficiency	17
Other genetic diseases	
Ornithine transcarbamylase (OTC) deficiency	18,19
Fatty acid oxidation disorders	20
Wolman disease/cholesterol ester storage disease	21
Wilson disease	22
Infection	
Human herpes virus 6	23,24
Toxin of *Bacillus cereus*	25
Hepatitis, cause unknown, probably viral	26
Superinfection of HDV on HBV	Historically, was called Labrea hepatitis in the Amazon[27] and Santa Marta hepatitis in northern south America[28] before the recognition of HBV/HDV
Acute hepatitis, B and C	29
Toxins	
Arsenic toxicity	30
Industrial solvents	31
Jamaican vomiting sickness (toxin from akee fruit)	32
Hornet sting	33
Medication effect	
Linezolid	34
Chloroform	35

(Continued)

TABLE 2.2 **Differential for Microvesicular Steatosis** (Continued)	
Cause	Comment/Representative Reference
L-asparaginase	Some cases will be predominately macrovesicular steatosis[36]
Amiodarone	[37,38]
Rye syndrome	[39]
Nucleoside analog reverse-transcriptase inhibitors used in HIV infection treatment	Some cases will be pure microvesicular steatosis. Others will have mixed micro- and macrovesicular steatosis.[40]
Valproate	[41]
High-dose tetracycline	
Cytosine arabinoside	[42]

In many of these diseases microvesicular steatosis is the major finding; in other cases, it is seen along with additional changes such as cholestasis, necrosis, or hepatitis.
HBV, hepatitis B virus; HDV, hepatitis D virus; HIV, human immunodeficiency virus.

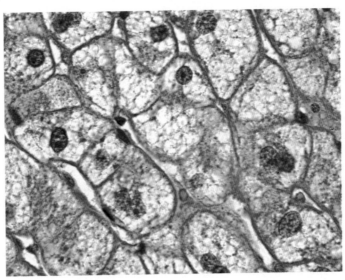

FIGURE 2.10 **Microvesicular steatosis.** The hepatocyte cytoplasm is filled with numerous small droplets of fat.

For clinical purposes, microvesicular steatosis is best diagnosed on H&E stains, not oil red O stains. Although older publications have recommended using oil red O stains on frozen sections,[10] this approach is now recognized as problematic. Extensive experience in evaluating donor liver biopsies at the time of transplant indicates that diffuse small-droplet fat is not uncommon in oil red O stains performed on healthy livers (Figures 2.11 and 2.12). Others have also shown that many different liver diseases,

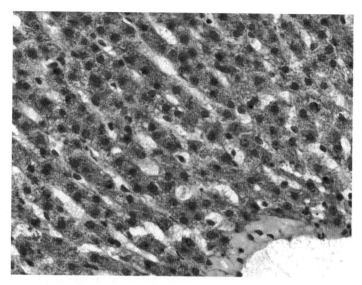

FIGURE 2.11 **Normal liver.** This liver shows no microvesicular fat on hematoxylin-eosin (H&E) stain.

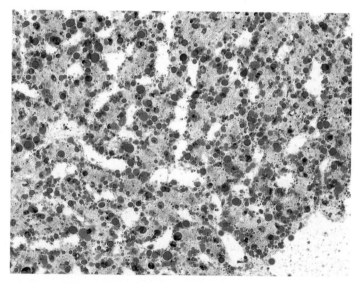

FIGURE 2.12 **Normal liver and oil red O stain.** An oil red O stain on a normal liver can demonstrate small- and intermediate-sized droplets of fat that were not visible on hematoxylin-eosin (H&E). This image is taken from the same field as shown in Figure 5.5.

ones that have nothing to do with the microvesicular steatosis pattern of injury, can show extensive small-droplet staining on the oil red O stain, with staining patterns that are very hard to distinguish from those of true microvesicular steatosis.[43] For this reason, diagnostic misadventures can result from making a diagnosis of microvesicular steatosis solely using the oil red O stain.

BILIARY OBSTRUCTIVE PATTERN

Main Features
Alkaline phosphatase predominant liver enzyme elevations.
Bile ductular proliferation that is variably prominent.
Mixed portal inflammation (neutrophils, lymphocytes, occasional eosinophils).

Additional Findings
Acute obstruction, but not always present
- Portal tract edema
- Lobular cholestasis

Chronic obstruction, but not always present
- Portal fibrosis
- Periductal onion-skin fibrosis
- Fibro-obliterative duct lesion
- Bile duct duplication
- Bile duct loss

Key Supporting Stains
CK7
Copper

Obstruction of large branches of the bile duct, such as the right, left, or common hepatic duct, as well as larger intrahepatic ducts, leads to a pattern of injury with bile ductular proliferation as a characteristic feature. Additional features can be seen depending on whether the obstruction is acute or chronic and depending on the degree of biliary obstruction.

With acute obstruction, the liver is only rarely biopsied because the clinical presentation in most cases is distinctive, with patients presenting with "biliary colic" or episodic acute right upper quadrant. When biopsied, the most striking findings are in the portal tracts, which demonstrate bile ductular proliferation, mixed lymphocytic and neutrophilic portal tract inflammation, and often portal tract edema (Figure 2.13). Scattered portal tract eosinophils are not uncommon. Although not dominant features, mild lymphocytosis of the bile ducts and occasional apoptotic bodies in the bile duct epithelium can also be seen. The bile duct proper may have neutrophils in the lumen if there is superimposed acute cholangitis. There also may be lobular, canalicular, or ductular cholestasis. In very severe cases, bile infarcts can develop, usually next to portal tracts.

Chronic biliary obstructive disease is most commonly biopsied in cases of primary sclerosing cholangitis, biliary stones, chronic pancreatic disease with duct stricturing, or anastomotic strictures after liver transplant, but there are many additional less common causes of biliary strictures or obstruction.

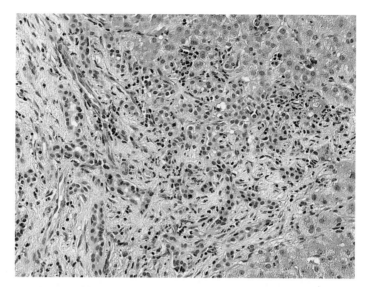

FIGURE 2.13 **Ductular reaction.** A ductular reaction is seen in this case of extrahepatic biliary obstruction and is composed of proliferating bile ducts and mixed inflammation with portal edema.

The biopsy results show predominately portal tract changes with bile ductular proliferation and often portal fibrosis. The ductular proliferation can be patchy and can vary in intensity but is usually milder than that seen with acute obstruction. Mild portal chronic inflammation is common, composed of lymphocytes and often admixed neutrophils. Portal tract edema, on the other hand, is absent. There are a number of uncommon findings that, when present, support a diagnosis of chronic biliary obstruction: bile duct duplication (not to be confused with bile ductular proliferation) (Figure 2.14, eFig. 2.1), ductopenia (Figure 2.15), cholate stasis with periportal copper deposition (Figure 2.16), onion-skin fibrosis (Figure 2.17), and fibro-obliterative duct lesions (Figure 2.18). In addition, if there is decompensated cirrhosis or extensive bile duct loss, the lobules can become cholestatic.

BLAND LOBULAR CHOLESTASIS

Main Features

Lobular cholestasis
No evidence of biliary obstruction
No significant lobular hepatitis
No ductopenia

Key Supporting Stains

CK7 (rules out ductopenia)

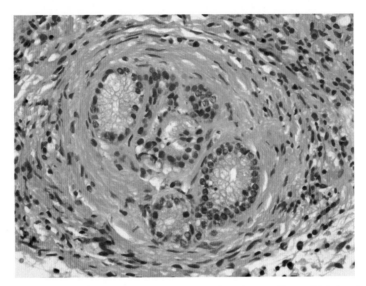

FIGURE 2.14 **Duct duplication.** In contrast to a ductular reaction, which has increased numbers of small ductules at the edge of the portal tract, this central duct appears to be duplicated.

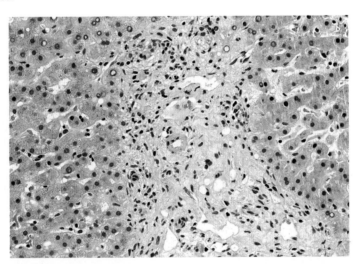

FIGURE 2.15 **Ductopenia.** No bile duct is seen in this portal tract in a case of ductopenia associated with Hodgkin lymphoma.

In general, lobular cholestasis can be classified into several distinct patterns of injury, each with its own differential: (1) acute biliary obstruction, (2) a moderately or severely active acute hepatitis that causes secondary cholestasis, (3) acute alcoholic hepatitis, (4) advanced ductopenia, (5) decompensated liver cirrhosis, or (6) the bland lobular cholestatic pattern of injury.

By definition, the bland lobular cholestatic pattern of injury should have little or no portal tract changes, little or no lobular inflammation,

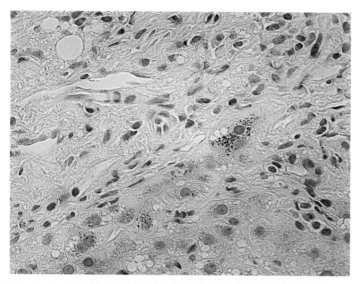

FIGURE 2.16 **Periportal copper in chronic cholestasis.** In this case of PBC, mild copper deposition is seen in the periportal hepatocytes.

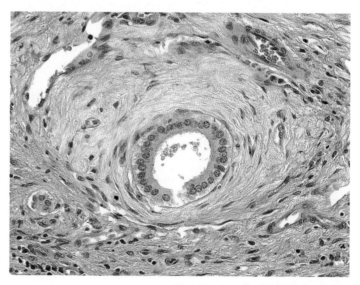

FIGURE 2.17 **Periductal or onion-skin fibrosis.** The bile duct is surrounded by an eccentric cuff of fibrosis.

no evidence of alcoholic hepatitis, and no ductopenia. The cholestasis is found predominately in the hepatocytes or the bile canaliculi (Figure 2.19). When associated with an acute clinical presentation, the bland lobular cholestasis pattern of injury usually resulted from drug-induced liver injury. Occasionally, acute viral hepatitis, such as hepatitis E virus (HEV) infection, can also show this same pattern of injury. Acute biliary obstruction

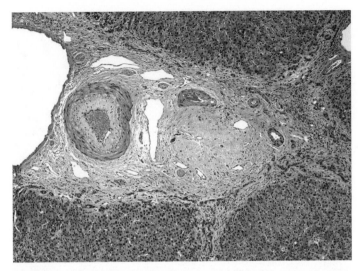

FIGURE 2.18 **Fibro-obliterative duct lesion**. The bile duct has been replaced by a fibrous scar in this case of primary sclerosing cholangitis.

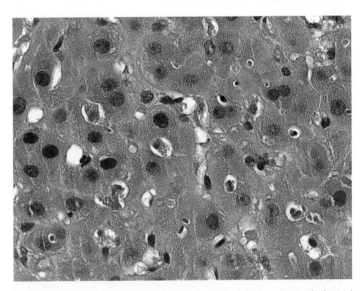

FIGURE 2.19 **Bland lobular cholestasis**. The hepatic lobules show cholestasis with no inflammation in this example of a drug reaction.

can have lobular cholestasis but is differentiated from the bland lobular cholestasis pattern by the presence of bile ductular proliferation. Likewise, a moderate to severe lobular hepatitis is often associated with lobular cholestasis, but the inflammatory changes provide a clear separation from the bland lobular cholestasis pattern. Additional causes for the bland lobular cholestasis pattern of injury are shown in Table 2.3; these are all either uncommonly biopsied, as the diagnosis is evident clinically, or uncommon causes.

TABLE 2.3	Differential for Bland Lobular Cholestasis

Most common cause in liver biopsy specimens
- Drug-induced liver injury

Rare causes, rarely biopsied

Paraneoplastic syndromes
- Lymphomas are most common
- Others include renal cell carcinoma (Stauffer syndrome)

PFIC disorders
- *ATP8B1* mutations (PFIC1); mutated protein is called FIC1
- *ABCB11* mutations (PFIC2); mutated protein is called BSEP
- *ABCB4* mutations (PFIC3); mutated protein is called MDR3

Thyroid disease (mild cholestasis in some patients, not usually biopsied)
- Hyperthyroid
- Hypothyroid

Clinically common causes, rarely biopsied

Patients in the intensive care unit

Sepsis

Debilitating chronic illnesses

Decompensated liver cirrhosis

Intrahepatic cholestasis of pregnancy

PFIC, progressive familial intrahepatic cholestasis.

DUCTOPENIA

Main Features

Bile duct loss.
Alkaline phosphatase levels should be disproportionately elevated.
Lobular cholestasis may or may not be present.

Additional Findings

Cholate stasis

Key Supporting Stains

CK7
Copper

Ductopenia (Figure 2.15) can occur in the context of chronic biliary obstruction or can be the primary pattern of liver injury. When it is the primary pattern of injury, there is typically little or no portal or lobular inflammation and no evidence of biliary tract obstruction. In either setting, the diagnosis is made in the same way. There are many potential causes (Table 2.4).

TABLE 2.4 **Differential for Bile Duct Loss**	
Etiology	Comment/Representative Reference
Primary chronic biliary tract disease	
Primary sclerosing cholangitis	
Primary biliary cirrhosis/cholangitis	
ABCB4/MDR3 deficiency	Including heterozygous mutations
Alagile syndrome	Can sometimes present in adults
Pediatric liver disease	
Paucity of intrahepatic bile ducts	Syndromic (eg, Alagile syndrome) or nonsyndromic
Neonatal hepatitis	Often subtle; keratin stain is very helpful. Duct loss does not always reach the full threshold of established ductopenia.
Biliary atresia	Usually not until there is advanced fibrosis
α1 Antitrypsin deficiency	
ITCH mutations with multiorgan autoimmune disease including autoimmune hepatitis	44
Secondary causes of chronic biliary tract disease	
Sarcoidosis	Granulomas in hilar lymph nodes can cause biliary obstruction; rarely there can also be granulomatous destruction of the bile ducts.
Intra-arterial chemotherapy	
Mast cell cholangitis	
Portal biliopathy	Chronic portal vein thrombosis and tissue remodeling obstructs large bile ducts
Extrahepatic bile duct obstruction	Any chronic extrahepatic biliary tract obstruction. Common causes include stones, strictures, pancreatic disease.
Infections	
Recurrent pyogenic cholangitis	
AIDS	Thought to result from chronic infection of the biliary tree; potential agents include *Cryptosporidium*, *Microsporidium*, cytomegalovirus, and *Cyclospora*.[45,46]
Drug-induced liver injury	Many different medications[47]
	Total parenteral nutrition
	Herbal remedies

TABLE 2.4 Differential for Bile Duct Loss (Continued)	
Etiology	Comment/Representative Reference
Paraneoplastic syndrome	
Lymphoma	Hodgkin disease[48]
	Peripheral T-cell lymphoma[49]
Carcinoma	
Transplant related	
Chronic allograft rejection	
Biliary anastomotic strictures	
Ischemic cholangiopathy resulting from hepatic artery thrombosis	
Bone marrow transplant related	Graft-versus-host disease, drug-induced liver injury
Idiopathic	

AIDS, acquired immunodeficiency syndrome.

As noted previously, a few of the smaller portal tracts can be missing a bile duct within a liver biopsy specimen and still be normal, so at least 50% of the portal tracts should have no bile ducts in order to qualify for ductopenia. The definition also assumes a reasonably sized liver biopsy specimen, with at least 10 portal tracts. For cases where bile ducts appear to be diminished, but the full threshold of 50% loss is not met, the pathology report can still indicate that early ductopenia may be present. CK7 stain should be used to both confirm the bile duct loss and to identify intermediate hepatocytes, which are invariably present in zone 1. Copper stains also commonly show positive results. Alkaline phosphatase level is always elevated and is always the predominantly elevated liver enzyme; aspartate transaminase (AST) and alanine transaminase (ALT) levels can be normal or mildly elevated.

PATTERNS OF NECROSIS

Main Features

Lobular necrosis.
May or may not be associated with lobular hepatitis

Key Supporting Stains

Trichrome, reticulin (may help in distinguishing bridging necrosis from bridging fibrosis)
Viral immunostains, based on pattern of necrosis

Necrosis patterns in liver biopsy specimens are generally subclassified according to their severity as *spotty, confluent, panacinar, submassive,* or *massive.* Mixed patterns are not uncommon, in which case the most severe pattern is used for classification. As another layer of information, necrosis can be classified as *zonal* or *azonal.*

Single or small clusters of dead hepatocytes are called *spotty necrosis.* Spotty necrosis can be seen in any part of the lobule and is common in many different types of acute and chronic hepatitis. In most hepatitic patterns of injury, the amount of apoptosis tends to covary with the degree of lobular hepatitis; the apoptosis in this setting is considered part of the hepatitic pattern of injury and not a separate pattern of injury. On the other hand, when there is little or no inflammation, then the spotty necrosis may be the predominant pattern of injury, engendering a differential of drug-induced liver injury, acute viral hepatitis, and ischemia.

Somewhat larger clusters of dead hepatocytes, involving at least three contiguous hepatocytes, are called *confluent necrosis* and are found in zone 3 as part of a hepatitic pattern of injury, usually in the setting of moderate to severe lobular hepatitis. Of course, the cutoff of three hepatocytes is used to compare and contrast with spotty necrosis and nobody expects (or wants) you to try to count the number of dead hepatocytes. Confluent necrosis can have distinct zonal patterns. The most common is zone 3, but rare cases have a zone 1 or zone 2 distribution; these zonal patterns are discussed in more detail in the *Bland Necrosis* section. Foci of confluent necrosis that do not follow a zonal pattern are called *azonal*; these necrotic foci are often rather large and can have inflammatory changes at their edges, a pattern that suggests active viral infection from herpes simplex virus (HSV), varicella-zoster virus (VZV), or adenovirus.

The next level of necrosis, in terms of severity, is bridging necrosis, where bands of necrosis connect central veins to central veins or portal tracts to portal tracts or portal tracts to central veins. The areas of bridging necrosis show loss of hepatocytes, condensed parenchyma, and varying degrees of inflammation. They can be easily mistaken for bands of bridging fibrosis, even after examination using the trichrome stain, as the condensed but nonfibrotic tissue in the areas of necrosis can stain light blue on trichrome stain.

In more severe injuries, the necrosis can extend to involve the entire lobule/acinus. A single necrotic lobule is almost never seen in isolation, so the term *panlobular necrosis* is used (synonyms: *panacinar necrosis, multiacinar necrosis*).

MASSIVE NECROSIS involves a large proportion of the tissue (greater than 75%). Livers with massive necrosis often show a thin rim of surviving hepatocytes hugging the portal tracts.

The term *submassive necrosis* is used in two distinct settings: first, where it refers to the relative amount of necrosis and is used essentially as a synonym for *panlobular necrosis*, and second where the term also incorporates a component of the time since necrosis; thus, the context of usage is important to understand the intent. In liver biopsy specimens, this term typically references the first definition, indicating that the areas of necrosis are severe but are less than massive. While there are no official definitions, a reasonable approach is to use the term *submassive necrosis* for cases with necrosis that involves more than 25% but less than 75% of the tissue specimen. In many of these cases, either *panacinar necrosis* or *submassive necrosis* would be the appropriate term.

The term *submassive necrosis,* when used in explanted livers, generally has a different meaning, indicating that there has been both severe liver necrosis and sufficient time for there to be at least some regeneration, with regenerative nodules interspersed within large areas of parenchymal collapse. In these cases, the liver did not fully recover from the severe injury (which could have been massive or submassive in terms of the initial extent) but there was time for at least partial liver regeneration. This pattern is seen often with transplants performed weeks to months after the initial acute, severe liver injury. The term *subacute necrosis* is also used in this context.

Bland Necrosis

Main Features

Lobular necrosis.
Lobular hepatitis is minimal or absent.
Azonal necrosis patterns should be examined for viral cytopathic effect.

Key Supporting Stains

Viral immunostains, based on pattern of necrosis

Bland necrosis is not accompanied by significant lobular hepatitis. Lobular cholestasis can be present but is typically not a dominant feature when the injury is acute, becoming more common in cases where there have been longer time intervals between the initial injury and the biopsy.

In some cases, the source of injury may be known and the biopsy was performed not for a causative diagnosis but to assess the amount of necrosis. In these cases, an estimate of necrosis to the nearest 10% is sufficient. If the biopsy specimen is obtained during a laparotomy, then remember that the surgeon may have sampled a circumscribed ischemic lesion and thus the biopsy may not be representative of the entire liver. If you know the biopsy was targeted to a focal lesion, then indicate so in the biopsy report.

Zone 3 Pattern

Differential for Zone 3 Pattern of Necrosis

- Drug reaction including acetaminophen
- Ischemia
- Various toxins

This pattern of injury is associated with toxic injuries; effects of some medication, such as acetaminophen; or ischemia. The hepatocyte necrosis can be limited to zone 3 or can be panacinar. In most cases, there is little or no portal or lobular inflammation (Figure 2.20). If there has been sufficient time between the injury and the biopsy, the portal tracts may have a significant bile ductular proliferation, which can extend into the areas of lobular necrosis, partially filling the areas of parenchymal collapse within the lobules. The surviving hepatocytes often show small and intermediate-sized fat droplets. An iron stain may show marked iron accumulation in the Kupffer cells, and, if a replacement ductular proliferation has developed, the small ductules filling up the lobules may show extensive iron staining.

Ischemia may also lead to a zone 3 pattern of necrosis or can reach the level of massive necrosis in severe cases. Very early ischemic injury can be challenging to recognize, as the hepatocytes may still be present and many, or even all, of the hepatocytes can still have their nuclei. The cytoplasm of the dead hepatocytes, however, will be more eosinophilic, leading to distinct color differences when compared with living

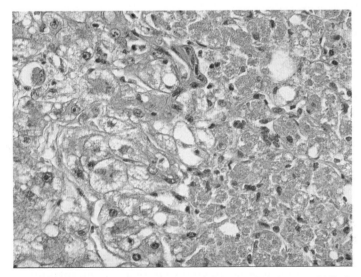

FIGURE 2.20 **Bland necrosis.** Acetaminophen toxicity has led to zone 3 lobular necrosis with no significant inflammation. The necrosis is on the right side of the image.

hepatocytes, typically best seen using lower power lenses such as a 4× or 10× lens. Areas of necrosis also lose the normal CD10 canalicular staining pattern very early after the ischemic insult. If the liver is cirrhotic, the ischemic injury pattern can sometimes lead to necrosis in the center of scattered cirrhotic nodules (Figure 2.21) or to massive necrosis in more severe cases.

Identifying the acute necrosis pattern of injury on frozen sections can be particularly difficult but, with careful attention, the cytoplasm of the hepatocytes will be noticeably more eosinophilic in the necrotic area and this can guide you to the proper diagnosis.

Zone 1 Pattern

Differential for Zone 1 Pattern of Necrosis

- Endotoxin release from *Proteus vulgaris*
- Ferrous iron toxicity
- Halothane toxicity (zone 3 necrosis is more typical)
- Acute hepatitis A viral (HAV) hepatitis
- Industrial chemicals such as allyl alcohol
- White phosphorus toxicity

A predominate zone 1 necrosis pattern is rare and, when present, often extends into zone 2 (Figure 2.22). With more extensive necrosis, the

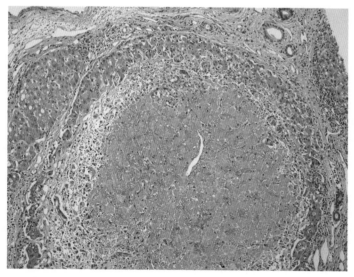

FIGURE 2.21 **Zone 3 necrosis in cirrhosis.** Ischemic necrosis led to central necrosis of cirrhotic nodules.

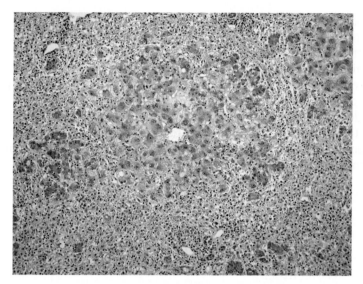

FIGURE 2.22 **Zone 1 pattern of necrosis.** The liver shows extensive necrosis with sparing of the zone 3 hepatocytes in this case associated with halothane use.

underlying zonal patterns can be challenging to identify and the overall pattern of zonality is often best assessed by looking for where the hepatocytes are still viable. Reported causes for zone 1 necrosis include halothane toxicity (more commonly causes zone 3 necrosis), ferrous iron toxicity, white phosphorus toxicity, endotoxin release from *Proteus vulgaris,* and some industrial chemicals such as allyl alcohol.

Zone 2 Pattern

Differential for Zone 2 Pattern of Necrosis

- Heavy metals such as beryllium
- Poisons
- Yellow fever virus

Selective zone 2 necrosis is also very rare. The differential includes rare poisons such as ngaione, heavy metals such as beryllium, and rare viral infections such as yellow fever virus infection. Of note, both the zone 1 and the zone 2 patterns of liver necrosis are sufficiently rare that many associations are based on data limited to case reports or small case series.

CYTOPLASMIC CHANGES

Diffuse Cytoplasmic Changes

Glycogen accumulation
- Glycogenic hepatopathy
- Glycogen storage disease
- Urea cycle defects

Iron accumulation
- Genetic hemochromatosis
- Secondary iron overload

Diffuse dense lipofuscin deposition
- Gilbert syndrome

Key Supporting Stains

Iron

Distinct Cytoplasmic Inclusions

Eosinophilic, often small, with multiple inclusions per hepatocyte
- α1-Antitrypsin (zone 1 mostly)
- Nonspecific inclusions in congestive hepatopathy (mostly zone 3, sparse)
- Other rare genetic disorders such as antithrombin III deficiency and antichymotrypsin deficiency
- Megamitochondria (any zone)

Light gray inclusions, typically large with inclusions one per hepatocyte
- Hepatitis B virus (HBV), ground glass
- Pseudoground glass, usually a medication effect
- Disulfiram (ETOH aversion therapy)
- LECT2, amyloid
- Fibrinogen storage disease (eosinophilic to light gray)
- Nonspecific fibrinogen inclusions
- Type IV glycogen storage disease (children)
- Lafora disease (children, teenagers)

Key Supporting Stains

PAS
PASD
HBsAg
α1-Antitrypsin
LECT2

Various diseases can lead to cytoplasmic changes within hepatocytes as the primary pattern of injury. Cytoplasmic changes can be diffuse, for example, in glycogenic hepatopathy, where hepatocytes have abundant glycogen accumulation. This pattern most commonly results from poorly controlled type I diabetes (Figure 2.23), but the differential can also include glycogen storage disease and urea cycle defects in infants and children. Other diffuse cytoplasmic changes include iron deposition and lipofuscin. Fatty and iron-associated liver diseases are further discussed in their own chapters.

A number of liver diseases can lead to distinct inclusions in the cytoplasm of hepatocytes. A useful approach is to divide the inclusions into two major types based on their morphology. Eosinophilic inclusions are usually small and are commonly seen as multiple, globular inclusions. The most common cause is the accumulation of α1-antitrypsin proteins, which are predominantly located in zone 1 hepatocytes (Figure 2.24) and are highlighted by PASD stains (Figure 2.25). Small and usually sparse eosinophilic inclusions can occasionally be seen in zone 3 hepatocytes in livers with chronic passive congestion (Figure 2.26); these represent a nonspecific accumulation of various proteins within lysosomes.[50] The inclusions can show positive staining for α1-antitrypsin in the setting of congestive liver disease,[50] but this finding represents a nonspecific accumulation and/or cross-reaction and not true α1-antitrypsin disease. Megamitochondria can sometimes enter the differential, but they tend to be smaller in size.

Large, single, pale-gray inclusions that fill up most of the cytoplasm are called *ground glass inclusions* when they occur in the setting of

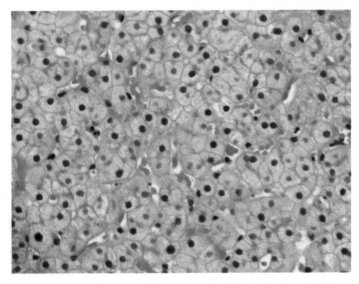

FIGURE 2.23 **Glycogenic hepatopathy.** A young patient with type 1 diabetes mellitus presented with an acute increase in liver enzyme levels. The hepatocytes show clearing of their cytoplasm.

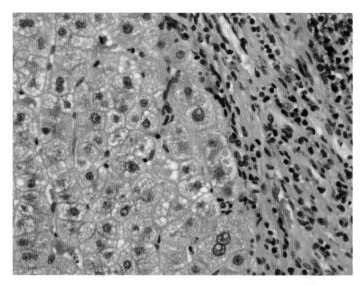

FIGURE 2.24 **A1AT (α1-antitrypsin) protein globules, hematoxylin-eosin (H&E).** Subtle, small globules are located in zone 1 hepatocytes.

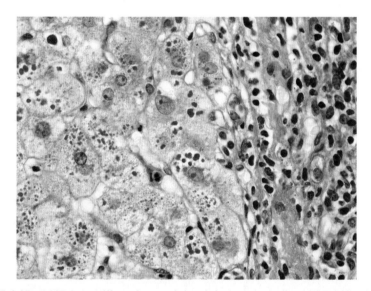

FIGURE 2.25 **A1AT (α1-antitrypsin) protein globules, periodic acid-Schiff with diastase (PASD).** The globules stand out on PASD stain.

chronic hepatitis B viral (HBV) infection (Figure 2.27); these inclusions will be strongly positive on hepatitis B surface antigen (HBsAg) immunostain. Histologically identical inclusions occur in patients who do not have HBV infection, but who are often immunosuppressed and taking many medications, a finding that represents a mild drug effect and is called

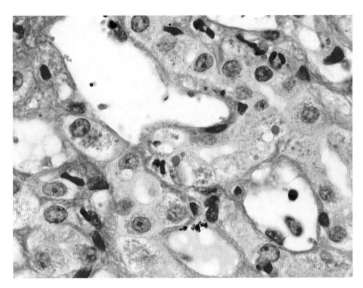

FIGURE 2.26 **Globules in congestive hepatopathy, periodic acid-Schiff with diastase (PASD).** These small globules can be positive by immunostains for A1AT (α1-antitrypsin) protein, but this is a nonspecific finding that does not indicate patients have *SERPINA1* mutations.

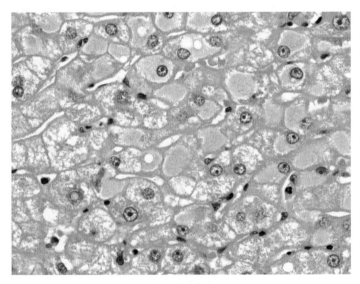

FIGURE 2.27 **Hepatits B virus (HBV) ground glass.** Numerous ground glass hepatocytes are present, with large amphophilic inclusions that fill the cytoplasm.

pseudoground glass inclusions or *pseudoground glass changes*[51] (Figure 2.28). Occasionally, identical pseudoground glass changes can be idiopathic and are found in patients who are not immunosuppressed and/or on multiple medications. Clinical testing or immunostains for HBsAg are important

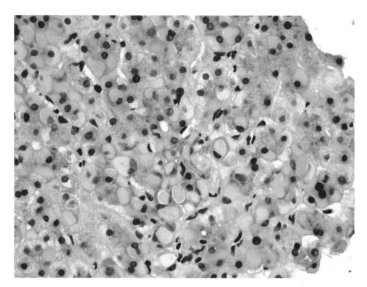

FIGURE 2.28 **Pseudoground glass change.** Scattered hepatocytes have large ampho-philic inclusions that fill the cytoplasm; biopsy is from an immunosuppressed patient taking many medications.

to rule out HBV infection before labeling a case as pseudoground glass change. Other very rare genetic diseases can lead to similar inclusions, including type IV glycogen storage disease, fibrinogen storage disease, and Lafora disease. The large, pale-gray inclusions in cases of ground glass and pseudoground glass change are all PAS-positive and are generally diastase sensitive (although diastase digestion can be variable even within a given biopsy specimen), with the exception of the inclusions in both fibrinogen storage disease and nonspecific fibrinogen-rich inclusions,[52] which are PAS-negative. Finally, the histologic findings in LECT amyloid can also show large gray to eosinophilic hepatocyte inclusions.[53]

VASCULAR DISEASE

Large Vein Obstruction

- Zone 3 predominant congestion
- Atrophy of zone 3 hepatocytes
- Note: some cases can have bile ductular proliferation in the portal tracts, mimicking biliary obstruction

Sinusoidal/Small-Vein Obstruction (Venoocclusive Disease/Sinusoidal Obstructive Syndrome)

- Zone 3 predominant congestion–"bridging congestion."
- Nodular regenerative hyperplasia (NRH) is often present.
- Fibrous obliteration of small central veins can be seen.

Portal Vein Disease

- Portal vein atrophy or loss.
- Portal vein herniation.
- Muscularization of portal vein wall.
- Nodular regenerative hyperplasia is often present.
- Lobular atrophy in severe cases.

Peliosis Hepatis

- Localized lesion of dilated sinusoids/cystic spaces

Key Supporting Stains

- Reticulin (helps identify nodular regenerative hyperplasia)
- CK7 (zone 3 intermediate hepatocytes can be seen in vascular outflow disease)

Vascular injury is discussed in detail in Chapter 13, but a useful conceptual framework is to classify vascular injury into one of several major patterns. While these patterns certainly may have some overlapping features, the differential largely is determined by the dominant pattern. The first major pattern is large-vein obstruction, such as with Budd-Chiari syndrome or chronic heart disease, where the main finding is that of congestive hepatopathy with dilated sinusoids (Figure 2.29). The zone 3 hepatocytes often show atrophy and there can be zone 3 pericellular fibrosis in chronic

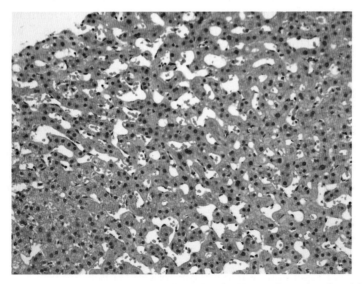

FIGURE 2.29 **Congestive hepatopathy.** The patient had known long-standing right-sided failure and the biopsy showed diffuse, mild to moderate zone 3 sinusoidal dilatation.

cases. CK7 may also show a zone 3 pattern of intermediate hepatocytes, which can be a helpful supporting stain in subtle or challenging cases. When there is more severe disease, the portal tracts may show a brisk bile ductular proliferation that mimics biliary obstruction.

A second pattern, called *venoocclusive disease* or the synonym *sinusoidal obstructive syndrome*, results from diffuse injury to medium- and small-sized central veins and/or the sinusoidal endothelial cells, leading to varying degrees of thrombosis and fibrosis of the central veins (Figure 2.30), usually combined with sinusoidal dilation and congestion and some degree of NRH. The thrombosed central veins can be sparse, however, and the histology is often dominated by the mild sinusoidal congestion and NRH. This pattern can be caused by chemotherapy, other medications or herbal remedies, or infection/inflammatory central vein injury. Clotting disorders can also lead to thrombosis of small- and medium-sized central veins; in this setting, however, the findings are typically focal, leading to localized vascular flow abnormalities and sometimes regenerative changes that can mimic a mass lesion.

Finally, chronic injury or loss of the portal veins also leads to liver pathology, which may include varying degrees of absence or scarring of the portal veins, portal vein herniation, NRH, or generalized liver atrophy. These findings are almost never all present in any given case, but the diagnosis is strengthened when more individual changes are seen and when the changes are multifocal or diffuse throughout the biopsy specimen. In chronic and more severe cases of portal vein thrombosis or loss, liver atrophy can be detected by imaging studies or at the time of surgery, with the

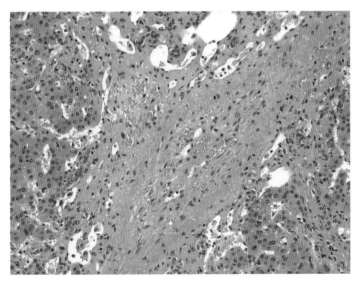

FIGURE 2.30 **Venoocclusive disease.** Several central veins showed fibrous scarring in this patient who received chemotherapy for colorectal carcinoma.

histologic correlate being portal tracts that are more closely approximated than in a normal liver.

Peliosis Hepatis

Diseases Associated With the Peliosis Hepatis

- Malignancy, for example, lymphoma, leukemia
- Chronic debilitating infections
  - Systemic lupus erythematosus
  - Chronic renal failure
  - Tuberculosis
  - Leprosy
  - AIDS (can be *Bartonella* related)
- Severe malnutrition
- Medications, most commonly oral contraceptives, androgens, and azathioprine

Peliosis hepatis is an uncommon pattern of injury, one defined by cyst-like spaces in the lobules that are filled with blood (Figure 2.31). The individual cyst-like structures can be microscopic or up to several centimeters in diameter. The areas of peliosis can be grossly confined to a localized region of the liver or can be more diffusely present throughout the parenchyma.

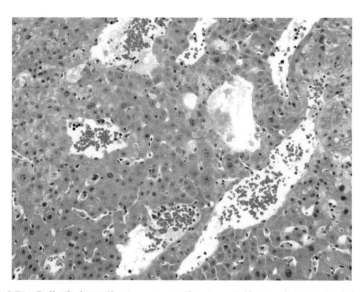

FIGURE 2.31 **Peliosis hepatis.** A young patient was taking androgens and developed hepatic lesions on imaging. Biopsy showed peliosis hepatitis, with cyst-like spaces ranging from small (shown) to large in size.

Often, the cyst-like spaces are not clearly interconnected with each other, but at their edges, they may communicate with the sinusoids. In most cases, the cyst-like spaces are not lined by endothelial cells but an endothelial lining can develop over time in larger lesions.

Of note, in some cases, peliosis is a systemic disease process, involving multiple organs, most often the spleen, bone marrow, and lymph nodes. Occasionally, the gastrointestinal (GI) tract, adrenal glands, and kidney are also involved.[54]

OTHER PATTERNS

Granulomas are discussed in Chapter 7 and amyloid is discussed in Chapter 17, on systemic diseases involving the liver.

Giant Cell Transformation Pattern

Giant cell transformation is a nonspecific reactive change seen within hepatocytes. When it is the dominant histologic finding, the diagnosis of giant cell hepatitis is made (Figure 2.32). Mild giant cell transformation, however, can be seen in a variety of other liver diseases where it is a nonspecific change and does not merit a separate diagnosis of giant cell hepatitis (Figure 2.33). The hepatocytes in giant cell transformation are generally nonproliferative and may result from the fusion of hepatocytes or from nuclear division without cytoplasmic division. As a focal or patchy mild change, it is most commonly seen in cholestatic conditions or chronic hepatitis C. The reason this pattern is seen in

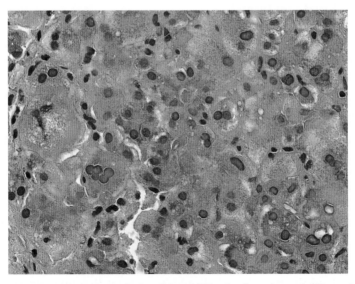

FIGURE 2.32 **Idiopathic adult giant cell hepatitis.** The liver showed diffuse cholestasis and giant cell transformation. No cause was identified.

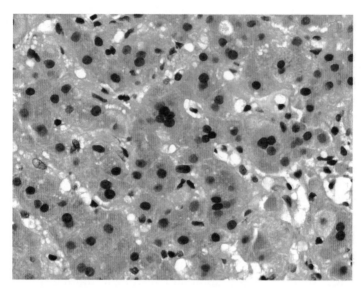

FIGURE 2.33 **Nonspecific giant cell transformation.** This transplant biopsy showed mild bland lobular cholestasis and had very focal giant cell transformation limited to single zone 3 region; this focal change, while striking, does not qualify for adult idiopathic giant cell hepatitis.

some individuals but not others remains obscure, but the findings can be persistent in follow-up biopsies. The differential for giant cell change is shown in Table 2.5.

FIBROSIS EVALUATION

Specimen Adequacy

Determining the amount of liver scarring, or fibrosis stage, is an important component of liver pathology in both clinical care and research settings. In general clinical parlance, "advanced fibrosis" indicates at least bridging fibrosis.

For clinical care, the pathologist should determine the adequacy of the specimen for fibrosis staging by examining the specimen and not by a ruler or by counting the number of portal tracts. For example, a small biopsy specimen that shows unequivocal cirrhosis is adequate for staging for clinical care, while larger biopsy specimens may be fragmented or be markedly inflamed or have other features that limit staging accuracy.

When it comes to staging accuracy, "the bigger, the better" certainly holds true for biopsy specimens. As a general rule of thumb, an adequate biopsy will typically have at least 10 portal tracts and be at least 1 cm in length.[86] The portal tracts do not have to be completely present to be counted, but enough of the portal tract should be present that you can reasonably determine if it is fibrotic. Smaller biopsy specimens tend to understage the

TABLE 2.5 Differential for Giant Cell Changes in Hepatocytes	
Cause	Comment/Representative Reference
Idiopathic adult giant cell hepatitis	[55]
In the settings below, the diagnosis is not "idiopathic giant cell hepatitis" but giant cell transformation in the setting of a different disease process. In these cases, the giant cell transformation does not have clinical relevance.	
Viral infections	
Chronic hepatitis C	Often in the setting of injection drug use, where changes can be persistent[56,57]
Hepatitis E	[58]
Nonhepatotropic viruses	CMV[59]
	EBV[60]
	HIV[61]
	HHV-6A[62] can also lead to giant cell changes in bile ducts[63]
	Possible novel paramyxovirus[64]
Other infections	
Syphilis	[65]
Cholestatic liver diseases	Various causes, most commonly seen in neonates and young children, such as neonatal hepatitis and PFIC disorders
Autoimmune diseases	The frequency is very rare in all these conditions
	Autoimmune hepatitis[55,66]
	Autoimmune hemolytic anemia[67]
	Graves disease[68]
	Immune thrombocytopenic purpura[69]
	PBC[70]
	Systemic lupus erythematosus[71]
	Ulcerative colitis[72,73]
	Connective tissue disorders[74]
	ITCH mutations with multiorgan autoimmune disease[44]
Drug-induced liver injury/herbal reaction	Overall, very rare[75-77]
Hematologic disorders	Non-Hodgkin lymphoma[55]
	Chronic lymphocytic leukemia[78]
	Necrobiotic xanthogranuloma[79]

(Continued)

TABLE 2.5 **Differential for Giant Cell Changes in Hepatocytes (Continued)**	
Cause	Comment/Representative Reference
Genetic causes (in addition to PFIC and related genetic disorders)	
	IGHMBP2 mutations[80]
	CYP27 A mutations[81]
	CYP7B1 mutations[81,82] [81]
	2MACR mutations[83]
	Mitochondrial DNA depletion syndrome[84]
	Mitochondrial phosphoenolpyruvate carboxykinase deficiency[85]
	Wilson disease[59]; very rare, limited to case reports and strength of association is unclear.

Please note that for many of the disease associations, the literature is limited to small numbers of case reports.
CMV, cytomegalovirus; EBV, Epstein-Barr virus; HHV-6A, human herpesvirus 6A; HIV, human immunodeficiency virus; PFIC, progressive familial intrahepatic cholestasis.

degree of inflammation and fibrosis.[87] For example, fibrosis can be patchy with early chronic liver disease, in particular in biliary tract diseases,[88] leading to understaging the fibrosis. On the other hand, fibrosis in cases of chronic viral hepatitis and fatty liver disease tends to be more uniform in early disease,[89-91] although some early cases can still show patchy fibrosis.[90] Fibrosis is typically evaluated using a trichrome stain or a Sirius Red stain. Increased fibrosis can be seen in the portal tracts or in the hepatic lobules, and the various patterns have separate differentials. Lobular fibrosis is most commonly seen in the setting of fatty liver disease, some drug-induced liver injuries, or chronic congestive hepatopathy, while portal-based fibrosis can be seen in chronic liver disease from essentially any cause.

Even on trichrome or other special stains, distinguishing no fibrosis from very early stages of fibrosis can be challenging. When fibrosis staging is complicated by inflammation, biliary proliferation, or other challenges, it can sometimes be appropriate to use terms such as "focal equivocal fibrosis." In general, however, cases with equivocal fibrosis are best classified as showing no fibrosis. This holds true for both formal staging systems and clinical care. In fact, most cases staged as "focal equivocal fibrosis" or with related terminology are classified as showing no fibrosis on expert review. Sometimes there can be lingering concern that someone else will look at the biopsy and decide there is focal mild fibrosis when you did not think so, or vice versa, which can make noncommittal terms such as "focal equivocal fibrosis" seem attractive. Such minor differences are not true discrepancies, however, and have no clinical impact, so they should not be a cause for concern.

Wedge Biopsy Specimen

Wedge biopsies are reliable for assessing liver fibrosis, except for those cases where the biopsy mostly stripped the capsule and sampled little or no underlying liver parenchyma, or in cases in which just a tiny bit of the anterior edge of the liver was sampled, showing mostly capsule without much underlying liver parenchyma.

Some pathologists are reluctant to provide a fibrosis stage on wedge biopsies, having been taught that wedge biopsies are undesirable because they overestimate fibrosis due to "subcapsular fibrosis." This notion extends back at least 100 years, being present in papers from the 1920s, but was addressed in a classic paper, published in 1967, in which the authors state after completing their study "We are thus unable to support the conclusion of Metzler (1925) and Enders (1926) that wedge biopsies in adults have a limited diagnostic value because subcapsular fibrous tissues leads to confusion between normal and fibrotic livers."[92]

It is true that the liver capsule is bright blue on Masson trichrome stain and that its interface with the liver parenchyma is not always perfectly smooth, but this is never a true diagnostic dilemma. As noted earlier, the anterior lip/edge of the liver often has a bit of fibrosis (Figure 2.34), but again there is very little risk that you will interpret this incorrectly.

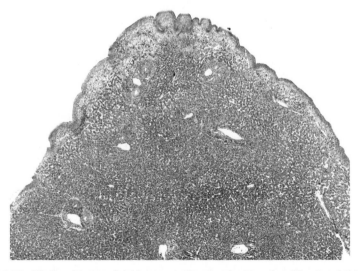

FIGURE 2.34 **Wedge biopsy, fat blue capsule of anterior edge.** The tip of this wedge biopsy shows mild nonspecific fibrosis, but fibrosis evaluation of the parenchyma is readily performed and reliable.

Thus, you can feel very comfortable staging the fibrosis on wedge liver biopsy specimens, using the same common sense and wisdom you apply to needle biopsy specimens. In fact, several studies have convincingly shown that wedge biopsies and needle biopsies provide essentially the same quality of information for grading and staging liver disease[93] or that wedge biopsies have a slight advantage because of their greater amount of tissue.[94]

Sinusoidal Fibrosis

The terms *sinusoidal fibrosis*, *perisinusoidal fibrosis*, and *pericellular fibrosis* are synonyms and are used interchangeably. The term *chicken-wire fibrosis* is sometimes used for its descriptive power, mostly in teaching environments. Pericellular fibrosis typically starts in zone 3 and is most often a result of fatty liver disease, but there are many additional, although uncommon, causes (Table 2.6). Central vein fibrosis is typically lumped in with pericellular fibrosis, as they generally occur together and have similar risk factors. In cases of congestive hepatopathy, however, the fibrosis can be primarily central vein based, sometimes leading to cases with central vein to central vein bridging fibrosis but relatively little pericellular or portal fibrosis.

Pericellular fibrosis shows irregular strands of interconnecting fibrosis extending along the sinusoids. A common approach, one used by the NASH-CRN staging system, is to classify pericellular fibrosis as mild when it is seen on trichrome, but not clearly present on H&E, and moderate when it is definitely visible on H&E (Figure 2.35). One common diagnostic challenge results from overstained trichrome stains, where livers with no fibrosis can be over-staged as having sinusoidal fibrosis. This can be remedied in most cases by repeating the staining. In addition, livers that have either significant hepatitis or significant cholestasis typically show Kupffer cell hyperplasia, and the hyperplastic Kupffer cells can stain light blue on trichrome stain, mimicking pericellular fibrosis. Finally, in some liver biopsies without true fibrosis, the sinusoids have small amounts of collagen detectable by trichrome stain, but the collagen is well organized and lacks the irregular meshlike pattern seen with true pericellular fibrosis (Figure 2.36).

Portal-Based Fibrosis and Fibrosis Progression

Portal-based fibrosis progresses through a stereotypical sequence of fibrosis stages, although progression is not linear over time. Fibrosis first begins as expansion of the portal tracts (portal fibrosis). In the portal fibrosis stage, not every portal tract will be fibrotic in any given case. In addition, the fibrosis may preferentially affect certain sized portal tracts, typically reflecting the location of the disease. For example, in chronic hepatitis C virus (HCV) infection, the largest portal tracts are often spared in very early portal fibrosis, which preferentially affects the small- and medium-sized portal tracts.

TABLE 2.6 Causes of Pericellular Fibrosis	
Cause	**Comment/Representative Reference**
Fatty liver disease	
Alcohol liver disease	
Nonalcoholic liver disease	
Vascular disease	
Chronic venous outflow obstruction	Examples include congestive heart disease, chronic Budd-Chiari syndrome, venoocclusive disease
Medications/toxin	
Drug effect	Methotrexate therapy is one example[95]
Total parenteral nutrition	More common if portal fibrosis is also present[47]
Vitamin A	[96]
Arsenic toxicity	[97,98]
Infections	
Visceral leishmaniasis	[99]
Fibrosing cholestatic hepatitis C or B	
Metabolic/genetic disorders	
Acid sphingomyelinase deficiency (Niemann-Pick disease type B)	[100]
Hyperpipecolic acidemia	[101]
Oxidative phosphorylation deficiency	[17]
Down syndrome	[102]
Unclassified copper overload syndromes	[103]
Miscellaneous conditions	
Idiopathic portal hypertension	[104]
Crohn disease	Rarely can be massive[105]
Diabetic hepatosclerosis	[106,107]
Neonatal giant cell hepatitis	[108]
Myelofibrosis	[109,110]
Idiopathic thrombocytopenic purpura	[111]

Diagnosing Fibrosis

How do you diagnose portal fibrosis? In most cases, the diagnosis is based on assessing the relative size of the portal area and the smoothness of the border between the portal tract and lobules. Assessing portal fibrosis based on the relative size of the portal tract requires some experience to have a

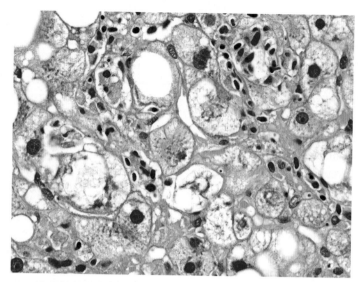

FIGURE 2.35 Pericellular fibrosis. As the pericellular fibrosis is visible on hematoxylin-eosin (H&E), it would be scored as moderate. Ballooned hepatocytes can also be appreciated in this case of steatohepatitis.

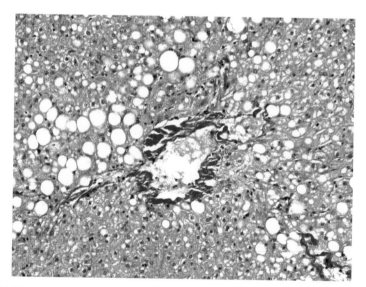

FIGURE 2.36 Normal liver with thick central vein collagen. The central vein has a thick collar of collagen, but in this case, it is normal. Note how the collagen is smooth and organized. The background liver shows steatosis.

sense of how much collagen should normally be present; the size of the portal tract has to be considered too, as larger portal tracts normally have considerably more collagen than medium-sized or smaller sized portal tracts.

In some cases, portal fibrosis is evidenced by a global expansion of the portal tract with relatively smooth borders (Figure 2.37). In other

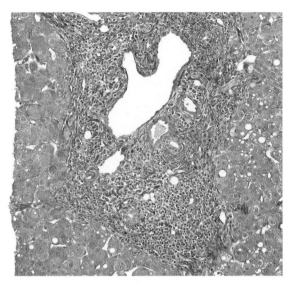

FIGURE 2.37   **Portal fibrosis.** This portal tract shows generalized expansion by fibrous tissue.

cases, the border of a fibrotic portal tract may be irregular and have slender fibrous extensions into the lobules (Figure 2.38), or the portal tract may have hepatocytes at the interface that are "trapped," or surrounded, by thin strands of fibrosis (Figure 2.39). As a general rule of thumb in chronic hepatitis, fibrosis of a few portal tracts is considered to be mild portal fibrosis, whereas fibrosis of half or more of the portal tracts is considered moderate portal fibrosis.

The next step in fibrosis progression, following portal fibrosis, is the development of bridging fibrosis (Figure 2.40). Bridging fibrosis is defined as abnormal fibrous tissue extending from portal tract to portal tract, portal tract to central vein, or central vein to central vein, but in the setting of portal based fibrosis, bridging fibrosis is usually from portal tract to portal tract or portal tract to central vein. When examining a two-dimensional tissue section via the microscope, bridging fibrosis appears as an irregular linear structure of various thicknesses, but in three dimensions, bridging fibrosis is actually an irregular membrane or sheet-like layer of fibrosis that tends to start at the branch points of portal tracts and fill the space in between them, much as the leather webbing of baseball glove extends between the thumb and forefinger of the baseball glove.[112]

There is no fully affirmed thickness that is required as part of the definition for a fibrous bridge. Thicker well-formed bridges are easily agreed upon by all, but very thin delicate strands of fibrosis, some of which may not be quite complete, are not as reproducibly classified. This is not an issue when providing a verbal report, but it can be more problematic when using some of the formal staging schemas. When using a verbal system,

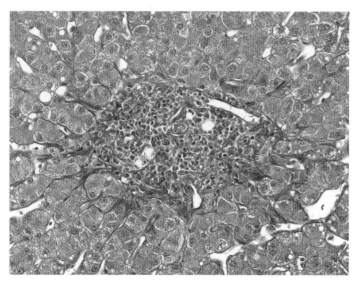

FIGURE 2.38 **Portal fibrosis with irregular fibrous extension.** This portal tract has numerous irregular spikelike extensions. The term periportal fibrosis is sometimes used to describe this pattern.

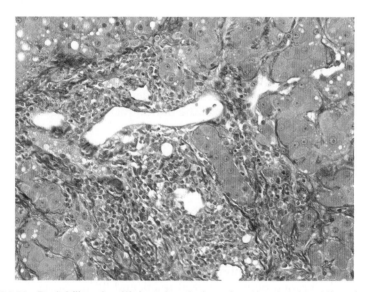

FIGURE 2.39 **Portal fibrosis with hepatocyte trapping.** Hepatocytes at the edge of the portal tract appear trapped in the fibrous tissue.

these cases are handled simply by stating that very thin fibrous structures are present, forming equivocal bridges.

Cirrhosis is defined as regenerative nodules of hepatocytes surrounded by bands of fibrosis. If the nodularity is not complete, that is, if the nodularity is present in some parts of the biopsy but not others, then the term "early cirrhosis" or "incomplete cirrhosis" is often used. Of the major

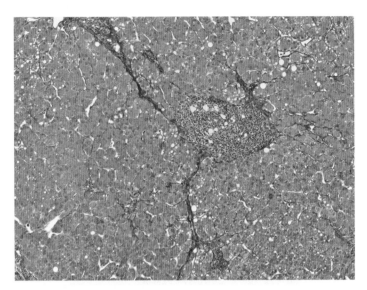

FIGURE 2.40   **Bridging fibrosis.** Thin fibrous bridges connect the portal tracts.

staging systems, only the Laennec system subdivides cirrhotic livers, using a three tier system of 4A, 4B, and 4C, subclassifying cirrhosis based on the thickness of the fibrous bands (please see Chapter 5 for details). With this system, the severity of cirrhosis predicts clinical parameters such as portal hypertension.[113]

Intralobular fibrosis is most typically called pericellular fibrosis or perisinusoidal fibrosis. This pattern of fibrosis is seen most often in fatty liver disease, both alcohol and nonalcohol related. The differential for a zone 3 pattern of pericellular and central vein fibrosis also includes chronic congestive liver disease as well as other rare entities shown in Table 2.6.

COMMON CHALLENGES IN FIBROSIS STAGING

Markedly Inflamed Portal Tracts

The presence of fibrosis can help refine the differential for clinically acute liver injury, as the presence of fibrosis indicates an underlying chronic liver disease that has a superimposed acute injury ie, acute on chronic liver disease—either a flare of a single disease, for example, with chronic hepatitis B or autoimmune hepatitis, or a new superimposed injury on a different underlying chronic liver disease. As an important pitfall, however, portal tracts can be markedly expanded by inflammation or bile ductular proliferation, all of it staining blue, giving a false impression of true portal fibrosis on trichrome stain (Figure 2.41).

Bridging Necrosis

The trichrome stain should also be interpreted cautiously in the setting of significant necrosis, as bridging necrosis can mimic bridging fibrosis. Bridging necrosis in the setting of acute liver injury that is only a few days

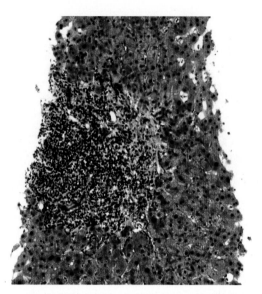

FIGURE 2.41 **Marked portal inflammation mimicking portal fibrosis.** This is an important diagnostic pitfall when staging liver biopsies.

old, for example, from acetaminophen toxicity, is generally not a problem because the areas of necrosis will contain dead hepatocytes. However, if there has been sufficient time for the hepatocytes to drop out and the parenchymal connective tissue to condense (Figure 2.42), then these areas of bridging necrosis will stain blue on trichrome and can closely mimic bridging fibrosis (Figure 2.43). In some cases, there can be regenerative liver nodules and the whole picture can closely mimic cirrhosis. In fact, over the years, this author has encountered several consult cases of fibrosis/cirrhosis "regression," where an early biopsy in the setting of a marked acute hepatitis was overinterpreted as showing advanced fibrosis, but a follow-up biopsy after resolution of the acute hepatitis showed no fibrosis. If you are just not sure about the fibrosis stage, it is best to state so. As one example, if a biopsy shows extensive necrosis and you are not sure if there is underlying mild fibrosis, but you are sure there is not cirrhosis, you might say, "fibrosis staging in the setting of extensive necrosis can be inaccurate, but there appears to be no evidence for established cirrhosis."

Fragmented Specimens

In general, a fragmented liver specimen is more commonly seen with advanced fibrosis.[114,115] Related to this, adequate (in terms of total tissue) but fragmented biopsy specimens tend to be associated with advanced fibrosis.[116] On the other hand, specimen fragmentation in biopsies with very little total tissue is much less meaningful. These are widely known observations, but there are some important caveats that are sometimes forgotten. First, some degree of specimen fragmentation is almost universally seen,

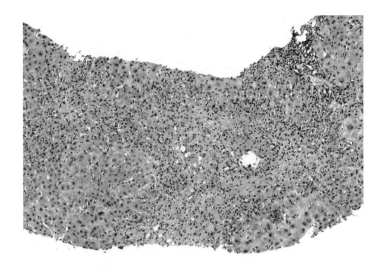

FIGURE 2.42 **Bridging necrosis.** This case of autoimmune hepatitis has bridging necrosis that extends across the middle of this image.

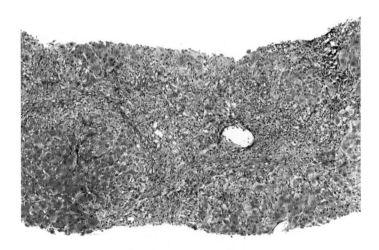

FIGURE 2.43 **Bridging necrosis.** On trichrome stain, the area of parenchymal collapse stains blue, mimicking bridging fibrosis.

regardless of the degree of fibrosis. Second, it is only the *very fragmented* specimens, in one study only specimens with >12 fragments,[114] that are strongly associated with advanced fibrosis or cirrhosis.

So, then, what should you do with a fragmented specimen? If you can confidently diagnose cirrhosis, then the specimen is adequate for fibrosis staging. If not, then first decide if the biopsy has enough total tissue to evaluate.

If it does, next determine the fibrosis stage using the method you choose, whether it be a verbal description or a formal staging system—but do not upgrade the fibrosis stage you put into the surgical pathology report solely because the specimen is fragmented. Instead, report out the fibrosis stage exactly as you see it on the slide, but indicate in a note that significantly fragmented specimens can sometimes underestimate the true fibrosis stage.

Fibrous Caps

"Fibrous caps" is a concept related to biopsy specimen fragmentation. Some of the nodules can have a rim of fibrous tissue that is referred to as a "fibrous cap" (Figure 2.44). Sometimes this fibrous cap can indicate bridging fibrosis or cirrhosis. This finding, however, should be approached carefully, especially if the fibrous caps are thin and are the only evidence for advanced fibrosis seen in the biopsy specimen; the "caps" in this situation do not provide strong evidence for bridging fibrosis. However, if the "caps" are thick and outline well-formed nodules, then this finding suggests at least bridging fibrosis and often cirrhosis.

Portal Tract Branch Points

Normal portal tracts branch as they extend deeper into the liver parenchyma. These branch points can mimic fibrous bridges if they are cut in parallel to the direction in which they are running. In most cases, the branch point is readily seen and there is little risk of confusion. In cases that are more challenging,

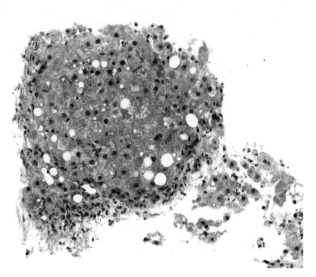

FIGURE 2.44 **Fibrous caps.** This badly fragmented specimen has a fibrous cap composed of a thin rim of collagen that mimics advanced fibrosis but was called inadequate for staging. A repeat biopsy showed no fibrosis.

other findings can further guide the fibrosis staging. For example, a normal portal tract cut along its axis will typically have vessels running along the length of portal area and will have smooth borders with the adjacent hepatocytes (Figure 2.45). In contrast, a fibrous bridge tends to be irregular at the interface with the lobules, tends to not have vessels running along the entire length, and is often inflamed. The entire context of the case is also very helpful; if the biopsy has no portal fibrosis, then bridging fibrosis is unlikely.

Advanced Fibrosis Without Well-Defined Nodularity

In rare biopsy specimens, the trichrome stain shows diffuse, severe lobular fibrosis, often accompanied by bridging fibrosis, but the liver does not show well-defined parenchymal nodularity (Figure 2.46). This pattern is most often seen when there is advanced fibrosis in the setting of active and significant alcohol use. This pattern—that of severe lobular fibrosis that is diffuse throughout the specimen—can be reported descriptively in the pathology report, but the findings are clinically equivalent to cirrhosis in terms of its association with portal hypertension. In these cases, the regenerative nodules of cirrhosis often develop only after the use of alcohol diminishes sufficiently for there to be sufficient hepatocyte regeneration.

NONINVASIVE MARKERS OF FIBROSIS

Commonly Available Noninvasive Tests for Liver Fibrosis

1. **Serum tests.** Based on a panel of serum markers, usually five or less, often combined with age and gender.
   Examples: FibroTest, APRI, Fibrosis-4.
   For example, the FibroTest uses this panel: α_2-macroglobulin, haptoglobin, γ-glutamyl transpeptidase (GGT), apolipoprotein A1, and total bilirubin.
2. **Standard imaging modalities**
   Examples: ultrasound, conventional or contrast-enhanced magnetic resonance imaging (MRI), computed tomography (CT).
   Features of cirrhosis can generally be thought of as falling into two categories: (1) direct findings such as a coarse liver texture, a nodular liver surface, and liver volume reduction; (2) indirect features such as portal hypertension, splenomegaly, ascites, and/or esophageal varices.
3. **Elastography.** Fibrosis is assessed by how fast ultrasound waves, or vibrations produced by a mechanical device, can pass through the liver—the faster they go, the stiffer the liver.
   • Ultrasound based; for example, FibroScan.
   • MRI based; for example, magnetic resonance elastography (MRE).

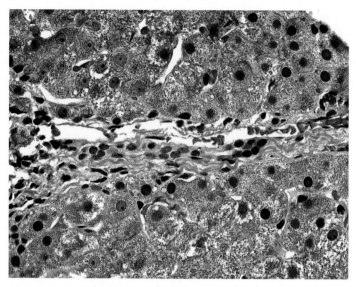

FIGURE 2.45 **Normal portal tract cut longitudinally.** Longitudinal sections of normal portal tracts can sometimes mimic bridging fibrosis.

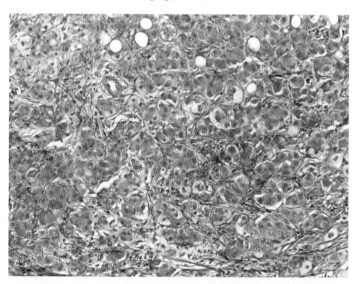

FIGURE 2.46 **Diffuse lobular fibrosis.** The patient had a long history of ethanol (ETOH) abuse and portal hypertension. The liver is not technically cirrhotic but shows diffuse severe pericellular fibrosis.

Clinical teams now commonly rely on noninvasive markers of fibrosis as their main tool for assessment of liver fibrosis in patients with known chronic liver disease, by using serologic assays, imaging, or liver stiffness tests. Biopsies are then performed only when there is a discrepancy between other clinical findings and the noninvasive test results, or there is clinical concern for additional disease processes. Overall, noninvasive tests perform well on both sides of the histologic fibrosis spectrum. They typically can accurately identify cases as having no fibrosis/minimal fibrosis or has having cirrhosis. Stages of fibrosis in between that of no fibrosis and cirrhosis, however, are not reliably classified by noninvasive markers of fibrosis.[117,118] In clinical practice, they are most commonly used to exclude advanced fibrosis/cirrhosis.[119] In general, elastographic methods are more accurate than blood-based assays,[120] but they can be technically difficult to perform in obese patients. Magnetic resonance (MR) elastography is even more accurate[121] and can be performed in obese patients, but is expensive.

In some cases, there can be significant discrepancies between the histologic stage of fibrosis and noninvasive test results. Changes that tend to "stiffen" the liver, such as congestive hepatopathy, severe hepatitis,[122] NRH, and sometimes moderate or severe steatosis/steatohepatitis,[122] can all lead to overstaging by noninvasive methodologies. Discrepancies in the other direction, where the noninvasive markers underestimate the amount of histologic fibrosis, also occur but are less common.[123]

FIBROSIS REGRESSION PATTERNS

For a very long time, cirrhosis was thought to be irreversible. This was changed when careful morphologic studies of liver biopsies, by Wanless and colleagues,[124] led to a paradigm shift when they reported that cirrhosis and fibrosis could regress if the agent of injury was removed. As is true for many innovative ideas, ones that lead to major changes in the way diseases are understood, these early reports were met with a great deal of skepticism. It is now widely accepted, however, that fibrosis can regress. In fact, full acceptance of this important notion has led some authors to suggest abandoning the term cirrhosis in favor of the term "advanced stage."[125]

Conceptually, as cirrhosis regresses, the thick fibrotic bridges that surround cirrhotic nodules become thin and eventually incomplete and, with enough time, can disappear. This regression of the fibrotic bridges surrounding cirrhotic nodules, plus active liver regeneration, transforms small cirrhotic nodules into larger nodules and eventually the nodularity regresses.

The histologic correlates of cirrhosis regression have been suggested to include the following features,[124] listed approximately from early to later findings: (1) minute regenerative nodules/isolated, small clusters of hepatocytes in fibrous bands, which reflect early regeneration; (2) perforated delicate fibrous bridges, which reflect reabsorption of the fibrous bridges (Figure 2.47); (3) closely approximated medium-sized portal tracts and central veins that are connected by very short and broad fibrous bridges (called *adhesions* or *parenchymal extinction lesion*[126]); (4) isolated thick collagen bundles in the lobules (Figure 2.48); (5) delicate spikes of fibrosis extending from portal tracts, for example, "periportal" fibrosis; and (6) remnants of

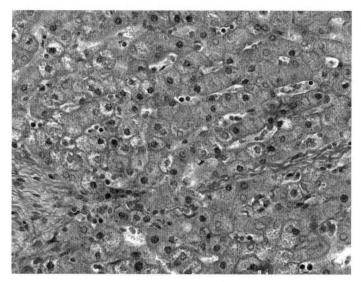

FIGURE 2.47 **Perforated delicate bridges.** This thin delicate fibrous bridge appears to be focally perforated.

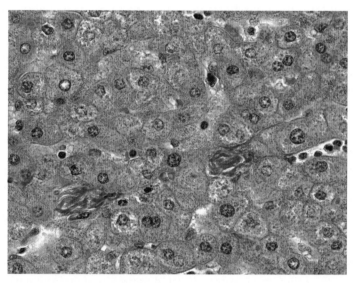

FIGURE 2.48 **Isolated thick collagen bundles.** A trichrome stain shows isolated bundles of thick collagen in the hepatic lobules.

portal tracts or central veins in an otherwise almost normal liver. Most of these findings are better seen on trichrome stains than H&E stains.

Studies have yet to firmly nail down the most accurate way to score features of fibrosis regression, but it is important to know that fibrosis can regress and the features listed earlier are currently thought to be potentially relevant to this important area of pathology. Ongoing challenges include a lack of data on the most specific and reproducible findings that indicate fibrosis regression. In addition, for most clinical cases, there is no reliable way to determine the "fibrosis direction arrow," which is critically important because the laying down of new fibrosis and reabsorption of old fibrosis is an ongoing, dynamic process; it is the balance of the two that determines whether or not fibrosis progresses or regresses. Research studies often benefit from having paired biopsy specimens, which provide information on the "fibrosis direction arrow," but this is rarely available in clinical cases.

Finally, clinical relevance has not been established. It seems reasonable that information on fibrosis regression would be clinically helpful, but this has not been demonstrated to date, with no studies providing a clear road map on how this information would be incorporated into clinical management, which is currently focused on removing or minimizing active injury.

On the other hand, the conventional fibrosis stage, regardless of the "fibrosis direction," remains clinically relevant because it predicts clinical outcomes.[127-129] Even in this setting, noninvasive markers of fibrosis have progressed to the point that they can guide clinical management of liver disease for many of the most common causes.

REFERENCES

1. Crawford AR, Lin XZ, Crawford JM. The normal adult human liver biopsy: a quantitative reference standard. *Hepatology*. 1998;28:323-331.

2. Kietzmann T. Metabolic zonation of the liver: the oxygen gradient revisited. *Redox Biol*. 2017;11:622-630.

3. Schmucker DL. Age-related changes in liver structure and function: implications for disease? *Exp Gerontol*. 2005;40:650-659.

4. Wlodzimirow KA, Eslami S, Abu-Hanna A, et al. Systematic review: acute liver failure—one disease, more than 40 definitions. *Aliment Pharmacol Ther*. 2012;35:1245-1256.

5. O'Grady JG, Schalm SW, Williams R. Acute liver failure: redefining the syndromes. *Lancet*. 1993;342:273-275.

6. Singhal A, Vadlamudi S, Stokes K, et al. Liver histology as predictor of outcome in patients with acute liver failure. *Transpl Int*. 2012;25:658-662.

7. Donaldson BW, Gopinath R, Wanless IR, et al. The role of transjugular liver biopsy in fulminant liver failure: relation to other prognostic indicators. *Hepatology*. 1993;18:1370-1376.

8. Miraglia R, Luca A, Gruttadauria S, et al. Contribution of transjugular liver biopsy in patients with the clinical presentation of acute liver failure. *Cardiovasc Intervent Radiol*. 2006;29:1008-1010.

9. Johnson K, Kotiesh A, Boitnott JK, et al. Histology of symptomatic acute hepatitis C infection in immunocompetent adults. *Am J Surg Pathol*. 2007;31:1754-1758.

10. Rolfes DB, Ishak KG. Acute fatty liver of pregnancy: a clinicopathologic study of 35 cases. *Hepatology*. 1985;5:1149-1158.

11. Uchida T, Kao H, Quispe-Sjogren M, et al. Alcoholic foamy degeneration—a pattern of acute alcoholic injury of the liver. *Gastroenterology*. 1983;84:683-692.

12. Tandra S, Yeh MM, Brunt EM, et al. Presence and significance of microvesicular steatosis in nonalcoholic fatty liver disease. *J Hepatol.* 2011;55:654-659.

13. Tesarova M, Mayr JA, Wenchich L, et al. Mitochondrial DNA depletion in Alpers syndrome. *Neuropediatrics.* 2004;35:217-223.

14. Mandel H, Hartman C, Berkowitz D, et al. The hepatic mitochondrial DNA depletion syndrome: ultrastructural changes in liver biopsies. *Hepatology.* 2001;34:776-784.

15. Holve S, Hu D, Shub M, et al. Liver disease in Navajo neuropathy. *J Pediatr.* 1999;135:482-493.

16. Krahenbuhl S, Kleinle S, Henz S, et al. Microvesicular steatosis, hemosiderosis and rapid development of liver cirrhosis in a patient with Pearson's syndrome. *J Hepatol.* 1999;31:550-555.

17. Bioulac-Sage P, Parrot-Roulaud F, Mazat JP, et al. Fatal neonatal liver failure and mitochondrial cytopathy (oxidative phosphorylation deficiency): a light and electron microscopic study of the liver. *Hepatology.* 1993;18:839-846.

18. Capistrano-Estrada S, Marsden DL, Nyhan WL, et al. Histopathological findings in a male with late-onset ornithine transcarbamylase deficiency. *Pediatr Pathol.* 1994;14:235-243.

19. Badizadegan K, Perez-Atayde AR. Focal glycogenosis of the liver in disorders of ureagenesis: its occurrence and diagnostic significance. *Hepatology.* 1997;26:365-373.

20. Rinaldo P, Yoon HR, Yu C, et al. Sudden and unexpected neonatal death: a protocol for the postmortem diagnosis of fatty acid oxidation disorders. *Semin Perinatol.* 1999;23:204-210.

21. Hulkova H, Elleder M. Distinctive histopathological features that support a diagnosis of cholesterol ester storage disease in liver biopsy specimens. *Histopathology.* 2012;60:1107-1113.

22. Sevenet F, Sevestre H, Masmoudi K, et al. Massive microvesicular steatosis and Wilson's disease. Article in French. *Gastroenterol Clin Biol.* 1988;12:764-765.

23. Chang YL, Parker ME, Nuovo G, et al. Human herpesvirus 6-related fulminant myocarditis and hepatitis in an immunocompetent adult with fatal outcome. *Hum Pathol.* 2009;40:740-745.

24. Aita K, Jin Y, Irie H, et al. Are there histopathologic characteristics particular to fulminant hepatic failure caused by human herpesvirus-6 infection? A case report and discussion. *Hum Pathol.* 2001;32:887-889.

25. Mahler H, Pasi A, Kramer JM, et al. Fulminant liver failure in association with the emetic toxin of Bacillus cereus. *N Engl J Med.* 1997;336:1142-1148.

26. Pereira FE, Musso C, Lucas Ede A. Labrea-like hepatitis in Vitoria, Espirito Santo State, Brazil: report of a case. *Rev Soc Bras Med Trop.* 1993;26:237-242.

27. Andrade ZA, Lesbordes JL, Ravisse P, et al. Fulminant hepatitis with microvesicular steatosis (a histologic comparison of cases occurring in Brazil–Labrea hepatitis–and in central Africa–Bangui hepatitis). *Rev Soc Bras Med Trop.* 1992;25:155-160.

28. Buitrago B, Popper H, Hadler SC, et al. Specific histologic features of Santa Marta hepatitis: a severe form of hepatitis delta-virus infection in northern South America. *Hepatology.* 1986;6:1285-1291.

29. Kobayashi K, Hashimoto E, Ludwig J, et al. Liver biopsy features of acute hepatitis C compared with hepatitis A, B, and non-A, non-B, non-C. *Liver.* 1993;13:69-72.

30. Verheij J, Voortman J, van Nieuwkerk CM, et al. Hepatic morphopathologic findings of lead poisoning in a drug addict: a case report. *J Gastrointestin Liver Dis.* 2009;18:225-227.

31. Redlich CA, West AB, Fleming L, et al. Clinical and pathological characteristics of hepatotoxicity associated with occupational exposure to dimethylformamide. *Gastroenterology.* 1990;99:748-757.

32. Hautekeete ML, Degott C, Benhamou JP. Microvesicular steatosis of the liver. *Acta Clin Belg.* 1990;45:311-326.

33. Weizman Z, Mussafi H, Ishay JS, et al. Multiple hornet stings with features of Reye's syndrome. *Gastroenterology.* 1985;89:1407-1410.

34. De Bus L, Depuydt P, Libbrecht L, et al. Severe drug-induced liver injury associated with prolonged use of linezolid. *J Med Toxicol.* 2010;6:322-326.

35. Lionte C. Lethal complications after poisoning with chloroform—case report and literature review. *Hum Exp Toxicol.* 2010;29:615-622.

36. Bodmer M, Sulz M, Stadlmann S, et al. Fatal liver failure in an adult patient with acute lymphoblastic leukemia following treatment with L-asparaginase. *Digestion.* 2006;74:28-32.

37. Puli SR, Fraley MA, Puli V, et al. Hepatic cirrhosis caused by low-dose oral amiodarone therapy. *Am J Med Sci.* 2005;330:257-261.

38. Lewis JH, Mullick F, Ishak KG, et al. Histopathologic analysis of suspected amiodarone hepatotoxicity. *Hum Pathol.* 1990;21:59-67.

39. Bove KE, McAdams AJ, Partin JC, et al. The hepatic lesion in Reye's syndrome. *Gastroenterology.* 1975;69:685-697.

40. Coghlan ME, Sommadossi JP, Jhala NC, et al. Symptomatic lactic acidosis in hospitalized antiretroviral-treated patients with human immunodeficiency virus infection: a report of 12 cases. *Clin Infect Dis.* 2001;33:1914-1921.

41. Scheffner D, Konig S, Rauterberg-Ruland I, et al. Fatal liver failure in 16 children with valproate therapy. *Epilepsia.* 1988;29:530-542.

42. Kirtley DW, Votaw ML, Thomas E. Jaundice and hepatorenal syndrome associated with cytosine arabinoside. *J Natl Med Assoc.* 1990;82:209, 213, 217-218.

43. Fraser JL, Antonioli DA, Chopra S, et al. Prevalence and nonspecificity of microvesicular fatty change in the liver. *Mod Pathol.* 1995;8:65-70.

44. Kleine-Eggebrecht N, Staufner C, Kathemann S, et al. Mutation in ITCH gene can cause syndromic multisystem Autoimmune disease with acute liver failure. *Pediatrics.* 2019;143(2):e20181554.

45. Hindupur S, Yeung M, Shroff P, et al. Vanishing bile duct syndrome in a patient with advanced AIDS. *HIV Med.* 2007;8:70-72.

46. Aldeen T, Davies S. Vanishing bile duct syndrome in a patient with advanced AIDS. *HIV Med.* 2007;8:70-72, 573-574.

47. Naini BV, Lassman CR. Total parenteral nutrition therapy and liver injury: a histopathologic study with clinical correlation. *Hum Pathol.* 2012;43:826-833.

48. Ballonoff A, Kavanagh B, Nash R, et al. Hodgkin lymphoma-related vanishing bile duct syndrome and idiopathic cholestasis: statistical analysis of all published cases and literature review. *Acta Oncol.* 2008;47:962-970.

49. Gill RM, Ferrell LD. Vanishing bile duct syndrome associated with peripheral T cell lymphoma, not otherwise specified, arising in a posttransplant setting. *Hepatology.* 2010;51:1856-1857.

50. Buglioni A, Wu TT, Mounajjed T. Immunohistochemical and ultrastructural features of hepatocellular cytoplasmic globules in venous outflow impairment. *Am J Clin Pathol.* 2019;152:563-569.

51. Wisell J, Boitnott J, Haas M, et al. Glycogen pseudoground glass change in hepatocytes. *Am J Surg Pathol.* 2006;30:1085-1090.

52. Zen Y, Nishigami T. Rethinking fibrinogen storage disease of the liver: ground glass and globular inclusions do not represent a congenital metabolic disorder but acquired collective retention of proteins. *Hum Pathol.* 2020;100:1-9.

53. Chandan VS, Shah SS, Lam-Himlin DM, et al. Globular hepatic amyloid is highly sensitive and specific for LECT2 amyloidosis. *Am J Surg Pathol.* 2015;39: 558-564.

54. Tsokos M, Erbersdobler A. Pathology of peliosis. *Forensic Sci Int.* 2005;149:25-33.
55. Devaney K, Goodman ZD, Ishak KG. Postinfantile giant-cell transformation in hepatitis. *Hepatology.* 1992;16:327-333.
56. Moreno A, Perez-Elias MJ, Quereda C, et al. Syncytial giant cell hepatitis in human immunodeficiency virus-infected patients with chronic hepatitis C: 2 cases and review of the literature. *Hum Pathol.* 2006;37:1344-1349.
57. Micchelli ST, Thomas D, Boitnott JK, et al. Hepatic giant cells in hepatitis C virus (HCV) mono-infection and HCV/HIV co-infection. *J Clin Pathol.* 2008;61:1058-1061.
58. Harmanci O, Onal IK, Ersoy O, et al. Postinfantile giant cell hepatitis due to hepatitis E virus along with the presence of autoantibodies. *Dig Dis Sci.* 2007;52:3521-3523.
59. Welte S, Gagesch M, Weber A, et al. Fulminant liver failure in Wilson's disease with histologic features of postinfantile giant cell hepatitis; cytomegalovirus as the trigger for both? *Eur J Gastroenterol Hepatol.* 2012;24:328-331.
60. Lau JY, Koukoulis G, Mieli-Vergani G, et al. Syncytial giant-cell hepatitis--a specific disease entity? *J Hepatol.* 1992;15:216-219.
61. Witzleben CL, Marshall GS, Wenner W, et al. HIV as a cause of giant cell hepatitis. *Hum Pathol.* 1988;19:603-605.
62. Potenza L, Luppi M, Barozzi P, et al. HHV-6A in syncytial giant-cell hepatitis. *N Engl J Med.* 2008;359:593-602.
63. Randhawa PS, Jenkins FJ, Nalesnik MA, et al. Herpesvirus 6 variant A infection after heart transplantation with giant cell transformation in bile ductular and gastroduodenal epithelium. *Am J Surg Pathol.* 1997;21:847-853.
64. Fimmel CJ, Guo L, Compans RW, et al. A case of syncytial giant cell hepatitis with features of a paramyxoviral infection. *Am J Gastroenterol.* 1998;93:1931-1937.
65. Mulder CJ, Cho RS, Harrison SA, et al. Syphilitic hepatitis uncommon presentation of an old scourge. *Mil Med.* 2015;180:e611-e613.
66. Ben-Ari Z, Broida E, Monselise Y, et al. Syncytial giant-cell hepatitis due to autoimmune hepatitis type II (LKM1+) presenting as subfulminant hepatitis. *Am J Gastroenterol.* 2000;95:799-801.
67. Maggiore G, Sciveres M, Fabre M, et al. Giant cell hepatitis with autoimmune hemolytic anemia in early childhood: long-term outcome in 16 children. *J Pediatr.* 2011;159:127-132.e1.
68. Harrison RA, Bahar A, Payne MM. Postinfantile giant cell hepatitis associated with long-term elevated transaminase levels in treated Graves' disease. *Am J Med.* 2002;112:326-327.
69. Shores D, Kobak G, Pegram LD, et al. Giant cell hepatitis and immune thrombocytopenic purpura: reversal of liver failure with rituximab therapy. *J Pediatr Gastroenterol Nutr.* 2012;55:e128-30.
70. Watanabe N, Takashimizu S, Shiraishi K, et al. Primary biliary cirrhosis with multinucleated hepatocellular giant cells: implications for pathogenesis of primary biliary cirrhosis. *Eur J Gastroenterol Hepatol.* 2006;18:1023-1027.
71. Cairns A, McMahon RF. Giant cell hepatitis associated with systemic lupus erythematosus. *J Clin Pathol.* 1996;49:183-184.
72. Labowitz J, Finklestein S, Rabinovitz M. Postinfantile giant cell hepatitis complicating ulcerative colitis: a case report and review of the literature. *Am J Gastroenterol.* 2001;96:1274-1277.
73. Protzer U, Dienes HP, Bianchi L, et al. Post-infantile giant cell hepatitis in patients with primary sclerosing cholangitis and autoimmune hepatitis. *Liver.* 1996;16:274-282.
74. Rauf M, Sen S, Levene A, et al. Giant cell hepatitis—a rare association with connective tissue disease. *Mediterr J Rheumatol.* 2019;30:224-227.

75. Moreno-Otero R, Trapero-Marugan M, Garcia-Buey L, et al. Drug-induced postinfantile giant cell hepatitis. *Hepatology*. 2010;52:2245-2246.

76. Fraquelli M, Colli A, Cocciolo M, et al. Adult syncytial giant cell chronic hepatitis due to herbal remedy. *J Hepatol*. 2000;33:505-508.

77. Schoepfer AM, Engel A, Fattinger K, et al. Herbal does not mean innocuous: ten cases of severe hepatotoxicity associated with dietary supplements from Herbalife products. *J Hepatol*. 2007;47:521-526.

78. Gupta E, Yacoub M, Higgins M, et al. Syncytial giant cell hepatitis associated with chronic lymphocytic leukemia: a case report. *BMC Blood Disord*. 2012;12:8.

79. Amer R, Pe'er J, Pappo O, et al. Necrobiotic xanthogranuloma associated with choroidal infiltration and syncytial giant cell hepatitis. *J Neuro Ophthalmol*. 2005;25:189-192.

80. Fanos V, Cuccu A, Nemolato S, et al. A new nonsense mutation of the IGHMBP2 gene responsible for the first case of SMARD1 in a Sardinian patient with giant cell hepatitis. *Neuropediatrics*. 2010;41:132-134.

81. Clayton PT, Verrips A, Sistermans E, et al. Mutations in the sterol 27-hydroxylase gene (CYP27A) cause hepatitis of infancy as well as cerebrotendinous xanthomatosis. *J Inherit Metab Dis*. 2002;25:501-513.

82. Dai D, Mills PB, Footitt E, et al. Liver disease in infancy caused by oxysterol 7 alpha-hydroxylase deficiency: successful treatment with chenodeoxycholic acid. *J Inherit Metab Dis*. 2014;37:851-861.

83. Setchell KD, Heubi JE, Bove KE, et al. Liver disease caused by failure to racemize trihydroxycholestanoic acid: gene mutation and effect of bile acid therapy. *Gastroenterology*. 2003;124:217-232.

84. Muller-Hocker J, Muntau A, Schafer S, et al. Depletion of mitochondrial DNA in the liver of an infant with neonatal giant cell hepatitis. *Hum Pathol*. 2002;33:247-253.

85. Clayton PT, Hyland K, Brand M, et al. Mitochondrial phosphoenolpyruvate carboxykinase deficiency. *Eur J Pediatr*. 1986;145:46-50.

86. Schiano TD, Azeem S, Bodian CA, et al. Importance of specimen size in accurate needle liver biopsy evaluation of patients with chronic hepatitis C. *Clin Gastroenterol Hepatol*. 2005;3:930-935.

87. Colloredo G, Guido M, Sonzogni A, et al. Impact of liver biopsy size on histological evaluation of chronic viral hepatitis: the smaller the sample, the milder the disease. *J Hepatol*. 2003;39:239-244.

88. Olsson R, Hagerstrand I, Broome U, et al. Sampling variability of percutaneous liver biopsy in primary sclerosing cholangitis. *J Clin Pathol*. 1995;48:933-935.

89. Abdi W, Millan JC, Mezey E. Sampling variability on percutaneous liver biopsy. *Arch Intern Med*. 1979;139:667-669.

90. Merriman RB, Ferrell LD, Patti MG, et al. Correlation of paired liver biopsies in morbidly obese patients with suspected nonalcoholic fatty liver disease. *Hepatology*. 2006;44:874-880.

91. Larson SP, Bowers SP, Palekar NA, et al. Histopathologic variability between the right and left lobes of the liver in morbidly obese patients undergoing Roux-en-Y bypass. *Clin Gastroenterol Hepatol*. 2007;5:1329-1332.

92. Petrelli M, Scheuer PJ. Variation in subcapsular liver structure and its significance in the interpretation of wedge biopsies. *J Clin Pathol*. 1967;20:743-748.

93. Padoin AV, Mottin CC, Moretto M, et al. A comparison of wedge and needle hepatic biopsy in open bariatric surgery. *Obes Surg*. 2006;16:178-182.

94. Rawlins SR, Mullen CM, Simon HM, et al. Wedge and needle liver biopsies show discordant histopathology in morbidly obese patients undergoing Roux-en-Y gastric bypass surgery. *Gastroenterol Rep (Oxf)*. 2013;1:51-57.

95. Ahern MJ, Kevat S, Hill W, et al. Hepatic methotrexate content and progression of hepatic fibrosis: preliminary findings. *Ann Rheum Dis.* 1991;50:477-480.

96. Nollevaux MC, Guiot Y, Horsmans Y, et al. Hypervitaminosis A-induced liver fibrosis: stellate cell activation and daily dose consumption. *Liver Int.* 2006;26:182-186.

97. Labadie H, Stoessel P, Callard P, et al. Hepatic venooclusive disease and perisinusoidal fibrosis secondary to arsenic poisoning. *Gastroenterology.* 1990;99:1140-1143.

98. Cowlishaw JL, Pollard EJ, Cowen AE, et al. Liver disease associated with chronic arsenic ingestion. *Aust N Z J Med.* 1979;9:310-313.

99. el Hag IA, Hashim FA, el Toum IA, et al. Liver morphology and function in visceral leishmaniasis (Kala-azar). *J Clin Pathol.* 1994;47:547-551.

100. Thurberg BL, Wasserstein MP, Schiano T, et al. Liver and skin histopathology in adults with acid sphingomyelinase deficiency (Niemann-Pick disease type B). *Am J Surg Pathol.* 2012;36:1234-1246.

101. Challa VR, Geisinger KR, Burton BK. Pathologic alterations in the brain and liver in hyperpipecolic acidemia. *J Neuropathol Exp Neurol.* 1983;42:627-638.

102. Inoue T, Kobayashi Y, Kusuda S. Unusual hepatic fibrosis in three cases of Down syndrome. Article in Japanese. *Rinsho Byori.* 1996;44:590-594.

103. Ramakrishna B, Date A, Kirubakaran C, et al. Atypical copper cirrhosis in Indian children. *Ann Trop Paediatr.* 1995;15:237-242.

104. Nakanuma Y, Tsuneyama K, Ohbu M, et al. Pathology and pathogenesis of idiopathic portal hypertension with an emphasis on the liver. *Pathol Res Pract.* 2001;197:65-76.

105. Bosma A, Meuwissen SG, Stricker BH, et al. Massive pericellular collagen deposition in the liver of a young female with severe Crohn's disease. *Histopathology.* 1989;14:81-90.

106. Harrison SA, Brunt EM, Goodman ZD, et al. Diabetic hepatosclerosis: diabetic microangiopathy of the liver. *Arch Pathol Lab Med.* 2006;130:27-32.

107. Latry P, Bioulac-Sage P, Echinard E, et al. Perisinusoidal fibrosis and basement membrane-like material in the livers of diabetic patients. *Hum Pathol.* 1987;18:775-780.

108. Torbenson M, Hart J, Westerhoff M, et al. Neonatal giant cell hepatitis: histological and etiological findings. *Am J Surg Pathol.* 2010;34:1498-1503.

109. Tsao MS. Hepatic sinusoidal fibrosis in agnogenic myeloid metaplasia. *Am J Clin Pathol.* 1989;91:302-305.

110. Roux D, Merlio JP, Quinton A, et al. Agnogenic myeloid metaplasia, portal hypertension, and sinusoidal abnormalities. *Gastroenterology.* 1987;92:1067-1072.

111. Lafon ME, Bioulac-Sage P, Grimaud JA, et al. Perisinusoidal fibrosis of the liver in patients with thrombocytopenic purpura. *Virchows Arch A Pathol Anat Histopathol.* 1987;411:553-559.

112. Hoofring A, Boitnott J, Torbenson M. Three-dimensional reconstruction of hepatic bridging fibrosis in chronic hepatitis C viral infection. *J Hepatol.* 2003;39:738-741.

113. Kim MY, Cho MY, Baik SK, et al. Histological subclassification of cirrhosis using the Laennec fibrosis scoring system correlates with clinical stage and grade of portal hypertension. *J Hepatol.* 2011;55:1004-1009.

114. Malik AH, Kumar KS, Malet PF, et al. Correlation of percutaneous liver biopsy fragmentation with the degree of fibrosis. *Aliment Pharmacol Ther.* 2004;19:545-549.

115. Poynard T, Halfon P, Castera L, et al. Variability of the area under the receiver operating characteristic curves in the diagnostic evaluation of liver fibrosis markers: impact of biopsy length and fragmentation. *Aliment Pharmacol Ther.* 2007;25:733-739.

116. Everhart JE, Wright EC, Goodman ZD, et al. Prognostic value of Ishak fibrosis stage: findings from the hepatitis C antiviral long-term treatment against cirrhosis trial. *Hepatology.* 2010;51:585-594.

117. Castera L, Pinzani M. Biopsy and non-invasive methods for the diagnosis of liver fibrosis: does it take two to tango? *Gut.* 2010;59:861-866.

118. Chin JL, Pavlides M, Moolla A, et al. Non-invasive markers of liver fibrosis: adjuncts or alternatives to liver biopsy? *Front Pharmacol*. 2016;7:159.

119. Loomba R, Adams LA. Advances in non-invasive assessment of hepatic fibrosis. *Gut*. 2020;69:1343-1352.

120. Sterling RK, King WC, Wahed AS, et al. Evaluating noninvasive markers to identify advanced fibrosis by liver biopsy in HBV/HIV Co-infected adults. *Hepatology*. 2020;71:411-421.

121. Xiao H, Shi M, Xie Y, et al. Comparison of diagnostic accuracy of magnetic resonance elastography and Fibroscan for detecting liver fibrosis in chronic hepatitis B patients: a systematic review and meta-analysis. *PLoS One*. 2017;12:e0186660.

122. Fraquelli M, Rigamonti C, Casazza G, et al. Etiology-related determinants of liver stiffness values in chronic viral hepatitis B or C. *J Hepatol*. 2011;54:621-628.

123. Kirk GD, Astemborski J, Mehta SH, et al. Assessment of liver fibrosis by transient elastography in persons with hepatitis C virus infection or HIV-hepatitis C virus coinfection. *Clin Infect Dis*. 2009;48:963-972.

124. Wanless IR, Nakashima E, Sherman M. Regression of human cirrhosis. Morphologic features and the genesis of incomplete septal cirrhosis. *Arch Pathol Lab Med*. 2000;124:1599-1607.

125. Hytiroglou P, Snover DC, Alves V, et al. Beyond "cirrhosis": a proposal from the International Liver Pathology Study Group. *Am J Clin Pathol*. 2012;137:5-9.

126. Wanless IR. The role of vascular injury and congestion in the pathogenesis of cirrhosis: the congestive escalator and the parenchymal extinction sequence. *Curr Hepatol Rep*. 2020;19:40-53.

127. Hagstrom H, Nasr P, Ekstedt M, et al. Fibrosis stage but not NASH predicts mortality and time to development of severe liver disease in biopsy-proven NAFLD. *J Hepatol*. 2017;67:1265-1273.

128. Angulo P, Kleiner DE, Dam-Larsen S, et al. Liver fibrosis, but no other histologic features, is associated with long-term outcomes of patients with nonalcoholic fatty liver disease. *Gastroenterology*. 2015;149:389-397 e10.

129. Limketkai BN, Mehta SH, Sutcliffe CG, et al. Relationship of liver disease stage and antiviral therapy with liver-related events and death in adults coinfected with HIV/HCV. *J Am Med Assoc*. 2012;308:370-378.

3

IMMUNOHISTOCHEMISTRY AND SPECIAL STAINS IN LIVER PATHOLOGY

ETERNAL LAWS OF SPECIAL STAINS AND IMMUNOHISTOCHEMISTRY

There are four fundamental, immutable laws governing the use of special stains in liver pathology. The wheels of time continually add new stains to the armamentarium used by liver pathologists to make diagnoses, while discarding less useful, older stains, but these laws are unchanging. The laws are worth knowing as they will help guide decisions about incorporating and using new testing within your practice. While first formulated for evaluating liver tumors,[1] they apply equally to medical liver pathology.

Law 1 *Special stains and immunostains should always be interpreted in conjunction with the hematoxylin and eosin (H&E) findings.* Immunohistochemical stains greatly extend the power of microscopy, increasing diagnostic sensitivity and specificity. Of note, however, this power is greatly diminished when immunohistochemical stains are used in isolation, or with only cursory examination of the H&E morphology. It cannot be overemphasized that the full synergistic value is achieved only when H&E findings are used together with immunohistochemical stains. Some readers might be tempted to dismiss Law 1 as being self-evident, yet, the literature is rich in papers that do not understand this Law or perhaps choose to ignore it. One example is papers that discuss sensitivity and specificity of markers for hepatocellular differentiation, without accounting for tumor grade, when the strong influence of tumor grade on both sensitivity and specificity is well documented. In other words, the best markers for hepatocellular differentiation will vary depending on whether tumors are well differentiated, moderately differentiated, or poorly differentiated; in fact, the same observation is equally true for immunostain markers in cholangiocarcinoma. Yet, most papers simply calculate sensitivity and specificity for their overall group of cases, ignoring the importance of stratifying for morphology (tumor grade in this example), obscuring the true strengths and weaknesses of different markers.

Law 2 *The sensitivity and specificity of immunostains invariably worsens as more studies are reported.* The first study is always the best. This is a natural consequence of science, since additional studies will examine more tumors and a wider range of different types of tumors, refining our understanding of how a new stain performs. This inevitably leads to diminished sensitivity and specificity for the new marker. In addition, the performance of stains will vary between different laboratories because they often use different commercial antibody clones and have different staining protocols, all contributing to the inevitable decline of the initially reported sensitivity and specificity. Over time, the data will coalesce for any given immunostain, establishing a true, stable sensitivity and specificity, but this process generally takes around 5 years.

A natural corollary is this: Early studies that report that the stain *de jour* is statistically better than established stains should be interpreted cautiously, at least in terms of making decisions on adding the new stain or dropping an old stain from your laboratory menu, especially in the first five or so years after a new stain is introduced.

Law 3 *If there is a discrepancy between the morphology and immunohistochemical findings, additional studies must be performed.* Many times, discrepancies between morphological findings and immunohistochemical findings can be resolved based on personal experience or known diagnostic pitfalls. When this is not the case, a choice to follow one discrepant result over another can be arbitrary and lead to confusion. In this setting, the morphology and the special stains should be reviewed to make sure they were interpreted correctly. If the problem remains unresolved, additional sections can be submitted on resection specimens, discrepant immunostains can be repeated, and other immunostains added to clarify the diagnosis.

Law 4 *A difficult case is the wrong time to use a stain you're not familiar with.* To confidently and skillfully use any stain, it is important to know how the stain performs in the full range of typical cases, as well as in less common situations. But that is just the first step, and it is equally important to know how the stain performs in other entities or tumors that enter the morphological differential. If you do not have this background experience then it is often best to review the results with somebody in your group, or an outside consultant, who does have the requisite experience. In addition, when you add a new stain to your laboratory menu, it is helpful to use it in conjunction with stains you already have, stains that address the same question as the new stain, in order to familiarize yourself with staining patterns and to assess its performance. Finally, it is best to use stains often enough to maintain your skills in their interpretation.

UP-FRONT STAINS

Medical liver biopsy specimens are often sectioned up front, by protocol and before histological examination, to include H&E stain(s), often two, as well as several additional up-front stains. There is variability between

TABLE 3.1	Routine Up-Front Stains in Medical Liver Pathology	
Stain	Use in Routine Practice	Major Purpose
H&E × 2	Every case	Tissue visualization
Trichrome (or similar)	Every case	Fibrosis assessment
Iron	Baseline biopsy, others as needed	Assess iron overload
PASD	Baseline biopsy, others as needed	Assess for alpha-1-antitrypsin globules
Reticulin	As needed based on H&E findings	Assess for nodular regenerative hyperplasia
PAS	As needed based on H&E findings	Assess hepatocyte inclusions

H&E, hematoxylin and eosin; PAS, periodic acid-Schiff; PASD, periodic acid-Schiff with diastase.

practices, but the most common panel of up-front special stains includes trichrome, iron, and periodic acid-Schiff with diastase (PASD) stains, with some laboratories extending this panel to include routine reticulin and periodic acid-Schiff (PAS) stains. There is no data on the optimal panel of stains and most pathologists will choose a panel based on their own personal preferences. For those rethinking their current approach, a reasonable method is shown in Table 3.1. Additional helpful stains are shown in Table 3.2, organized by the ways in which they are most commonly used.

TRICHROME STAIN OVERVIEW. Lower stages of fibrosis are hard to see on H&E, so trichrome stains (or similar stains such as Sirius Red), are helpful for evaluating fibrosis. A trichrome stain, however, is not always needed in a few specific situations: (1) the liver shows established cirrhosis on H&E; (2) follow-up biopsies are performed to assess treatment response and are performed soon after the initial biopsy (days to weeks).

The trichrome stain is so named because it uses three dyes, staining collagen blue (or green), smooth muscle red, and nuclei black (Figures 3.1 and 3.2). The Sirius red stains collagen red; it also stains amyloid red. There are several other less commonly used collagen stains. For example, with the van Gieson stain, collagen is stained red, smooth muscle yellow, and nuclei are black. Often, the van Gieson stain is combined with the Verhoeff elastic stain, called an elastic-van Gieson stain, which will add an additional color for elastic tissue: blue-black.

The results of trichrome stains can be reported using descriptive terms, such as portal fibrosis, bridging fibrosis, cirrhosis, etc., or with a formal staging system. In many cases, using both can be a helpful way to accurately convey what the biopsy shows (please see Chapter 4 for more details).

IRON STAIN OVERVIEW. Lower grades of iron deposition in the liver are easily overlooked on H&E stains but are nicely highlighted by the Perls iron stain

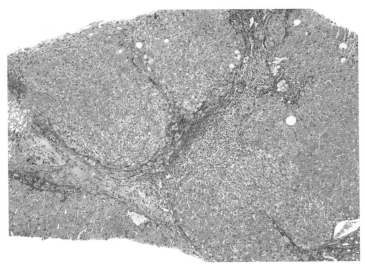

FIGURE 3.1 **Trichrome stain.** Bands of fibrosis are highlighted in this case of cirrhosis.

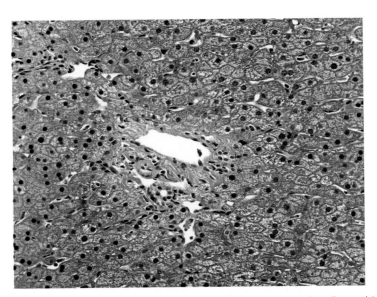

FIGURE 3.2 **Trichrome stain.** At high power, the hepatocytes red, collagen blue, and hepatocyte nuclei black.

(or similar iron stains). Positive staining is seen as bright, blue granules of hemosiderin in the cytoplasm of cells (Figure 3.3). As a caveat, the Perls iron stain can show a light, cytoplasmic, blue-blush in hepatocytes, but this represents ferritin, not hemosiderin, and can be ignored (Figure 3.4).

Routine iron stains are not always necessary, as there are other reasonable approaches on when to perform an iron stain. For example, iron

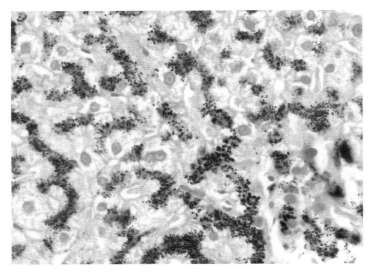

FIGURE 3.3 **Perls iron stain.** This liver biopsy is from a patient with C282Y homozygous *HFE* mutations. There are diffuse and severe deposits of iron in the hepatocytes, identified by the granular blue staining.

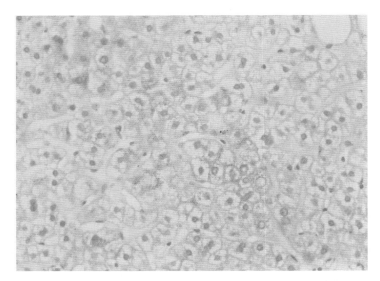

FIGURE 3.4 **Perls iron stain.** Ferritin shows a light blue cytoplasmic staining.

stains could be ordered when there is visible pigment on H&E that suggests iron, or if the serum ferritin is significantly elevated (>1000 µg/L), or transferrin saturation is 45% or greater. Such an approach would certainly miss some cases of low-grade iron deposition, but this is offset by the knowledge that minimal to mild iron accumulation has no clinical significance in the vast majority of cases.

TABLE 3.2	Stains for Specific Purposes	
Purpose	First-Line Special Stains	Supplemental Stains/ Methods
Assess for normal pattern of liver	• CK7 (bile ducts)	
	• CD31 (periportal sinusoids)	
	• Glutamine synthetase (zone 3 hepatocytes)	
	• Reticulin (plate thickness)	
	• Ki67 (low-proliferation rate, less than 1%)	
Cytoplasmic pigments		
Iron	• Perls	
Lipofuscin	• Fontana-Masson	
Copper	• Rhodanine	Orcein
Bile	• Halls (rarely needed)	
Cytoplasmic inclusions in hepatocytes		
A1AT protein	• PASD	
Ground-glass inclusions	• HBsAg	Orcein
	• PAS/PASD	Fibrinogen
		LECT2
Mallory hyaline	• Ubiquitin	
	• P62	
	• CK8/18	
Specific disease/disease patterns		
Amyloid	• Congo Red	Mass spectrophotometry
Autoimmune hepatitis	• IgG, IgM (to distinguish from PBC)	
	• PASD (inclusions in Kupffer cells)	
Chronic cholestatic liver disease	• CK7 (periportal interme- diate hepatocytes)	
	• Copper	
PBC	• Additional levels	CD1a
	• CK7	IgG, IgM
	• copper	
IgG4 disease	• IgG, IgM	

(Continued)

TABLE 3.2 Stains for Specific Purposes (Continued)		
Purpose	**First-Line Special Stains**	**Supplemental Stains/ Methods**
Chronic vascular outflow disease	• CK7 (zone 3 intermediate hepatocytes) • Trichrome (zone 3 fibrosis) • Reticulin (nodular regenerative hyperplasia can be present)	
Granulomas	• AFB • GMS	Polarize to rule out foreign material
Viral infections	• CMV, HSV, adenovirus, EBV, etc	
Bacterial infections	• Gram (for gram-positive organisms) • Brown and Hops (for gram-negative organisms) • Ziehl-Neelsen (*M. tuberculosis*) • Fite (leprosy) • PAS (Whipple)	
Fungal infections	• GMS	PAS

AFB, acid-fast bacteria; CMV, cytomegalovirus; EBV, Epstein-Barr virus; GMS, Grocott methenamine silver; HSV, herpes simplex virus; PBC, primary biliary cholangitis; PAS, periodic acid-Schiff; PASD, periodic acid-Schiff with diastase.

For clinical purposes, the amount of iron can be reported either descriptively (minimal, mild, moderate, marked), along with the location of the iron deposition, or can be reported out using a numerical system (please see Chapter 15).

RETICULIN STAIN OVERVIEW. In medical liver biopsies, reticulin stains are used mostly to assess for nodular regenerative hyperplasia (NRH); their use in tumor biopsies is discussed in Chapter 21. NRH most often results from blood flow abnormalities that lead to parenchymal nodularity without fibrosis, where the nodularity is caused by areas of compressed hepatocytes surrounded by normal to plump-sized hepatocytes. The diagnosis of NRH is easily made when the findings are well-developed, but there is a continuum of changes and subtle cases of possible NRH benefit from confirmation with a reticulin stain. Of note, reticulin stains performed in injured,

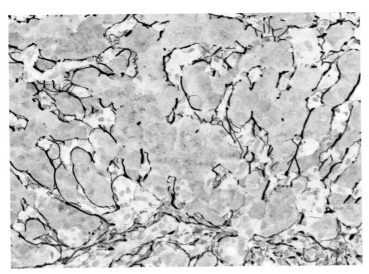

FIGURE 3.5 **Reticulin stain.** There is focal plate thickening in this case of acute hepatitis with active liver regeneration.

reactive livers never look quite normal, but the lack of a completely normal reticulin stain should not be equated with NRH; instead, a diagnosis of NRH requires there to be compatible findings on both H&E and reticulin stain. In other words, if you do not see some evidence of parenchymal nodularity on the H&E, then a diagnosis of NRH based on the reticulin alone should be considered carefully. Also, by definition, there should be no evidence for advanced fibrosis, although mild portal fibrosis and/or mild pericellular fibrosis can occasionally be seen. Another useful cross-check is the liver enzyme elevation patterns, as most cases of NRH have a disproportionate elevation in alkaline phosphatase levels.

Reticulin stains can lose the normal staining pattern when there is marked liver regeneration, leading to thickening of the hepatic plates (Figure 3.5) or in areas of macrovesicular steatosis, where there can be physiological reduction in the amount of reticulin (Figure 3.6).

Reticulin stains are occasionally used in a second setting. Some pathologists find the reticulin stain helpful to distinguish bridging necrosis from bridging fibrosis. Bridging necrosis leads to closely approximated reticulin fibers (Figure 3.7), resulting from hepatocyte necrosis and collapse of the normal reticulin meshwork; while bridging fibrosis will have less striking reticulin deposits (Figure 3.8). These patterns, however, take some experience to be interpreted accurately. For this reason, most pathologists use the combined findings of the H&E and trichrome to distinguish bridging necrosis from bridging fibrosis. Of course, the clinical setting is also helpful, as bridging necrosis is associated with acute-onset, moderate-to-severe elevations in liver enzymes.

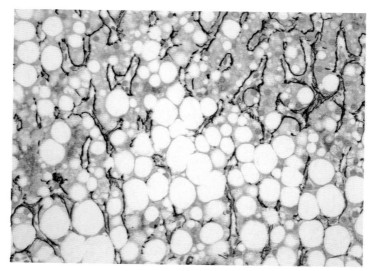

FIGURE 3.6 **Reticulin stain.** In this liver with marked macrovesicular steatosis, there are areas of reduced reticulin staining.

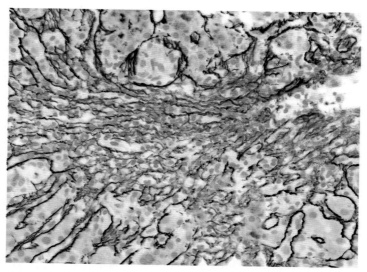

FIGURE 3.7 **Reticulin stain.** Bridging necrosis leads to compression of the residual reticulin fibers.

PAS. The PAS stain without diastase highlights glycogen in hepatocytes (Figure 3.9), but that aspect of the stain is not diagnostically useful, other than when evaluating rare cases of hepatocyte inclusions. On the other hand, some pathologists like the stain for its ability to identify foci of lobular necrosis, which stand out in negative relief against the background, intact PAS-positive hepatocytes (Figure 3.10).

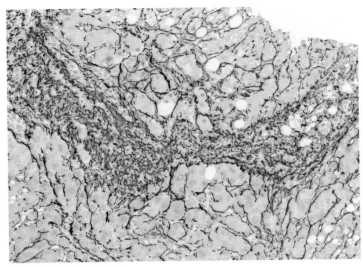

FIGURE 3.8   **Reticulin stain.** Bridging fibrosis shows relatively fewer reticulin fibers. The collagen stains a light gray, in contrast to the black staining for reticulin, but there is enough overlap that interpretation can sometimes be challenging.

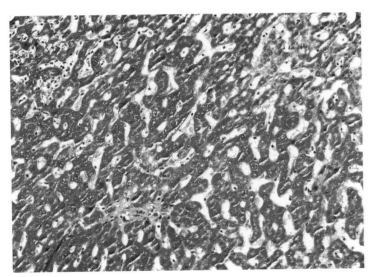

FIGURE 3.9   **Periodic Acid-Schiff (PAS) stain.** There is bright hepatocellular cytoplasmic staining in this normal liver biopsy.

PASD OVERVIEW. The PASD stain is used to screen for intrahepatic globules of alpha-1-antitrypsin protein (Figure 3.11), which can be easily overlooked on H&E but are nicely highlighted with the PASD stain. PASD stains will also highlight small cytoplasmic globules in Kupffer cell in the setting of autoimmune hepatitis (Figure 3.12), primary biliary cholangitis (PBC), or

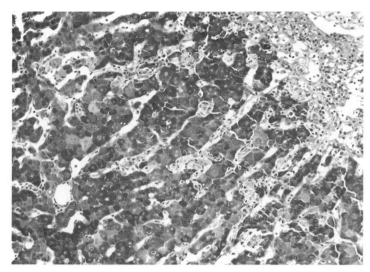

FIGURE 3.10 **Periodic Acid-Schiff (PAS) stain.** The lobular inflammation stands out in relief from the background PAS staining of the hepatocytes.

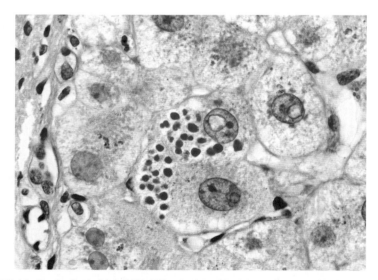

FIGURE 3.11 **Periodic Acid-Schiff with Diastase (PASD) stain.** Cytoplasmic inclusions of alpha-1-antitrypsin protein are highlighted.

other diseases with hypergammaglobulinemia; the small globular inclusions are composed of immunoglobulins. Finally, PASD stains also highlight macrophages in areas of prior or ongoing lobular inflammation (Figure 3.13). This finding can be helpful in biopsies that appear histologically almost normal, supporting a resolving hepatitis pattern of injury. Sometimes these small Kupffer cell aggregates can suggest a granuloma, but they will be PASD-positive, in contrast to typical epithelioid granulomas (Figure 3.14).

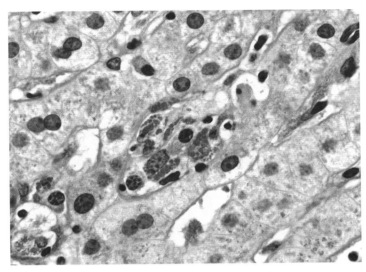

FIGURE 3.12   **Periodic Acid-Schiff with Diastase (PASD) stain.** The Kupffer cells have small inclusions in this case of autoimmune hepatitis.

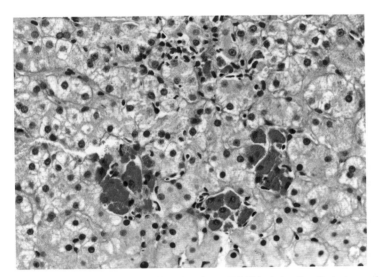

FIGURE 3.13   **Periodic Acid-Schiff with Diastase (PASD) stain.** Small clusters of lobular macrophages stand out in this biopsy with a resolving hepatitis pattern of injury.

Globules of alpha-1-antitrypsin protein are most commonly seen with the Z allele (MZ or ZZ), but livers with the S allele (MS or SS) can occasionally develop globules,[2-5] in particular in the setting of other concomitant liver diseases. Of note, finding PASD-positive globules in hepatocytes does not mean the patient has alpha-1-antitrypsin deficiency, as that distinction is made by serum levels of alpha-1-antitrypsin protein, and most

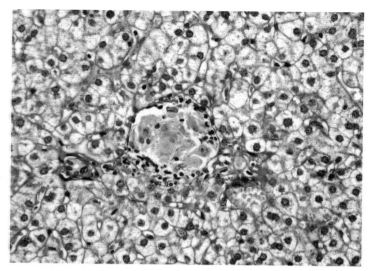

FIGURE 3.14 **Periodic Acid-Schiff with Diastase (PASD) stain.** The small granuloma is PASD-negative.

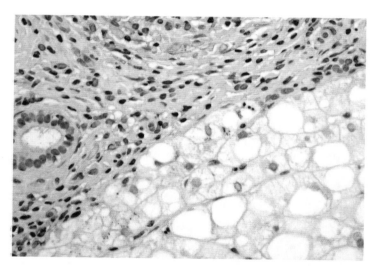

FIGURE 3.15 **Rhodanine stain.** The red-brown granules seen on this stain represent lyso-somal accumulation of copper; image is from a biopsy with early changes of primary biliary cholangitis (PBC).

of the patients identified by screening with PASD stains have heterozygous mutations and do not have clinical alpha-1-antitrypsin deficiency.

COPPER STAINS OVERVIEW. A positive Rhodanine copper stain shows small, discrete, red-brown granules in hepatocyte cytoplasm, primarily in zone 1 hepatocytes (Figure 3.15). The stain detects copper metal that has been deposited in lysosomes but does not stain copper that is located in the cell cytosol. In early Wilson disease, copper is first deposited in the cytosol, with little or no deposits in the lysosomes. For this reason, the Rhodanine stain can be negative in early Wilson disease.

The Rhodanine stain is also used to detect copper deposition in cases of chronic cholestatic liver disease, as discussed below. Regardless of the reason for using the Rhodanine stain, sections should be cut at 10 microns to optimize the detection of copper.

SHIKATA ORCEIN/VICTORIA BLUE. Both of these stains have similar staining properties and are popular as up-front stains in many parts of the world, though not so much in the United States of America (USA). Some laboratories favor the Victoria blue over the orcein for technical ease of performance. The stains serve three major purposes. First, they reliably stain copper-binding proteins (brown for orcein, blue for Victoria blue), which is codeposited along with copper metal in lysosomes of hepatocytes, leading to similar staining properties as the Rhodanine stain. Secondly, these stains will highlight the ground glass inclusions found in some patients with chronic hepatitis B; the inclusions staining dark brown/blue, respectively. This role has lessened considerably with the availability of more specific HBsAg immunostains and the widespread use of hepatitis B virus (HBV) serological testing. Finally, both of these stains will highlight elastic fibers, which can be helpful in cases of bridging necrosis, since elastic fibers are absent in areas of bridging necrosis for the first several weeks following the injury but then slowly get deposited in areas of parenchymal collapse. Thus, the staining patterns can then help distinguish bridging necrosis from bridging fibrosis and serve as an approximate timescale of when the severe liver injury occurred.

RUBEANIC ACID. Copper granules stain blue-black with the rubeanic acid stain, and the hepatocyte cytoplasm stains pink. This stain is used in a similar fashion to the Rhodanine stain.

STAINS HELPFUL IN THE EVALUATION OF INJURY PATTERNS

Stains to See If Liver Is Normal/Nearly Normal

In some cases, special stains are useful when the H&E is almost normal, to ensure there are no subtle abnormalities. A cytokeratin 7 (CK7) can ensure bile ducts are present and can also identify subtle bile ductular proliferation, intermediate hepatocytes in zone 1 that would suggest chronic cholestatic liver disease, or intermediate hepatocytes in zone 3 that would suggest subtle vascular outflow disease.

Additional stains can also help identify subtle vascular flow abnormalities. A glutamine synthetase normally stains a thin rim of zone 3 hepatocytes (Figure 3.16), while abnormal vascular flow can lead to either aberrant complete loss of staining or aberrant blotchy staining that does

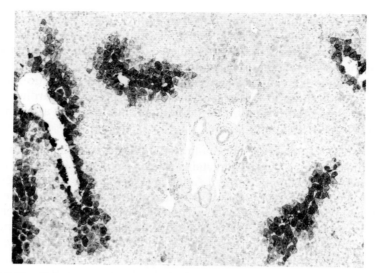

FIGURE 3.16 **Glutamine synthetase.** The zone 3 hepatocytes stain strongly and brightly. There is no staining in hepatocytes in zones 1 or 2.

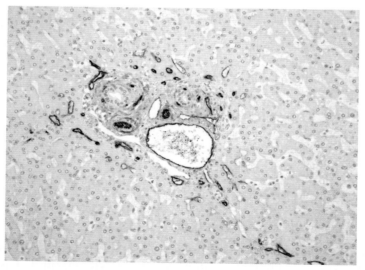

FIGURE 3.17 **CD34.** The normal staining pattern shows vessels in the portal tracts and a few sinusoids in zone 1 are positive.

not correlate with a zone 3 pattern. Vascular flow changes can also lead to abnormal CD34 staining (Figure 3.17), with extension of the normal zone 1 staining pattern into zones 2 and 3. A reticulin will show regular, well-organized thin cords and trabeculae in the normal liver, but in cases of NRH, the stain highlights areas of compressed hepatocytes.

Finally, a Ki-67 can help confirm a normal liver. The normal, quiescent liver has a proliferation rate of less than 1%, while a proliferative rate that is clearly above normal indicates active hepatocyte regeneration, even if the biopsy otherwise looks almost normal or shows only mild nonspecific changes, suggesting recovery from recent or ongoing injury. The Ki-67 stain can sometimes be useful in the opposite setting too, where there is a known clinical or histological source of significant liver injury. In this setting, the Ki-67 is expected to be significantly elevated above baseline; if it is not, this suggests impaired liver regeneration, a phenomenon most commonly seen in the elderly.

CHRONIC CHOLESTATIC LIVER DISEASE

Several stains are particularly helpful for confirming chronic cholestatic liver disease by identifying cholate stasis or ductopenia. If there is obvious chronic cholestatic liver disease, stains can are also helpful to evaluate for bile duct loss.

DUCTOPENIA. Ductopenia is best assessed using keratin stains and several will due, including CK AE1/AE3, CK19, and CK7. CK7 is in many ways preferred, as it will do double duty, also identifying intermediate hepatocytes. To diagnose ductopenia, look for the absence of a least 50% of the bile ducts in a biopsy that has at least 10 portal tracts. True loss of bile ducts will correlate with disproportionately elevated serum alkaline phosphatase levels; if that is not the case, it is best to back-off of a definitive diagnosis of ductopenia.

In the pediatric patient population, the differential for liver biopsies with paucity of intrahepatic bile ducts includes Alagille syndrome. In the normal liver, the bile canaliculi are mature and express CD10 by age of about 2 years. In children with Alagille syndrome, however, there can be persistent lack of CD10 that extends into older age groups.[6]

CHOLATE STASIS. The CK7 and the Rhodanine copper stain are useful for identifying subtle evidence of chronic cholestasis in noncirrhotic livers; once a liver is cirrhotic, however, positive stains lose their specificity for chronic cholestatic liver disease. On the other hand, their sensitivity increases and cirrhosis from chronic cholestatic liver disease is almost always positive for copper and shows intermediate hepatocytes; their absence would argue against chronic cholestatic liver disease as a cause of the cirrhosis.

Copper is excreted from the liver via bile, but, when there is chronic cholestasis from any cause, copper can be retained, accumulating in the lysosomes of periportal hepatocytes. The staining can be very focal, so the copper stain should be examined carefully.

CK7 normally stains the bile ducts and bile ductules but not the hepatocytes. With chronic cholestasis, however, zone 1 hepatocytes can become CK7-positive, and when they do, they are called intermediate hepatocytes (Figure 3.18). As an important caveat, it is important to look carefully at where the intermediate hepatocytes are located, as CK7-positive hepatocytes can be located in zone 3 when there is congestive hepatopathy.[7]

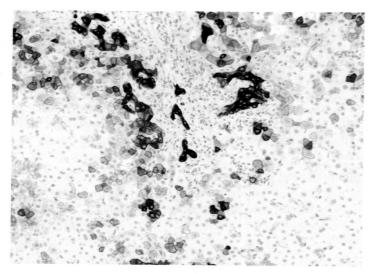

FIGURE 3.18 **CK7 and intermediate hepatocytes.** The bile ductules stain strong and bright, while the intermediate hepatocytes are also positive.

There is no great data set looking at the length or intensity of chronic cholestasis needed before hepatocytes are positive for copper and/or CK7. Nonetheless, experience indicates that intermediate hepatocytes are often seen on liver biopsies before copper accumulation is found. On the other hand, there are cases that have the opposite pattern (copper-positive, CK7 negative) so, in general, it is best to use both stains to evaluate for subtle changes of chronic cholestatic liver disease.

INHERITED CHRONIC CHOLESTATIC LIVER DISEASES. Additional immunostains are available at some medical centers for BSEP and MDR3. Progressive familial intrahepatic cholestasis type 2 (PFIC2) is caused by germline mutations in *ABCB11*, which encodes the bile salt export pump (BSEP) protein. Loss of canalicular staining for BSEP in pediatric liver samples can suggest PFIC2 in the right histological and clinical setting but are not entirely sensitive nor specific, so must be confirmed by sequencing studies.[8-10] Similarly, PFIC3 is caused by mutations in *ABCB4*, which encodes multiple drug resistance 3 protein (MDR3), and MDR3 immunostains that show a loss of canalicular staining can suggest *ABCB4* mutations in the right clinical context, but again must be confirmed by sequencing studies. Since these conditions are very rare and genetic testing is required anyway, immunostains to confirm these disorders are not widely available.

AUTOIMMUNE CONDITIONS OF THE LIVER

AUTOIMMUNE HEPATITIS. Autoimmune hepatitis typically has portal chronic inflammation that is enriched for plasma cells. If immunostains are applied to subtype the plasma cells, they will show a predominance of IgG-positive, with fewer IgM-positive plasma cells. In contrast, the portal tracts in cases of PBC typically have similar or greater numbers of IgM-positive plasma cells, compared to IgG.[11] This pattern reflects the serum findings, where autoimmune hepatitis shows primarily serum IgG elevations, with normal levels or milder elevations in IgM, while PBC shows disproportionate elevations in serum IgM over IgG levels in most cases. Of note, immunophenotyping the plasma cells is helpful for the very focused differential of autoimmune hepatitis versus PBC and not in any other setting. For example, immunostains will not distinguish autoimmune hepatitis from a plasma cell–rich drug reaction, or from a plasma cell–rich viral hepatitis. In addition, IgG and IgM immunostains have not been well-studied in establishing a diagnosis of autoimmune hepatitis-PBC overlap syndrome.

PBC. In cases where there is clinical concern for PBC, but H&E findings are not clear, additional stains can help support the diagnosis. As a first step, the findings in early PBC can be patchy and missed in the first set of H&E sections, so additional H&E levels will sometimes show more classic portal tract changes. In addition, CK7 and Rhodanine, or other copper stains, can identify evidence of chronic cholestasis, even when the biopsy findings are very mild and nonspecific. While these stains do not prove the diagnosis is PBC, they are supportive of chronic cholestatic liver disease when positive. Immunostains for CD1a can also be helpful in some cases of PBC, as dendritic cells in the inflamed bile ducts can be positive.[12]

IgG4 DISEASE. Increased levels of IgG4-positive plasma cells can support the diagnosis of IgG4 disease. A common cut-off is 10 or more positive plasma cells in a 40× field,[13] or that 40% of the IgG-positive plasma cells are of the IgG4 subtype, but these cut-offs have to be used with H&E findings and some common sense. Please see IgG4 disease section for more details.

AMYLOIDOSIS

The diagnosis of amyloidosis is made using a Congo red stain. Once there is a firm diagnosis of amyloid, then the clinical team will often want the amyloid subtyped. There are two basic approaches for amyloid subtyping: immunostains and mass spectrophotometry. Immunostains for subtyping amyloid are often available at tertiary care centers. In most cases, they consist of a limited panel that focuses on the most common types of amyloid. Nonetheless, available immunostains include kappa and lambda light chains, AA amyloid, amyloid P component, LECT2, fibrinogen, lysozyme, prealbumin, apolipoprotein A1, lambda light chain–derived peptide antibodies, and transthyretin, although not all stains are available at all centers. Mass spectrophotometry has many advantages over immunostaining for amyloid subtyping,[14] including greater sensitivity, greater specificity, the need for less tissue, and ability to detect rare forms of amyloid; thus, this method is now preferred in most medical centers.

MALLORY HYALINE/BALLOON CELLS

Mallory hyaline (also known as Mallory-Denk bodies) is readily identified on H&E and immunostains are not necessary for clinical care. Mallory hyaline is composed of misfolded aggregates of ubiquitinated cytokeratin filaments and other associated proteins, so they can be highlighted with a number of different stains, including ubiquitin, p62, CK8/18, and CK19. Mallory hyaline is most commonly seen in ballooned hepatocytes and CK8/18 will further highlight the ballooned hepatocytes in negative relief, as the ballooned hepatocytes typically lose the diffuse cytoplasmic staining seen in nonballooned hepatocytes.[15]

INFECTIONS

BACTERIAL STAINS. Gram stains and other general bacterial stains are used primarily to identify organisms in hepatic abscesses; they are not always necessary in this setting, as the diagnosis of a hepatic abscess is sufficient in most cases for treatment decisions. Most abscesses are not knowingly resected unless they are refractory to therapy, but if the diagnosis is known or strongly suspected ahead of time, tissue should be submitted for culture. Mixed bacterial and fungal abscess are not uncommon, so fungal culture/stains can also be helpful. In terms of bacterial stains, gram-positive organisms are blue on the Gram-Weigert stain, while bacteria that do not stain are assumed to be gram-negative. Of note, some acid-fast bacteria (AFB) can stain red. With the Brown-Hopps stain, gram-positive organisms stain blue and gram-negative organisms stain red.

TROPHERYMA WHIPPLEI infections (Whipple disease) is only rarely seen in liver specimens, but infected foamy macrophages are located in the portal tracts and lobules and are highlighted by PAS stains.

FUNGAL STAINS. The Grocott methenamine silver (GMS) stain identifies fungi; the stain is also positive in some bacteria but the size and the morphology will help identify organisms as fungal. In most laboratories, the GMS stain tends to be a bit dirty, so is should be examined carefully; true organisms have regularity to their morphology that is not seen with the background nonspecific staining. Some pathologists prefer the PAS stain when looking for fungi, with the caveat that dead fungi are often PAS negative.

ACID FAST BACTERIAL STAINS. The most commonly used AFB stain is the Ziehl-Neelsen stain (organisms red, background blue), but the Kinyoun stain also works well (organisms red, background green). Mycobacterial organisms are typically sparse in cases of mycobacterium tuberculosis, so the AFB stain should be examined carefully. If the clinical setting is suspicious for tuberculosis, then repeating the AFB stain should be considered. Polymerase chain reaction (PCR) detection can also be helpful, although is not available in all centers and there are sensitivity issues because of the sparsity of organisms, so the AFB stains should still be performed. A modified Ziehl-Neelsen stain, called the Fite stain, uses gentler staining conditions to identify the more fragile bacterial walls of *M. leprae* (leprosy), Nocardia, and Rhodococcus.

SILVER STAINS. Silver stains, such as Warthin-Starry, have historically been used to assess for syphilis but immunostains are much more sensitive and specific, as silver stains are usually dirty, making them hard to read. The Warthin-Starry stain can also detect *Bartonella henselae*, the organism that causes cat-scratch disease and bacterial peliosis in the liver.

VIRAL STAINS. A number of stains can detect viral infections; their staining pattern will depend on the targeted antigen, but below are the most commonly used stains, with the most common staining patterns:

- Hepatitis B infection: HBsAg (cytoplasmic) and HBcAg (nuclear)
- Cytomegalovirus (CMV): Cytoplasmic/nuclear. The nuclear staining is often darker and can be seen without cytoplasmic staining
- Herpes simplex virus (HSV): Cytoplasmic/nuclear
- Adenovirus: Cytoplasmic/nuclear
- Epstein-Barr virus (EBV): EBV-LMP (cytoplasmic); EBER (nuclear)
- Human herpesvirus-8 (HHV8): Nuclear
- Parvovirus: Cytoplasmic

ADDITIONAL HISTOCHEMICAL STAINS

FONTANNA-MASSON. Fontanna-Masson stains lipofuscin with a granular black pattern (Figure 3.19).

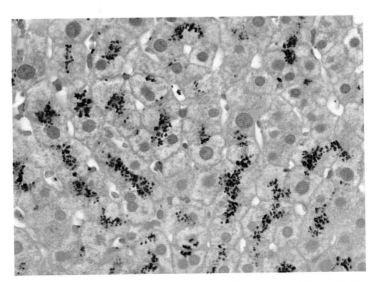

FIGURE 3.19 **Fontanna-Masson.** Lipofuscin stains with a granular black pattern.

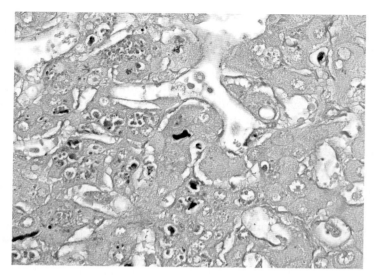

FIGURE 3.20 **Hall bile stain.** The bile stains a dark green color.

HALL BILE STAIN. Also called Hall bilirubin stain, this stain highlights bile with a dark green color (Figure 3.20), but it is rarely used in surgical pathology of the liver, since the H&E findings are sufficient to recognize bile and, in equivocal cases, serum bilirubin levels should be checked anyway.

OIL RED O STAIN. This stain was used in times-past on frozen tissue to identity neutral fat, which stains bright red. Historically, for example, it was used when evaluating donor livers for fat. The stain, however, was never user-friendly, as it tends to be dirty and even normal hepatocytes can be Oil Red O–positive, so its use often led to over-estimating the amount of fat in donor livers.

Over the years, some authors have also advocated its use to identify microvesicular steatosis, but the H&E findings are sufficient, and actually better, for making the diagnosis and Oil Red O stains are not needed. As with donor liver biopsies, Oil Red O can be challenging to interpret in this setting too, as it stains normal hepatocytes that do not have microvesicular steatosis; most clinical cases do not have frozen tissue anyway.

Today, the stain is most often used in either cell culture studies or animal studies, where it retains some usefulness because staining can be directly compared to control groups. Also, the Oil Red O stain has found at least two other uses: generating the red color smoke found in some pyrotechnics and developing latent fingerprints from porous surfaces such as paper. These are probably better uses for this stain anyway.

PHOSPHOTUNGSTIC ACID-HEMATOXYLIN STAIN (PTAH). In liver pathology, this stain is rarely needed, but it will highlight megamitochondria in hepatocytes with a blue-black color (Figure 3.21); it also stains fibrin blue. Pseudoground glass hepatocyte inclusions can be positive in a subset of cases.

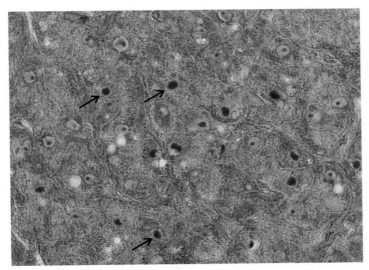

FIGURE 3.21 **Phosphotungstic acid-hematoxylin stain.** The megamitochondria stain a blue-black color; a few of the many megamitochondria in this image are indicated by arrows.

SUDAN BLACK. This stain, like Oil Red O, is no longer used in surgical pathology of the liver. It had similar performance characteristics to Oil Red O but stained neutral fat black and not red.

ADDITIONAL USEFUL IMMUNOSTAINS

C4D. This stain is used to assess for antibody-mediated rejection. While not necessary for use in clinical cases, apoptotic hepatocytes are often C4d-positive and a subset of cases with glycogen pseudoground glass are C4d-positive.

CD68. Kupffer cells are strongly CD68-positive. The KP1 clone also stains lysosomes. Normal hepatocytes are either negative or focally and very lightly positive, but most fibrolamellar carcinomas and a subset of conventional hepatocellular carcinomas show stronger, diffuse staining.

CD10. This stain identifies bile canaliculi of normal hepatocytes. Historically, CD10 was used as a marker of hepatocellular differentiation, but newer generations of stains for hepatocellular differentiation are more sensitive and specific.

In most medical liver biopsies, identifying the bile canaliculi is not necessary, but in rare cases, it can be useful. For example, the normal CD10 staining pattern can be lost in patients with Alagille syndrome greater than 2 years of age.[6] In addition, in livers with lobular ischemic or toxic necrosis, the hepatocytes lose their canalicular staining pattern before the hepatocytes are obviously necrotic.

CD34. In the normal liver, CD34 stains only sinusoids in zone 1. In response to high arterial blood flow, the sinusoids become more diffusely positive for CD34.

SMOOTH MUSCLE ACTIN. Smooth muscle actin is often used in research studies to identify stellate cell activation. In the normal liver, there is little or no staining for smooth muscle actin within the sinusoids. When activated by liver injury, however, the stellate cells express smooth muscle actin. Overall, this stain has more value in research studies than in clinical care. It has been used as an adjunct to help support a diagnosis of stellate cell hyperplasia from vitamin A excess, but it is nonspecific in that setting and does not appear to be diagnostically useful.

REFERENCES

1. Torbenson MS, Zen Y, Yeh MM, et al. *Tumors of the Liver.* American Registry of Pathology; 2018:xv, 449.

2. Hodges JR, Millward-Sadler GH, Barbatis C, et al. Heterozygous MZ alpha 1-antitrypsin deficiency in adults with chronic active hepatitis and cryptogenic cirrhosis. *N Engl J Med.* 1981;304:557-560.

3. Gourley MF, Gourley GR, Gilbert EF, et al. Alpha 1-antitrypsin deficiency and the PiMS phenotype: case report and literature review. *J Pediatr Gastroenterol Nutr.* 1989;8:116-121.

4. Kelly JK, Taylor TV, Milford-Ward A. Alpha-1-antitrypsin Pi S phenotype and liver cell inclusion bodies in alcoholic hepatitis. *J Clin Pathol.* 1979;32:706-709.

5. Millward-Sadler GH. Alpha-1-antitrypsin deficiency and liver disease. *Acta Med Port.* 1981;(suppl 2):91-102.

6. Byrne JA, Meara NJ, Rayner AC, et al. Lack of hepatocellular CD10 along bile canaliculi is physiologic in early childhood and persistent in Alagille syndrome. *Lab Invest.* 2007;87:1138-1148.

7. Pai RK, Hart JA. Aberrant expression of cytokeratin 7 in perivenular hepatocytes correlates with a cholestatic chemistry profile in patients with heart failure. *Mod Pathol.* 2010;23:1650-1656.

8. El-Guindi MA, Sira MM, Hussein MH, et al. Hepatic immunohistochemistry of bile transporters in progressive familial intrahepatic cholestasis. *Ann Hepatol.* 2016;15:222-229.

9. Wendum D, Barbu V, Rosmorduc O, et al. Aspects of liver pathology in adult patients with MDR3/ABCB4 gene mutations. *Virchows Arch.* 2012;460:291-298.

10. Evason K, Bove KE, Finegold MJ, et al. Morphologic findings in progressive familial intrahepatic cholestasis 2 (PFIC2): correlation with genetic and immunohistochemical studies. *Am J Surg Pathol.* 2011;35:687-696.

11. Daniels JA, Torbenson M, Anders RA, et al. Immunostaining of plasma cells in primary biliary cirrhosis. *Am J Clin Pathol.* 2009;131:243-249.

12. Graham RP, Smyrk TC, Zhang L. Evaluation of Langerhans cell infiltrate by CD1a immunostain in liver biopsy for the diagnosis of primary biliary cirrhosis. *Am J Surg Pathol.* 2012;36:732-736.

13. Culver EL, Chapman RW. IgG4-related hepatobiliary disease: an overview. *Nat Rev Gastroenterol Hepatol.* 2016;13:601-612.

14. Vrana JA, Gamez JD, Madden BJ, et al. Classification of amyloidosis by laser microdissection and mass spectrometry-based proteomic analysis in clinical biopsy specimens. *Blood.* 2009;114:4957-4959.

15. Guy CD, Suzuki A, Burchette JL, et al. Costaining for keratins 8/18 plus ubiquitin improves detection of hepatocyte injury in nonalcoholic fatty liver disease. *Hum Pathol.* 2012;43:790-800.

4

THE ALMOST NORMAL LIVER BIOPSY

OVERVIEW

One of the persistent challenges in liver pathology is generating a diagnosis and differential for biopsies that histologically appear almost normal but were performed for elevations in liver enzymes. Overall, the almost-normal-liver biopsy makes up about 5% of all medical liver cases submitted for extramural consultations.[1] In some cases, the enzyme elevations can be fairly dramatic, in contrast to the minimal findings on liver biopsy. In these cases, there may be a very mild nonspecific portal or lobular chronic inflammation, or perhaps minimal fatty change, but not findings that seem adequate to explain the elevated liver enzymes. What to do?

Because the biopsy findings are so mild and nonspecific, the differential becomes very long, often so long that it is essentially meaningless. There is, however, hope! In many cases, a diagnosis can still be made (Table 4.1) by using a careful, systematic approach (Table 4.2), one designed to reveal even subtle and easily overlooked diagnoses.

The first step is to review all available clinical information, laboratory findings, and imaging findings. Knowing the clinical indication for the liver biopsy is particularly important, as it allows you to write a useful report, perhaps even a great report, one that includes all of the pertinent negatives. For example, a patient with systemic lupus erythematous, high serum antinuclear antibody (ANA) titers, and low but chronic elevations in aspartate transaminase (AST) and alanine transaminase (ALT) may undergo liver biopsy to rule out autoimmune hepatitis. In this setting, the biopsy often shows minimal nonspecific inflammation and mild reactive changes, which your report will undoubtedly clearly indicate; your report, however, becomes even more valuable to the clinical team when it specifically states that there is no evidence for autoimmune hepatitis and no fibrosis, a statement that alleviates concern over a smoldering autoimmune hepatitis that would need treatment to prevent fibrosis/cirrhosis of the liver.

The second step of this systemic approach is to examine the biopsy specimen at low power, a step that identifies the dominant histological

TABLE 4.1 Systematic Approach to the Almost Normal Liver Biopsy

Factors	Comments
History	
Indication for biopsy	This can really help focus the histological evaluation and allow you to address the clinical questions
Imaging findings	Hepatomegaly? Vascular flow changes? Steatosis? Biliary tract disease?
Laboratory tests	The predominant enzyme pattern can help guide evaluation of the biopsy
Liver Architecture	
Low-power view	Rule out nodular regenerative hyperplasia, sinusoidal dilatation
Liver Structures	
Bile ducts	Rule out ductopenia, subtle duct proliferation
Portal veins	Rule out portal vein atrophy, loss, muscularization
Hepatic arteries	Rule out amyloid
Hepatocytes	Rule out inclusions, apoptosis, endoplasmic reticulum proliferation, pigments such as iron or copper
Sinusoids	Rule out amyloid, light chain deposition disease, diabetic sclerosis, stellate cell hyperplasia, Kupffer cell hyperplasia, abnormal cell infiltrates
Central veins normal	Rule out veno-occlusive disease

pattern of injury. In the almost normal liver biopsy, there should be no significant inflammation, fatty change, or ductular proliferation, but examination at low power also helps exclude subtle changes of nodular regenerative hyperplasia (NRH) or sinusoidal dilatation.

The next step is examining the liver at medium and high power, looking for subtle changes. Here too, it is best to be systematic. There are many different approaches, but one good method is to follow the blood flow: Start in the portal tracts, move through the lobules, and end at the central veins. Make sure that all of the normal constituents of the liver are present and normal in appearance: Bile ducts, portal veins, and hepatic artery. Examine the hepatocytes for inclusions or other cytoplasmic changes and for increased apoptosis. Check to make sure the central veins are normal, with no inflammation or fibrosis. Supplement this careful histological examination with special stains, including a reticulin stain (another check for NRH), iron stain, and periodic acid-Schiff with diastase (PASD) stain.

Many of these cases benefit further from being set aside and taking a second look the next day. If there is still no reasonable histological explanation for the clinical, imaging, or laboratory findings, then sharing the biopsy

TABLE 4.2 The Differential for an Almost Normal Liver Biopsy Can Include These Conditions

Diagnoses	Major Findings
Alpha-1 antitrypsin deficiency	Periportal hepatic globules–in infants, the globules may be small and poorly formed, or even absent
Amyloid	Acellular deposits in sinusoids or vessels
Celiac disease	Mild nonspecific inflammatory changes
Crohn disease of the small bowel	Mild nonspecific inflammatory changes
Cystic fibrosis	Patchy areas of bile ductular proliferation and fibrosis. May also see nodular regenerative hyperplasia.
Ferroportin disease	Moderate iron deposits, Kupffer cells ≫ hepatocytes, in a person with low or normal transferrin saturation levels, but high serum ferritin
Glycogenic hepatopathy	Enlarged, swollen pale hepatocytes in a person with poorly controlled diabetes
Glycogen psuedoground glass	Large amphophilic hepatocyte inclusions in immunosuppressed patient on many medications
Hemochromatosis	Moderate to marked hepatocellular iron
Hepatoportal sclerosis	Loss or atrophy of portal veins; often accompanied by nodular regenerative hyperplasia
Hypervitaminosis A	Can be very subtle! Enlarged vacuolated stellate cells
Mitochondrial injury	Microvesicular steatosis
Nodular regenerative hyperplasia	Distinct nodularity to the liver parenchyma, but without significant fibrosis; best seen on low-power magnification
Sickle cell hepatopathy	Dilated sinusoids, sickled red blood cells, Kupffer cell iron
Small bowel bacterial overgrowth	Mild nonspecific inflammatory changes
Thyroid disease	Mild cholestasis with hyperthyroidism
	Fatty change (maybe minimal) with hypothyroidism
Wilson disease	Mild fatty change, sometimes with disproportionately prominent glycogenated nuclei

with others can sometimes be helpful. In some of the most difficult cases, the diagnosis becomes evident only after an iterative process between the clinical teams and the pathologists, where the histology findings are discussed with the clinician, during which time the clinician also shares relevant clinical, laboratory, and or imaging findings that were not previously made known to the pathologist. Next, both groups go back and reexamine the case in light of the new information—the pathologist looks again at the biopsy, the clinician may reexamine the patient or take additional history, or the radiologist may revisit the imaging findings. A subsequent joint discussion in most cases can establish a firm diagnosis, or a focused differential, or point to the further lines of investigation that may be needed. The discussions are often best included as part of regular QA conferences, when they are available.

The specific entities in Table 4.2 are discussed in detail in the relevant sections of this book, but this table provides a useful compilation of subtle biopsy findings to exclude when the biopsy looks almost normal. The next section of this chapter is devoted to highlighting some of the entities that do not fit well anywhere else in the book. The last section in this chapter discusses the differential in the almost normal, nonfibrotic liver when all of the potential causes discussed in this chapter have been carefully excluded. Cryptogenic cirrhosis is considered in a separate chapter.

In terms of nomenclature, there is not a great term yet for the almost-normal liver specimen. The term *nonspecific reactive hepatitis* has roots that go back at least 50 years[2] and is sometimes used as a synonym, but historically, this term has incorporated a much wider range of histological abnormalities, including mild nonspecific chronic hepatitis, mild changes suggestive of biliary obstruction, and is sometimes used for the changes seen with celiac disease.[3] Given the lack of a clear definition and its inconsistent usage, *nonspecific reactive hepatitis* is not a great synonym for the almost-normal liver biopsy specimen.

LIVER ENZYMES

As a preface, AST, ALT, ALP, and GGT are not liver function tests per se (in contrast to albumin and prothrombin, which are), so the most technically correct terminology for them is *liver enzymes*.[4]

When evaluating liver enzymes, the predominant pattern is what matters. For example, hepatitic diseases show disproportion elevations in AST and ALT versus ALP and vice versa for biliary tract disease. The precise AST to ALT ratio is not that important unless you are a medical student preparing to be grilled during general medicine rounds; we all learned in medical school that AST:ALT ratio is 2× or greater in alcohol-related liver disease but of course clinical reality is much more complicated, with many exceptions.[5] For those who are still interested in this ratio (formally called the De Ritis ratio), it might be fun to know that some disciplines continue to incorporate this ratio in their research, mostly epidemiologists studying large populations. For example, it turns out that if you are middle-aged and eat too fast, your AST:ALT ratio will be lowered; in fact, to reduce this risk of a low AST:ALT ratio, it has been suggested you can moderate your eating speed.[6]

Liver Enzymes

- ALT (also known as SGPT)
  - Produced in hepatocytes
  - Reasonably specific for hepatocytes; only low concentrations in other organs
- AST (also known as SGOT)
  - There are two isoenzymes; the standard laboratory assays detect the total amount and does not distinguish between the isoenzymes
    - Mitochondrial isoenzyme: produced in hepatocytes
    - Cytosolic isoenzyme: present in kidney, heart, skeletal muscle
  - Levels generally parallel ALT
- Alkaline Phosphatase (ALP)
  - A group of multiple isoenzymes; most laboratory findings can fractionate to determine liver, intestinal, or bone origin
  - Liver isoenzyme is produced in bile ducts and bile canaliculi
  - Biliary obstruction or other injury leads to increased synthesis in the injured ducts, which leak into the blood
  - Other isoenzymes are found in the intestine, bone, kidney, and placenta
- Gamma-glutamyl transferase (GGT)
  - In the liver, GGT is found in microsomes of the hepatocytes and cholangiocytes
  - GGT is also found in the kidney, pancreas, and intestine
  - GGT is elevated in biliary tract disease; combined disproportionate rise of ALP and GGT is very common and reasonably specific for biliary obstruction
    - GGT and ALP patterns are particularly important in pediatric cholestatic liver disease
  - GGT is also elevated in other liver injuries including drug reactions and alcoholic liver disease

ALP predominant patterns suggest biliary tract disease, but the extended differential includes less common entities such as granulomatous diseases, NRH, and sinusoidal infiltrative processes. Unusually low levels of ALP are very rare, but the differential includes generalized malnutrition, hypothyroidism, vitamin deficiency (especially vitamin C, zinc), pernicious anemia, and Wilson disease.[7] Finally, if the biopsy looks normal and there is a disproportionate elevation in alkaline phosphatase, then nonhepatic causes should also be considered (Table 4.3).

ISOLATED ALKALINE PHOSPHATASE LEVELS. Isolated ALP levels can result from ductopenia, NRH, granulomatous diseases, and various sinusoidal infiltrative processes. One study of hospitalized patients found the following etiologies for patients with isolated ALP levels: Malignancy (20%), congestive

TABLE 4.3 Nonhepatic Causes of Persistent Elevations in Serum Alkaline Phosphatase Levels

Causes	Example
Physiological	Adolescence
	Pregnancy
Bone disease	Healing fracture
	Rickets
	Osteomalacia
Renal failure	
Heart failure	
Endocrine disease	Thyroid disease Parathyroid disease
Malignancy	Osteosarcoma
	Renal cell carcinoma
	Lymphoma
	Leukemia

heart failure (16%), benign bone disease (8%), hyperthyroidism (2%), end-stage renal disease (5%), or unknown (27%).[8] This same study found that in 50% of patients, the ALP levels normalized within a year. Finally, a small subset of patients with the metabolic syndrome, usually older-aged women that have minimal to mild fatty liver disease on biopsy, can also present with isolated ALP elevations.[9] Of course, elevated ALP is not always from liver disease. As a potential clue, if the ALP is elevated, but GGT levels are normal, this points to nonliver causes.[10]

ISOLATED HYPERBILIRUBINEMIA. This finding (elevated bilirubin with normal ALP levels) is very rarely an indication for liver biopsy but is not uncommon after major surgeries. In nonhospitalized patients, isolated direct hyperbilirubinemia can be seen with the Dubin-Johnson or Rotor syndrome; in contrast, isolated indirect hyperbilirubinemia suggests recent trauma, hemorrhage, or blood transfusion. If these common causes are excluded, then the differential may include Gilbert syndrome or Crigler-Najjar syndrome.[11]

ISOLATED HYPERAMMONEMIA. In noncirrhotic patients, isolated elevations in serum ammonia levels are rare. In the pediatric population, the differential includes urea cycle defects.[12] Drug effects, in particular valproate, can also lead to isolated hyperammonemia.[13] In patients with liver transplants, vascular abnormalities can lead to isolated hyperammonemia, such as anastomotic strictures of the portal or hepatic veins or patent portosystemic shunts.[14] Rare cases of shunting, sometimes fatal, have also been reported after gastric bypass surgery.[15]

PORTAL TRACT CHANGES

The portal tracts should be examined for changes to the bile ducts, including ductopenia, periductal fibrosis, duct duplication, or subtle ductular proliferation. CK7 is helpful because it can highlight any bile duct loss, subtle bile ductular proliferation, and intermediate hepatocytes. A copper stain is also useful to evaluate for detecting subtle chronic cholestatic liver disease.

The portal veins should be examined for changes including portal vein muscularization, thrombosis, herniation, atrophy, or loss. Portal vein changes can be tricky, as they are particularly easy to overcall when the biopsy is essentially normal. There is a natural tendency for thresholds for abnormal findings to drop the longer we look at a biopsy. The diagnosis of portal vein abnormalities is strengthened when multiple different types of portal vein changes are identified and each is present in multiple portal tracts. There is no well-established cut-off for determining portal vein atrophy or portal vein loss, but the changes should reasonably diffuse to be diagnostically useful. If the changes are still present on deeper levels, this can also make the diagnosis more convincing. NRH, while not always present, also strengthens the diagnosis of portal vein abnormalities.

HEPATIC ARTERY CHANGES. Hepatic artery pathology is very rare, so it is easy to get out of the habit of carefully examining them. The most common diagnostically significant finding is amyloid deposition. Rare cases of amyloid involving the liver have amyloid deposition that is exclusively, or nearly so, located in the hepatic arteries. This can be very subtle and is best brought out by Congo red stain. A more common but incidental finding, one that can mimic amyloid deposition, is hepatic artery arteriolosclerosis, which is seen in elderly patients with hypertension and/or diabetes[16] but is Congo red–negative.

HEPATOCYTE CHANGES

In the context of the almost normal liver biopsy differential, hepatocyte changes usually fall into one of a few categories, including increased apoptosis, cytoplasmic changes, or cell size variability. In terms of cytoplasmic changes, hepatocytes can show diffuse changes: glycogen accumulation in the setting of glycogenic hepatopathy, endoplasmic reticulum proliferation as a medication effect, or mild cholestasis. Inclusions can range from small eosinophilic structures, such as megamitochondria, to larger inclusions that fill the entire cytoplasm.

INCREASED APOPTOSIS. Increased apoptosis can be very subtle as an isolated finding, with a differential that mostly includes intermittent ischemia and drug effects. In cases of ischemia, the scattered apoptotic bodies can be accompanied by increased mitotic figures in nearby hepatocytes; this pattern was first worked out in the setting of liver transplantation[17] but can be

Hepatocyte Changes

- Increased apoptosis
- Resolving hepatitis pattern
- Cytoplasmic changes
  - Glycogen accumulation
  - Induced hepatocytes
  - Cholestasis
- Cytoplasmic inclusions–primarily small and eosinophilic
  - Megamitochondria
  - Alpha-1 antitrypsin protein
  - Alpha-1 antichymotrypsin
  - Reactive globules
- Cytoplasmic inclusions–primarily larger and amphophilic
  - Ground-glass inclusions from HBsAg
  - Pseudoground glass, usually a medication effects
  - Other rare genetic conditions such as Lafora bodies, dysfibrinogenemia
- Changes in hepatocyte size
  - NRH
  - Other rare conditions

seen in nontransplanted livers too. The very earliest manifestations of acute viral hepatitis C and B show a similar pattern of scattered lobular apoptosis with little or no inflammation, a pattern once again was first worked out in the transplant setting, but holds true in other settings as well.[18]

The "Resolving Hepatitis Pattern"

This pattern of injury is most commonly seen with acute idiosyncratic drug-induced liver injury, where the agent was removed (by the patient, family physician, etc) some weeks prior to seeing a hepatologist and having a liver biopsy. The biopsy shows minimal or no inflammation, while the lobules and sometimes the portal tracts have scattered, small clusters of pigmented macrophages, which represents the "clean-up" efforts responding to prior liver injury (Figure 4.1). A Ki-67 will often demonstrate a mild but definite increase in proliferation (normal quiescent liver <1%). Acute self-limited viral hepatitis can also have a resolving hepatitis pattern.

GLYCOGEN ACCUMULATION. Diffuse glycogen is seen most commonly in the setting of glycogenic hepatopathy, but similar patterns are found in glycogen storage diseases. Small discrete foci of glycogen enriched hepatocytes, called glycogen storage foci, are incidental findings that would not explain abnormal liver enzymes.

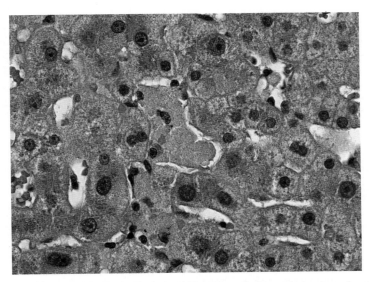

FIGURE 4.1 **Lobular macrophages.** A small cluster of pigmented macrophages marks the site of prior injury in this biopsy that otherwise had no significant histological findings.

INDUCED ENDOPLASMIC RETICULIN PROLIFERATION. This change is manifested in hepatocytes that have distinctly amphophilic changes to their cytoplasm (Figure 4.2). The changes do not lead to well-defined inclusions, in contrast to glycogen pseudoground glass, but also represent a drug effect. The hepatocyte cytoplasm in many cases is distinctly "two-toned," as the cytoplasm will be divided into two separate and distinctive colors. This change can be seen with a number of different medications.

MINIMAL BLAND LOBULAR CHOLESTASIS. This finding is most commonly seen with drug reactions, but there is a longer differential (Chapter 2, Table 2.3). In some cases, the cholestasis will be so mild that it is only evident after carefully searching, prompted by a history of chronic mild bilirubin elevations. You can also do stains that confirm chronic mild cholestatic liver disease. A copper stain can show copper deposition in periportal hepatocytes—the positivity can be very focal and mild, so you have to look carefully (Figure 4.3). A CK7 immunostain, which is typically negative in hepatocytes, will also commonly show mild staining in the setting of chronic cholestasis (Figure 4.4). In congestive hepatopathy from heart disease, the CK7 positivity can show a zone 3 distribution,[19] but in early cholestatic diseases, the pattern will be zone 1.

PROMINENT MEGAMITOCHONDRIA. Megamitochondria are commonly seen as an incidental finding in the setting of fatty liver disease and various chronic cholestatic liver diseases. In this case, however, we are discussing cases that lack any significant fat or cholestatic changes and the main finding is that of prominent hepatocyte megamitochondria. Overall, this

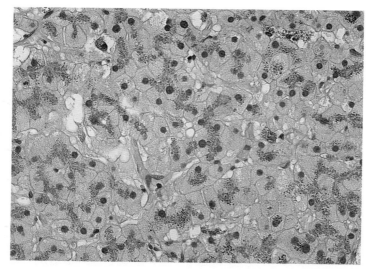

FIGURE 4.2　**Induced hepatocytes.** The hepatocytes show a distinctive cytoplasmic amphophilic changed caused by smooth endoplasmic reticulin proliferation. In this case, the liver also has abundant lipofuschin, which gets pushed to the side and accentuates the findings.

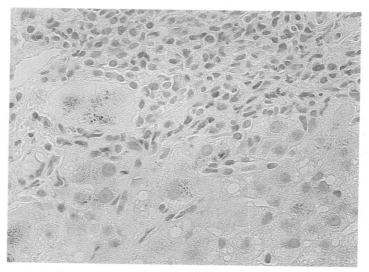

FIGURE 4.3　**Copper in chronic cholestasis.** A copper stain demonstrates periportal copper deposition in this case of chronic cholestasis.

finding is nonspecific and is only rarely seen as an isolated finding. In adults, this pattern can be associated with drug effects, though typically there will also be other findings of drug-induced liver injury.[20] In children, this pattern can be associated with the earliest changes of inherited mitochondrial diseases, or with various defects of the urea cycle, or with other

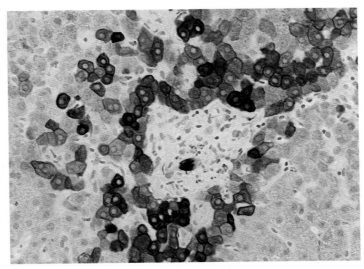

FIGURE 4.4 **CK7 immunostain in chronic cholestasis.** An immunostain for CK7 shows staining of the periportal hepatocytes in this case of early primary biliary cholangitis (PBC).

inherited metabolic abnormalities such as lysinergic protein intolerance and hypermethioninemia.[21]

GROUND-GLASS, PSEUDOGROUND GLASS, AND RELATED CHANGES. Ground-glass changes/inclusions result from hepatitis B virus (HBV) and are discussed in the chapter on viral hepatitis. Pseudoground glass change is discussed in detail in the chapter on drug-induced liver injury. Inherited causes of inclusions are discussed in the chapter on genetic diseases.

Briefly, the main finding is that of large amphophilic to slightly eosinophilic inclusions in hepatocytes. In many cases, the changes are striking and rather diffuse and thus easy to identify, but in some cases, the findings can be focal and more subtle. These inclusions are typically PAS positive and most represent either chronic HBV infection with ground-glass inclusions or medication effects with pseudoground glass inclusions.

Rarely, the inclusions can be PAS-negative. PAS-negative inclusions can be isolated findings, seen in an almost normal liver, or present in the setting of other acute or chronic liver diseases. In most cases, the PAS negative inclusions appear to be a nonspecific reactive change.[22] In a very small subset of cases, however, the inclusions represent fibrinogen storage disease; these patients typically have histories of bleeding or thrombotic abnormalities.

Finally, nonspecific reactive globules can be seen in zone 3 hepatocytes in the setting of chronic vascular congestion.[23] The globules are typically PASD-positive and can cross-react with immunostains for alpha-1 antitrypsin, but patients do not have alpha-1 antitrypsin mutations.

LOBULAR DISARRAY. Lobular disarray can be subjective when very mild but refers to lobules that no longer show the normal, largely parallel organization of hepatocytes into thin trabecula. The pattern of lobular disarray is very nonspecific for etiology but results from hepatocellular regeneration following many different sorts of lobular injury. When this pattern is seen in isolation, without ongoing active injury, the differential is broad but the most likely explanation is resolving hepatitis or low-grade chronic ischemia. Scattered hepatocytes with large cell change can also be seen in some cases, especially with chronic ischemia.

CHANGES IN HEPATOCYTE SIZE. NRH can lead to subtle changes in hepatocyte size, with thin bands of smaller-sized hepatocytes, usually in zone 3, surrounding nodules of normal-sized hepatocytes, giving the parenchyma a nodular appearance on low power. The findings can be further accentuated with a reticulin stain.

Other rare conditions, such as hyperviscosity syndrome, can show more heterogeneous variation in hepatocyte size, often accompanied by lobular disarray, presumably due to low-grade ischemia (Figure 4.5). The hyperviscosity syndrome can be seen in a wide variety of conditions, including multiple myeloma, Waldentrom macroglobulinemia, and polycythemia vera. Autoimmune diseases such as Sjögren syndrome, systemic lupus erythematosus, or rheumatoid arthritis, can also be associated with the hyperviscosity syndrome.

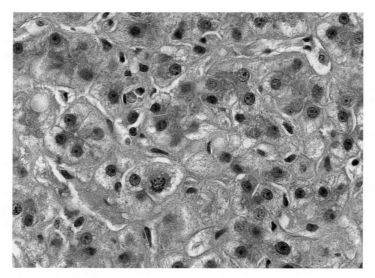

FIGURE 4.5 **Hyperviscosity syndrome.** The lobules show lobular disarray with occasional apoptotic bodies and mitotic figures.

SINUSOIDAL CHANGES

Sinusoidal dilation and congestion can be important clues to vascular out-flow abnormalities. The sinusoidal dilation usually has a zone 3 prominence and is typically diffuse. There may be zone 3 or central vein fibrosis in chronic vascular outflow disease, but many times fibrosis will not be evident. Other causes of sinusoidal dilatation include drug-induced liver injury.

In most cases, the hematoxylin and eosin (H&E) findings are sufficient to make the diagnosis, but there are many cases in which the sinusoidal dilatation is subtle or equivocal. In some of these cases, the sinusoidal dilatation is truly present, but there is no clinical or imaging evidence for vascular outflow disease and no relevant medication history. In these cases, the differential includes systemic inflammatory diseases, infectious granulomatous diseases, autoimmune diseases, and paraneoplastic effects from carcinomas in other organs.[24,25] Autoimmune conditions that can be associated with mild sinusoidal dilatation include the antiphospholipid syndrome[26] and rheumatoid arthritis.[27] As a caveat, subtle sinusoidal dilation can also be seen with rapid blood volume expansion and a wide variety of other conditions. In fact, very mild sinusoidal congestion often lacks any diagnostic value and is sometimes over-interpreted. If the biopsy also shows zone 3 hepatocyte atrophy, this can increase the confidence that the findings indicate true disease. The atrophy can be highlighted with a reticulin stain in many cases. A CK7 immunostain can also be helpful to look for zone 3 intermediate hepatocytes. For cases without atrophy or intermediate hepatocytes, the congestion or sinusoidal dilatation has to be reasonably more than is seen in most biopsies to be diagnostically useful, which can take experience to comfortably recognize.

THE DIFFERENTIAL FOR THE ALMOST NORMAL LIVER BIOPSY

This section focuses on those biopsies which show no fibrosis and are histologically essentially normal, with all of the subtle findings discussed above excluded. Overall, approximately 5% of biopsies performed for unexplained liver enzyme elevations fall into this category and will have at most only mild nonspecific changes, in other words an "almost normal" appearance. This frequency does not include protocol biopsies (for example, in transplant patients or as part of research studies). These "almost normal" biopsies will have no more than minimal portal or lobular lymphocytic inflammation and no other significant finding. Of these cases, approximately 80% are biopsied for mild chronic elevations in liver enzymes and the remaining 20% for unexplained ascites.[28]

While data is limited, studies suggest a probable or definite cause can be found in 20% to 50% of cases, based on careful correlation with current and subsequent laboratory and clinical findings (Table 4.2).[28,29]

- In 15% of cases, the patients will have known systemic autoimmune conditions at the time of the biopsy, such as systemic lupus erythematosus or rheumatoid arthritis. In these cases, the liver enzyme elevations appear to be a manifestation of systemic disease. The biopsies often show minimal lymphocytic portal inflammation, but the clinical, laboratory, and biopsy findings do not support a diagnosis of autoimmune hepatitis.
- In 10% of cases, patients will subsequently develop a more typical autoimmune hepatitis, PBC, or sarcoidosis involving the liver.
- Another 10% of cases are associated with obesity and metabolic syndrome, despite the lack of fat on the biopsy. In many of these cases, very mild patchy fat is evident on imaging studies but presumably was not sampled on the biopsy.
- In about 10% of cases, individuals with obesity and metabolic syndrome can simply lack fat in the liver, although they often have minimal, nonspecific chronic inflammation in the portal tracts.
- Another 5% of "almost normal biopsies" are seen in the setting of chronic inflammatory conditions of the gut, many of which were undiagnosed at the time of the liver biopsy.
- In up to 5% of cases, patients have risk factors for hepatic ischemia, but the injury is insufficient to cause a typical ischemic injury pattern with zone 3 necrosis, instead there is only mild nonspecific changes on biopsy.
- For those patients in whom no cause is identified at the time of biopsy, or by the subsequent clinical course, the hepatic enzymes will self-normalize in 50% of cases, while the remaining 50% will continue to have mild unexplained elevations in liver enzymes for many years.

REFERENCES

1. Torbenson MS, Arnold CA, Graham RP, et al. Identification of key challenges in liver pathology: data from a multicenter study of extramural consults. *Hum Pathol.* 2019;87:75-82.
2. Schaffner F, Popper H. Nonspecific reactive hepatitis in aged and infirm people. *Am J Dig Dis.* 1959;4:389-399.
3. Volta U. Pathogenesis and clinical significance of liver injury in celiac disease. *Clin Rev Allergy Immunol.* 2009;36:62-70.
4. Kwo PY, Cohen SM, Lim JK. ACG clinical guideline: evaluation of abnormal liver chemistries. *Am J Gastroenterol.* 2017;112:18-35.
5. Botros M, Sikaris KA. The de ritis ratio: the test of time. *Clin Biochem Rev.* 2013;34:117-130.

6. Ozaki E, Ochiai H, Shirasawa T, et al. Eating quickly is associated with a low aspartate aminotransferase to alanine aminotransferase ratio in middle-aged adults: a large-scale cross-sectional survey in Japan. *Arch Public Health.* 2020;78:101.

7. Siddique A, Kowdley KV. Approach to a patient with elevated serum alkaline phosphatase. *Clin Liver Dis.* 2012;16:199-229.

8. Lieberman D, Phillips D. "Isolated" elevation of alkaline phosphatase: significance in hospitalized patients. *J Clin Gastroenterol.* 1990;12:415-419.

9. Pantsari MW, Harrison SA. Nonalcoholic fatty liver disease presenting with an isolated elevated alkaline phosphatase. *J Clin Gastroenterol.* 2006;40:633-635.

10. Slaunwhite D, Tuggey RL, Reynoso G. A supplement to alkaline phosphatase fractionations: utilization of gamma-glutamyl transpeptidase and hydroxyproline assays. *Ann Clin Lab Sci.* 1978;8:117-121.

11. Shroff H, Maddur H. Isolated elevated bilirubin. *Clin Liver Dis.* 2020;15:153-156.

12. Acikalin A, Disel NR, Direk EC, et al. A rare cause of postpartum coma: isolated hyperammonemia due to urea cycle disorder. *Am J Emerg Med.* 2016;34(7):1324.e3-4.

13. Wadzinski J, Franks R, Roane D, et al. Valproate-associated hyperammonemic encephalopathy. *J Am Board Fam Med.* 2007;20:499-502.

14. Belenky A, Igov I, Konstantino Y, et al. Endovascular diagnosis and intervention in patients with isolated hyperammonemia, with or without ascites, after liver transplantation. *J Vasc Interv Radiol.* 2009;20:259-263.

15. Fenves A, Boland CR, Lepe R, et al. Fatal hyperammonemic encephalopathy after gastric bypass surgery. *Am J Med.* 2008;121:e1-e2.

16. Balakrishnan M, Garcia-Tsao G, Deng Y, et al. Hepatic arteriolosclerosis: a small-vessel complication of diabetes and hypertension. *Am J Surg Pathol.* 2015;39:1000-1009.

17. Liu TC, Nguyen TT, Torbenson MS. Concurrent increase in mitosis and apoptosis: a histological pattern of hepatic arterial flow abnormalities in post-transplant liver biopsies. *Mod Pathol.* 2012;25(12):1594-1598.

18. Saxena R, Crawford JM, Navarro VJ, et al. Utilization of acidophil bodies in the diagnosis of recurrent hepatitis C infection after orthotopic liver transplantation. *Mod Pathol.* 2002;15:897-903.

19. Pai RK, Hart JA. Aberrant expression of cytokeratin 7 in perivenular hepatocytes correlates with a cholestatic chemistry profile in patients with heart failure. *Mod Pathol.* 2010;23:1650-1656.

20. Itoh S, Yamaba Y, Matsuo S, et al. Sodium valproate-induced liver injury. *Am J Gastroenterol.* 1982;77:875-879.

21. Gaull GE, Bender AN, Vulovic D, et al. Methioninemia and myopathy: a new disorder. *Ann Neurol.* 1981;9:423-432.

22. Zen Y, Nishigami T. Rethinking fibrinogen storage disease of the liver: ground glass and globular inclusions do not represent a congenital metabolic disorder but acquired collective retention of proteins. *Hum Pathol.* 2020;100:1-9.

23. Klatt EC, Koss MN, Young TS, et al. Hepatic hyaline globules associated with passive congestion. *Arch Pathol Lab Med.* 1988;112:510-513.

24. Kakar S, Kamath PS, Burgart LJ. Sinusoidal dilatation and congestion in liver biopsy: is it always due to venous outflow impairment? *Arch Pathol Lab Med.* 2004;128:901-904.

25. Bruguera M, Aranguibel F, Ros E, et al. Incidence and clinical significance of sinusoidal dilatation in liver biopsies. *Gastroenterology.* 1978;75:474-478.

26. Saadoun D, Cazals-Hatem D, Denninger MH, et al. Association of idiopathic hepatic sinusoidal dilatation with the immunological features of the antiphospholipid syndrome. *Gut.* 2004;53:1516-1519.

27. Laffon A, Moreno A, Gutierrez-Bucero A, et al. Hepatic sinusoidal dilatation in rheumatoid arthritis. *J Clin Gastroenterol*. 1989;11:653-657.

28. Czeczok TW, Van Arnam JS, Wood LD, et al. The almost-normal liver biopsy: presentation, clinical associations, and outcome. *Am J Surg Pathol*. 2017;41:1247-1253.

29. Strasser M, Stadlmayr A, Haufe H, et al. Natural course of subjects with elevated liver tests and normal liver histology. *Liver Int*. 2016;36:119-125.

5

ACUTE AND CHRONIC VIRAL HEPATITIS

GRADING AND STAGING BIOPSIES WITH CHRONIC VIRAL HEPATITIS

Historically, one of the most common liver biopsy specimens was those performed in the setting of known chronic viral hepatitis, either hepatitis C virus (HCV) or hepatitis B virus (HBV), which were obtained to determine the amount of inflammation (grade) and fibrosis (stage). This indication for biopsy has diminished significantly with the development of highly effective antiviral therapies and the advent of noninvasive markers of fibrosis, which can identify patients with minimal or no fibrosis and those with advanced fibrosis. In contrast, today, most biopsies in patients with known chronic HCV or HBV are performed to evaluate for possible concomitant liver disease.

The Knodell score was the first formal numerical system for scoring active injury and fibrosis in chronic hepatitis. It gives numbers for the amount of inflammation in the portal tracts, the interface (or piecemeal necrosis, which included bridging necrosis and panacinar necrosis), the hepatic lobules, and fibrosis. The numbers are then added, with higher scores indicating greater liver injury.[1] This paper revolutionized the study of chronic viral hepatitis because it allowed statistical analysis of biopsy data and provided potential endpoints in clinical studies. It was soon realized, however, that combining fibrosis and inflammation into a single system was not optimal and a number of grading and staging systems were quickly proposed over the next several years, including the Scheuer system, the Batts-Ludwig system, the Ishak system, and the METAVIR system. Other systems have been proposed, but these four are the most commonly used for clinical research. Each system has its own merits and fan base. At this point, there is no compelling data to suggest one system is superior to another. They score similar components of the inflammation (portal, interface, lobular) and all share the same conceptual framework for fibrosis evaluation (no fibrosis, portal fibrosis, bridging fibrosis, cirrhosis), but with each system subdividing and scoring these main categories of inflammation and fibrosis somewhat differently. Tables 5.1-5.7 provide a summary of the main staging systems, along with the grading system for Ishak and Batts-Ludwig systems. Overall, the METAVIR and the Ishak scoring system are the most commonly used in research studies. Table 5.8 provides a "Rosetta stone" for translating the various fibrosis stages from one system into another system.

TABLE 5.1	Ishak Grading System[2]	
Score	Definition	Comments
Interface activity[a]		Interface activity can also be seen along fibrous bridges or fibrous rims of cirrhotic nodules
0	Absent	
1	Mild: focal, few portal areas	Less than 50% of portal tracts; not continuous around any portal tract
2	Mild/Moderate: focal, most portal areas	50% or more of portal tracts; not continuous around any portal tract
3	Moderate: continuous around less than 50% of portal tracts	Continuous has been variably interpreted, but should involve most of the interface, ie, at least 50% of the interface for any given portal tract
4	Severe: continuous around more than 50% of portal tracts	
Confluent necrosis[b]		Confluent necrosis is defined as at least three adjacent necrotic hepatocytes. Usually, there is more than that
0	Absent	
1	Focal	
2	Zone 3, some areas	Less than 50% of central veins
3	Zone 3, most areas	
4	Zone 3 necrosis plus occasional portal to central bridging necrosis	Original intent was to score only portal to central bridging, but this can be hard to determine. So, in practice any bridging necrosis is given at least a 4
		Of note, bridging necrosis is not seen with chronic hepatitis unless there is a superimposed injury (or flare of activity in HBV)

TABLE 5.1	Ishak Grading System[2] (Continued)	
Score	Definition	Comments
5	Zone 3 necrosis plus multiple portal to central bridging necrosis	Not seen with chronic hepatitis unless there is a superimposed injury (or flare of activity in HBV)
6	Panacinar or multiacinar necrosis	Not seen with chronic hepatitis unless there is a superimposed injury (or flare of activity in HBV)
Lobular inflammation		Includes lobular inflammation, acidophil bodies
		Score with a 10× lens
0	Absent	
1	Mild: focal, few portal areas	One focus or less per 10× field
2	Mild/Moderate: focal, most portal areas	2-4 foci per 10× field
3	Moderate: continuous around less than 50% of portal tracts	5-10 per 10× field
4	Severe: continuous around more than 50% of portal tracts	More than 10 per 10× field
Portal inflammation		
0	Absent	
1	Mild, some or all portal tracts	
2	Moderate, some or all portal tracts	
3	Moderate/marked, all portal tracts	
4	Marked, all portal tracts	

HBV, hepatitis B virus.
[a]Also called periportal interface hepatitis.
[b]You may not see the necrotic hepatocytes, but instead, see areas of dropout.

The inflammatory grade can be determined by adding up the individual scores for inflammation in the portal tracts, interface activity, and lobular inflammation, leading to a composite inflammatory grade. Not all systems, however, use all three categories of inflammation. For example, the Scheuer, METAVIR, and Batts-Ludwig systems rely on interface activity

TABLE 5.2	Ishak Fibrosis Staging System
Stage	**Definition**
0	No fibrosis
1	Portal fibrosis of some portal tracts
2	Portal fibrosis of most portal tracts (50% or more of portal tracts)
3	Portal fibrosis with occasional bridging fibrosis
4	Portal fibrosis with marked bridging fibrosis
5	Marked bridging fibrosis with occasional nodules (incomplete cirrhosis)
6	Cirrhosis, probable or definite

Note: Original paper.[2]

TABLE 5.3	Batts-Ludwig Grading System	
Stage	**Definition**	**Comment**
0	No activity	Portal inflammation only
1	Minimal activity	Portal tracts: Variable
		Interface activity: up to focal, minimal
		Lobular activity: minimal
2	Mild activity	Portal tracts: Variable
		Interface activity: up to mild, involving some or all portal tracts
		Lobular activity: up to mild
3	Moderate activity	Portal tracts: Variable
		Interface activity: moderate, involving all portal tracts
		Lobular activity: moderate
4	Marked activity	Portal tracts: Variable
		Interface activity: severe
		Lobular activity: severe ± confluent necrosis

Note 1: Original paper.[3]
Note 2: Portal inflammation is not included in the grade. The highest inflammation for interface activity and lobular activity drives the score. For example, marked portal chronic inflammation with mild interface activity and moderate lobular activity is scored as grade 3.

and lobular activity to determine the inflammatory grade. The Ishak grading system is summarized in Table 5.1, and the Batts-Ludwig grading system is summarized in Table 5.3. The inflammation in these three areas of the liver (portal tracts, interface activity, and lobular), all covary in chronic viral hepatitis, with portal inflammation and interface activity having the strongest association.[9] In other words, as portal inflammation increases, the amount

TABLE 5.4	Batts-Ludwig Staging System
Stage	**Definition**
0	No fibrosis
1	Portal fibrosis
2	Periportal fibrosis with no more than rare fibrous septa
3	Septal fibrosis
4	cirrhosis

Note 1: Original paper.[3]
Note 2: Periportal fibrosis is used to describe portal fibrosis with irregular, short, spike-like fibrous extensions that do not reach the level of full fibrous bridges.
Note 3: Stage 2 fibrosis allows rare bridging fibrosis.

TABLE 5.5	METAVIR Fibrosis Staging System
Stage	**Definition**
0	No fibrosis
1	Portal fibrosis without septa (bridging fibrosis)
2	Portal tract fibrosis with rare septa (bridging fibrosis)
3	Numerous septa (bridging fibrosis) without cirrhosis
4	Cirrhosis

Note: Original paper.[4]

TABLE 5.6	Scheuer Staging System
Stage	**Definition**
0	No fibrosis
1	Portal fibrosis
2	Periportal fibrosis or bridging fibrosis, but with intact architecture
3	Fibrosis with architectural distortion but no obvious cirrhosis
4	Probable or definitive cirrhosis

Note 1: Original paper.[5]
Note 2: Periportal fibrosis is used to describe portal fibrosis with irregular, short, spike-like fibrous extensions that do not reach the level of full fibrous bridges.

TABLE 5.7	Laennec Staging System
Stage	Definition
0	No definite fibrosis
1	Minimal fibrosis (no septa or rare thin septum; may have portal expansion or mild sinusoidal fibrosis)
2	Mild fibrosis (occasional thin septa)
3	Moderate fibrosis (moderate thin septa; up to incomplete cirrhosis
4A	Mild cirrhosis, definite or probable; most septa are thin; one broad septum allowed
4B	Moderate cirrhosis (at least two broad septa; no very broad septa and less than half of the biopsy composed of minute nodules)
4C	Severe cirrhosis (at least one very broad septum or more than half of the biopsy composed of minute nodules)

Note 1: Original papers.[67]
Note 2: The term "broad septum" indicates a septal thickness less than the size of the hepatocellular nodule and "very broad septum" as being thicker than the size of nodule.

of interface activity also increases. Lobular inflammation, while still associated with the other two, is less tightly linked. This observation provides some support for systems that do not incorporate portal inflammation into the final grade; yet, it also seems apparent that cases with marked portal inflammation but mild interface activity are unlikely to be "the same" as cases with mild portal inflammation and mild interface activity.

Chapter 1 discusses the pros and cons of using formal grading and staging systems in your clinical pathology reports. The full discussion will not be repeated here, but perhaps it is worthwhile restating a few of the key points: (1) use a formal grading/staging system if you or your clinical team find them useful, but do not forget that formal systems are simply a communication tool and not a substitute for the pathology itself; (2) many formal grading/staging system were originally designed for research studies and are most useful in that setting; any additional value over traditional pathology descriptions for routine patient care has not been identified to date and is unlikely to be identified in the future (this may be a surprise to some readers, but is true!); (3) the formal grading/staging systems use words and numbers as synonyms, so while "METAVIR stage 1 fibrosis" does sound more impressive than "portal fibrosis," they are in fact the same thing; (4) grading and staging schemas do not create a "universal" system that eliminates interpretive variability—in fact, each of the formal systems introduces another layer of potential interpretive variability; (5) if you do use a formal system, please state in the clinical report which one you are using, and use it exactly as described in the original paper that defined the system—this would not be the time to demonstrate your individuality and creativity by "improving the system" with personal changes, even if they are brilliant.

TABLE 5.8 Fibrosis Rosetta Stone

Brief Description	Ishak[2] (MHAI)	METAVIR[4]	Batts-Ludwig[3]	Desmet[5]	Scheuer[8]	Knodell[1] (HAI)
None	0	0	0	0	0	0
Mild portal fibrosis	1	1	1	1	1	1
Moderate portal fibrosis	2	1	1 or 2	1	1 or 2	1
Bridging fibrosis	3	2	2	2 or 3[b]	2	3[a]
Extensive bridging with nodularity	4	3	3	2 or 3	3	3
Early cirrhosis	5	3	3	3	3	3
Cirrhosis	6	4	4	4	4	4

HAI, histology activity index; MHAI, modified histology activity index.
[a]Requires two or more portal to portal or portal to central bridges (ie, one bridge is still considered stage 2, though in common practice this guideline was often not followed).
[b]Stage 3 requires portal to central bridging fibrosis, though in practice stage 3 is commonly used for extensive bridging fibrosis.

For those who would like to read more about fibrosis staging systems, an excellent, thoughtful, and thorough article has been published by Goodman.[10] Another excellent article has been published by Guido et al.[11] There are other fine review articles, but I would recommend these two articles as good places to start. Regardless of the approach you decide to use, all liver pathology reports should indicate the amount of fibrosis/fibrosis stage, which is best determined by using special stains, such as the Masson trichrome or Sirius red.

When grading fibrosis, there are several pitfalls to avoid. These pitfalls are discussed and illustrated in Chapter 2 and are important to know. These pitfalls are not unique to viral hepatitis and can be encountered when staging fibrosis that occurs in any of the major causes of chronic hepatitis, including viral hepatitis, autoimmune hepatitis, fatty liver disease, and drug-induced liver injury (DILI). Of these diagnostic pitfalls, the two most common are (1) marked portal expansion by inflammation or bile ductular proliferation that leads to over-staging of portal fibrosis and (2) areas of bridging necrosis or panacinar necrosis that mimic bridging fibrosis, also leading to over-staging.

RISK FACTORS FOR FIBROSIS PROGRESSION

The risk factors for fibrosis progression have been most extensively studied in chronic HCV, but the general principles are broadly applicable. Major risk factors for fibrosis progression include fibrosis on a prior biopsy, male gender, older age at first infection, length of infection, HIV coinfection,[12] HBV coinfection,[13] and additional coexisting liver diseases, such as fatty liver disease[14] from the metabolic syndrome or from alcoholic liver disease. On the other hand, an increased risk for fibrosis progression is less clear when the patient does not have risk factors for the metabolic syndrome or a history of alcohol use, and the fatty liver disease instead appears to be caused solely by hepatitis C itself, principally viral genotype 3.[15] Iron overload that is moderate or marked also likely increases the risk for fibrosis progression.[16] Likewise, alpha-1-antitrypsion mutations can increase the risk for fibrosis progression. Interestingly, fibrosis progression is not linear overtime but progresses more rapidly with advanced fibrosis. For example, progression from portal fibrosis to bridging fibrosis takes considerably longer, on average, than progression from bridging fibrosis to cirrhosis.

HEPATITIS A

Hepatitis A virus (HAV) is an RNA virus transmitted primarily through the oral-fecal route, but sexual transmission and blood-borne transmission are also possible. It was first visualized by electron microscopy in 1973.[17] While an effective vaccine for HAV has been available since the 1990s, it is still an important cause of acute hepatitis. The virus is very stable at room temperatures and is resistant to low pH, allowing it to survive well in the environment. Several of the world's largest known epidemics of HAV have been associated with eating raw seafood.[18,19] The viral incubation period is 2 to 7 weeks. Overall, less than 30% of infected children will be symptomatic, while up to 80% of infected adults will have symptomatic hepatitis. Also, individuals with chronic liver disease, such as chronic HCV or HBV, have a higher risk of fulminant hepatitis and fatality when superinfected with HAV. HAV does not cause chronic hepatitis per se, but it can recur in the liver allograft of patients who are transplanted for fulminant HAV.[20,21] Acalculous cholecystitis is found at presentation in about 1/3 of symptomatic patients.[22]

Biopsies are rarely performed in patients with acute HAV because the diagnosis can be made by serological studies. Overall, biopsies in the setting of HAV are more common when there is a relapsing course or a prolonged cholestatic course, both of which are discussed in more detail below.

Histological Findings

Acute HAV infection shows a hepatitic pattern of injury with varying degrees of lobular and portal inflammation. In many cases, the portal inflammation is more striking than the lobular hepatitis.[23,24] The portal infiltrates can also be plasma cell rich.[24,25] The lobular hepatitis can have a zone 3 predominate pattern in some cases.[24,25] Kupffer cell hyperplasia is common and erythrophagocytosis can be present. In liver biopsies with marked hepatitis, the lobules may be cholestatic and the portal tracts can show bile ductular proliferation, usually mild. Rare cases of acute HAV with fibrin ring granulomas have been reported.[26] HAV also causes fulminant liver failure, representing 3% of all cases of acute liver failure in the United States of America (USA)[27]; biopsies are not commonly performed but show marked inflammation and massive liver necrosis.

Overall, there are no histological findings that will allow you to distinguish acute HAV from other causes of acute hepatitis, including other viruses, DILI, or autoimmune hepatitis. As noted above, acute HAV can have prominent plasma cells in the portal tracts, so do not overinterpret this histological finding as being diagnostic of autoimmune hepatitis. Fibrosis is not a component of acute HAV and, when convincingly present, indicates that there is an additional underlying liver disease, with superimposed acute HAV. The diagnosis of acute HAV is made by antibody studies (hepatitis A IgM positivity) or by polymerase chain reaction (PCR) for Hepatitis A RNA.

Atypical Clinical Courses

In most individuals, HAV infection is self-limited and the laboratory and biopsy findings return to normal, although mild nonspecific inflammatory changes may persist in the liver for up to a year following the acute hepatitis.[28] On the other hand, it is important to know that about 10% to 20% of patients have atypical courses for their hepatitis.[29] One of these atypical courses is called *relapsing HAV*. In these cases, an individual diagnosed with acute HAV will appear to recover based on clinical findings, but then will have a relapse of the hepatitis, which is typically milder than at the initial presentation.[29] The most common time interval between the first and second hepatitis enzyme peaks is 4 to 7 weeks. This pattern of relapsing HAV is well documented, but is uncommon, and thus, may lead to clinical uncertainty over the cause of the second bout of hepatitis, and then to a liver biopsy. The pathology in relapsing HAV typically shows mild to moderate portal and lobular hepatitis without specific features. There may be mild lobular cholestasis. Rarely, the hepatitis can be granulomatous.[30]

A second unusual clinical course is prolonged cholestasis after HAV infection. In most individuals, the bilirubin returns to normal within about 4 weeks after initial presentation. In about 2% of patients, however, there can be prolonged elevations in bilirubin.[31] Biopsies show residual and often mild portal and lobular lymphocytic inflammation along with mild lobular cholestasis (eFigs 5.1 and 5.2). Features of biliary obstruction are not present and the cholestasis is typically intrahepatic and canalicular.

HEPATITIS B

HBV is a partially double-stranded DNA virus. High levels of HBV virions can be present in many different body fluids. In those parts of the world where HBV infection is endemic, mother to neonate transmission is common. In contrast, in portions of the world where HBV infection is uncommon within the population, most infections occur in adults through injection drug use or sex. Acute HBV infection has very different outcomes depending on the age of the infected person; neonates have a 90% risk of developing chronic HBV, versus adults who have about a 5% chance of progressing to chronic HBV.

To help manage the different phases of infection, patients with chronic HBV are clinically categorized into those with immunotolerant HBV, chronic HBV, inactive HBV carrier state, and resolved HBV (Table 5.9).[32] Occult HBV is an additional category, wherein HBsAg is undetectable in the serum, but HBV DNA is present in the blood or liver tissues. This information on clinical categories will not help you at the microscope, but it is the main conceptual framework around which clinicians and researchers organize clinical care and research studies, so it can be useful to know as you discuss cases with your colleagues and as you read the literature. Of note, the clinical categories of HBV infection do not correlate very well with histological findings, nor are there consistent correlates between viral load and histological findings.

TABLE 5.9 Clinical Terms Used to Describe HBV Infections

Clinical and Laboratory Findings	Biopsy Findings[a]
Immunotolerant phase • HBsAg-positive >6 mo • HBeAg-positive • DNA levels $10^{5\text{-}12}$ • AST/ALT levels normal or near normal.	Minimal to mild chronic hepatitis Fibrosis is typically absent, occasionally mild
Chronic hepatitis B (AKA immunoactive phase) • HBsAg-positive >6 mo • Can be HBeAg-positive or negative • DNA levels >10^5 when HBeAg-positive • DNA levels may be lower if HBeAg-negative • AST/ALT levels show persistent or intermittent elevations.	Mild to moderately active chronic hepatitis; may be severe, especially if there is an HBV flare Fibrosis varies from none to advanced
Inactive HBsAg carrier state (AKA nonreplicative phase) • HBsAg-positive >6 mo • HBeAg-negative; HBeAb-positive • DNA levels <10^4 • Normal or near normal ALT/AST levels	Minimal or mild chronic hepatitis Fibrosis varies from none to advanced
Resolved hepatitis B • Previous known history of acute or chronic HBV or serum HBcAb positivity ± HBsAb positivity • HBsAg-negative • Serum HBV DNA negative • Normal ALT/AST	No or minimal chronic inflammation Fibrosis varies from none to advanced
Occult hepatitis B (some classify this as a sub-type of resolved hepatitis B) • HBsAg-negative ± HBcAb positivity ± HBsAb positivity • Serum HBV DNA-positive at very low levels or HBV DNA-positive in liver tissue • ALT/ST normal or minimal elevated (may still have enzyme flares).	No or minimal chronic inflammation; Immunostains for HBsAg may show rare positive cells Fibrosis varies from none to advanced

ALT, alanine aminotransferase; AST, aspartate aminotransferase; HBV, hepatitis B virus.
[a]Note: Biopsy findings for any category can vary widely, but "typical" findings are listed in this section.
Adapted from 2009 AASLD Guidelines, but with some modifications to biopsy findings and addition of the occult HBV category.

Likewise, histological findings and serum alanine aminotransferase (ALT) levels do not correlate well. For example, individuals with low or normal ALT levels may still have significant inflammation and fibrosis in liver biopsy specimens.[33,34] Nonetheless, there are a few broad correlates that have been observed. First, individuals in the immunotolerant phase of chronic HBV tend to show minimal or mild inflammation and no or mild fibrosis.[35] Second, the overall amount of inflammation typically decreases after HBeAg seroconversion, an observation best seen in studies that examine paired biopsies.

Acute Hepatitis B

Patients with acute HBV are rarely biopsied because the diagnosis can be made by serological studies and serum PCR for HBV nucleic acids. Biopsies can be encountered when clinical testing is incomplete or the results are ambiguous.

In acute HBV, the portal tracts show mild to moderate portal lymphocytic inflammation; the portal inflammation can also be plasma cell rich in some cases. The lobules show moderate to marked lymphocytic inflammation, hepatocyte swelling, and scattered apoptotic bodies. Kupffer cells are typically prominent and there may be cholestasis, especially when there is severe lobular hepatitis, or in older patients. When there is more severe hepatitis, areas of confluent or bridging necrosis may be seen. Do not look for HBV ground glass inclusions—they are present only in cases of chronic HBV.[36-38] Immunostains for HBsAg are typically either negative or only focally positive in very early acute infections.[39]

Chronic Hepatitis B

The number of biopsies in patients with chronic HBV has dropped significantly over the past decade. Today, most biopsies are performed to rule out additional disease processes; only rarely is the biopsy performed specifically to evaluate the degree of inflammation or the stage of fibrosis in patients with chronic HBV, the latter indication largely replaced by noninvasive testing.

Most cases with chronic HBV show a hepatitic pattern of injury, with findings that are not specific because there is significant overlap with other causes of chronic hepatitis, such as HCV, autoimmune hepatitis, and DILI. The overall body of literature indicates that lymphoid aggregates and bile duct lymphocytosis are somewhat less common in chronic HBV, compared to chronic HCV, an observation that is interesting but not diagnostically useful.

PORTAL TRACT CHANGES. Chronic HBV typically shows mild to moderate portal chronic inflammation. The portal inflammation will be predominately lymphocytic and discrete lymphoid aggregates may be present in

10% to 20% of cases.[40] Interface activity is common, varying from minimal to moderate, and only rarely severe. Interface activity, of note, is etiologically nonspecific and can be seen with variable prominence in chronic hepatitis from any cause, where it generally parallels the overall degree of portal inflammation. In approximately 10% of cases, a rare portal tract may show a duct-centered lymphoid aggregate along with mild bile duct lymphocytosis and reactive bile duct epithelial changes (Poulsen lesion).[40]

LOBULAR CHANGES. Approximately 80% of cases will have lobular inflammation that ranges from minimal to mild, with most of the remaining cases showing moderate lobular inflammation. Marked lobular hepatitis is unusual outside of the setting of an HBV flare, HDV superinfection, or an additional hepatitic injury to the liver, one superimposed on the background of chronic HBV. In all cases, the lobular inflammation is predominately lymphocytic. Kupffer cells are often prominent when there is moderate or marked lobular inflammation.

Rarely, hepatocytes in cases of HBV can have nuclear inclusions that are called "sanded glass" nuclei (Figure 5.1). These nuclear inclusions are most commonly seen in individuals with high–viral replication levels[41-44] and will stain-positive for HBcAg by immunostain. They are not specific to HBV, however, as similar inclusions can be seen in patients with HBV/hepatitis D virus (HDV) infection[45] and in patients without HBV, where they appear to be incidental findings. Of note, the HBcAg immunostain will also stain-positive many hepatocyte nuclei that do not show sanded glass changes. Immunostains for HBcAg may also stain the cytoplasm of hepatocytes in some cases, a finding that is dependent to some degree on

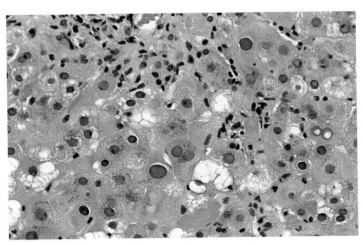

FIGURE 5.1 **Sanded glass nuclei.** The hepatocyte nuclei show red, homogenous inclusions that represent hepatitis B core antigen.

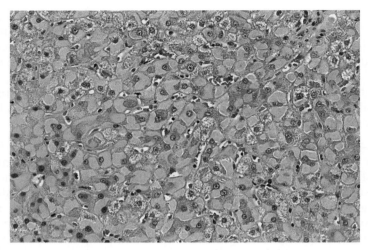

FIGURE 5.2 **Hepatitis B ground glass cytoplasm.** In some cases of chronic hepatitis B, the viral surface antigens accumulate in the cytoplasm and can be seen as amphophilic inclusions that fill the cytoplasm.

the antibody used for immunohistochemistry and perhaps on the HBeAg status. A cytoplasmic staining pattern has also been linked to higher overall grades of inflammation.[42-44] Rarely, the nuclei of bile duct epithelial cells will also stain-positive for HBcAg.

In a subset of cases with long-standing chronic HBV, the hepatocytes can show ground glass cytoplasmic inclusions (Figure 5.2). Ground glass inclusions are more common and more famous than sanded glass nuclei and are composed of HBsAg located within the smooth endoplasmic reticulum of the hepatocyte cytoplasm. Molecular studies have found that the viral proteins in ground glass inclusions are highly mutated,[46] perhaps preventing their normal release. The accumulation of viral proteins can also interfere with secretion of other cellular proteins, which also accumulate and contribute to the ground glass appearance.[47] Ground glass change usually takes decades to develop and is not found in acute HBV infection. Ground glass hepatocytes can be stained with Shikata orcein stain and with Victoria blue, but most centers now use immunostains. In most cases, the smooth endoplasmic reticulum proliferation that causes the ground glass change can also be enriched in glycogen molecules, and thus will be periodic acid–Schiff (PAS)-positive. Very similar inclusions can be seen as a medication effect in patients who are HBV-negative, a finding called *pseudoground glass change.*[48]

Immunostains for HBsAg will strongly stain ground glass hepatocytes, as well as many hepatocytes that do not have ground glass change on hematoxylin and eosin (H&E) stains. In fact, most hepatocytes that are HBsAg-positive by immunostain do not have ground glass changes. Positive hepatocytes can have several different staining patterns, the

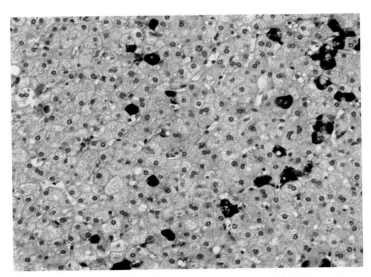

FIGURE 5.3 **Type I HBsAg stain pattern.** Scattered positive cells are seen.

most common being called type 1 (Figure 5.3, eFig 5.3) and type 2 (Figure 5.4A and B, eFig 5.4). Type 2 has a stronger connection to tumor genesis,[49] but staining patterns do not need to be specifically indicated in liver pathology reports. Other less common staining patterns include membranous staining and distinctive course granular cytoplasmic staining (eFigs 5.5 and 5.6).

One of the important features about the biology of chronic HBV is that there can be flares of increased viral replication, leading to episodes of increased liver injury. Flares are often defined as aspartate aminotransferase (AST)/ALT elevations more than 2× the baseline value and more than 10× the upper limit of normal. In most cases, these flares are recognized clinically as part of the natural history of HBV infection and are not biopsied. When they are biopsied, the liver shows either an acute hepatitis pattern or an acute on chronic hepatitis pattern, with moderately to markedly active lobular hepatitis, often with foci of zone 3 confluent necrosis. In some cases, there may be bridging necrosis or panacinar cell necrosis. The differential for an HBV flare should always include HDV superinfection as well as DILI.

GRANULOMAS AND HEPATITIS **B.** About 1% to 2% of biopsies for chronic HBV will have small epithelioid granulomas without polarizable material.[50,51] Extensive clinical and pathology work-ups are typically negative,[50] although it is probably still important to examine the granulomas with acid-fast bacilli (AFB) and Grocott methenamine silver (GMS) stains. The etiology of these small idiopathic granulomas is unclear but their significance is typically minimal; they can be persistent on follow biopsies but do not appear to contribute to increased fibrosis.

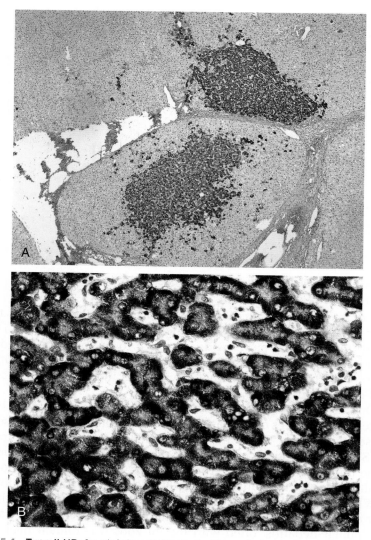

FIGURE 5.4 **Type II HBsAg staining pattern.** Positive cells form discrete aggregates (4A) and on higher power have accentuated staining at the cell periphery (4B).

LIVER CELL DYSPLASIA. The hepatocytes in chronic HBV can show large cell change or small cell change, findings sometimes called large cell dysplasia and small cell dysplasia, respectively. Both of these findings are more common in chronic HBV than in other chronic liver diseases, but they are not unique to HBV. These changes are most commonly seen in livers with advanced fibrosis. Small cell change refers to small discrete aggregates of hepatocytes with relatively little cytoplasm but otherwise near-normal nuclear and cytoplasmic cytology. In contrast, large cell change is defined by aggregates of hepatocytes with normal to abundant amounts of cytoplasm and a normal or near-normal N:C ratio but with sometimes striking nuclear changes that include hyperchromasia, mild pleomorphism, and occasional multinucleation. Both of these findings have been linked to higher hepatocellular carcinoma risk, with small cell change having a greater risk than large cell change.

HEPATOCYTE ONCOCYTOSIS. Rarely, biopsies can show distinctive nodules of hepatocytes with cytoplasmic oncocytic change (eFig 5.7), a finding that is not specific for chronic HBV but seems to be more common in chronic HBV than in other diseases. This finding is most commonly found in cirrhotic livers, but can also be seen in noncirrhotic livers, typically in individuals with long-standing chronic HBV infection. The significance of this finding remains unclear and it does not need to be mentioned in the pathology report.

IMMUNOSTAINS. Immunostains for HBsAg or HBcAg are not necessary for routine grading and staging of disease. They can be helpful for establishing a diagnosis of HBV when laboratory testing is not available or is equivocal. Immunostain patterns have some broad correlates with the clinical category of disease (clinical categories of HBV disease are summarized in Table 5.9) and with the degree of inflammation, but are not incorporated into current treatment guidelines. Briefly, in the immunotolerant phase, there tends to be little lobular inflammation, lots of HBcAg positivity in hepatocyte nuclei (eFig 5.8), and strong HBsAg staining of hepatocytes, often with a membranous pattern. In the inactive carrier stage, HBcAg nuclear staining tends to be sparse or sometimes negative, while HBsAg staining is still evident but ranges from rare scattered hepatocytes to large numbers of cells. Distinct, circumscribed aggregates of HBsAg-positive hepatocytes tend to be more common in the inactive carrier state when there also is advanced fibrosis.

Fibrosing Cholestatic Hepatitis B

Fibrosing cholestatic HBV is a rare form of infection seen in immunosuppressed patients, typically those with organ transplants and high levels of immunosuppression. Fibrosing cholestatic HBV is only rarely encountered anymore because of improvements in immunosuppression and drugs that inhibit HBV replication. In classic cases, the liver shows marked lobular cholestasis with hepatocyte ballooning degeneration, moderate ductular proliferation in the portal tracts, and pericellular and portal fibrosis on trichrome stain. The ductular proliferation often suggests obstructive biliary tract disease and biliary tract obstruction should be ruled out as part of the workup for such cases. The pericellular fibrosis is often more prominent in zone 1. The inflammatory changes tend to be mild despite the marked ongoing liver injury. Viral DNA levels are significantly elevated above baseline and the pathology is thought to result from direct viral toxicity due to the high–viral replication levels. There can be rapid progression to cirrhosis.

Cases with these classic histological findings and typical clinical history are usually easy to recognize. This constellation of classic findings, however, represents the end of a spectrum of findings and you may encounter cases with less striking changes. For example, there are cases of cholestatic HBV in immunosuppressed patients who may lack the fibrosis and portal tract changes of classic fibrosing cholestatic HBV, but whose lobular cholestasis improves significantly with reduced immunosuppression.

HEPATITIS D

HDV is an RNA virus that only infects hepatocytes that are already infected by HBV. The HDV virus "commandeers" the viral coat made by HBV to package its own nucleic acids. Perinatal transmission of HDV is rare and the most common transmission routes are similar to those seen with adult HBV infections. Acute HDV infection occurs in two main settings: coinfection, where acute HBV and HDV are transmitted together and infect the liver simultaneously, or superinfection, where HDV infects a liver that already has chronic HBV infection. Adult patients with acute coinfection of HBV and HDV tend to clear the infections (as do most adults with acute HBV monoinfection). In contrast, adult patients with superinfection are more likely to develop chronic HDV infection and are at greater risk for fibrosis progression and hepatocellular carcinoma.

At the histological level, there are no findings that are unique to HDV infection (Figure 5.5). With coinfection, the biopsy typically shows moderate to marked lobular hepatitis, often with confluent or bridging necrosis. With superinfection, the biopsy will show the ordinary changes of chronic

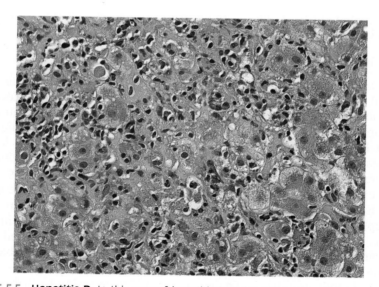

FIGURE 5.5 **Hepatitis D.** In this case of hepatitis B and D coinfection, there is a marked hepatitis with mild lobular cholestasis, but these findings are not specific for hepatitis D coinfection.

hepatitis B, although the lobular activity tends to be moderate to marked in severity.[52] Recent exposure to risk factors, or an unexplained flare of hepatitis, are the most important diagnostic clues. Laboratory results are also helpful, as HBV DNA levels are elevated above their baseline in a flare of chronic HBV, while in a case of HDV superinfection, the increased liver enzymes are not accompanied by a significant increase in HBV viral DNA levels.[53]

In some parts of the South America, superinfection with HDV has been associated with a high risk for acute liver failure; in these cases, the biopsies showed a microvesicular pattern of steatosis and in some cases had numerous acidophil bodies (extensive eosinophilic necrosis).[54-56]

Immunostains for HDV are not available at most centers and the diagnosis in most cases is established by laboratory studies. In general, testing for IgG or IgM antibodies is performed first, followed by confirmatory RNA testing usingPCR.[57]

HEPATITIS C

Acute Hepatitis C

Acute hepatitis C viral (HCV) infection is rarely biopsied because in most cases the acute infection causes no or mild clinical symptoms. In elderly patients, however, acute HCV can be symptomatic and is occasionally biopsied.[58] In this setting, the liver typically shows a cholestatic hepatitis pattern, with moderate to marked lobular inflammation and moderate lobular cholestasis.[58] The portal tracts contain mild to moderate lymphocytic inflammation and, with more severe activity, the portal tracts can also show a ductular reaction, with proliferating bile ductules and mixed portal inflammation. The bile ductular proliferation can closely mimic biliary tract obstructive disease,[58] but the presence of the moderate to marked lobular inflammation will typically protect you from this diagnostic pitfall. In some cases, the histological findings can resemble that of DILI, with bland lobular cholestasis and only very mild inflammatory changes. Rare cases of fulminant liver failure from acute HCV have also been reported.[59]

Chronic Hepatitis C

While most of the literature on chronic HCV has come from the study of adult biopsies, the findings of chronic HCV in children are essentially the same.[60] Of note, children with perinatal acquisition of HCV can have advanced fibrosis, despite a relatively short time of infection.

PORTAL TRACT FINDINGS. The inflammation in the portal tracts is typically mild (~30% of cases) or moderate (~65% of cases) and only occasionally marked (~5% of cases).[61] In most biopsy specimens, there will be fairly diffused portal chronic inflammation that is at least minimal in all portal

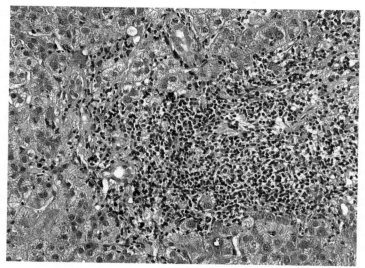

FIGURE 5.6 **Interface activity.** This case of chronic hepatitis C shows marked portal chronic inflammation along with interface activity.

tracts and maybe moderate or marked in the medium-sized and larger portal tracts. Lymphoid aggregates may be present in the portal tracts, sometimes complete with germinal centers, but this finding is not specific for chronic HCV and you should not overinterpret lymphoid aggregates as having any special significance.

Interface activity is also common with chronic HCV (Figure 5.6). Overall, the degree of interface activity correlates with the amount of portal chronic inflammation. Interface activity has received a great deal of attention over the years, as it was an important part of an older classification system for chronic hepatitis, wherein cases were classified into "chronic aggressive hepatitis" and "chronic persistent hepatitis."[62] This older classification system is no longer in use because it was not very reproducible and is no longer clinically relevant, but it played a major role in early attempts to classify chronic hepatitis and understand why some cases of chronic hepatitis progress to fibrosis/cirrhosis and some do not.[63] Interface inflammation played an important role in this early classification system and continues to have a key role in grading disease activity today.

On the other hand, interface activity has no special significance that makes it more important than portal inflammation or lobular inflammation—it is simply one histological feature that is convenient to examine when providing semiquantitative information on the amount of active injury in a liver specimen; it is usually combined with lobular and (often) portal inflammation. In this regard, HCV infected hepatocytes are not specifically localized in the portal/lobular interface,[64] so interface activity does not reflect immune activity directed against virally infected hepatocytes—at least no more so than inflammation elsewhere in the lobules.

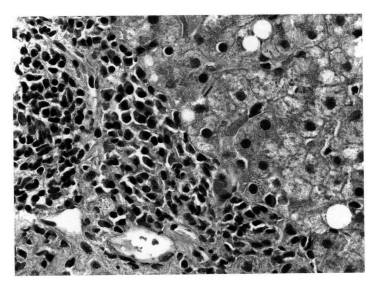

FIGURE 5.7 **Portal tract plasma cells in hepatitis C virus (HCV).** In this case of chronic hepatitis C, there is a mild prominence in portal tract plasma cells, but there were no other clinical or laboratory findings to indicate an additional component of autoimmune hepatitis.

In most cases, the portal inflammation is primarily lymphocytic with only occasional plasma cells, while in rare cases, plasma cells can be more prominent (Figure 5.7), a finding that can also be associated with low-level autoantibody titers.[65] It is important, however, to not overinterpret this finding as indicating that an additional component of autoimmune hepatitis is present. In fact, in cases of chronic HCV with mildly prominent portal plasma cells, the inflammatory changes resolve with antiviral therapy, leaving behind no evidence for an underlying autoimmune hepatitis.[66] Of course, autoimmune hepatitis can very rarely co-occur with chronic HCV, but a true autoimmune hepatitis is most clearly diagnosed when there is striking plasma cell–rich portal inflammation, moderate to marked lobular activity, often with lobular plasma cells, along with moderate to higher titer serum autoantibodies, as well as elevated serum IgG levels. Low-level autoantibody titers are not very useful and mostly confuse the situation, as they can also be found in patients with many inflammatory diseases of the liver, ranging from fatty liver disease to chronic viral hepatitis, as well as in the general population.

The bile ducts can show focal, mild lymphocytosis and reactive epithelial changes in 20% to 30% of cases (Figure 5.8).[67] These lesions are also called Poulsen lesions or Poulsen-Cristoffersen lesions, in particular when they are associated with a lymphoid aggregate. Some studies report a much higher frequency of these bile duct lesions, but they are probably using a more generous definition of lymphocytosis and injury. These bile duct changes are more common in chronic HCV than chronic HBV[40] and may be associated with mildly higher alkaline phosphatase levels

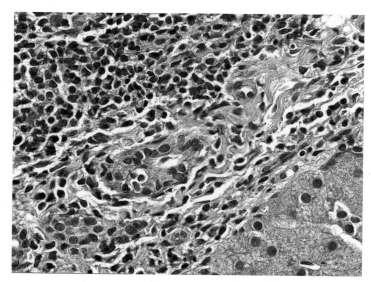

FIGURE 5.8 **Bile duct lymphocytosis.** This case of chronic hepatitis C shows mild bile duct lymphocytosis with reactive epithelial changes.

and/or gammaglutamyltranspeptidase (GGT) levels, as well as more portal inflammation, portal lymphoid aggregates, and more advanced fibrosis.[67-69] Nonetheless, they do not have any true clinical or histological significance and, while fun to identify, they do not need to be specifically mentioned in the pathology report.

In about 2% of liver explants, the bile ducts can show biliary intraepithelial neoplasia (BilIN).[70] The dysplasia typically affects the small- and medium-sized bile ducts, ones that are only rarely sampled on needle biopsies but can be sampled with wedge biopsies or larger specimens. Cirrhosis from chronic HCV is an important risk factor for intrahepatic cholangiocarcinoma and these dysplastic foci may be precursor lesions (Figure 5.9).

LOBULAR FINDINGS. The lobules most commonly show minimal or mild chronic inflammation (~55% of cases), less often moderate chronic inflammation (~40% of cases) and only rarely severe inflammation (less than 5% of cases). In fact, if you have a biopsy with marked lobular hepatitis, it is good practice to check the liver enzymes to see if there has been a recent flare of enzymes. If there has been, this strongly suggests an additional liver injury superimposed upon the chronic HCV, since liver enzymes in chronic HCV can wax and wane a bit, but never flare. For example, this additional injury might be a drug reaction or superinfection with HBV.[71,72]

With the exception of some cases of recurrent HCV after liver transplantation, chronic HCV does not show lobular cholestasis. If there is lobular cholestasis, then there likely is an additional disease process that has been superimposed on chronic HCV.

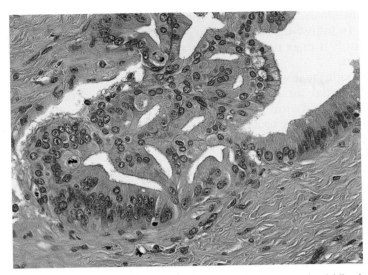

FIGURE 5.9 **Hepatitis C with bile duct dysplasia**. This medium-sized bile duct shows biliary intraepithelial neoplasia (BilIN) 3.

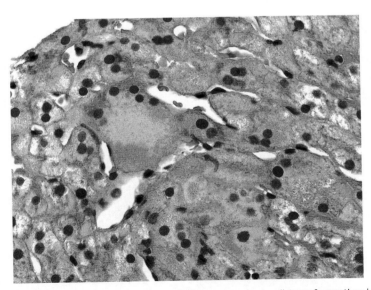

FIGURE 5.10 **Giant cell change**. Giant cell change or giant cell transformation is seen in these zone 3 hepatocytes in an individual with chronic hepatitis C.

Within the hepatic lobules, focal giant cell transformation of zone 3 hepatocytes occasionally may be observed (Figure 5.10). This finding is most commonly seen in the setting of injection drug use, but the etiology is unclear.[73] It may be an unknown viral infection or an unusual reactive change. Giant cell transformation can be seen with either HIV/HCV coinfection or with HCV monoinfection.[58,74] This finding is not associated with cholestasis, the degree of lobular inflammation, or the degree of fibrosis. In follow-up biopsies, the giant cell transformation is commonly persistent.[73] It does not need to be specifically mentioned in the pathology report.

Hepatic steatosis is relatively common in patients with chronic HCV. The differential for the fatty change includes the metabolic syndrome,[14] drug effect,[14] and viral genotype 3[75]; the histological findings do not provide any reliable way to identify the cause of the fat. Individuals with HCV genotype 3 and the metabolic syndrome are particularly likely to have fat in the biopsy specimen.

The portal veins and/or the central veins can show a mild venulitis in chronic HCV or HBV; one study reported this lesion in 42% of HCV biopsies and 7% of HBV biopsies,[76] but the findings are typically so mild and innocuous that they come to one's attention only when you are specifically looking for them and so are seen considerably less often in actual clinical practice. The venulitis may have lymphocytes attached to the luminal surface of the endothelium or may have a cuff of lymphocytes immediately underneath the endothelium (Figure 5.11). The presence of these changes tends to correlate with the overall severity of the hepatitis,[77] but at this point, venulitis does not have any independent clinical significance.

Immunohistochemistry for HCV to date has not been diagnostically useful. There have been abstracts and papers showing HCV immunopositivity in liver biopsies,[64] some of them quite convincing, but none have been widely reproduced and none have become clinically useful in the practice of diagnostic surgical pathology.

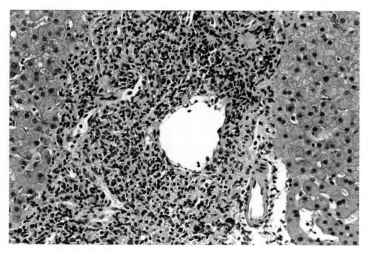

FIGURE 5.11 **Hepatitis C with venulitis.** There is marked portal inflammation and mild to moderate portal venulitis in this case of chronic hepatitis C.

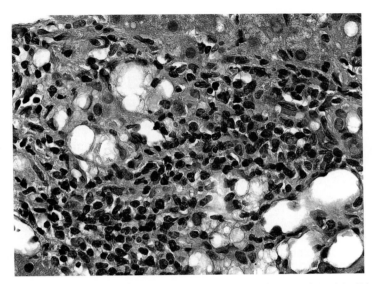

FIGURE 5.12 **Lipogranuloma.** A lipogranuloma is seen in the portal tract in this case of chronic hepatitis C.

HEPATITIS C AND GRANULOMAS. About 20% of liver biopsies with chronic HCV will have lipogranulomas.[78] Lipogranulomas can represent either mineral oil or lipid droplets released from hepatocytes in the setting of fatty liver disease. Mineral oil is a commonly used food additive in the developed world. Histologically they look similar and may be associated with focal fibrosis (Figure 5.12), but are otherwise an incidental finding with no clinical significance.

In about 1% of biopsies performed for staging and grading chronic HCV, small epithelioid granulomas are found in either the portal tracts (Figure 5.13) or less commonly the lobules.[79,80] Rare studies have reported granulomas in up to 10% of biopsies,[51] but results from subsequent and larger studies have been in the 1% range; this does not include foreign body granulomas,[79] which typically will have polarizable material. AFB and GMS stains are routinely negative, although it is still prudent to do them. There is no clinical significance to these granulomas; they are often present in subsequent liver biopsies of the same patient but are not associated with the degree of portal or lobular inflammation or risk for fibrosis progression.

Fibrosing Cholestatic Hepatitis C

Fibrosing cholestatic HCV is a rare form of infection most commonly seen in individuals with liver transplants, high levels of immunosuppression, and high levels of viral replication, often with viral RNA levels that are greater than 30 million. Fibrosing cholestatic HCV is most commonly seen

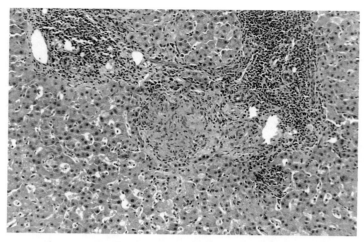

FIGURE 5.13 **Granuloma.** A small epithelioid granuloma is seen in a case of chronic hepatitis C. No cause was identified.

within the first year after transplant, with most cases occurring between 1 and 5 months.[81] The pathology is essentially identical to that described for fibrosing cholestatic HBV. The liver shows marked lobular cholestasis with hepatocyte swelling, ductular proliferation in the portal tracts, and pericellular and portal fibrosis on trichrome stain. The pericellular fibrosis is often more prominent in the periportal areas. The four elements that go into the histological pattern of fibrosing cholestatic HCV (cholestasis, hepatocyte swelling, ductular proliferation, and fibrosis) can be present in varying degrees. The inflammatory changes are typically mild despite the marked ongoing liver injury. The pathology is thought to result from direct viral toxicity and there can be rapid progression to cirrhosis.

As discussed in the section on HBV, fibrosing cholestatic HCV represents the end of a spectrum of findings and you may encounter cases whose findings are not as striking as those seen in fully developed cases. For example, there are cases of cholestatic HCV in immunosuppressed patients who lack the fibrosis and the portal tract changes of typical fibrosing cholestatic HCV but whose lobular cholestasis disappears with reduced immunosuppression. Other causes of lobular cholestasis also need to be excluded before reaching a diagnosis of fibrosing cholestatic hepatitis C, such as DILI and biliary obstruction.[81]

Hepatitis C and Autoimmune Hepatitis Overlap Syndrome

Occasional patients will have both autoimmune hepatitis as well as chronic HCV. These cases are rare and can engender some confusion on both the clinical and pathological side. There are no specific pathological findings that will tell you when both diseases are present, but, in general, the findings tend to be a composite of typical chronic HCV and typical autoimmune hepatitis. In comparison to chronic HCV alone, cases with both diseases have moderate or greater portal inflammation, typically moderately prominent portal plasma cells, and moderate or severe lobular hepatitis. In rare cases, there may be bridging necrosis or panacinar necrosis. The presence of bridging necrosis or panacinar necrosis is very unusual for chronic HCV alone and should always trigger concern for an additional disease process. Interface activity is typically present in HCV/autoimmune hepatitis overlap syndrome, but its mere presence is not very informative, as it is also present in most cases of chronic HCV alone.

Additional serological findings are needed to confirm a diagnosis of combined chronic HCV and autoimmune hepatitis, including moderate or higher levels of autoantibodies and elevated serum IgG levels. Of the autoantibody tests, smooth muscle antibodies with anti-actin specificity, combined with antinuclear antibodies (ANA) positivity, are most helpful.[82]

Low-level autoantibodies by themselves are not informative as they can be seen in the general population as well as in individuals with chronic liver inflammation from any cause, including chronic HCV. For example, about 15% of individuals with chronic HCV alone will have ANA antibodies, 34% smooth muscle antibodies, and 0.5% anti- liver/kidney microsomal (LKM) antibodies.[83]

Liver biopsies are helpful in this setting to rule out concomitant autoimmune hepatitis. Once autoimmune hepatitis has been excluded, there is no clinical significance for positive serological autoantibodies. Studies have carefully examined the histological findings in patients with chronic HCV and mild nonspecific elevations in autoantibodies but without true autoimmune hepatitis. These studies found this group of patients is enriched for female gender, may have slightly higher liver enzymes and slightly more inflammation on liver biopsy,[65,82,84] and the portal inflammation tends to have slightly more prominent plasma cells.[65] Historically, this group of patients was sometimes referred to as "chronic HCV with autoimmune features," but this is not a distinct histological or clinical entity[85] and the term should no longer be used. This group of patients responds to anti-HCV medication in the usual fashion and does not have underlying residual autoimmune hepatitis after antiviral therapy.

HEPATITIS E

Hepatitis E virus (HEV) is a small RNA virus that causes both sporadic and epidemic disease, the latter typically as a water-borne illness in developing nations. In the setting of epidemic disease, the fatality rate is about 5%, with pregnant women at higher risk. HEV is also an uncommon but important cause of clinical hepatitis in the industrialized world, including the USA, Europe, and other developed nations. The epidemic disease in developing nations is caused by HEV genotypes 1 and 2, while sporadic cases in industrialized nations (often called endemic or "autochthonous" in the literature) are caused by genotype 3.[86] Interestingly, serology studies indicate that 20% of the USA adult population have been exposed to HEV,[87] albeit subclinically. The source of exposure is only rarely identified in sporadic cases, but known risk factors include eating wild game[88] and undercooked pork.[86] Older adults are at the highest risk for symptomatic acute HEV infections,[86] where acute infection can clinically and histologically mimic other causes of acute hepatitis, including DILI.[89]

Acute HEV

The histology of acute HEV can vary from an almost normal liver to fulminant hepatitis. Most sporadic cases show minimal to moderate hepatitis, with immunocompetent patients tending to show more inflammation than immunosuppressed patients.[90] Epidemic cases can show more severe hepatitis, including massive liver necrosis.

In patients with underlying liver diseases, such as fatty liver disease, who also have sporadic acute HEV hepatitis, the underlying liver disease can sometimes dominate the histology findings. In these cases, the most important clue is typically not the histology but instead the clinical findings of an unexplained flare in liver enzymes or the sudden onset of new symptoms not readily attributable to the underlying liver disease; the histology findings tend to look fairly typical for the underlying liver disease, often showing only subtly increased lobular hepatitis and apoptosis.

In cases of acute HEV infection alone, biopsies tend to show a lobular predominant, lymphocytic hepatitis, which can be cholestatic.[91-93] The degree of inflammation varies considerably, from minimal to marked; moderate and severe cases also commonly show a mild bile ductular reaction (Figures 5.14 and 5.15). The clinical and histological findings are

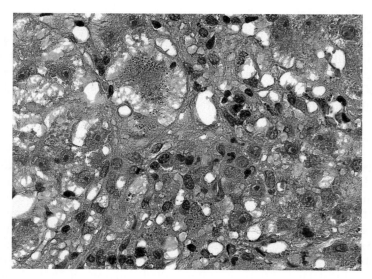

FIGURE 5.14 **Hepatitis E.** This case of acute hepatitis E infection showed lobular cholestasis and disarray, but relatively little inflammation.

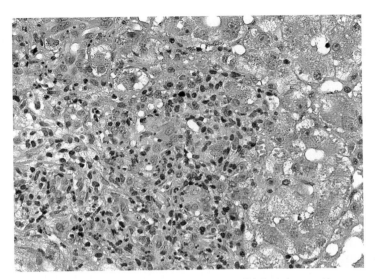

FIGURE 5.15 **Hepatitis E.** The portal tracts showed a mild ductular reaction.

indistinguishable from DILI or other viral causes of acute or chronic hepatitis.[89,94] One useful clue, although it is present in only a subset of cases, is finding neutrophils in the sinusoidal infiltrates,[91,93] since this finding is unusual for most other causes of acute hepatitis. Overall, your best ally for making the diagnosis is the combined picture of an acute onset, unexplained hepatitis, often in an elderly individual, with a biopsy showing a hepatitic pattern of injury, often with cholestasis.

Chronic Hepatitis E

Chronic HEV occurs primarily in immunosuppressed patients,[95] in particular, those with solid organ transplants,[96,97] but also in persons with HIV infection, hematological malignancies, or receiving chemotherapy for various types of cancer.[86,95] Rare cases of chronic HEV have been reported in patients without obvious immunosuppression.[95]

In individuals with a liver transplant, chronic HEV can be associated with an unexplained chronic hepatitis pattern of injury.[98] In general, biopsies show a hepatitic pattern of injury and do not mimic acute cellular rejection; retrospective studies indicate that few cases of HEV are misinterpreted as rejection.[99] The best clue, again, is that of an unexplained acute hepatitis or chronic hepatitis that does not respond to optimization of immunosuppressant levels in patients where HCV, HBV, and DILI have been excluded.

Confirmatory Tests

The locally available tests to confirm a diagnosis of HEV vary but, in general, IgG and IgM antibodies appear in the serum right before the onset of increased liver enzymes. IgM antibodies are detectable for 3 to 12 weeks after acute infection, while IgG antibodies are detectable for many years and probably for life. Testing for HEV RNA and stool testing are also available at some medical centers. Immunostains for HEV that work in paraffin-embedded tissues are also available in a few specialized medical centers.[94,100]

OTHER CAUSES OF VIRAL HEPATITIS

Cytomegalovirus (CMV)

Cytomegalovirus (CMV) hepatitis is relatively rare and is essentially always seen in immunosuppressed individuals. The biopsy findings are often mild and nonspecific, with only mild to moderate nonspecific portal chronic inflammation with mild lobular lymphocytic inflammation (Figure 5.16).[101] In some cases, a potential histological clue can be patchy clusters of neutrophils, or "mini-microabscesses" located in the lobules (Figure 5.17).[101] This finding is not specific for CMV infection,[102,103] and most cases with mini-microabscesses will be negative for CMV on immunostain. The presence of numerous lobular mini-microabscesses is more likely to be CMV infection than finding one or two. Nonetheless, it is common practice to do a CMV stain, even if only a single mini-microabscess is seen, if the patient is immunosuppressed.

Viral inclusions are not seen on H&E stains in many cases, so it is best to do CMV immunostains whenever you are suspicious, even if you see no inclusions. When inclusions are present, they can be seen in hepatocytes, endothelial cells, or bile ducts (Figures 5.18 and 5.19).

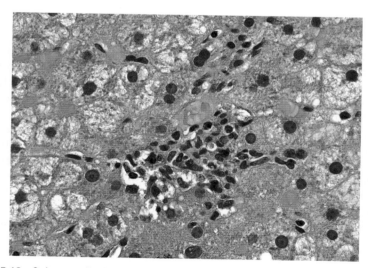

FIGURE 5.16 **Cytomegalovirus (CMV) infection.** In some cases of mild CMV hepatitis, the only biopsy findings will be nonspecific inflammation. In this liver allograft biopsy specimen, there was only mild patch lobular hepatitis.

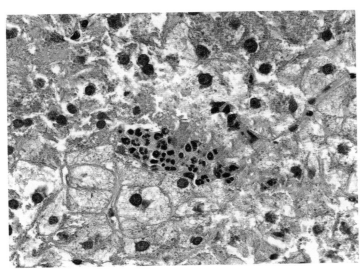

FIGURE 5.17 **Microabscesses in cytomegalovirus (CMV) infection.** The sinusoids contain a small cluster of neutrophils. This finding is a potential clue to possible CMV hepatitis in immunosuppressed patients but is neither sensitive nor specific.

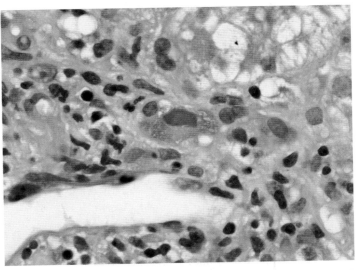

FIGURE 5.18 **Cytomegalovirus (CMV) nuclear inclusion.** A red nuclear inclusion is seen in this CMV-infected cell.

Herpes Simplex Virus (HSV)

Herpes simplex virus (HSV) hepatitis is rare and usually seen in immunosuppressed individuals. The pathology findings typically show distinct, circumscribed areas of hepatocyte necrosis, termed "punched-out" necrosis.

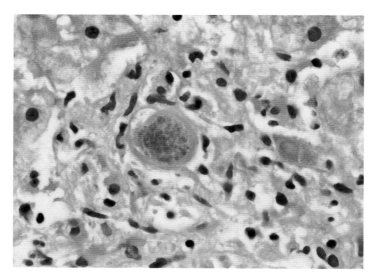

FIGURE 5.19 **Cytomegalovirus (CMV) cytoplasmic inclusion.** This CMV-infected cell has striking granular basophilic cytoplasmic inclusions.

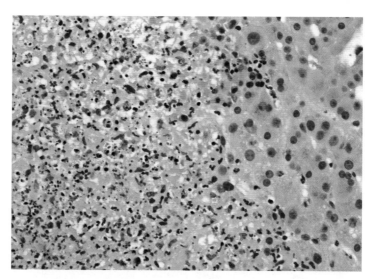

FIGURE 5.20 **Herpes simplex virus hepatitis.** A discrete, "punched-out" foci of inflammatory necrosis is present.

These areas of necrosis can vary in size from that of 5 to 10 hepatocytes to large panacinar areas of necrosis (Figure 5.20, eFig 5.9). The overall prognosis depends on the amount of necrosis, with those cases showing only small focal areas of necrosis having a good prognosis.[104] Viral cytopathic effect can be seen as diffuse amphophilic nuclear inclusions that completely fill the nucleus or as discrete eosinophilic inclusions in an empty appearing nucleus with a rim of marginated chromatin (Cowdry type A). Multinucleated hepatocytes can also be observed. Viral cytopathic changes are typically most evident in the viable hepatocytes adjacent to the necrotic areas. An immunostain for HSV is very helpful to make the diagnosis.

Adenovirus (ADV)

Adenovirus (ADV) hepatitis is very rare and usually seen in immunosuppressed patients. Infections are usually fatal. The histological findings on biopsies vary but the most common pattern is that of extensive hepatocyte necrosis with no strong zonal distribution. The areas of necrosis may be well circumscribed and limited to several hundred hepatocytes in milder cases or may show necrosis involving most of the biopsy. There is typically mild lymphocytic inflammation at the edges of the necrosis, but the necrosis is substantially out of proportion to the amount of inflammation. The viable hepatocytes at the edges of the necrotic areas can show viral cytopathic changes, with enlarged nuclei containing dark-purple, smudgy chromatin (Figure 5.21). The viable hepatocytes can also show fatty change, with both small and large droplets of fat. Immunostain confirmation should be performed as extensively necrotic livers often have reactive nuclear changes that can mimic viral inclusions.

Epstein Barr-Viral Hepatitis (EBV)

Epstein-Barr virus (EBV) hepatitis can be encountered in immunosuppressed patients as well as immunocompetent individuals, most commonly in young adults. The liver shows a lobular predominant pattern of

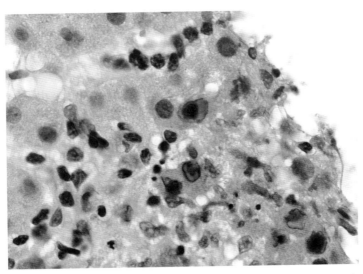

FIGURE 5.21 **Adenovirus hepatitis.** Small inflammatory foci are present at the edge of the biopsy core. The hepatocytes at the edge of the foci show dark, smudgy nuclei.

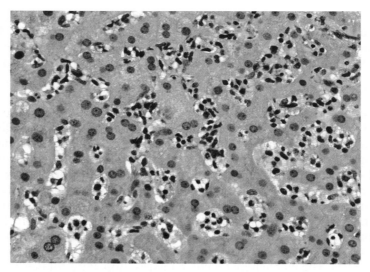

FIGURE 5.22 **Epstein-Barr Virus hepatitis.** The lobules show striking lymphocytosis, with relatively little hepatocyte injury.

hepatitis, with numerous lymphocytes in the sinusoids (Figure 5.22, eFig 5.10). However, there are typically few or no acidophil bodies and the degree of hepatocyte injury is disproportionally low given the amount of lobular inflammation. The lymphocytes can be larger and somewhat more reactive in their appearance than normal lymphocytes. Their appearance in the sinusoids has been called "beaded" because of the lines of back-to-back lymphocytes within the sinusoids, but this pattern is neither sensitive nor specific for EBV hepatitis. Small epithelioid and fibrin ring granulomas can also be seen. The diagnosis is confirmed by either Epstein-Barr encoding region (EBER) or EBV–latent membrane protein (LMP) stains.

Enteric Viruses

Echovirus is an enteric virus that most commonly causes disease in children and infants, although rare cases have also been reported in immunosuppressed adults.[105,106] There can be a high mortality rate. Severe cases of echovirus hepatitis show diffuse hemorrhagic necrosis of the liver and adrenal glands.[107] The virus appears to target endothelial cells and can have a veno-occlusive disease pattern.

Coxsackievirus B virus (an enterovirus closely related to echovirus) can also cause hepatitis.[108-111] The histological findings have only rarely been reported, but one case report described a mild hepatitic pattern of injury with mixed portal inflammation (lymphocytes, neutrophils), mild lobular hepatitis, moderate numbers of apoptotic hepatocytes, and numerous hepatocyte mitotic figures.[108] An earlier case study reported a cholestatic hepatitis pattern of injury with mixed portal inflammation but also described bile duct lymphocytosis and injury.[112]

COVID-19

The histological findings tend to be nonspecific, with mild nonspecific portal and lobular inflammation and often mild zone 3 sinusoidal dilatation.[113,114] Occasional granulomas can also be seen.[114] Fatty change is common, including cases with a zone 1 distribution of macrovesicular steatosis. The steatosis can represent preexisting fatty liver disease, but, at least in some cases, appears to develop during the course of the COVID-19 infection; the etiology is still unclear and could represent malnutrition, steroid therapy, or potentially be causally related to the viral infection[114] Another study identified similar findings of mild inflammation and fatty change, but also emphasized histiocyte-rich inflammation with fat droplets in the portal tracts, resembling lipogranulomas, but positive for COVID-19 on immunostain; this same study also found widespread fibrin thrombi and ischemic type zone 3 necrosis.[115]

Other Viruses

There are a large number of viruses that can cause hepatitis that cannot be discussed here because of space limitations. Many of these viral infections are rare or are have strong geographic associations. For example, the annual incidence of Lassa virus infection in West Africa is up to 500,000 individuals, but Lassa virus infection is very rare in most other parts of the world. Other viruses cause hepatitis as part of systemic illness that includes the liver. These viruses include dengue fever (Figure 5.23), yellow fever virus, Ebola virus, and Marburg virus. The list is much longer, but this should suffice to make the point that there are many known viruses

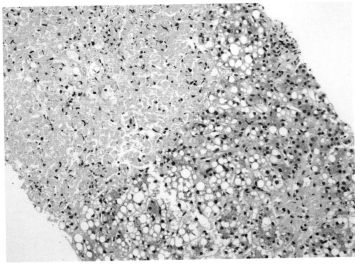

FIGURE 5.23 **Dengue Fever.** The biopsy shows striking zone 3 necrosis in a background of fatty liver disease.

that can cause hepatitis. With the great amount of international travel and immigration in the modern world, these rare viruses are potentially going to be more relevant in patients with acute hepatitis of unknown cause. Finally, there are almost certainly some unknown viruses that can also cause hepatitis. In fact, new potential hepatitic viruses continue to be described.[116]

ADULT GIANT CELL HEPATITIS

Adult giant cell hepatitis is also referred to as *post-infantile giant cell hepatitis* or as *syncytial giant cell hepatitis* and denotes a pattern of injury that can be seen with multiple different etiologies. An infectious etiology is suspected in some cases because the disease can recur following liver transplantation and cause progressive fibrosis.[117-119] In a few cases, viruses have been directly implicated, including HHV-6A,[120] CMV,[121] HEV,[122] and EBV.[123] In HHV-6A, the bile ducts can also undergo giant cell transformation.[124] The differential includes many different entities (Table 5.4, Chapter 5).

The histological findings fall into two main categories. The first is when giant cell transformation of hepatocytes is the main pattern of injury in adult biopsies, where the giant cell transformation is moderate to marked and is a dominant part of the histology. It is typically accompanied by mild to occasionally moderate lymphocytic inflammation in the portal tracts and minimal to mild lobular hepatitis, often with mild lobular cholestasis (Figure 5.24). This pattern is classically referred to as *adult giant cell hepatitis* and has a broad differential that includes DILI and viral hepatitis,

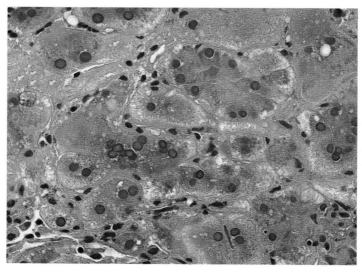

FIGURE 5.24 **Adult giant cell hepatitis.** This adult giant cell hepatitis shows marked giant cell transformation of hepatocytes, cholestasis, and mild lobular inflammation.

although most cases are idiopathic. The overall fibrosis risk has not been well characterized and presumably depends on the etiology. When a specific etiology can be identified or strongly suggested, then that should be clearly indicated.

In the second setting, there is mild giant cell transformation, a minor finding in the background of changes otherwise typical for a known disease. For example, chronic HCV can have mild giant cell transformation of zone 3 hepatocytes in biopsies that are otherwise typical for chronic HCV.[74,123] The giant cell change is not associated with the inflammatory grade or fibrous stage but is often seen on subsequent biopsies.[123] As a second example, chronic cholestasis from many different causes can lead to focal giant cell transformation of hepatocytes. In these cases, the giant cell transformation is a nonspecific reactive change and does not need to be mentioned in the pathology report. If it is mentioned, the report should clarify that the giant cell transformation is a mild and incidental finding.

In the neonate population, cholestatic or hepatitic injury patterns frequently leads to giant cell transformation, a pattern historically called neonatal giant cell hepatitis. In this setting, the giant cell transformation can result from many different etiologies and does not suggest a specific etiology or differential. Thus, this pattern has largely been folded into the more general entirety of *neonatal hepatis*; see Chapter 12 for more detail.

REFERENCES

1. Knodell RG, Ishak KG, Black WC, et al. Formulation and application of a numerical scoring system for assessing histological activity in asymptomatic chronic active hepatitis. *Hepatology*. 1981;1:431-435.
2. Ishak K, Baptista A, Bianchi L, et al. Histological grading and staging of chronic hepatitis. *J Hepatol*. 1995;22:696-699.
3. Batts KP, Ludwig J. Chronic hepatitis. An update on terminology and reporting. *Am J Surg Pathol*. 1995;19:1409-1417.
4. The French METAVIR Cooperative Study Group. Intraobserver and interobserver variations in liver biopsy interpretation in patients with chronic hepatitis C. The French METAVIR Cooperative Study Group. *Hepatology*. 1994;20:15-20.
5. Desmet VJ, Gerber M, Hoofnagle JH, et al. Classification of chronic hepatitis: diagnosis, grading and staging. *Hepatology*. 1994;19:1513-1520.
6. Wanless IR, Sweeney G, Dhillon AP, et al. Lack of progressive hepatic fibrosis during long-term therapy with deferiprone in subjects with transfusion-dependent beta-thalassemia. *Blood*. 2002;100:1566-1569.
7. Kim MY, Cho MY, Baik SK, et al. Histological subclassification of cirrhosis using the Laennec fibrosis scoring system correlates with clinical stage and grade of portal hypertension. *J Hepatol*. 2011;55:1004-1009.
8. Scheuer PJ. Classification of chronic viral hepatitis: a need for reassessment. *J Hepatol*. 1991;13:372-374.
9. ter Borg F, ten Kate FJ, Cuypers HT, et al. A survey of liver pathology in needle biopsies from HBsAg and anti-HBe positive individuals. *J Clin Pathol*. 2000;53:541-548.
10. Goodman ZD. Grading and staging systems for inflammation and fibrosis in chronic liver diseases. *J Hepatol*. 2007;47:598-607.

11. Guido M, Mangia A, Faa G. Chronic viral hepatitis: the histology report. *Dig Liver Dis.* 2011;43(suppl 4):S331-S343.

12. Sulkowski MS, Mehta SH, Torbenson MS, et al. Rapid fibrosis progression among HIV/hepatitis C virus-co-infected adults. *AIDS.* 2007;21:2209-2216.

13. Perumalswami PV, Bini EJ. Epidemiology, natural history, and treatment of hepatitis B virus and hepatitis C virus coinfection. *Minerva Gastroenterol Dietol.* 2006;52:145-155.

14. Sulkowski MS, Mehta SH, Torbenson M, et al. Hepatic steatosis and antiretroviral drug use among adults coinfected with HIV and hepatitis C virus. *AIDS.* 2005;19:585-592.

15. Bugianesi E, Salamone F, Negro F. The interaction of metabolic factors with HCV infection: does it matter? *J Hepatol.* 2012;56(suppl 1):S56-S65.

16. Torbenson M. Iron in the liver: a review for surgical pathologists. *Adv Anat Pathol.* 2011;18:306-317.

17. Feinstone SM, Kapikian AZ, Purceli RH. Hepatitis A: detection by immune electron microscopy of a viruslike antigen associated with acute illness. *Science.* 1973;182:1026-1028.

18. Pontrelli G, Boccia D, DI Renzi M, et al. Epidemiological and virological characterization of a large community-wide outbreak of hepatitis A in southern Italy. *Epidemiol Infect.* 2008;136:1027-1034.

19. Halliday ML, Kang LY, Zhou TK, et al. An epidemic of hepatitis A attributable to the ingestion of raw clams in Shanghai, China. *J Infect Dis.* 1991;164:852-859.

20. Eisenbach C, Longerich T, Fickenscher H, et al. Recurrence of clinically significant hepatitis A following liver transplantation for fulminant hepatitis A. *J Clin Virol.* 2006;35:109-112.

21. Gane E, Sallie R, Saleh M, et al. Clinical recurrence of hepatitis A following liver transplantation for acute liver failure. *J Med Virol.* 1995;45:35-39.

22. Bura M, Michalak M, Chojnicki MK, et al. Viral hepatitis A in 108 adult patients during an eight-year observation at a single center in Poland. *Adv Clin Exp Med.* 2015;24:829-836.

23. Abe H, Beninger PR, Ikejiri N, et al. Light microscopic findings of liver biopsy specimens from patients with hepatitis type A and comparison with type B. *Gastroenterology.* 1982;82:938-947.

24. Okuno T, Sano A, Deguchi T, et al. Pathology of acute hepatitis A in humans. Comparison with acute hepatitis B. *Am J Clin Pathol.* 1984;81:162-169.

25. Teixeira MR Jr, Weller IV, Murray A, et al. The pathology of hepatitis A in man. *Liver.* 1982;2:53-60.

26. Yamamoto T, Ishii M, Nagura H, et al. Transient hepatic fibrin-ring granulomas in a patient with acute hepatitis A. *Liver.* 1995;15:276-279.

27. Taylor RM, Davern T, Munoz S, et al. Fulminant hepatitis A virus infection in the United States: incidence, prognosis, and outcomes. *Hepatology.* 2006;44:1589-1597.

28. Kryger P, Christoffersen P. Liver histopathology of the hepatitis A virus infection: a comparison with hepatitis type B and non-a, non-b. *J Clin Pathol.* 1983;36:650-654.

29. Shin EC, Jeong SH. Natural history, clinical manifestations, and pathogenesis of hepatitis A. *Cold Spring Harb Perspect Med.* 2018;8:a031708.

30. Inuzuka S, Ueno T, Tateishi H, et al. A patient with hepatic granuloma formation and angiotensin-converting enzyme production by granuloma cells during clinical relapse of hepatitis A. *Pathol Int.* 1994;44:391-397.

31. Petrov AI, Vatev NT, Atanasova MV. Cholestatic syndrome in viral hepatitis A. *Folia Med (Plovdiv).* 2012;54:30-35.

32. Lok AS, McMahon BJ. Chronic hepatitis B: update 2009. *Hepatology.* 2009;50:661-662.

33. Lesmana CR, Gani RA, Hasan I, et al. Significant hepatic histopathology in chronic hepatitis B patients with serum ALT less than twice ULN and high HBV-DNA levels in Indonesia. *J Dig Dis*. 2011;12:476-480.

34. Gobel T, Erhardt A, Herwig M, et al. High prevalence of significant liver fibrosis and cirrhosis in chronic hepatitis B patients with normal ALT in central Europe. *J Med Virol*. 2011;83:968-973.

35. Andreani T, Serfaty L, Mohand D, et al. Chronic hepatitis B virus carriers in the immunotolerant phase of infection: histologic findings and outcome. *Clin Gastroenterol Hepatol*. 2007;5:636-641.

36. Deodhar KP, Tapp E, Scheuer PJ. Orcein staining of hepatitis B antigen in paraffin sections of liver biopsies. *J Clin Pathol*. 1975;28:66-70.

37. Winckler K, Junge U, Creutzfeldt W. Ground-glass hepatocytes in unselected liver biopsies. ultrastructure and relationship to hepatitis B surface antigen. *Scand J Gastroenterol*. 1976;11:167-170.

38. Thomsen P, Clausen PP. Occurrence of hepatitis B-surface antigen in a consecutive material of 1539 liver biopsies. *Acta Pathol Microbiol Immunol Scand A*. 1983;91:71-75.

39. Su IJ, Kuo TT, Liaw YF. Hepatocyte hepatitis B surface antigen. Diagnostic evaluation of patients with clinically acute hepatitis B surface antigen-positive hepatitis. *Arch Pathol Lab Med*. 1985;109:400-402.

40. Rozario R, Ramakrishna B. Histopathological study of chronic hepatitis B and C: a comparison of two scoring systems. *J Hepatol*. 2003;38:223-229.

41. Serinoz E, Varli M, Erden E, et al. Nuclear localization of hepatitis B core antigen and its relations to liver injury, hepatocyte proliferation, and viral load. *J Clin Gastroenterol*. 2003;36:269-272.

42. Son MS, Yoo JH, Kwon CI, et al. Associations of expressions of HBcAg and HBsAg with the histologic activity of liver disease and viral replication. *Gut Liver*. 2008;2:166-173.

43. Milani S, Ambu S, Patussi V, et al. Serum HBV DNA and intrahepatic hepatitis B core antigen (HBcAg) in chronic hepatitis B virus infection: correlation with infectivity and liver histology. *Hepatogastroenterology*. 1988;35:306-308.

44. Ramakrishna B, Mukhopadhya A, Kurian G. Correlation of hepatocyte expression of hepatitis B viral antigens with histological activity and viral titer in chronic hepatitis B virus infection: an immunohistochemical study. *J Gastroenterol Hepatol*. 2008;23:1734-1738.

45. Moreno A, Ramon y Cajal S, Marazuela M, et al. Sanded nuclei in delta patients. *Liver*. 1989;9:367-371.

46. Wang HC, Wu HC, Chen CF, et al. Different types of ground glass hepatocytes in chronic hepatitis B virus infection contain specific pre-S mutants that may induce endoplasmic reticulum stress. *Am J Pathol*. 2003;163:2441-2449.

47. Schirmacher P, Schauss D, Dienes HP. Intracellular accumulation of incompletely processed transforming growth factor-alpha polypeptides in ground glass hepatocytes of chronic hepatitis B virus infection. *J Hepatol*. 1996;24:547-554.

48. Wisell J, Boitnott J, Haas M, et al. Glycogen pseudoground glass change in hepatocytes. *Am J Surg Pathol*. 2006;30:1085-1090.

49. Su IJ, Wang HC, Wu HC, et al. Ground glass hepatocytes contain pre-S mutants and represent preneoplastic lesions in chronic hepatitis B virus infection. *J Gastroenterol Hepatol*. 2008;23:1169-1174.

50. Tahan V, Ozaras R, Lacevic N, et al. Prevalence of hepatic granulomas in chronic hepatitis B. *Dig Dis Sci*. 2004;49:1575-1577.

51. Goldin RD, Levine TS, Foster GR, et al. Granulomas and hepatitis C. *Histopathology*. 1996;28:265-267.

52. Verme G, Amoroso P, Lettieri G, et al. A histological study of hepatitis delta virus liver disease. *Hepatology*. 1986;6:1303-1307.

53. Genesca J, Jardi R, Buti M, et al. Hepatitis B virus replication in acute hepatitis B, acute hepatitis B virus-hepatitis delta virus coinfection and acute hepatitis delta superinfection. *Hepatology*. 1987;7:569-572.

54. Andrade ZA, Lesbordes JL, Ravisse P, et al. Fulminant hepatitis with microvesicular steatosis (a histologic comparison of cases occurring in Brazil—Labrea hepatitis—and in central Africa—Bangui hepatitis). *Rev Soc Bras Med Trop*. 1992;25:155-160.

55. Bensabath G, Hadler SC, Soares MC, et al. Hepatitis delta virus infection and Labrea hepatitis. Prevalence and role in fulminant hepatitis in the Amazon Basin. *J Am Med Assoc*. 1987;258:479-483.

56. Buitrago B, Popper H, Hadler SC, et al. Specific histologic features of Santa Marta hepatitis: a severe form of hepatitis delta-virus infection in northern South America. *Hepatology*. 1986;6:1285-1291.

57. Pascarella S, Negro F. Hepatitis D virus: an update. *Liver Int*. 2011;31:7-21.

58. Johnson K, Kotiesh A, Boitnott JK, et al. Histology of symptomatic acute hepatitis C infection in immunocompetent adults. *Am J Surg Pathol*. 2007;31:1754-1758.

59. Kanzaki H, Takaki A, Yagi T, et al. A case of fulminant liver failure associated with hepatitis C virus. *Clin J Gastroenterol*. 2014;7:170-174.

60. Badizadegan K, Jonas MM, Ott MJ, et al. Histopathology of the liver in children with chronic hepatitis C viral infection. *Hepatology*. 1998;28:1416-1423.

61. Bedossa P, Poynard T. An algorithm for the grading of activity in chronic hepatitis C. The METAVIR Cooperative Study Group. *Hepatology*. 1996;24:289-293.

62. De Groote J, Desmet VJ, Gedigk P, et al. A classification of chronic hepatitis. *Lancet*. 1968;2:626-628.

63. Torbenson M, Washington K. Pathology of liver disease: advances in the last 50 years. *Hum Pathol*. 2020;95:78-98.

64. Mensa L, Perez-del-Pulgar S, Crespo G, et al. Imaging of hepatitis C virus infection in liver grafts after liver transplantation. *J Hepatol*. 2013;59:271-278.

65. Yee LJ, Kelleher P, Goldin RD, et al. Antinuclear antibodies (ANA) in chronic hepatitis C virus infection: correlates of positivity and clinical relevance. *J Viral Hepat*. 2004;11:459-464.

66. Putra J, Schiano TD, Fiel MI. Resolution of HCV-autoimmune hepatitis overlap syndrome with antiviral TreatmentA paired liver biopsy study. *Am J Clin Pathol*. 2019;152:735-741.

67. Giannini E, Ceppa P, Botta F, et al. Steatosis and bile duct damage in chronic hepatitis C: distribution and relationships in a group of Northern Italian patients. *Liver*. 1999;19:432-437.

68. Hwang SJ, Luo JC, Chu CW, et al. Clinical, virological, and pathological significance of hepatic bile duct injuries in Chinese patients with chronic hepatitis C. *J Gastroenterol*. 2001;36:392-398.

69. Kaji K, Nakanuma Y, Sasaki M, et al. Hepatitic bile duct injuries in chronic hepatitis C: histopathologic and immunohistochemical studies. *Mod Pathol*. 1994;7:937-945.

70. Torbenson M, Yeh MM, Abraham SC. Bile duct dysplasia in the setting of chronic hepatitis C and alcohol cirrhosis. *Am J Surg Pathol*. 2007;31:1410-1413.

71. Mehta SH, Netski D, Sulkowski MS, et al. Liver enzyme values in injection drug users with chronic hepatitis C. *Dig Liver Dis*. 2005;37:674-680.

72. Kannangai R, Vivekanandan P, Netski D, et al. Liver enzyme flares and occult hepatitis B in persons with chronic hepatitis C infection. *J Clin Virol*. 2007;39:101-105.

73. Micchelli ST, Thomas D, Boitnott JK, et al. Hepatic giant cells in hepatitis C virus (HCV) mono-infection and HCV/HIV co-infection. *J Clin Pathol*. 2008;61:1058-1061.

74. Moreno A, Perez-Elias MJ, Quereda C, et al. Syncytial giant cell hepatitis in human immunodeficiency virus-infected patients with chronic hepatitis C: 2 cases and review of the literature. *Hum Pathol.* 2006;37:1344-1349.

75. Negro F. Hepatitis C virus-induced steatosis: an overview. *Dig Dis.* 2010;28:294-299.

76. Lory J, Zimmermann A. Endotheliitis-like changes in chronic hepatitis C. *Histol Histopathol.* 1997;12:359-366.

77. Yeh MM, Larson AM, Tung BY, et al. Endotheliitis in chronic viral hepatitis: a comparison with acute cellular rejection and non-alcoholic steatohepatitis. *Am J Surg Pathol.* 2006;30:727-733.

78. Zhu H, Bodenheimer HC Jr, Clain DJ, et al. Hepatic lipogranulomas in patients with chronic liver disease: association with hepatitis C and fatty liver disease. *World J Gastroenterol.* 2010;16:5065-5069.

79. Snyder N, Martinez JG, Xiao SY. Chronic hepatitis C is a common associated with hepatic granulomas. *World J Gastroenterol.* 2008;14:6366-6369.

80. Ozaras R, Tahan V, Mert A, et al. The prevalence of hepatic granulomas in chronic hepatitis C. *J Clin Gastroenterol.* 2004;38:449-452.

81. Narang TK, Ahrens W, Russo MW. Post-liver transplant cholestatic hepatitis C: a systematic review of clinical and pathological findings and application of consensus criteria. *Liver Transpl.* 2010;16:1228-1235.

82. Cassani F, Cataleta M, Valentini P, et al. Serum autoantibodies in chronic hepatitis C: comparison with autoimmune hepatitis and impact on the disease profile. *Hepatology.* 1997;26:561-566.

83. Clifford BD, Donahue D, Smith L, et al. High prevalence of serological markers of autoimmunity in patients with chronic hepatitis C. *Hepatology.* 1995;21:613-619.

84. Hsieh MY, Dai CY, Lee LP, et al. Antinuclear antibody is associated with a more advanced fibrosis and lower RNA levels of hepatitis C virus in patients with chronic hepatitis C. *J Clin Pathol.* 2008;61:333-337.

85. Czaja AJ, Carpenter HA. Histological findings in chronic hepatitis C with autoimmune features. *Hepatology.* 1997;26:459-466.

86. Hoofnagle JH, Nelson KE, Purcell RH. Hepatitis E. *N Engl J Med.* 2012;367: 1237-1244.

87. Thomas DL, Yarbough PO, Vlahov D, et al. Seroreactivity to hepatitis E virus in areas where the disease is not endemic. *J Clin Microbiol.* 1997;35:1244-1247.

88. Legrand-Abravanel F, Kamar N, Sandres-Saune K, et al. Characteristics of autochthonous hepatitis E virus infection in solid-organ transplant recipients in France. *J Infect Dis.* 2010;202:835-844.

89. Davern TJ, Chalasani N, Fontana RJ, et al. Acute hepatitis E infection accounts for some cases of suspected drug-induced liver injury. *Gastroenterology.* 2011;141: 1665-1672.e1-9.

90. Lenggenhager D, Pawel S, Honcharova-Biletska H, et al. The histologic presentation of hepatitis E reflects patients' immune status and pre-existing liver condition. *Mod Pathol.* 2020;34:233-248.

91. Malcolm P, Dalton H, Hussaini HS, et al. The histology of acute autochthonous hepatitis E virus infection. *Histopathology.* 2007;51:190-194.

92. Moucari R, Bernuau J, Nicand E, et al. Acute hepatitis E with severe jaundice: report of three cases. *Eur J Gastroenterol Hepatol.* 2007;19:1012-1015.

93. Peron JM, Danjoux M, Kamar N, et al. Liver histology in patients with sporadic acute hepatitis E: a study of 11 patients from South-West France. *Virchows Arch.* 2007;450:405-410.

94. Lenggenhager D, Weber A. Clinicopathologic features and pathologic diagnosis of hepatitis E. *Hum Pathol.* 2020;96:34-38.

95. Ankcorn M, Said B, Morgan D, et al. Persistent hepatitis E virus infection across England and Wales 2009-2017: demography, virology and outcomes. *J Viral Hepat.* 2021;28:420-430.

96. Kamar N, Selves J, Mansuy JM, et al. Hepatitis E virus and chronic hepatitis in organ-transplant recipients. *N Engl J Med.* 2008;358:811-817.

97. Pischke S, Suneetha PV, Baechlein C, et al. Hepatitis E virus infection as a cause of graft hepatitis in liver transplant recipients. *Liver Transpl.* 2010;16:74-82.

98. Haagsma EB, van den Berg AP, Porte RJ, et al. Chronic hepatitis E virus infection in liver transplant recipients. *Liver Transpl.* 2008;14:547-553.

99. Darstein F, Hauser F, Mittler J, et al. Hepatitis E is a rare finding in liver transplant patients with chronic elevated liver enzymes and biopsy-proven acute rejection. *Transplant Proc.* 2020;52:926-931.

100. Gupta P, Jagya N, Pabhu SB, et al. Immunohistochemistry for the diagnosis of hepatitis E virus infection. *J Viral Hepat.* 2012;19:e177-e183.

101. Lautenschlager I, Halme L, Hockerstedt K, et al. Cytomegalovirus infection of the liver transplant: virological, histological, immunological, and clinical observations. *Transpl Infect Dis.* 2006;8:21-30.

102. MacDonald GA, Greenson JK, DelBuono EA, et al. Mini-microabscess syndrome in liver transplant recipients. *Hepatology.* 1997;26:192-197.

103. Lamps LW, Pinson CW, Raiford DS, et al. The significance of microabscesses in liver transplant biopsies: a clinicopathological study. *Hepatology.* 1998;28:1532-1537.

104. Kusne S, Schwartz M, Breinig MK, et al. Herpes simplex virus hepatitis after solid organ transplantation in adults. *J Infect Dis.* 1991;163:1001-1007.

105. Nicolini LA, Canepa P, Caligiuri P, et al. Fulminant hepatitis associated with echovirus 25 during treatment with ocrelizumab for multiple sclerosis. *JAMA Neurol.* 2019;76:866-867.

106. Lefterova MI, Rivetta C, George TI, et al. Severe hepatitis associated with an echovirus 18 infection in an immune-compromised adult. *J Clin Microbiol.* 2013;51:684-687.

107. Wang J, Atchison RW, Walpusk J, et al. Echovirus hepatic failure in infancy: report of four cases with speculation on the pathogenesis. *Pediatr Dev Pathol.* 2001;4:454-460.

108. Moreau B, Bastedo C, Michel RP, et al. Hepatitis and encephalitis due to Coxsackie virus A9 in an adult. *Case Rep Gastroenterol.* 2011;5:617-622.

109. David JJ, Dietz FR, Jones MM. Coxsackie-B monarthritis with hepatitis. A case report. *J Bone Joint Surg Am.* 1993;75:1685-1686.

110. Thapa J, Koirala P, Gupta TN. Coxsackie B virus infection as a rare cause of acute renal failure and hepatitis. *Kathmandu Univ Med J.* 2018;16:100-102.

111. Gregor GR, Geller SA, Walker GF, et al. Coxsackie hepatitis in an adult, with ultrastructural demonstration of the virus. *Mt Sinai J Med.* 1975;42:575-580.

112. Sun NC, Smith VM. Hepatitis associated with myocarditis. Unusual manifestation of infection with Coxsackie virus group B, type 3. *N Engl J Med.* 1966;274:190-193.

113. Tian S, Xiong Y, Liu H, et al. Pathological study of the 2019 novel coronavirus disease (COVID-19) through postmortem core biopsies. *Mod Pathol.* 2020;33:1007-1014.

114. Lagana SM, Kudose S, Iuga AC, et al. Hepatic pathology in patients dying of COVID-19: a series of 40 cases including clinical, histologic, and virologic data. *Mod Pathol.* 2020;33:2147-2155.

115. Zhao CL, Rapkiewicz A, Maghsoodi-Deerwester M, et al. Pathological findings in the postmortem liver of COVID-19 patients. *Hum Pathol.* 2021;109:59-68.

116. Xu B, Zhi N, Hu G, et al. Hybrid DNA virus in Chinese patients with seronegative hepatitis discovered by deep sequencing. *Proc Natl Acad Sci U S A.* 2013;110:10264-10269.

117. Nair S, Baisden B, Boitnott J, et al. Recurrent, progressive giant cell hepatitis in two consecutive liver allografts in a middle-aged woman. *J Clin Gastroenterol.* 2001;32:454-456.

118. Lerut JP, Claeys N, Ciccarelli O, et al. Recurrent postinfantile syncytial giant cell hepatitis after orthotopic liver transplantation. *Transpl Int.* 1998;11:320-322.

119. Pappo O, Yunis E, Jordan JA, et al. Recurrent and de novo giant cell hepatitis after orthotopic liver transplantation. *Am J Surg Pathol.* 1994;18:804-813.

120. Potenza L, Luppi M, Barozzi P, et al. HHV-6A in syncytial giant-cell hepatitis. *N Engl J Med.* 2008;359:593-602.

121. Welte S, Gagesch M, Weber A, et al. Fulminant liver failure in Wilson's disease with histologic features of postinfantile giant cell hepatitis; cytomegalovirus as the trigger for both? *Eur J Gastroenterol Hepatol.* 2012;24:328-331.

122. Harmanci O, Onal IK, Ersoy O, et al. Postinfantile giant cell hepatitis due to hepatitis E virus along with the presence of autoantibodies. *Dig Dis Sci.* 2007;52:3521-3523.

123. Lau JY, Koukoulis G, Mieli-Vergani G, et al. Syncytial giant-cell hepatitis--a specific disease entity? *J Hepatol.* 1992;15:216-219.

124. Randhawa PS, Jenkins FJ, Nalesnik MA, et al. Herpesvirus 6 variant A infection after heart transplantation with giant cell transformation in bile ductular and gastroduodenal epithelium. *Am J Surg Pathol.* 1997;21:847-853.

6

OTHER INFECTIONS OF THE LIVER

This chapter discusses nonviral infections that involve the liver. There are so many organisms that can infect the liver that they cannot all be reasonably covered in this chapter. Instead, the focus is on the most common organisms encountered in routine biopsy specimens, and even then, most of these are very rare. Echinococcal and amebic cysts are typically not biopsied but are reviewed for completeness and because many times our clinical colleagues will ask if a biopsy that shows an abscess could represent a parasitic cyst.

BACTERIAL ABSCESS

Liver abscesses can be bacterial, fungal, or parasitic. In adults, bacterial (or pyogenic) abscesses are the most common. Risk factors include immunosuppression, diabetes mellitus, and chronic biliary tract disease.[1,2] Bacterial abscesses can also be associated with cancer, primarily of the biliary tree or pancreas,[3] as well as of the colon, even if there has not been metastatic disease to the liver.[4]

Hepatic abscesses are primarily caused by enteric bacteria. In adults, the most common organisms are streptococcal or *Pseudomonas* species; in many cases, abscesses are polymicrobial. Mixed bacterial and fungal abscesses are also common. In children, most hepatic abscesses are due to *Staphylococcus aureus*.[5]

The bacteria get into the liver mainly via one of these mechanisms: biliary tract obstruction (~50%); via the portal venous system as it drains other gastrointestinal (GI) tract organs that have bacterial infections, in particular appendicitis (~30%); direct extension from abdominal infection (~5%); hepatic artery seeding (rare); penetrating liver trauma (rare); and cryptogenic (frequency varies a lot in different studies).[3]

Most hepatic abscesses are not biopsied, as clinical histories and imaging studies can make the diagnosis, and the diagnosis is then confirmed by an appropriate response to antibiotic therapy (or surgical drainage when necessary). Some abscesses, however, are concerning for neoplasms by imaging studies and go on to liver biopsy; most of these are later-stage abscesses that have had partial resolution and become substantially fibrotic.

Liver biopsies of these later-stage abscesses typically show a fibrotic rind of tissue composed of mixed inflammation, compressed portal tracts with bile ductular proliferation, and varying amounts of fibrosis (Figure 6.1). The abscess itself is typically a mixture of inflammation, with neutrophils, lymphocytes, and plasma cells, and varying amounts of fibrosis. In many cases, the biopsy sample will also include necrotic tissue/inflammatory exudate in the center of the lesion (Figure 6.2), in which case stains for fungal organisms or bacteria can sometimes help identify the cause of the abscess (Figure 6.3). In time, if the abscess heals, it can transform into an inflammatory pseudotumor composed of mostly chronic inflammation and fibrosis.

ACTINOMYCOSIS. Actinomyces is part of the normal flora of the oral cavity, GI tract, and female genital tract. Actinomycosis abscesses in the liver typically result from the spread of infection originating in other organs, although apparently isolated liver abscesses can also be seen. Infections in the liver can form mass lesions that are single (2/3 of cases) or multiple and often mimic hepatic tumors on imaging studies.[6] Many cases are first diagnosed on liver biopsy. The organism is of relatively low pathogenicity, so symptoms are usually mild and nonspecific. Most patients are immunocompetent, and there is about a 2:1 male predominance.[6]

Biopsy results of mass lesions caused by actinomycosis are fundamentally similar to those of other pyogenic abscesses, typically showing a rind of inflamed/compressed liver, a middle layer of inflamed fibrotic tissue, and, depending on sampling, a central area of necrosis. *Actinomyces* can

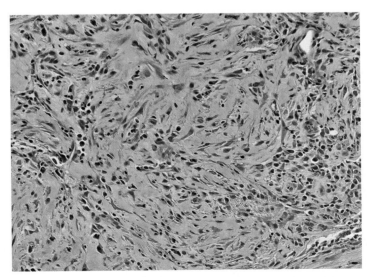

FIGURE 6.1 **Edge of abscess.** This biopsy is from the edge of a hepatic abscess and shows inflamed fibrous tissue. The inflammation is primarily lymphocytic but also has numerous plasma cells and scattered neutrophils.

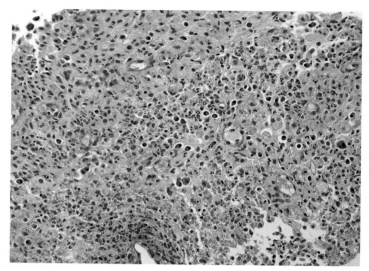

FIGURE 6.2 **Necrotic debris in an abscess.** In this biopsy of an abscess, an area of necrotic fibrinoinflammatory debris can be seen in the lower half of the image.

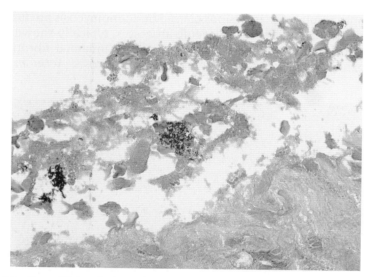

FIGURE 6.3 **Gram-Weigert stain.** Clusters of gram-positive cocci are seen in the necrotic debris of this abscess.

grow in large colonies within the areas of necrosis, appearing as large purple matts on hematoxylin-eosin (H&E) stain, surrounding or associated with sulfur granules (Figure 6.4); this finding is diagnostic of *Actinomyces*. *Actinomyces* is a gram-positive, filamentous bacteria that can have hypha-like structures that may mimic fungal organisms. The organisms are

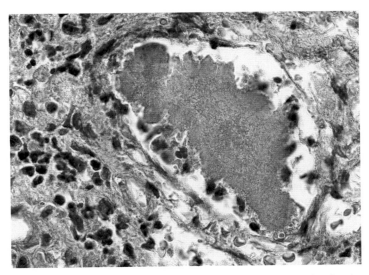

FIGURE 6.4 **Hepatic *Actinomyces*.** The filamentous bacteria are growing in a large colony or "sulfur granule."

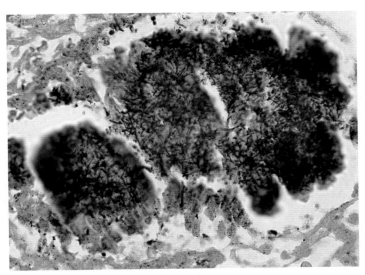

FIGURE 6.5 **Hepatic *Actinomyces*.** The filamentous bacteria are positive in Gomori methenamine silver (GMS) stain.

positive on Gomori methenamine silver (GMS) stain (Figure 6.5), which further adds to the potential for confusion with fungi, but the bacteria will be noticeably thinner. GMS or bacterial stains are most likely to show organisms in cases with fibrinoinflammatory exudate and/or central necrosis. About one-third of infections are polymicrobial, so you might see additional organisms on bacterial stains. If the biopsy sample includes mostly inflamed fibrotic tissue, the findings can closely resemble an inflammatory pseudotumor.

OTHER PATTERNS OF BACTERIAL INFECTION

Bacterial infections that primarily involve the GI tract often secondarily involve the liver. In these cases, biopsies of the liver are usually not needed for clinical diagnosis or management, so they are only rarely encountered in surgical pathology, unless patients have unusual presentations or complicated clinical settings. These enterically centered infections tend to have similar histologic patterns of injury when they involve the liver, with a central theme of mild to moderate Kupffer cell hyperplasia, plus or minus actual granulomas. In most cases, the Kupffer cell hyperplasia is also accompanied by Kupfer cell aggregates, which can be prominent, sometimes forming small nodules. The background liver commonly shows additional mild nonspecific portal and lobular lymphocytic inflammation; the liver may also have other findings depending on the underlying liver disease(s), including fatty liver disease or biliary tract disease.

In general, the patterns of injury for any given bacterial infection show significant overlap with other bacterial infections, so they are not specific. Some interesting broad patterns, however, have been reported and are summarized in Table 6.1, with the caveat that these are culled from literature that is mostly case reports and small case series, spread out over many decades, and are not from studies designed to directly examine similarities and differences between these various infections. The histologic differential for these patterns typically is that of drug-induced liver injury and acute viral hepatitis.

Syphilis

Syphilis is caused by *Treponema pallidum*; it is an infection that can be widely disseminated in the body and can involve the liver. Syphilis is rarely encountered in surgical pathology of the liver, as most cases are diagnosed by serologic studies. The liver can be involved in both congenital infection and acquired infection. Most cases seen today are acquired because of routine maternal testing, which has largely eliminated congenital transmission in many parts of the world.

The histologic findings in congenital syphilis were described many years ago, with essentially no recent data, but studies reported mild sinusoidal lymphocytosis with diffuse sinusoidal fibrosis and organisms that were easily identified on Warthin-Starry staining. Other congenital patterns include neonatal hepatitis[7] and paucity of intrahepatic bile ducts.[8]

The histologic findings in acquired syphilis vary all the way from an almost normal liver biopsy pattern to pseudotumors of the liver.[9,10] The biopsy findings in most cases are mild and nonspecific, with mild nonspecific portal and lobular chronic inflammation and mild Kupffer cell hyperplasia.[10,11]

TABLE 6.1 Bacterial Infections of the Liver

Bacterial Infection	Source of Infection	Additional Risk Factors for Infection	Presentation: Histologic Patterns
Leptospirosis	Rodent urine, most cases from tropical climates	Exposure to fresh water such as drinking unpurified water or swimming	1. Hepatitis, usually with systemic symptoms: lobular cholestasis, mild portal and lobular lymphocytic inflammation, and diffuse Kupffer cell hyperplasia. There may be small clusters of sinusoidal Kupffer cells. 2. Fulminant hepatic failure: extensive zone 3 hemorrhagic necrosis (rare).
Listeriosis (*Listeria monocytogenes*)	Contaminated foods such as milk, cheese, raw vegetable, undercooked meats; and seafood	Immunosuppression, including persons who are very young or very old. Pregnancy is another risk factor.	1. Hepatitis, usually with systemic symptoms: scattered small microabscesses in the lobules, measuring 1-3 mm diameter. The microabscesses commonly show a central core of necrosis/neutrophils and a rim of macrophages. Larger epithelioid granulomas may be present. 2. Mass lesion: hepatic abscess.
Salmonella hepatitis (*Salmonella typhi* or *Salmonella paratyphi*)	Oral-fecal route, from contaminated food and water. Humans are the only known natural reservoir		1. Hepatitis, usually with systemic symptoms: diffuse Kupffer cell hyperplasia. There can be mild to moderate sinusoidal lymphocytosis that suggests EBV hepatitis. 2. Later cases can show "typhoid nodules", granuloma-like nodules in the lobules 3. Mass lesion: hepatic abscess.
Tularemia (*Francisella tularensis*)	• Tick and deerfly bites • Handling infected animal carcasses • Exposure to contaminated water • Inhaling contaminated soil		1. Hepatitis, usually with systemic symptoms: scattered microabscesses of 1-3 mm diameter with a central core of necrosis/neutrophils and rim of macrophages. More typical epithelioid granulomas can also be seen. 2. Mass lesion: hepatic abscess.
Whipple disease (*Tropheryma whipplei*)	Unknown, presumably environmental exposure, probably oral-fecal route	Male gender; exposure to raw sewage	Numerous PAS-positive foamy macrophages that can involve the lobules and the portal tracts. Epithelioid granulomas may also be seen.

EBV, Epstein-Barr virus; PAS, periodic acid-Schiff.

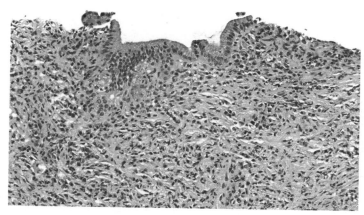

FIGURE 6.6 **Syphilis.** This biopsy showed mild nonspecific portal inflammation, with the exception of one medium- to large-sized bile duct that had a dense cuff of plasma-cell-rich inflammation and occasional neutrophils in the epithelium.

Uncommonly, the biopsy can show a more significant hepatitis, which can be rich in plasma cells, mimicking autoimmune hepatitis.[12] Occasional epithelioid granulomas may also be seen. As another uncommon pattern, some biopsies show plasma-cell-rich inflammation that is focused on a large duct, in the background of an otherwise almost normal liver biopsy (Figure 6.6). The inflamed bile duct often has neutrophils in the epithelium but does not have the typical features of ascending cholangitis, with no duct dilatation, no attenuation of the epithelium, and no large plugs of neutrophils in the lumen. There can be patchy bile ductular proliferation, and the overall findings can mimic primary sclerosing cholangitis, both histologically and by imaging.[13]

In rare cases, late syphilis can lead to mass lesions in the liver that mimic malignancies on imaging studies. These mass lesions can be further classified as either inflammatory pseudotumors[14] or gummas.[15] While both are rare, inflammatory pseudotumors are more common of the two. Syphilitic inflammatory pseudotumors are histologically indistinguishable from other causes of inflammatory pseudotumors, showing inflamed fibrous tissue, with the inflammation composed of lymphocytes, plasma cells (variable prominent), and often small numbers of eosinophils and neutrophils (Figure 6.7).[14] In contrast, gummas look similar to an abscess or a large necrotizing granuloma, with necrosis in the center and a surrounding rim of inflamed fibrous tissue that is often histiocyte rich and may include Langerhans-type giant cells. The center of the lesion can have small islands of dead hepatocytes that appear "mummified," "floating" in the necrotic debris.

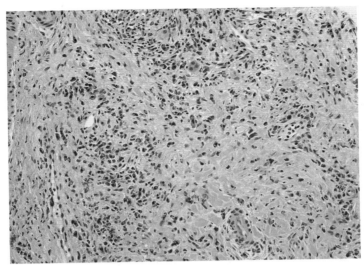

FIGURE 6.7 **Syphilis, inflammatory pseudotumor.** The patient had a mass lesion on imaging that was suspicious for malignancy. The biopsy shows an inflammatory pseudo-tumor that had focally dense plasma-cell-rich inflammation, as shown in this image. An immunostain for *Treponema pallidum* was positive.

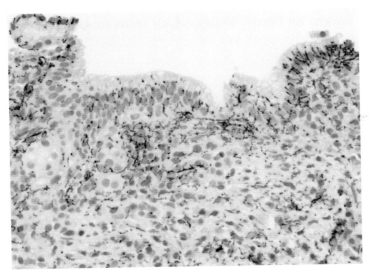

FIGURE 6.8 **Syphilis, immunostain.** The immunostain nicely highlights the organism. Same case as Figure 6.6.

For all these different patterns, a diagnosis can be strongly sup-ported by visualizing the organisms; immunostains are preferred over silver stains, for their ease of interpretation and better sensitivity (Figure 6.8). On the other hand, many of the *T. pallidum* immunostains are not entirely specific, as they can also show positive result with other spirochetes; for this reason, serologic testing is important to confirm the diagnosis.

Whipple Disease

Whipple disease is caused by *Tropheryma whipplei*, a gram-positive organism that is most likely spread by the oral-fecal route. For example, persons working with raw sewage have a high exposure rate, although symptomatic infections are rare.[16,17] In fact, most people who have the organism in their GI tract are asymptomatic.[16,18] The disease classically presents with arthralgia, abdominal pain, weight loss, and diarrhea.

The liver can be involved with systemic disease, but to date, isolated infections of the liver have not been reported. The histologic findings are broadly similar to those seen in other organs, with foamy macrophage infiltrates in the portal tracts and lobules (Figures 6.9 and 6.10). The macrophages tend to form small, discrete clusters. Epithelioid granulomas have also been reported and these can be negative for organisms on periodic acid-Schiff (PAS) stain.[19,20] The liver commonly shows a mild nonspecific lymphocytic hepatitis, along with mild nonspecific Kupffer cell hyperplasia.[21,22] PAS-positive macrophages can also be seen in the muscular walls of arteries (arteriopathy) in multiple organs, including the liver. The larger branches of the hepatic arteries are more commonly involved but are usually not present on needle biopsy, which tends to sample smaller portal tracts.[23]

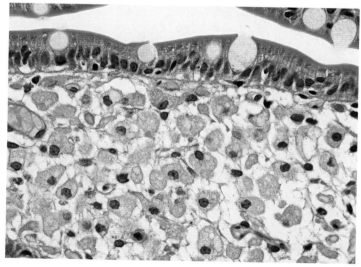

FIGURE 6.9 **Whipple disease.** This image is from the small bowel and shows numerous foamy macrophages.

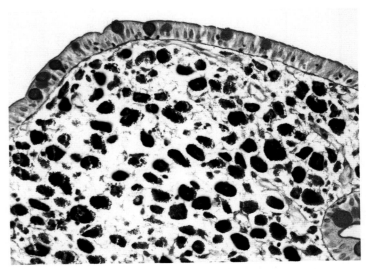

FIGURE 6.10 **Whipple disease, periodic acid-Schiff (PAS) stain.** The foamy macrophages are strongly PAS positive; same case as the preceding image.

TICK-BORNE DISEASES

Ticks can transmit a variety of infections, including protozoan, bacterial, and viral. While the liver is never the primary site of infection, it is a common site of secondary involvement for tick-borne diseases, especially with bacterial infections. In fact, liver disease has been reported in at least a few cases for all known tick-borne infections.[24] In these cases, there can be clinical liver disease, including jaundice, hepatomegaly, and elevated liver enzyme levels. GI manifestations are also common at clinical presentation and typically dominate the clinical presentation, including nausea, vomiting, abdominal pain, and diarrhea.

Almost all diagnoses are made using histories of possible or likely exposure, clinical examination, and serologic findings. Biopsies are only rarely performed, so histologic descriptions are limited, but what is available is summarized in Table 6.2. As an overview, the histologic changes range from mild nonspecific inflammatory changes to predominately cholestatic changes. Tularemia and Q fever can also cause granulomatous inflammation and are discussed in Chapter 7. The three tick-borne diseases that are most likely to cause liver dysfunction are discussed individually in the following sections.

ROCKY MOUNTAIN SPOTTED FEVER is caused by *Rickettsia rickettsii*, an organism transmitted by the wood tick and the dog tick. The organism infects endothelial cells throughout the body, including the liver. Rocky Mountain spotted fever is a serious illness that can be life-threatening. Early clinical symptoms (in the first 2-3 days of illness) are often associated with the

TABLE 6.2	**Tick-Borne Diseases**				
Infection	Organism	Source of Infection	Infected Cell	Organism Identification in Tissue	Histologic Patterns
Lyme disease	*Borrelia burgdorferi* or *Borrelia mayonii*; spirochetes	Tick bites. *Ixodes scapularis* (deer tick, also known as black-legged tick); *Ixodes pacificus* (Western black-legged tick)	Endothelial cells	Spirochetes have been seen on Dieterle silver stains and/or immunostains in some studies.[25-27]	**Hepatitic pattern with Kupffer cell hyperplasia** • Mild lobular hepatitis; predominately lymphocytic but can have admixed neutrophils.[24,25] • Kupffer cell hyperplasia. • Granulomatous hepatitis in rare cases.[27-29]
Rocky Mountain spotted fever	*Rickettsia rickettsii*, gram-negative intracellular bacteria	Tick bites. *Amblyomma americanum* (lone star tick), *Dermacentor variabilis* (American dog tick), and *Dermacentor andersoni* (Rocky Mountain wood tick)	Endothelial cells	Giemsa stain, not very sensitive	**Portal based inflammation with lobular cholestasis** • Mild to moderate portal inflammation with mixed lymphocytes and neutrophils.[30,31] Portal tract neutrophilia can be prominent. • Portal vein vasculitis and fibrin thrombi sometimes present. • Lobular cholestasis, Kupffer cell hyperplasia, and sometimes prominent erythrophagocytosis.

Disease	Organism	Source/Vector	Cell type	Diagnosis	Histology
Tularemia	*Francisella tularensis*, gram-negative coccobacillus	Rodents, rabbits, and deerfly or tick bites (*A. americanum*, *D. andersoni*, and *D. variabilis*), aerosolization of organisms in the soil	Monocytes/macrophages	Gram stain. However, organisms are only rarely found by tissue stain.[24]	**Hepatitic pattern with cholestasis and microabscesses** • Mild lobular inflammation and cholestasis. • Small abscesses, 1-2 mm in size. These show a necrotic center surrounded by a thin rim of mixed neutrophils, lymphocytes, and macrophages.[32-35] • A subset shows noncaseating epithelioid granulomas.[35]
Anaplasmosis and ehrlichiosis	*Anaplasma phagocytophilum* and *Ehrlichia chaffeensis*, respectively, are both obligate intracellular bacteria	Black-legged tick and Western black-legged tick (anaplasmosis) Lone star tick (ehrlichiosis)	Monocytes or granulocytes	Peripheral blood smears with cytoplasmic morulae in monocytes or granulocytes	**Lobular cholestasis; some also show scattered large lobular foci of lymphocytes/histiocytes** • Lobular cholestasis, mild Kupffer cell hyperplasia, and mild nonspecific lobular inflammation. • Lobules can show discrete foci of lymphocytes and macrophages (often 50-100 cells in size) associated with hepatocyte necrosis and drop out[36,37]; not always present.

GI tract and include anorexia, nausea, vomiting, and diarrhea. The classic findings of fever, headache, and rash, often take longer to develop. Risk factors for severe disease include older age, male gender, and glucose-6-phosphate dehydrogenase deficiency,[38] which is most commonly seen in persons of African and Mediterranean descent. Delayed initiation of doxycycline therapy is also a risk factor for death.[39]

Symptomatic individuals often have elevated liver enzyme levels and hepatomegaly. The histologic findings are mainly found in the portal tracts and show inflammation composed of mixed lymphocytes and neutrophils. The organisms infect the endothelium, and this can result in portal vein vasculitis as well as fibrin thrombi in portal or central veins. The vasculitis can be largely lymphocytic or can have a neutrophilic component. Vasculitis also affects the stomach, pancreas, and small and large intestine and can lead to significant clinical symptoms. A small subset of individuals also develop significant cholestasis. Liver biopsies in this setting show predominately cholestasis with mild nonspecific inflammatory changes.[40] In fatal cases, examination of liver tissue has demonstrated prominent sinusoidal erythrophagocytosis as well as inflammatory changes that predominately involve the portal tracts.[30,31]

LYME DISEASE is caused by a spirochete, *Borrelia burgdorferi*. Patients tend to present with nonspecific clinical findings, most of them GI in nature, such as anorexia, nausea, and vomiting. About 75% of persons will at some point have the classic erythema migrans rash ("bull's-eye rash"), which typically takes about a week to develop, but can take up to a month in some cases. Mild elevations in liver enzyme levels are often present.[41,42] Elevated bilirubin levels are rare but have been reported.[43]

The histologic findings are variable but generally show a mild to moderate hepatitic pattern of injury.[25] The lobular infiltrates can contain neutrophils as well as lymphocytes. In one reported case of Lyme disease, the liver biopsy showed large necrotizing granulomas with palisading histiocytes and multinucleated giant cells.[28]

EHRLICHIOSIS and anaplasmosis (anaplasmosis was formerly known as human granulocytic ehrlichiosis) are both tick-borne diseases caused by rickettsia-like bacteria that are transmitted by the lone star tick. The organisms are obligate intracellular bacteria that infect white blood cells. The diseases lead to liver dysfunction in greater than 80% of cases, although in most cases the liver dysfunction is mild and transitory, limited largely to aminotransferase elevations.[24] Some patients become jaundiced and the livers show lobular cholestasis, which can be marked in severe cases, and is often associated with a diffuse Kupffer cell hyperplasia. The inflammation is typically mild but individual foci of inflammation can be larger than those seen in other causes of hepatitis, forming scattered discrete aggregates of lymphocytes and macrophages (often 50-100 cells in size) that are associated with hepatocyte necrosis and drop out.[36] Larger areas of confluent necrosis have also been reported.[36]

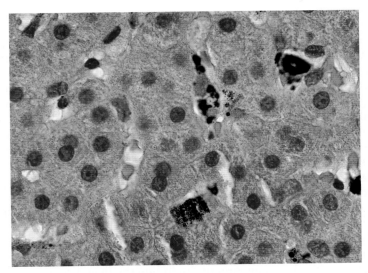

FIGURE 6.11 **Hemozoin or malarial pigment.** This biopsy was from a patient with unexplained liver enzyme level elevations. The pigment suggested the need for further workup for malaria, which was positive.

MALARIAL INFECTION

Malaria is rarely seen as a new infection within the United States, Canada, and Europe, but because of the increasingly global nature of medicine, as well as large population shifts from endemic areas to nonendemic areas, it is worthwhile knowing the pathologic findings. The liver findings can be mild and subtle, even with fatal cases.[44,45] Malarial organisms are generally not seen.[44] The liver shows mild sinusoidal congestion and Kupffer cell hyperplasia with distinctive brown-black malarial pigment in the sinusoidal Kupffer cells and/or portal tract macrophages (Figure 6.11, eFig 6.1). This malarial pigment is also called *hemozoin* and results from the hemophagocytosis of damaged, parasitized red blood cells. The pigment can be seen in about 75% of liver specimens that have active malarial infection,[46] but it is not permanent and will disappear about a month or so after clearance of the infection,[47,48] although the precise time to clearance of pigment has not been well worked out. In some cases, patients can be jaundiced and biopsies will show an additional component of lobular cholestasis. Inflammatory changes range from none to moderate, but as many individuals have comorbid conditions, such as chronic viral hepatitis, a significant component of hepatitis should prompt evaluation for additional causes of liver injuries.

ECHINOCOCCOSIS

Echinococcosis is a tape worm infection in humans and is also known as hydatid disease. There are three main patterns of infection: cystic, multilocularis (or alveolar), and neotropical (https://www.cdc.gov/dpdx/echinococcosis/index.html).

Cystic Echinococcosis

Cystic echinococcosis is caused by *Echinococcus granulosus,* a parasite that has a worldwide distribution but tends to be seen in regions with significant animal husbandry that involves grazing animals, such as raising sheep, goats, or cattle, especially if the farmer/rancher also has working dogs (which serve as the definitive host). This form of the disease is also called *unilocular echinococcosis*, but, of note, the liver can actually have multiple cysts. These cysts are separate from each other, however, in contrast to the multilocularis form, which tends to have fibrotic/necrotic mass(es) composed of multiple smaller cysts.

As is true for many parasites, the life cycle of *Echinococcus* is complicated. For *E. granulosus*, dogs (and wolves) are the definitive host, and they become infected when they eat the viscera of infected livestock. Once the parasites complete their life cycle in the definitive host, the animals then shed parasite eggs in their stool, leading to human infections when contaminated food or water is consumed. Once humans are infected, parasitic cysts can involve many organs, including the liver, brain, heart, kidney, lung, and spleen. Liver cysts are slow growing and can be very large at clinical presentation. Most cases are diagnosed by imaging studies followed by confirmation with serologic studies. Biopsies are generally not performed, as a ruptured cyst (a rare potential complication of biopsy) carries a risk of anaphylactic shock.

Hydatid cysts are basically parasitic abscesses. Cystic echinococcosis classically has three histologic layers (Figure 6.12). An outer layer

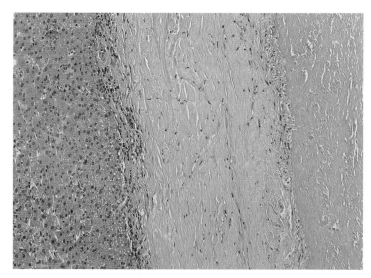

FIGURE 6.12 **Cystic echinococcosis.** This image is from the wall of a resected hydatid cyst. The hepatocytes are seen on the far left. In the middle of the image is the paucicellular and hyalinized outer wall of the pericyst. The middle layer and germinal layer (on the right) blend together in this case.

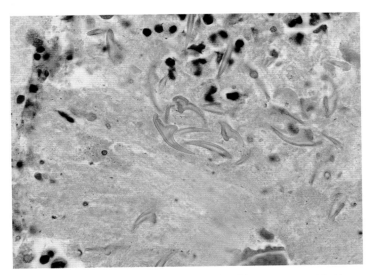

FIGURE 6.13   **Cystic echinococcosis.** A cluster of hooklets are present in the grungy cystic fluid.

is composed of a paucicellular and often hyalinized layer of fibrosis, with relatively little inflammation (sometimes called the outer pericyst). Occasional calcifications can be present. The middle layer is acellular and is often thin and amphophilic on H&E stain, while the inner layer (also called the germinal layer) contains the larval stage of the parasite. In many cases, especially with dead organisms, the only clearly identifiable layer may be the outer layer. The cyst fluid in the center can be hemorrhagic and is grungy appearing on H&E stain; careful examination often reveals remnants of dead parasites such as hooklets (Figure 6.13), scolices, and calcospherites.

Echinococcus multilocularis

Echinococcus multilocularis infections typically cause a multilocularis pattern. Infection is strongly associated with human exposure to wild animals, in particular, the red fox (which serves as the definitive host), and has a geographic range that is somewhat restricted to North America, central and northern Europe, and northern Asia. Other animals, including dogs and wolves, however, are also suitable hosts for *E. multilocularis* infection.

E. multilocularis infection of the liver forms mass lesions that can appear solid by imaging and gross examination, with only small microscopic cysts scattered throughout a larger mass lesion, which is composed of fibrotic and sometimes necrotic material (Figure 6.14). The classic three cyst layers can be present, but often the cysts walls are very degenerated and can be

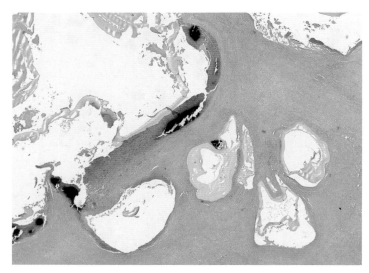

FIGURE 6.14 *Echinococcosis multilocularis*. This large mass was resected for a suspected malignancy, but instead it showed multiple small cysts embedded in dense fibrosis, with focal calcifications.

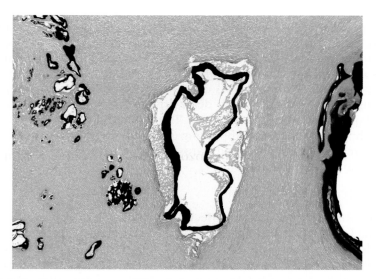

FIGURE 6.15 *Echinococcus multilocularis*, Gomori methenamine silver (GMS). The parasitic cysts pop out on GMS stain.

easily missed without performing special stains. The germinal layer of all types of echinococcosis-causing organisms, including degenerating forms, can be highlighted by trichrome, PAS, or GMS stain (Figure 6.15).[49] The germinal layer, when sufficiently well preserved, often appears laminated on GMS stain (Figure 6.16).

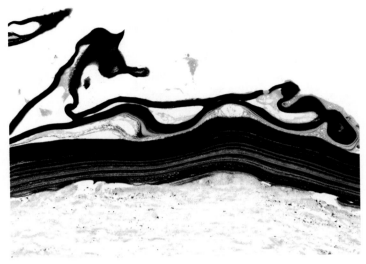

FIGURE 6.16 *Echinococcus multilocularis*, Gomori methenamine silver (GMS). The germinal layer is laminated.

Neotropical Echinococcosis

This form of infection, which is sometimes called polycystic echinococcosis, is the rarest type and is reported primarily in South America and Central America. Neotropical echinococcosis is caused by *Echinococcus vogeli*, which usually leads to a true polycystic infection, or *Echinococcus oligarthra*, which tends to form a single cyst. The histologic findings are similar to that of *E. multilocularis*.

Entamoeba histolytica

ENTAMOEBA HISTOLYTICA is a protozoan that is transmitted by the oral-fecal route and mainly causes intestinal disease. Overall, there is an estimated 40 million cases of *E. histolytica* colitis per year, and 2% of these patients will develop liver abscesses identified by imaging studies.[50] Amebic liver abscesses are rarely encountered in surgical pathology in the western world, where bacterial abscesses predominate, but in other parts of the world, amebic abscesses can be more numerous than bacterial abscesses.[51] For unclear reasons, amebic liver abscesses are 10 times more common in men than in women.[51] Histologically, they look essentially like pyogenic abscesses (Figure 6.17), but sometimes they can also have granulomatous inflammation of the cyst wall. Organisms can be easily missed when sparse but resemble histiocytes with a central dotlike karyosome (Figure 6.18). Many organisms will also have red blood cells in their cytoplasm.[52]

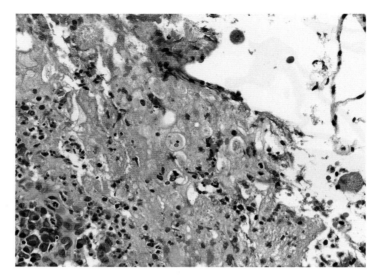

FIGURE 6.17 *Entamoeba histolytica* abscess. The center of the abscess shows necrotic debris. A few organisms can be seen.

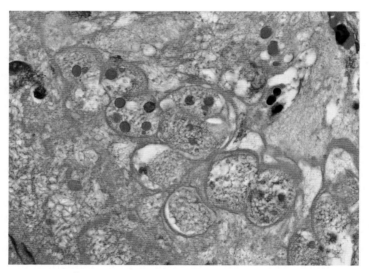

FIGURE 6.18 *Entamoeba histolytica* abscess. On high power, the organisms resemble foamy macrophages. Diagnostic clues include the presence of a central dotlike karyosome and red blood cells in the cytoplasm.

REFERENCES

1. Lee KT, Wong SR, Sheen PC. Pyogenic liver abscess: an audit of 10 years' experience and analysis of risk factors. *Dig Surg*. 2001;18:459-465; discussion 65-66.
2. Kubovy J, Karim S, Ding S. Pyogenic liver abscess: incidence, causality, management and clinical outcomes in a New Zealand cohort. *N Z Med J*. 2019;132:30-35.

3. Huang CJ, Pitt HA, Lipsett PA, et al. Pyogenic hepatic abscess. Changing trends over 42 years. *Ann Surg*. 1996;223:600-607; discussion 7-9.

4. Qu K, Liu C, Wang ZX, et al. Pyogenic liver abscesses associated with nonmetastatic colorectal cancers: an increasing problem in Eastern Asia. *World J Gastroenterol*. 2012;18:2948-2955.

5. Mishra K, Basu S, Roychoudhury S, et al. Liver abscess in children: an overview. *World J Pediatr*. 2010;6:210-216.

6. Kanellopoulou T, Alexopoulou A, Tanouli MI, et al. Primary hepatic actinomycosis. *Am J Med Sci*. 2010;339:362-365.

7. Shet TM, Kandalkar BM, Vora IM. Neonatal hepatitis – an autopsy study of 14 cases. *Indian J Pathol Microbiol*. 1998;41:77-84.

8. Sugiura H, Hayashi M, Koshida R, et al. Nonsyndromatic paucity of intrahepatic bile ducts in congenital syphilis. A case report. *Acta Pathol Jpn*. 1988;38:1061-1068.

9. Wright DJ, Berry CL. Letter: liver involvement in congenital syphilis. *Br J Vener Dis*. 1974;50:241.

10. Terry SI, Hanchard B, Brooks SE, et al. Prevalence of liver abnormality in early syphilis. *Br J Vener Dis*. 1984;60:83-86.

11. Pareek SS. Liver involvement in secondary syphilis. *Dig Dis Sci*. 1979;24:41-43.

12. Khambaty M, Singal AG, Gopal P. Spirochetes as an almost forgotten cause of hepatitis. *Clin Gastroenterol Hepatol*. 2015;13:A21-A22.

13. Wallace HE, Harrison LC, Monteiro EF, et al. The Great Pretender: early syphilis mimicking acute sclerosing cholangitis. *Frontline Gastroenterol*. 2015;6:178-181.

14. Hagen CE, Kamionek M, McKinsey DS, et al. Syphilis presenting as inflammatory tumors of the liver in HIV-positive homosexual men. *Am J Surg Pathol*. 2014;38:1636-1643.

15. Gaslightwala I, Khara HS, Diehl DL. Syphilitic gummas mistaken for liver metastases. *Clin Gastroenterol Hepatol*. 2014;12:e109-e110.

16. Fenollar F, Trani M, Davoust B, et al. Prevalence of asymptomatic Tropheryma whipplei carriage among humans and nonhuman primates. *J Infect Dis*. 2008;197:880-887.

17. Schoniger-Hekele M, Petermann D, Weber B, et al. Tropheryma whipplei in the environment: survey of sewage plant influxes and sewage plant workers. *Appl Environ Microbiol*. 2007;73:2033-2035.

18. Amsler L, Bauernfeind P, Nigg C, et al. Prevalence of Tropheryma whipplei DNA in patients with various gastrointestinal diseases and in healthy controls. *Infection*. 2003;31:81-85.

19. Torzillo PJ, Bignold L, Khan GA. Absence of PAS-positive macrophages in hepatic and lymph node granulomata in Whipple's disease. *Aust N Z J Med*. 1982;12:73-75.

20. Saint-Marc Girardin MF, Zafrani ES, Chaumette MT, et al. Hepatic granulomas in Whipple's disease. *Gastroenterology*. 1984;86:753-756.

21. Cho C, Linscheer WG, Hirschkorn MA, et al. Sarcoidlike granulomas as an early manifestation of Whipple's disease. *Gastroenterology*. 1984;87:941-947.

22. Viteri AL, Stinson JC, Barnes MC, et al. Rod-shaped organism in the liver of a patient with Whipple's disease. *Dig Dis Sci*. 1979;24:560-564.

23. James TN. The protean nature of Whipple's disease includes multiorgan arteriopathy. *Trans Am Clin Climatol Assoc*. 2001;112:196-214.

24. Zaidi SA, Singer C. Gastrointestinal and hepatic manifestations of tickborne diseases in the United States. *Clin Infect Dis*. 2002;34:1206-1212.

25. Goellner MH, Agger WA, Burgess JH, et al. Hepatitis due to recurrent Lyme disease. *Ann Intern Med*. 1988;108:707-708.

26. Duray PH, Steere AC. Clinical pathologic correlations of Lyme disease by stage. *Ann N Y Acad Sci.* 1988;539:65-79.

27. Middelveen M, McClain S, Bandoski C, et al. *Granulomatous hepatitis associated with chronic Borrelia burgdorferi infection: a case report.* In: *Biology and Environmental Science Faculty Publications Volume Paper 33,* 2014.

28. Zanchi AC, Gingold AR, Theise ND, et al. Necrotizing granulomatous hepatitis as an unusual manifestation of Lyme disease. *Dig Dis Sci.* 2007;52:2629-2632.

29. Chavanet P, Pillon D, Lancon JP, et al. Granulomatous hepatitis associated with Lyme disease. *Lancet.* 1987;2:623-624.

30. Adams JS, Walker DH. The liver in Rocky Mountain spotted fever. *Am J Clin Pathol.* 1981;75:156-161.

31. Jackson MD, Kirkman C, Bradford WD, et al. Rocky mountain spotted fever: hepatic lesions in childhood cases. *Pediatr Pathol.* 1986;5:379-388.

32. Case records of the Massachusetts General Hospital. Weekly clinicopathological exercises. Case 22-2001. A 25-year-old woman with fever and abnormal liver function. *N Engl J Med.* 2001;345:201-205.

33. Gourdeau M, Lamothe F, Ishak M, et al. Hepatic abscess complicating ulceroglandular tularemia. *Can Med Assoc J.* 1983;129:1286-1288.

34. Ortego TJ, Hutchins LF, Rice J, et al. Tularemic hepatitis presenting as obstructive jaundice. *Gastroenterology.* 1986;91:461-463.

35. Lamps LW, Havens JM, Sjostedt A, et al. Histologic and molecular diagnosis of tularemia: a potential bioterrorism agent endemic to North America. *Mod Pathol.* 2004;17:489-495.

36. Sehdev AE, Dumler JS. Hepatic pathology in human monocytic ehrlichiosis. Ehrlichia chaffeensis infection. *Am J Clin Pathol.* 2003;119:859-865.

37. Sosa-Gutierrez CG, Solorzano-Santos F, Walker DH, et al. Fatal monocytic ehrlichiosis in woman, Mexico, 2013. *Emerg Infect Dis.* 2016;22:871-874.

38. Walker DH, Hawkins HK, Hudson P. Fulminant Rocky Mountain spotted fever. Its pathologic characteristics associated with glucose-6-phosphate dehydrogenase deficiency. *Arch Pathol Lab Med.* 1983;107:121-125.

39. Regan JJ, Traeger MS, Humpherys D, et al. Risk factors for fatal outcome from rocky mountain spotted Fever in a highly endemic area-Arizona, 2002-2011. *Clin Infect Dis.* 2015;60:1659-1666.

40. Ramphal R, Kluge R, Cohen V, et al. Rocky Mountain spotted fever and jaundice. Two consecutive cases acquired in Florida and a review of the literature on this complication. *Arch Intern Med.* 1978;138:260-263.

41. Horowitz HW, Dworkin B, Forseter G, et al. Liver function in early Lyme disease. *Hepatology.* 1996;23:1412-1417.

42. Kazakoff MA, Sinusas K, Macchia C. Liver function test abnormalities in early Lyme disease. *Arch Fam Med.* 1993;2:409-413.

43. Edwards KS, Kanengiser S, Li KI, et al. Lyme disease presenting as hepatitis and jaundice in a child. *Pediatr Infect Dis J.* 1990;9:592-593.

44. Rupani AB, Amarapurkar AD. Hepatic changes in fatal malaria: an emerging problem. *Ann Trop Med Parasitol.* 2009;103:119-127.

45. Whitten R, Milner DA Jr, Yeh MM, et al. Liver pathology in Malawian children with fatal encephalopathy. *Hum Pathol.* 2011;42:1230-1239.

46. Kochar DK, Singh P, Agarwal P, et al. Malarial hepatitis. *J Assoc Physicians India.* 2003;51:1069-1072.

47. Lowenthal MN, Hutt MS. Malarial pigment. *Br Med J.* 1969;2:635.

48. Day NP, Pham TD, Phan TL, et al. Clearance kinetics of parasites and pigment-containing leukocytes in severe malaria. *Blood*. 1996;88:4694-4700.

49. Atanasov G, Benckert C, Thelen A, et al. Alveolar echinococcosis-spreading disease challenging clinicians: a case report and literature review. *World J Gastroenterol*. 2013;19:4257-4261.

50. Arellano-Aguilar G, Marin-Santillan E, Castilla-Barajas JA, et al. A brief history of amoebic liver abscess with an illustrative case. *Rev Gastroenterol Méx*. 2017;82:344-348.

51. Roediger R, Lisker-Melman M. Pyogenic and amebic infections of the liver. *Gastroenterol Clin North Am*. 2020;49:361-377.

52. Mokhtari M, Kumar PV. Amebic liver abscess: fine needle aspiration diagnosis. *Acta Cytol*. 2014;58:225-228.

7

GRANULOMATOUS DISEASE

> **Key Points for Interpreting Biopsies That Have Granulomas**
> - Correlate with clinical findings.
> - Are the granulomas part of the disease process or an incidental finding?
> - Do they have necrosis or any other distinctive findings?
> - Are they centered on a specific structure in the liver?
> - Examine under polarized light for foreign material.
> - Examine acid-fast bacteria (AFB) and Grocott-Gomori methenamine–silver nitrate (GMS) stains, as indicated by clinical and histologic findings.
> - Use the best terminology in the pathology report to describe the findings.

GENERAL APPROACH TO GRANULOMAS

Granulomas are seen in approximately 4% of liver biopsy specimens.[1,2] They are associated with a heterogeneous set of disorders, but when an etiology is identified, the most common etiology are primary biliary cholangitits/cirrhosis (PBC), sarcoidosis, infection, drug effect, autoimmune conditions, and idiopathic (Table 7.1). Interestingly, idiopathic granulomas make up the single largest group of granulomas (35%), a consistent observation in studies for many decades. Livers with idiopathic granulomas tend to have both mild and nonprogressive diseases, and currently there is no data to suggest these granulomas are significant contributors to morbidity or mortality.

Also of note, what is known today about mapping granulomas to specific etiologies has been largely known for decades; in this area of diagnostic pathology, we have been on a knowledge plateau for a very long time. For this reason, review articles and book chapters from decades ago can still be relevant today. The biggest advance seems to be efforts at adopting more uniform terminology.

As shown in Table 7.1, PBC and sarcoidosis are consistently two of the most common etiologies of granulomas seen in liver biopsy specimens.

TABLE 7.1	**Etiologies for Hepatic Granulomas**	
Cause	Approximate Frequency (%)	Comment
PBC	45	Frequency depends on the study population, with higher frequencies in populations of northern European ethnicity
Idiopathic	35	
Sarcoidosis	10	
Infection	5	Frequency of infectious granulomas varies
Drugs	3	
Other (e.g., paraneoplastic, etc.)	2	

Note: The frequency of different causes varies somewhat but generally are as shown.[1,3-6] Presented data is mostly from the United States, the United Kingdom, and Europe. Studies from other parts of the world often have fewer cases of primary biliary cirrhosis/cholangitis (PBC) and sarcoidosis but more infection-associated granulomas.[7].

In most of the published literature, however, studies collected data from sequential biopsies to determine the frequency and etiology of granulomas. In many (most?) of these case series, the diagnosis of PBC or sarcoidosis was known or strongly suspected clinically before the biopsy. Thus, there is very little data on the frequency or etiologies for cases of *unsuspected* granulomas in liver biopsy specimens, but, in my experience, unsuspected granulomas tend to be either idiopathic (when sparse and not part of a broader injury pattern) or caused by infections or drug reactions.

Most granulomas do not directly involve specific anatomic structures, such as bile ducts or blood vessels, but when this does occur, it can provide important clues to the etiology (Table 7.2).

DEFINITION. Granulomas are well-delineated clusters of epithelioid histiocytes. If multiple granulomas are present then you can use the term *granulomas* or *granulomata*, depending on how sophisticated you feel that day. Granulomas are typically round to ovoid and often have intermixed lymphocytes (Figure 7.1). Different morphologic variants, described in more detail later, can provide clues to the differential diagnosis; they are not going to be specific for etiology, however, unless you find organisms or foreign material.

Granulomas can be part of a systemic disease process, where granulomas involved many different organ systems, or can be limited to the liver. This distinction cannot be made by histologic findings alone and clinical correlation is important. Some conditions, such as PBC, are discussed in more detail in separate sections of the book.

Terminology for Granulomas

- Granuloma: cluster of epithelioid histiocytes.
- Granulomatous disease: a disease in which granulomas are a common or characteristic finding.
- Granulomatous hepatitis: a brisk lobular hepatitis, typically moderate or severe, associated with lobular granulomas.
- Granulomatous inflammation: a focal inflammatory lesion that has loose clusters of histiocytes.
- Microgranuloma: an older term that is best to not use; a better term is *Kupffer cell aggregate.*

TABLE 7.2 Granulomas Associated With Anatomic Structures	
Anatomic Structure	**Most Common Etiologies**
Bile duct	PBC with a florid duct lesion (most common)
	Drug reaction (uncommon)
Portal veins or central veins	Sarcoidosis[8]
	Schistosomiasis
	Drug reaction
	Histoplasmosis
	Bacterial infection[9]
Hepatic artery	ANCA-associated vasculitis
	Polyarteritis nodosa
	Giant cell arteritis

ANCA, antineutrophil cytoplasmic autoantibody; PBC, primary biliary cirrhosis.

At the practical level of diagnostic pathology, the etiology of granulomas is usually not evident by histology alone. Nonetheless, there can be clues that will help you weigh the differential from more likely to less likely and this information can be very helpful to your clinical colleagues. Remember that simply listing a generic differential for granulomas in your surgical pathology report is not terribly helpful, as that generic differential is already known to most physicians, having been mastered by them in medical school.

Granulomas vary in size, with most granulomas in the liver being either small or medium sized. Sometimes this question arises: what is the minimum size acceptable for a granuloma? A good rule of thumb is that if the focus in question is so small or disorganized that you are not sure if it is a granuloma, then it is probably not a granuloma. Counting histiocytes is not much fun and is not recommended, but for the record, a common (but arbitrary) cutoff is often set at five (or sometimes seven) epithelioid

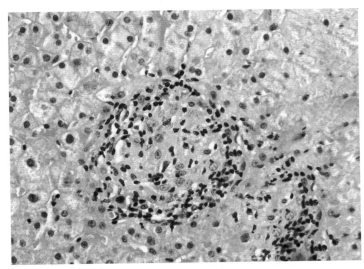

FIGURE 7.1 **Granuloma, epithelioid.** The granuloma is well circumscribed and composed of epithelioid histiocytes with admixed lymphocytes.

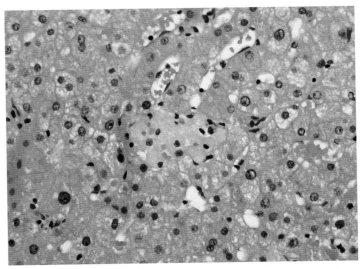

FIGURE 7.2 **Kupffer cell aggregate.** The lobules show small Kupffer cell aggregates in this case of resolving hepatitis.

histiocytes. A common reason for nomenclature uncertainty is small clusters of sinusoidal histiocytes/Kupffer cell aggregates in the setting of an active or resolving lobular hepatitis. These are not true granulomas but instead can be called *Kupffer cell aggregates* (Figure 7.2). An older term, *microgranuloma*, is discouraged because they are not "granulomas that are micro in size" but instead represent a different physiologic process. Kupffer cell aggregates represent sites of recent injury that are undergoing repair/remodeling/cleanup, whereas a true granuloma represents an immune response to a persistent antigen that cannot be quickly cleared by the body. True granulomas are typically periodic acid-Schiff with diastase (PASD) negative, whereas Kupffer cell aggregates are PASD positive. Even if you do not find the differences in biology sufficiently convincing to drop the use of the term *microgranuloma*, the term still is best avoided for practical reasons because it creates confusion with true granulomas, by both clinicians and patients.

Granulomatous disease is used to describe diseases that commonly have granulomas as part of the typical histologic findings, such as PBC, sarcoidosis, common variable immunodeficiency, and some infections, such as tuberculosis and fungal infections, and some parasites. On the other hand, there are many diseases that occasionally have granulomas, but the granulomas are not a consistent or typical part of the findings. For example, chronic hepatitis C virus (HCV) infection, chronic hepatitis B (HBV) infection, and fatty liver disease can all have small granulomas in about 1% of biopsy specimens,[10,11] but none of these are considered granulomatous diseases. In fact, referring to such cases as granulomatous hepatitis or granulomatous disease in your biopsy report can lead to clinical confusion. A better approach is to diagnose the chronic liver disease (such as chronic viral hepatitis or fatty liver disease) in the usual way and then mention that, as an additional finding, there are small, incidental epithelioid granulomas.

GRANULOMATOUS HEPATITIS refers to cases that show a hepatitic pattern of injury, plus granulomas. The granulomas are usually in the lobules, but they can be present in both the lobules and the portal tracts, and are typically multiple. As mentioned earlier, a small percentage of cases of chronic viral hepatitis, fatty liver disease, and many other etiology of chronic hepatitis can have rare, small incidental granulomas; these types of cases are not classified as granulomatous hepatitis. The differential for granulomatous hepatitis is primarily infection versus drug-induced liver injury.

GRANULOMATOUS INFLAMMATION as a term can overlap conceptually with *granulomatous hepatitis*, but the term *granulomatous inflammation* is generally used to describe a focal lesion, one located in either the portal tracts or the lobules, where there is inflammation associated with a poorly formed granuloma, the granuloma typically consisting of a loose aggregate of histiocytes. In general, the term *poorly formed granuloma* is used when there is a cluster of histiocytes that is not sharply demarcated like a true granuloma. The histiocytes are less epithelioid and often have foamy cytoplasm, in contrast to true granulomas, which are composed of a well-demarcated cluster of epithelioid histiocytes.

SYSTEMATIC APPROACH TO GRANULOMAS

Different types of granulomas have distinct but overlapping differentials. A systematic approach is very helpful, and you will comfortably handle most liver biopsies that have granulomas. Several broad principles can be helpful to quickly get you into the most likely differential.

PRINCIPLE 1. IMPORTANCE OF CLINICAL AND LABORATORY CORRELATES. Clinical or laboratory findings are often not available or are not informative, but they are worth seeking in difficult cases, as they can be very helpful. Useful clinical history includes potential occupational or hobby exposures, travel history, medication use, tick-bite history, injection drug use, or immunosuppression.

Occupations Associated With Hepatic Granulomas

- Silicosis: jobs such as sandblasting[12] and working with dry cement[13]
- Copper sulfate: mildew prevention in agriculture[14]
- Animal husbandry (brucellosis)
- Veterinarian (various animal-transmitted infections)

Hobbies Potentially Associated With Hepatic Granulomas

- Hunting, trapping (tick-bite exposure, alveolar echinococcosis)
- Spelunking (histoplasmosis, leptospirosis)
- Hiking (tick-bite exposure)
- Pet birds (psittacosis)

PRINCIPLE 2. DECIDE IF GRANULOMAS ARE THE MAIN FINDINGS IN THE BIOPSY OR PART OF A LARGER DISEASE PATTERN. It is helpful to decide if the liver disease is primarily a result of the granulomas, or if the granulomas are one part of a larger pattern of injury. For example, in sarcoidosis, the granulomas are often the primary manifestation of the disease seen on liver biopsy. As another example, in tuberculosis, granulomas can be the only significant histologic finding. As a contrasting example, granulomas in PBC, when present, are but one component of a typically larger disease pattern.

PRINCIPLE 3. GRANULOMA MORPHOLOGY AND LOCATION. Granulomas that have central necrosis are most likely infectious in origin (Figure 7.3). Look carefully for organisms, such as those causing schistosomiasis, and perform fungal stains and acid-fast stains on all cases with necrotizing granulomas. You should do fungal and acid-fast bacteria (AFB) stains even if you see parasitic organisms in some of the granulomas on

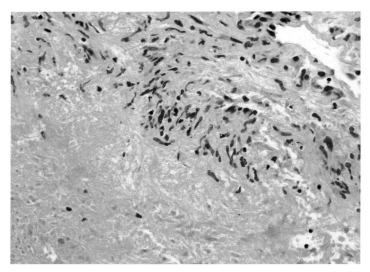

FIGURE 7.3 **Necrotizing granuloma.** This consult case showed necrotizing granulomas in an individual with acute-onset hepatitis. The findings are strongly suspicious for organisms, even though no organisms were seen on special stains.

hematoxylin-eosin (H&E), as multiple infections can coexist. In suspicious cases, it can be helpful to do a second set of AFB and GMS stains on deeper cut sections. Organism stains show negative results in many necrotizing granulomas, but your report should still convey that the granulomas are suspicious for infection. Rarely, large granulomas from other diseases, such as sarcoidosis, can have central hyalinization that mimics necrosis. In these cases, the hyalinized center is typically fibrinoid and brightly eosinophilic but is without the "dirty" nuclear and cellular debris seen in most necrotizing granulomas. Rare cases of large, noninfectious, but necrotizing, granulomas might occur in the liver, at least they have been reported in the literature, but they are always a diagnosis of exclusion.

Epithelioid granulomas should be polarized (Figures 7.4 and 7.5)—the H&E findings alone can sometimes indicate the presence of foreign material, but in other cases the correct diagnosis is achieved only after polarization. While you will polarize a whole lot of granulomas before you find a positive one, it is still an important part of the workup.

Outside of cases where granulomatous inflammation directly involves a blood vessel or a bile duct, the overall location of the granulomas, whether they are in the portal tracts, lobules, or both, does not provide a strong clue to the etiology.

PRINCIPLE 4. CLASSIC SARCOIDOSIS PATTERN. The most common sarcoidosis pattern is one where granulomas are the primary finding in the biopsy, with little or no inflammation, fatty change, or biliary tract disease. The

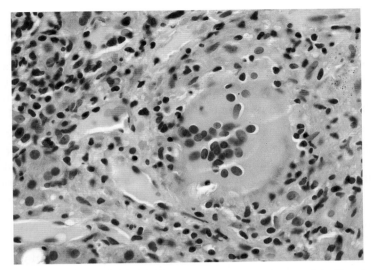

FIGURE 7.4 **Foreign body granuloma.** In this liver biopsy from an injection-drug-using individual, granulomas with foreign material are seen.

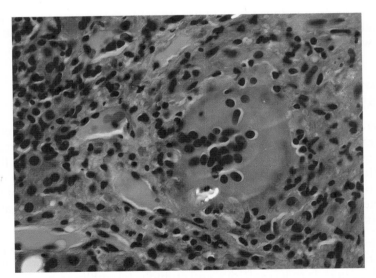

FIGURE 7.5 **Foreign body granuloma, polarization.** The foreign material polarizes (same field as preceding image).

granulomas can be located in the portal tracts or the lobules, but tend to be mostly in the portal tracts. The granulomas often appear to be of "varying ages," including older fibrotic granulomas as well as plump, fresh epithelioid granulomas. A diagnosis of sarcoidosis is never made on biopsy alone.

PRINCIPLE 5. GRANULOMATOUS BILIARY TRACT DISEASE HAS A LIMITED DIFFER-ENTIAL. Granulomatous biliary tract disease, where granulomas/granulomatous inflammation is directly associated with active bile duct injury, is most likely to be PBC or drug-induced liver injury. Parasitic infections of the biliary tree can also cause granulomatous biliary tract disease, but they are hardly ever encountered in liver biopsy specimens. Sarcoidosis has rarely been reported to have granulomas directly causing bile duct injury.

PRINCIPLE 6. GRANULOMATOUS HEPATITIS HAS A LIMITED DIFFERENTIAL. Granulomatous hepatitis shows moderate or marked lobular hepatitis and usually results from infection or drug-induced liver injury. The list of potential drugs that can cause granulomas is huge and ever growing and there is little point in trying to memorize them all. It is better for patient care to look up the medications that are being used by a patient in an actively maintained database—online sources are probably the best. Nonetheless, there are some drugs that are well known for causing granulomatous hepatitis and it can be useful to have a few of them tucked away in your memory: allopurinol, hydralazine, isoniazid, nitrofurantoin, and phenytoin.

PRINCIPLE 7. ACUTE-ONSET GRANULOMATOUS HEPATITIS. Cases of granulomatous liver disease presenting as acute-onset hepatitis are almost always an infection or drug-induced liver injury. In some cases, patients can present with febrile disease, which is mostly seen with infections but also sometimes with drug effects.

MORPHOLOGIC TYPES OF GRANULOMAS AND THEIR DISEASE CORRELATES

EPITHELIOID GRANULOMAS are the most common type of granuloma encountered in liver pathology. These granulomas are defined by an aggregate of histiocytes that has sharp borders, separating the granuloma from the surrounding tissue. Granulomas are typically amphophilic to slightly eosinophilic on low and medium power, with most being small to medium in size. Admixed lymphocytes are common. They are typically PASD negative, in contrast to Kupffer cell aggregates, which are PASD positive.

CASEATING GRANULOMAS. The term *caseating* or *caseation* is a gross pathology term derived from the Latin word for cheese, *caseus*, and is used to describe a nodule that is soft, dry, and crumbly, resembling a hunk of cheese. The term *caseating* is also commonly used to describe the corresponding microscopic findings, which show "dirty necrosis," with nuclear debris and dead cellular material in the center of a granuloma. Some authors prefer to use the term *caseating* only for gross findings and *necrotizing* for the microscopic findings, but overall, they tend to be used interchangeably.

Caseating/necrotizing granulomas are almost always infectious in origin. Necrosis typically involves a reasonably sized area of the granuloma; by way of contrast, it is not uncommon to see tiny areas, of a few cells in

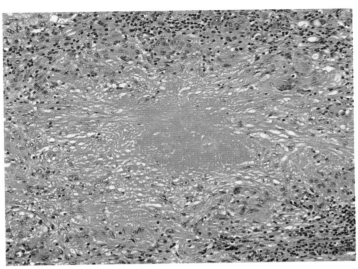

FIGURE 7.6 **Hyalinized granuloma.** This large sarcoidal granuloma shows central hyalinization but does not show necrosis.

size, in the center of a large granuloma that show increased eosinophilia, but these foci are not caseating necrosis. In fact, many reports of necrotizing granulomas associated with noninfectious causes fall into this category of tiny foci of fibrinous hyalinization, which does not represent true caseation. In other cases, large granulomas can have central degeneration and hyalinization (Figure 7.6), a finding unfortunately often called fibrinoid necrosis; this pattern is also not biologically equivalent to true caseating necrosis.

Rare cases of sarcoidal granulomas with true necrosis have been reported, but it is important to be very cautious before believing a caseating granuloma is not infectious. Sarcoidal granulomas with necrosis tend to be very large and are hardly ever sampled on liver biopsy, which instead typically samples small- or medium-sized granulomas. Sarcoidal granulomas sufficiently large to become necrotic are more common in lymph nodes of the lung.

Fibrin Ring Granulomas

The centers of fibrin ring granulomas contain a single large droplet of fat, which is surrounded by an eosinophilic fibrin ring of varying thickness, and then an outermost layer of macrophages. In the most ideal examples, a layer of histiocyte nuclei can also be seen between the fat and the fibrin ring (Figure 7.7).

Fibrin ring granulomas were first described in Q fever but can be seen in a wide range of conditions (Table 7.3). Other findings in the rest of the biopsy can provide clues to the possible etiology, but in most cases

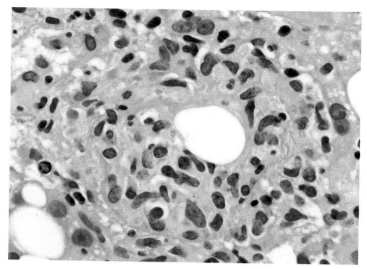

FIGURE 7.7 **Fibrin ring granuloma.** There is a central droplet of fat. The next layer is composed of histiocytes and a few lymphocytes, then there is a thin pink layer of fibrin, followed by an outer layer of histiocytes.

TABLE 7.3   Causes of Fibrin Ring Granulomas
Cause
Infection
Cytomegalovirus[1]
Hepatitis A[15,16]
Epstein-Barr virus[17]
Chronic hepatitis C[18]
Coxiella burnetii (Q fever)[19,20]
Boutonneuse fever (*Rickettsia conorii*)[21]
Toxoplasmosis[21]
Leishmaniasis[22,23]
Disseminated *Staphylococcus epidermidis*[24]
Medications
Allopurinol[23,25,26]
Checkpoint inhibitors (cancer therapy)[27]
Others
Giant cell arteritis[28]
Hodgkin disease[21]
Lupus and *Staphylococcus aureus* sepsis[29]
Idiopathic[30]

the etiology is determined by serologic testing or other laboratory testing. Fibrin ring granulomas are most commonly associated with infection or drug effect and that should be conveyed in the pathology report, even if an etiology is not clear at the time the pathology report is released.

While the morphology is distinctive, fibrin ring granulomas are almost always associated with an acute hepatitis that is superimposed on a background of fatty liver disease; thus, in most cases, the distinctive morphology probably reflects the cleanup of dead hepatocytes that contained fat and not much more than that. Rare cases of fibrin ring granulomas have been reported in livers that have no or minimal fat, however, so there may be additional mechanisms.[27]

FIBROTIC GRANULOMAS are exactly that—granulomas that have elicited fibrotic responses. Fibrotic granulomas tend be medium to large in size, noncaseating, and epithelioid. Most often, they are actually composed of an aggregate of smaller coalesced and fibrotic granulomas, with fibrosis involving the entire aggregate, extending around and within the individual granulomas (Figure 7.8; eFig. 7.1). Overall, most granulomas with this fibrotic morphology result from sarcoidosis. Fibrotic granulomas can also be seen with schistosomiasis, but they tend to be smaller and do not form distinct aggregates. In addition, large, single, fibrotic granulomas can represent old histoplasmosis or other infections; in many of these cases, there can be central hyalinization that should not be mistaken for necrosis. In time, some of these old granulomas are completely converted to fibrous scars.

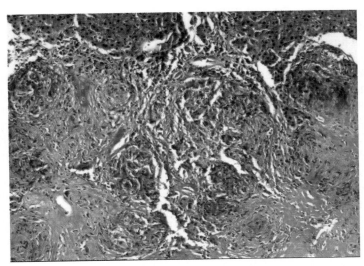

FIGURE 7.8 **Sarcoidosis, trichrome stain.** Fibrosis extends into and through the granuloma. A cuff of fibrosis can be seen with many long-standing granulomas, but fibrosis extending through the granulomas is more common with sarcoidosis.

FLORID DUCT LESIONS. A florid duct lesion is a medium-sized bile duct that is cuffed and infiltrated by lymphocytes, all of which is surrounded by ill-defined aggregates of macrophages. The duct epithelium is injured, often appearing disheveled, and has reactive changes. In rare cases, well-formed epithelioid granulomas are also present in the portal tract, but generally not as part of the florid duct lesion itself. The differential for florid duct lesions is essentially PBC (large majority of cases) versus drug-induced liver injury.

Foreign Body Granulomas. Foreign-Body-Type Granulomas

- Silica (usually occupational)[31]
- Beryllium
- Injection drug use (talc granulomas usually)[32]
- Prior surgery[33]
- Embolization therapy
- Worn prosthetic joints[34]
- Worn dental prostheses (porcelain material)[35]
- Silicone breast implants[36]
- Food (pulse granulomas)[37]

Foreign body granulomas in the liver can result from many different causes (eFigs. 7.2 and 7.3). Talc granulomas from injection drug use are usually incidental findings in patients with chronic HCV or HBV infection (Figures 7.9 and 7.10); they are not as commonly seen in practice today, as the clinical need for liver biopsies to manage chronic viral hepatitis has diminished. Other potential causes include prior abdominal surgery, interventional radiology procedures such as tumor embolization, and joint replacements (Figure 7.11). In some cases, the cause is not clear from the available history. The diagnosis is made by either seeing the foreign material on H&E stain (not all foreign material polarizes) or polarizing the granuloma and identifying the birefringent material. Exposure to heavy metals, such as beryllium, can also lead to granulomas, although granulomas are more commonly found in the lungs or skin than in the liver.

LIPOGRANULOMAS, sometimes also called *lipid granulomas*, are commonly encountered in surgical pathology specimens. They are composed of poorly formed clusters of macrophages with foamy cytoplasm and variously sized droplets of fat/lipid (Figure 7.12; eFig. 7.4). Most lipogranulomas are located in portal tracts next to portal veins, or are located next to central veins.[38] Lipogranulomas, especially when located in zone 3, may be associated with focal fibrosis, but by themselves do not affect fibrosis progression in chronic liver disease.

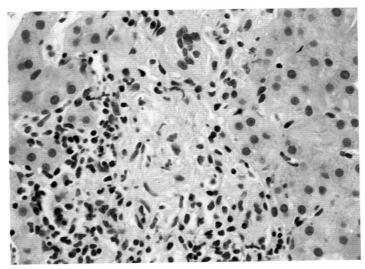

FIGURE 7.9 **Foreign body granuloma.** This liver biopsy, from a person with a history of injection drug use, shows talc granulomas.

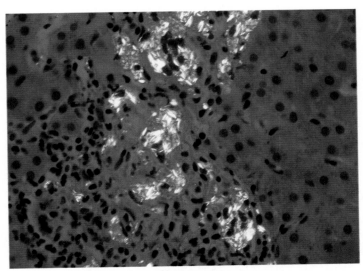

FIGURE 7.10 **Foreign body granuloma, polarization.** Polarization of the same field as seen in the preceding image shows the needle-shaped structures of talc.

Lipogranulomas appear to have two separate etiologies; they were first described in association with the ingestion of mineral oil, a commonly used food additive,[39,40] but in the current practice of surgical pathology, they are most commonly seen in fatty liver disease[41,42] and chronic HCV infection.[41] In the latter two disease settings, they have a frequency of

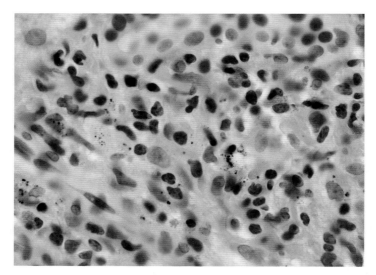

FIGURE 7.11 **Foreign body granuloma, titanium**. Brown-black pigment is seen, consistent with titanium. The patient had a history of a knee replacement.

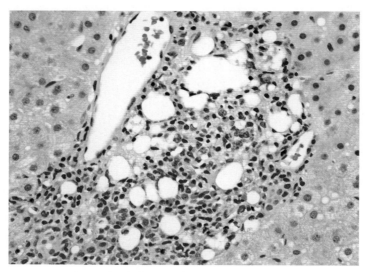

FIGURE 7.12 **Lipogranuloma**. The portal tract shows a loose collection of lymphocytes and macrophages, with many of the macrophages having fat droplets.

about 10%.[41,43] The histologic findings do not readily distinguish between the etiologies, but that is fine because the most important points to know are that they should not be mistaken for conventional granulomas, have no clinical significance, and do not need to be mentioned in the surgical pathology report.

GRANULOMAS ASSOCIATED WITH INFECTIONS

Granulomas can be seen with bacterial infections, viral infection, fungal infection, and parasites (Table 7.4). For the most part, there are no specific histologic findings that will allow confident diagnosis for the cause of the granulomas on H&E stain, with the exception of finding parasitic organisms. For this reason, organism stains are critical tools for evaluating granulomas. Specific infections are discussed in the following sections, but two important points should be kept in mind. First, infections do not always "read the book" and there can be substantial overlap for the histologic findings between different infectious organisms. Second, evaluating granulomas in the liver can be challenging, but doubly so if clinical findings are not incorporated into the histologic evaluation.

TABLE 7.4 Infections Associated With Granulomas
Cause
Fungal infections
Aspergillus
Candida
Cryptococcus neoformans
Cryptococcus gattii
Coccidioidomycosis[44]
Histoplasmosis
Mucor
Viral infections
Epstein-Barr virus[17]
Chronic hepatitis C[18]
Hepatitis A[15,16]
Hepatitis E
Cytomegalovirus[1]
Bacterial infections
Bartonella henselae[1]
Brucellosis
Chlamydia psittaci (zoonotic infection from birds)[45]
Coxiella burnetii (Q fever)[19,20]
Listeria[1]
Nocardiosis[46]
Psittacosis (caused by *C. psittaci*, mostly through exposure of pet birds)[47]
Rhodococcus equi
Rickettsia conorii (boutonneuse fever)[21]

(Continued)

TABLE 7.4	Infections Associated With Granulomas (Continued)
Cause	
Salmonella	
Staphylococcus epidermidis[24]	
Tularemia	
Yersinia pseudotuberculosis[1]	
Whipple disease	
Bacterial spirochetes	
Borrelia burgdorferi (Lyme disease)[48]	
Treponema pallidum (syphilis)[49]	
Mycobacteria	
Mycobacterium tuberculosis	
Mycobacterium leprae	
Mycobacterium avium-intracellulare	
Protozoa	
Toxoplasma gondii (toxoplasmosis)[21]	
Leishmaniasis[22,23]	
Parasites	
Schistosomiasis	
Giardia in the gastrointestinal tract[50]	

BARTONELLA HENSELAE. This bacterium had its name changed a few times; older names no longer in use include Afipia felis and Rochalimaea henselae. The early genus name of Afipia was awarded to honor the Armed Forces Institutes of Pathology, where the organism was first cultured.[51]

BARTONELLA HENSELAE is the cause of cat-scratch disease, a disease described in 1950 by Robert Debré, a French pediatrician, who reported self-limited regional lymphadenopathy in patients following cat scratches.[52,53] In most cases of cat-scratch disease, a localized infection results from the scratch, leading to infection of the lymph nodes draining that area of the skin. A very small subset of individuals, often children and teenagers, can develop disseminated disease that may involve the liver. Affected individuals typically are immunocompetent and present with systemic findings of fever, weight loss, and malaise. Liver lesions are frequently multiple and can resemble tumors on imaging studies.[54] The hilar lymph nodes are also commonly enlarged,[54] further mimicking potential metastatic disease.

Biopsies, when they "read the book," show irregular geographic areas of neutrophilic inflammation admixed with necrotic fibroinflammatory

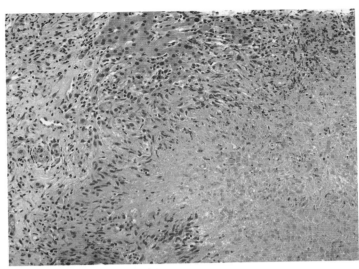

FIGURE 7.13 **Bartonella**. Palisading histiocytes surround an area of irregular, geographic necrosis.

debris, all surrounded by an inner layer of histiocytes and a second outer layer of lymphocytes (Figure 7.13). In the most perfect cases, the histiocytes that form the cuff surrounding the areas of central necrosis will show a somewhat vague nuclear alignment or "palisading." The lesion can also have an additional outer layer created by a thick fibrous rim surrounding the entire lesion. This overall classic set of findings is best seen on wedge biopsies. Immunostains for organisms (Warthin-Starry or Steiner) can be helpful. Organisms are usually (or at least most confidently) identified in small clumps, but also can be found as single organisms. Areas of necrosis are usually the best hunting ground to find the organisms. Special stains are positive in only one-third of cases,[55] and the diagnosis relies on serologic studies more than histochemical stains. *B. henselae* can also cause peliosis hepatis.[56] Finally, silver stains can have a lot of background, so it can be very helpful to review a positive control to refresh your memory of the organism's morphology before you evaluate the stain.

BRUCELLOSIS. *Brucella* is named after Sir David Bruce, who isolated the organism in 1887 from British soldiers who died from "Malta fever." In 1905, the source of infection was identified as goat milk and cheese by the Maltese physician Themistocles Zammit.[57] Today, brucella infection is rare and most commonly seen in individuals working with livestock. There is generally a 2- to 4-week latency period. Infection is transmitted to humans most often by aerosol from infected animals. Human to human transmission is rare. Infections can also occur after ingesting undercooked contaminated foods, unpasteurized milk, or unpasteurized cheese. Laboratory infection has also been reported and should be considered in laboratory workers who develop unexplained infection-type symptoms.[58]

Affected individuals generally present with fevers, headaches, arthralgia, and malaise. The fevers are typically acute in onset but can wax and wane in intensity. Hepatomegaly and lymphadenopathy are commonly present. Liver biopsy specimens range in their findings from nonspecific inflammatory changes (most common) to granulomatous hepatitis. The granulomas are noncaseating and can range all the way from poorly formed granulomas to discrete, well-formed epithelioid granulomas. The frequency of granulomas varies considerably in different studies, ranging from 10% to 100% of cases, likely because of different time intervals from infection to biopsy and because of different sources of infection, as granulomas may be less common in *Brucella melitensis* (source: goat and sheep) compared with *Brucella abortus* (source: bovine).[59-62] Organisms are generally not evident on special stains but can be seen if an abscess develops; *Brucella* is a gram-negative coccobacilli.

LISTERIOSIS. The genus *Listeria* is named in honor of Sir Joseph Lister, a British surgeon who pioneered early antiseptic methods in surgery, using phenol to sterilize surgical instruments and to clean wounds. The mouthwash Listerine is named in his honor. Interestingly, Lister's father (Joseph Jackson Lister) was a physicist who made important contributions to the development of microscopes.

Listeria monocytogenes is primarily a foodborne pathogen. The bacterium is remarkably sturdy; it can grow at 0 °C and is considerably resistant to freeze-thaw cycles as well as heat. Common contaminated foods include unpasteurized milk; cheese, particularly soft cheese; raw vegetables; and raw and smoked meats. While infection is not particularly common, outbreaks occur every year throughout the world, including the United States. For example, the CDC (https://www.cdc.gov/) lists outbreaks in the United States in 2020 from deli meats and enoki mushrooms; in 2019 from hard-boiled eggs, deli meats, and cheeses; and in 2018 from deli ham and other pork products.

There are approximately 1600 infections per year in the United States, with a death rate of 15%. Listeriosis most commonly affects neonates, immunocompromised persons, pregnant women (about 30% of all cases), or the elderly (about 50% of all cases). The primary site of infection is the small intestine. The histologic findings with hepatic involvement vary, but typically there are scattered microabscesses (small clusters of neutrophils within the sinusoidal) as well as small, epithelioid granulomas. Larger, epithelioid granulomas can be occasionally found. The organism is a short pleomorphic gram-positive rod, but organisms are typically sparse and hard to find on special stains.

MYCOBACTERIUM TUBERCULOSIS (MTB) was first identified in 1882 by Robert Koch (whose Koch postulates laid the foundation for modern microbiology).

The infection is spread by aerosolization, usually by coughing or sneezing. The organism primarily causes respiratory tract disease, but in a subset of individuals the liver is involved. If the pulmonary vein becomes eroded and organisms directly access the pulmonary veins, miliary tuberculosis to the liver can develop.

In one autopsy study, hepatic granulomas were found in approximately 40% of individuals with MTB infection. The granulomas were caseating in 60%, noncaseating in 25%, and "atypical" in 15% of cases.[63] In 20% of cases, there was secondary obstructive biliary tract disease caused by enlarged, granulomatous hilar lymph nodes that compressed the extrahepatic bile ducts. In MTB cases that did not have granulomas, the liver often showed mild fatty change and nonspecific chronic inflammation. Fibrosis was relatively uncommon, being found in 15% of all cases, with 7% of the livers showing bridging fibrosis or cirrhosis.[63] Of note, biopsy-based studies typically find a lower rate of granulomatous disease than autopsy-based studies.

MTB granulomas are typically small to medium in size (Figure 7.14). The organisms are identified on AFB stains as small, red rods, usually with very few organisms present (Figure 7.15). Because the organisms are almost always sparse, a repeat AFB stain on deeper levels can sometimes be helpful. Other clinical and laboratory findings can help arrive at a diagnosis in those cases where organisms are not seen.

Tuberculomas, or large aggregates of granulomas causing a pseudotumors, have been reported.[64] Histologically, the granulomas in tuberculomas can show extensive central caseating necrosis, often with a rim of giant cells. The tuberculomas can also show broad bands of fibrosis.

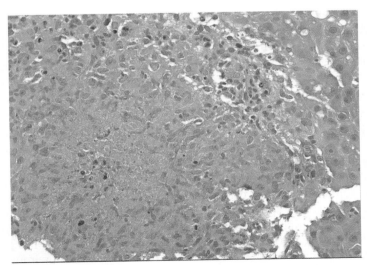

FIGURE 7.14 **Necrotizing granuloma, *Mycobacterium tuberculosis*.** This medium-sized granuloma shows central necrosis.

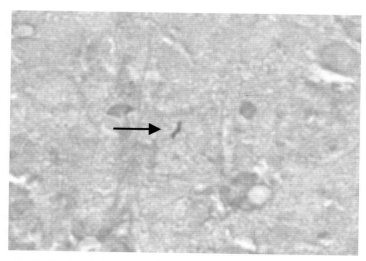

FIGURE 7.15 **Necrotizing granuloma, *Mycobacterium tuberculosis*, acid-fast stain.** Rare organisms are seen on acid-fast stain (*arrow*).

MYCOBACTERIUM CHIMAERA is an uncommon infection associated with open-heart surgery, where the mycobacteria colonize the heart valve prostheses and/or vascular grafts. In some patients, the infection can then disseminate and involve the liver.[65] The organism is slow growing and patients often do not present with symptoms until a year or so after surgery (median of 14 months); common symptoms are fever and weight loss. Despite this, the infection is challenging to treat and there can be a high mortality rate.

The liver biopsies typically show Kupffer cell hyperplasia with ill-defined aggregates of Kupffer cells, occasional Langerhans type giant cells in the sinusoids, and sometimes larger, non-necrotizing, epithelioid granulomas (Figure 7.16).[66] There can also be mild lobular cholestasis, sometimes subtle, and changes of vascular outflow disease, such as sinusoidal dilation and congestion.[66]

MYCOBACTERIUM AVIUM-INTRACELLULARE COMPLEX. This infection occurs primarily in individuals with significant immunosuppression, most commonly with end-stage HIV infection. Well-formed epithelioid granulomas are uncommon, outside of rare cases in immunocompetent individuals. Instead, most cases show aggregates of foamy macrophages in the sinusoids and portal tracts. The foamy macrophages are quite distinctive, but are not specific, and other infections that can manifest with similar findings include *Mycobacterium leprae*, *Rhodococcus equi*, and Whipple disease. With *Mycobacterium avium-intracellulare* infection, an AFB stain typically shows large numbers of organisms in immunosuppressed individuals but only rare to absent organisms in immunocompetent individuals.

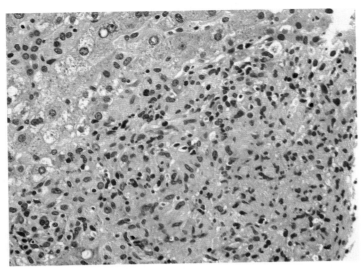

FIGURE 7.16 *Mycobacterium chimaera.* A large epithelioid, noncaseating granuloma is seen.

MYCOBACTERIUM LEPRAE. Leprosy (or Hansen disease) is a mycobacterial disease long recognized for its dreaded chronic, deforming disease. The primary injury is to the skin and peripheral nerves. The routes of transmission are not completely clear but appear most likely to be aerosolization. Reservoirs of infection include primates and some armadillo species. Liver involvement is classified as either lepromatous leprosy or as tuberculoid leprosy. Lepromatous leprosy has scattered, small aggregates of foamy histiocytes in the lobules (Figure 7.17) and portal tracts, typically with numerous organisms on Fite stain (Figure 7.18), while tuberculoid leprosy shows epithelioid granulomas, and organisms are often hard to find on acid-fast stains. There is significant variation in the relative frequency of lepromatous versus tuberculoid leprosy in different parts of the world. For example, tuberculoid leprosy is common in India and Africa, while lepromatous leprosy is more common in Mexico. This may reflect genetic differences in patients, environmental differences, or different species of *Mycobacterium.*[67]

BACILLUS CALMETTE-GUÉRIN. Vaccination with bacillus Calmette-Guérin (BCG) is common in many countries with high endemic rates of MTB, as vaccination is safe in immunocompetent persons and prevents early-life MTB infections, miliary MTB, and meningeal forms of MTB. Rarely, patients with undiagnosed immunodeficiency will get the vaccination and develop either local/regional infections (BCGitis) or disseminated disease (BCGosis), which can involve the liver.[68]

    Intravesicular BCG is commonly used to treat transitional cell carcinoma of the bladder, where it causes inflammation and scarring that destroys the carcinoma. In a small subset of individuals (about 4%), the

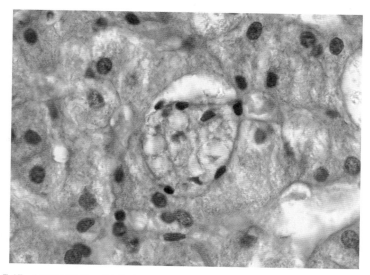

FIGURE 7.17 **Leprosy.** Small lobular aggregates of foamy macrophages are seen in this case of leprosy involving the liver.

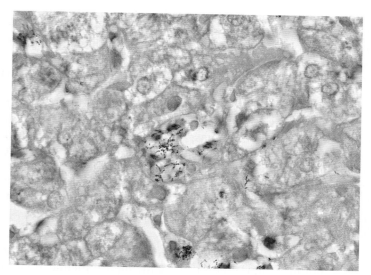

FIGURE 7.18 **Leprosy, Fite stain.** The organisms show a delicate beaded staining pattern.

organisms escape the bladder and cause disseminated infections,[69] which can involve the liver. Patients commonly present with fever and may have elevated liver enzyme levels and jaundice.[63,70] Liver biopsies typically show scattered, small, noncaseating granulomas (Figure 7.19; eFig. 7.5) in the lobules and portal tracts, with minimal to mild portal and lobular lymphocytic

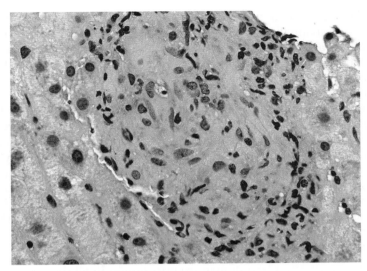

FIGURE 7.19 **Granuloma from bacillus Calmette-Guérin (BCG) therapy.** After BCG therapy for bladder cancer, the patient presented with fevers and elevated liver enzyme levels;
a biopsy showed granulomas.

inflammation. The organisms can be identified by AFB stains; if the AFB
stain results are negative and the clinical history is suspicious, then PCR
testing can be helpful. Patients are treated with a combination of antituber-
culosis drugs and steroids.[69]

SALMONELLA hepatitis is caused by either Salmonella *typhi* or S*almonella
paratyphi*. Infected patients can have sustained fevers, malaise, and delirium. The name is derived from the Greek word *typhos*, literally meaning a
stupor, smoke, or vapor of the mind, a term that captures the delirium that
often accompanies severe cases of typhoid fever.

Typhoid fever is an ancient disease that is thought to be the cause of
many historically important outbreaks, or plagues. For example, a plague
in Athens in 430 BC killed almost one-third of the population, including the great statesman Pericles, who was leading Athen's war efforts
against Sparta. Recent studies also suggest William Henry Harrison, the
9th President of the United States, died from typhoid fever in 1841, after
only 1 month in office, with exposure coming through contaminated water
supplies in Washington, DC.[71]

Long before the bacteria causing typhoid fever was identified (reported
in 1880 by Karl Joseph Eberth, a German microbiologist and pathologist
at the University of Zurich), the disease was thought to be likely infectious
and to be spread by contaminated water. While there are still 10 to 20
million cases of typhus per year worldwide, the disease has been mostly
eliminated in wealthier countries through the combination of improved
sanitation, chlorinated water supplies, and vaccination.

Most salmonella infections are gastrointestinal focused, but 10% to 20% of individuals also have liver disease. The liver disease manifests primarily as jaundice, with normal or mild elevations in serum aspartate transaminase (AST), alanine transaminase (ALT), and alkaline phosphatase levels.[72]

Histologically, salmonella hepatitis shows a generalized lobular Kupffer cell hyperplasia, often accompanied by mild nonspecific inflammatory changes and mild lobular cholestasis.[73,74] The Kupffer cells can focally aggregate into granuloma-like nodules called "typhoid nodules." The nodules are composed of histiocytes with admixed lymphocytes and sometimes show erythrophagocytosis; they can have a panlobular distribution or show a zone 3 predilection.[75] The lobules also show mild lymphocytic inflammation and occasional acidophil bodies. Lobular cholestasis, as well as mild hepatocyte ballooning, is often seen. The portal tracts can show increased numbers of macrophages as well as mild nonspecific inflammation.

TICK-BORNE DISEASES. Granulomas are uncommon in all the tick-borne diseases and, when present, hardly ever the dominant histologic findings. On the other hand, granulomas can be seen in most of the tick-borne diseases, especially Lyme disease, ehrlichiosis, and tularemia (discussed separately later). In most cases, the granulomas are poorly formed but they also can be epithelioid and can rarely show central necrosis. The liver also commonly shows mild nonspecific lobular and portal lymphocytic inflammation. A true granulomatous hepatitis pattern is uncommon but has been reported in Lyme disease.[2,76]

Q fever is not transmitted directly by ticks but is maintained in the tick population and spreads to humans via domesticated animals including sheep, goats, and cattle. Unpasteurized milk and cheese can cause hepatitis, while aerosolization of contaminated soil can lead to pneumonia. Fibrin ring granulomas have been linked to Q fever, but not all cases have them and there are many other known causes (Table 7.3).

TULAREMIA. This infection is caused by *Francisella tularensis*, a gram-negative coccobacillus that is transmitted to humans from small mammals, such as rodents and rabbits, as well as tick bites (*Amblyomma americanum* and *Dermacentor andersoni* and *Dermacentor variabilis*). Skinning rabbits or rodents is a common risk factor for infection. Domestic cats that have eaten infected rodents can also transmit the infection to humans. Tularemia is not transmitted from humans to humans. The disease has a bimodal, seasonal epidemiologic pattern, with a peak in the summer due to tick bites and a peak in the winter due to rabbit/rodent exposure. In the United States, the southeast and southwest account for the majority of reported cases.

The organism was first isolated in 1912 by GW McCoy of the US Public Health Services. However, the disease was well known anciently, and some propose it to be the etiologic agent for the "Hittite plague."[77]

The incubation period is on average 3 to 5 days but can range from 1 to 14 days. The disease has been classified into an ulceroglandular variant and a typhoidal variant. The ulceroglandular variant disease tends to be more localized, while the typhoidal pattern has more disseminated disease, often with pneumonia, and has a worse prognosis.[78] Histologic descriptions are limited because of the rarity of the disease, but there is hepatic involvement in more than three-fourths of cases. Infections cause small abscesses mixed with occasional areas that are granulomatous.[79] The abscesses can be up to 1 to 2 mm in size and have central areas of necrosis and fibroinflammatory exudates, all surrounded by a thin rim of mixed neutrophilic and lymphocytic inflammation. The hepatic parenchyma outside the small abscesses typically shows mild nonspecific inflammatory changes and sometimes mild to moderate lobular cholestasis. Mild nonspecific sinusoidal dilatation can also be seen.

WHIPPLE DISEASE. Whipple disease was first identified in 1907 by George Hoyt Whipple, an American pathologist who performed an autopsy on a 37-year-old missionary-physician who died of an unknown disease. He termed the disease "lipodystrophia intestinalis" for the accumulation of fat-like granular material (foamy histiocytes) in the intestine and lymph nodes and speculated the disease was infectious in origin.

Histologically, well-formed granulomas are rare in Whipple disease; instead, the primary finding is loose aggregates of PAS-positive, foamy macrophages in the sinusoids and portal tracts. When present, true epithelioid granulomas are often negative for organisms on PAS stains. Mild nonspecific chronic inflammation is also common and may reflect gastrointestinal mucosal disease, leading to increased amounts of foreign antigens in the portal circulation.

Fungal Infections, General Patterns

There are many different fungal infections that can involve the liver, usually as disseminated disease. Nonetheless, there are three basic patterns of histologic changes. In the first pattern, patients typically have an acute presentation that may include fevers and other systemic symptoms. The liver biopsy shows a granulomatous hepatitis pattern, with a moderate to marked lobular hepatitis that also has numerous, often poorly formed granulomas. The differential is mostly infection and drug-induced liver injury. In the second pattern, patients are asymptomatic and the biopsy is performed for elevated liver enzyme levels, showing occasional epithelioid granulomas as the main histologic finding, along with mild nonspecific portal and lobular inflammation. The third pattern shows old fibrotic granulomas that are incidental findings in specimens, often resections, taken for another reason.

HISTOPLASMOSIS is caused by *Histoplasma capsulatum*. The organism is found in soil, in particular soil that is contaminated by bird or bat droppings. Infection is caused by inhalation, and it is most common in the Ohio River valley and the lower Mississippi River valley. Most exposed individuals do not develop symptoms, but those who do can have flulike symptoms or nonspecific upper respiratory tract disease. Some individuals develop chronic cavitary lung disease. Spread outside the lungs can lead to fibrosing mediastinitis, lymphadenopathy, ulcers in the gastrointestinal tract, and hepatomegaly. Healing granulomas often undergo calcification.

In liver biopsy specimens, the most common finding is lymphohistiocytic inflammation in the portal tracts and Kupffer cell hyperplasia in the sinusoids.[80] The sinusoids can also appear congested when there is striking Kupffer cell hyperplasia. Well-formed granulomas are typically few in number, are round in profile, are noncaseating, are surrounded by a rim of lymphocytic inflammation, and may have a rim of fibrosis. They can be located in both the portal tracts and the lobules. Immunosuppressed patients can also present with an acute-onset hepatitis and show a granulomatous hepatitis pattern of injury (Figure 7.20). Occasionally, organisms are seen on H&E, but GMS stains are the best way to identify them (Figure 7.21). The organisms are 1 to 4 μm in diameter and can be single organisms (most common) or found in small grapelike clusters; budding is uncommon. Also, of note, organisms are much more often seen in individuals with active clinical symptoms, while organisms are sparse or absent in most cases with incidental granulomas, those found in liver biopsies performed for other clinical indications.

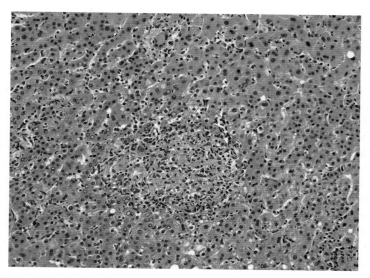

FIGURE 7.20 **Histoplasmosis.** A granulomatous hepatitis pattern is seen in this patient with Crohn disease who presented with acute-onset hepatitis.

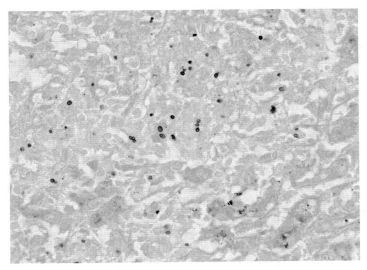

FIGURE 7.21 **Histoplasmosis, Grocott-Gomori methenamine–silver nitrate (GMS) stain.** Organisms can be seen in this case of granulomatous hepatitis caused by *Histoplasma capsulatum*.

CRYPTOCOCCUS NEOFORMANS hepatitis is typically seen only in immunosuppressed individuals. Well-formed granulomas are uncommon, but poorly formed granulomas as well as lobular aggregates of foamy histiocytes can be seen. The yeast is 4 to 6 µm in diameter and has a thick capsule that can be stained with a PAS stain. Budding yeast are not uncommon. *Cryptococcus gattii* is a different species, most commonly seen in tropical parts of Australia, Papua New Guinea, and Africa, as well as the British Columbia province of Canada. This species can infect immunocompetent individuals. The morphology looks very similar to that of *C. neoformans* on biopsy.

CANDIDA, ASPERGILLUS, AND MUCOR. These fungal infections may cause frank abscesses in immunosuppressed individuals, often when there are anatomic/surgical abnormalities of the biliary tree. The organisms are best seen on silver stains or PAS stains and the diagnosis is made in the usual way. Many of the abscesses will be mixed fungal and bacterial abscesses.

Schistosomiasis

Schistosomiasis is caused by several species of trematodes. Freshwater snails are an intermediate host, transmitting the parasite to humans who drink or swim in contaminated water. Thus, it is sometimes called "snail disease." The disease is found in many parts of the world, including the Middle East, tropical Africa, Southeast Asia, the Caribbean, and portions of South America. Schistosomiasis is endemic in a large number of developing countries. Also, the disease is increasingly seen in Europe, Canada, the United States, and other developed countries because of immigration and travel.

After penetrating the skin or intestinal mucosa, the trematodes migrate to the portal veins, where they mate and secrete thousands of eggs. The eggs can become trapped in the portal veins and hepatic parenchyma, where they elicit an inflammatory response. The adult worms are rarely if ever seen on liver biopsy; instead, the diagnosis is usually made when eggs, or portions thereof, are identified (Figures 7.22 and 7.23). Speciation of schistosomiasis is often challenging on liver biopsy, and I usually resist the temptation. Stool samples are a better method in my experience.

Portal vein sclerosis can develop in long-standing disease, where it can be the dominant histologic finding. The portal vein sclerosis can lead to a pattern of fibrosis characterized by rounded, chunky, markedly fibrotic portal tracts, a pattern sometimes called "Symmers fibrosis" or *pipestem fibrosis*. The biopsy may show vague nodularity with changes of nodular regenerative hyperplasia. In other cases with known disease, the biopsy may show only mild nonspecific inflammatory changes and portal vein fibrosis, but be negative for parasite eggs due to sampling.

Viral Infections

As a general rule, granulomas are uncommon in viral infections and are not the typical presentation for any viral infection. Granulomas, however, have been well documented in Epstein-Barr virus (EBV) hepatitis,

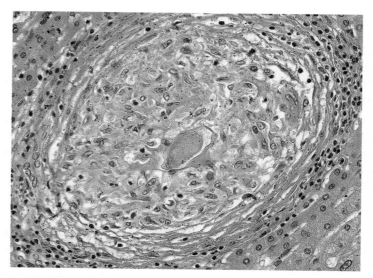

FIGURE 7.22 **Schistosomiasis, low power.** A granuloma is seen associated with a parasitic egg. Many times, the linear refractile edge of the egg is the most distinctive feature on low power.

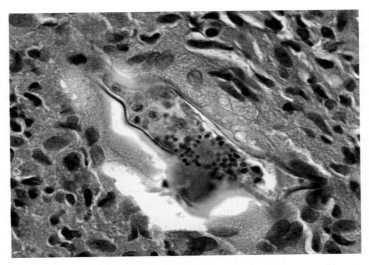

FIGURE 7.23 **Schistosomiasis, high power.** Additional details of a parasitic egg.

cytomegalovirus (CMV) hepatitis, hepatitis A virus (HAV) infection, and hepatitis E virus (HEV) infection. The granulomas can be epithelioid or fibrin ring but are never caseating.

About 1% of individuals with chronic HCV or chronic HBV infection will have occasional small, epithelioid, non-necrotizing granulomas.[11,81] The granulomas can be in the lobules or portal tracts. They are not associated with increased amounts of chronic inflammation or increased fibrosis risk and their significance is unclear, but there seems to be either no clinical significance or next-to-no clinical significance. Their cause is also unclear. All things considered, however, they appear to be incidental and are not part of the disease process of chronic viral hepatitis.

Sarcoidosis

Sarcoidosis is a systemic disease of unknown cause but is widely thought to be a granulomatous response to an unknown antigen in patients with permissible genetics, probably connected to infection in some manner. Symptoms are generally vague and a diagnosis can be delayed for many years. Current studies show most patients present in their mid-40s to early 50s,[82] which is later than earlier studies that reported peak ages of presentation between 20 and 45 years. Men tend to present earlier than women. Sarcoidosis can be found in all races, although the prevalence is highest in Scandinavia, particularly Sweden and Iceland. The disease, however, tends to be more indolent in Caucasians and more aggressive in those with African ancestry. Sarcoidosis can be associated with other autoimmune conditions including celiac disease. Smoking has a protective effect, whereas obesity increases the risk of clinical disease.[82]

Granulomas can be present in many different organ systems, most commonly the lungs, lymph nodes, and liver. Overall, the liver shows histological involvement in approximately 75% of cases. In the majority of these patients, however, liver function is only minimally affected. Even when there is clinically evident disease (about 10%-20% of patients), the disease is mild and severe liver disease is rare, occurring in less than 1% of patients.

There are four main patterns of sarcoidal involvement of the liver.[83] The first pattern is by far the most common and shows scattered, mainly portal granulomas that vary in age, with some showing fibrosis. The fibrosis extends into and through the granulomas, instead of being solely a fibrous rim around the granuloma (Figures 7.24 and 7.25). Rarely, Schaumann bodies and/or asteroid bodies (Figure 7.26) can be found, but they are not specific for sarcoidosis. Lobular epithelioid granulomas can also be seen (Figure 7.27). While this pattern of epithelioid granulomas with fibrosis is typical of sarcoidosis, correlation with other clinical and laboratory findings is important to secure the diagnosis; a diagnosis should not be made by histologic examination alone.

A second, rare pattern shows both granulomas and chronic obstructive biliary tract disease. In these cases, hilar lymphadenopathy obstructs the extrahepatic bile ducts, leading to obstructive biliary tract disease. The biopsies show varying degrees of ductular proliferation, portal fibrosis, and ductopenia.

In a third even rarer pattern, the sarcoidosis shows a striking involvement of the portal veins, with portal granulomatous venulitis and loss of portal veins.[8,83] The lobules can also show changes of nodular regenerative hyperplasia.

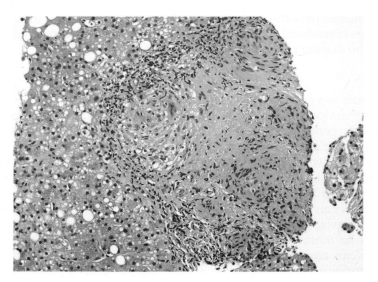

FIGURE 7.24 **Sarcoidosis.** Epithelioid granulomas are present in the portal tracts.

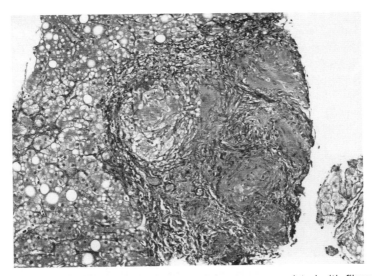

FIGURE 7.25 **Sarcoidosis, trichrome.** The granulomas are associated with fibrosis (same case as the preceding image).

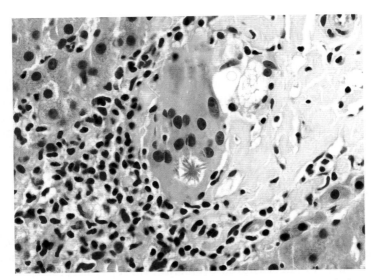

FIGURE 7.26 **Sarcoidosis, asteroid body.** Asteroid bodies are fun to see but are not specific for sarcoidosis.

As a fourth, super-rare pattern, patients can present with mass lesions that often mimic a tumor on imaging. Biopsy of the mass shows a nodule of confluent and fibrotic granulomas, a finding called a "sarcoidoma" to emphasize the masslike presentation.

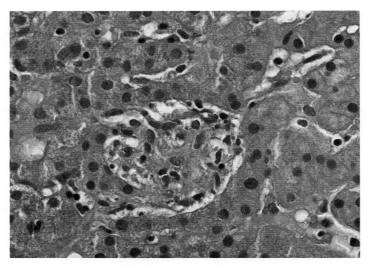

FIGURE 7.27 **Sarcoidosis, lobular granuloma.** A small epithelioid lobular granuloma without fibrosis can be seen.

Finally, exceedingly rare cases of sarcoidosis have been reported that have bile duct inflammation and injury leading to a florid duct type lesion that resembles PBC.[83] Often, however, it is not clear from reported cases in the literature if this is a true sarcoidosis pattern or if the patient actually has PBC or a drug reaction. In this setting, examination of the rest of the biopsy will typically point in the right direction—as sarcoidosis is unlikely if the rest of the biopsy shows features that are not typical for sarcoid. In any case, this pattern remains rare and incompletely defined, and a florid duct lesion is still most likely to be PBC or a drug reaction.

OTHER DISEASES WITH GRANULOMAS

ACUTE CELLULAR REJECTION. Rare cases have been reported of acute cellular rejection with granulomatous features.[2,84] In one report, the granulomas co-occurred with other typical features of acute cellular rejection and disappeared after successful antirejection therapy, suggesting the granulomatous inflammation was part of the rejection process.[2] This pattern of acute cellular rejection, however, remains incompletely defined. Of note, and this is important, other causes such as infection should be carefully excluded, even if there is coexisting acute cellular rejection. Overall, the majority of granulomas seen in the transplanted liver are not associated with acute cellular rejection[84] but instead have the usual differential of infection, drug effect, and recurrent disease (such as sarcoidosis or PBC).

CELIAC DISEASE. Protocol liver biopsies in the setting of celiac disease usually show mild nonspecific inflammatory changes, but occasionally also demonstrate small portal or lobular epithelioid granulomas. AFB and GMS stains should be performed, but their results are typically negative. Of note, celiac disease is associated with an increased frequency of both sarcoidosis and PBC, so features of these diseases should be sought both clinically and histologically. It is well known clinically that celiac disease can have mild transaminase level elevations, so most biopsies are performed when there are additional clinical or laboratory findings, such as moderate levels of liver enzyme elevations or jaundice. These biopsies performed for clinical reasons, in contrast to protocol biopsies, will be enriched for other diseases including PBC, sarcoidosis, autoimmune hepatitis, and primary sclerosing cholangitis.

CHRONIC GRANULOMATOUS DISEASE. This is an inherited immunodeficiency, which can be X-linked or autosomal recessive, leading to neutrophils that are unable to produce normal levels of hydrogen peroxide, resulting in recurrent bacterial and fungal infections. Patients have biochemically evident liver disease in about 35% of cases,[85] but liver biopsies are not a major part of clinical management, being performed only to evaluate unusual liver-related laboratory or imaging findings. On biopsy, the liver shows epithelioid granulomas in 75% of cases,[86] typically without necrosis, in a background of mild nonspecific portal lymphocytic inflammation. Other findings can include changes suggestive of chronic, large bile duct obstruction—including fibro-obliterative duct lesions, as well as portal venopathy and nodular regenerative hyperplasia.[86] Frank liver abscesses can sometimes form.[87]

COMMON VARIABLE IMMUNODEFICIENCY (CVID) can lead to granulomas in the liver (Figure 7.28).[88] The biopsies also show mild portal chronic inflammation without plasma cells and mild to focally moderate lobular lymphocytic inflammation.[88] The granulomas are usually small, noncaseating, and epithelioid.[88] Some livers may also show nodular regenerative hyperplasia.[89] In 5% to 10% of cases, the granulomatous disease affects multiple organ systems and is essentially indistinguishable from sarcoidosis, both clinically and histologically. For example, lung hilar adenopathy and elevated serum ACE levels are commonly found in both diseases. In fact, sarcoidosis may be the working clinical diagnosis before a diagnosis of CVID is made and some, but not all, authors believe that granulomatous CVID is a manifestation of sarcoidosis in the CVID population. In rare cases, granulomatous CVID can be associated with persistent febrile illness that responds to steroid therapy.[90]

CROHN DISEASE can rarely cause granulomas in the liver (Figure 7.29).[3,91-93] Most individuals with Crohn disease and abnormal liver enzyme levels, however, will have changes of primary sclerosing cholangitis, fatty liver disease, or a mild nonspecific hepatitis on liver biopsy.

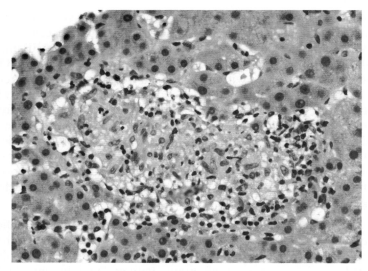

FIGURE 7.28 **Common variable immunodeficiency.** A large epithelioid granuloma with admixed lymphocytes is seen.

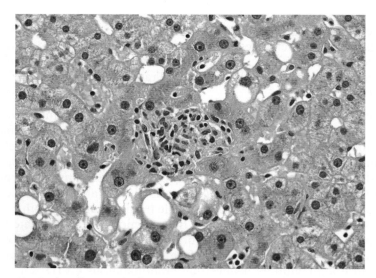

FIGURE 7.29 **Crohn disease.** The liver showed mild fatty change and occasional small non-necrotizing epithelioid granulomas.

PBC. Granulomas are a well-known component of the histology of PBC. PBC is discussed in more detail in Chapter 11. The granulomas can be well-formed, epithelioid granulomas that are located in the portal tracts or the lobules.

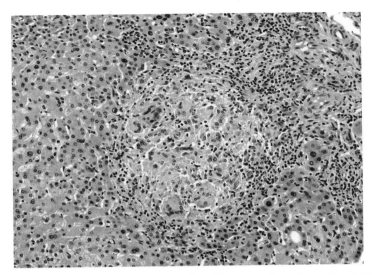

FIGURE 7.30 **Colon cancer, granuloma.** A liver biopsy confirmed metastatic colon adenocarcinomas. Granulomas were present in the background liver.

GRANULOMAS AND NEOPLASMS

Granulomas can be associated with tumors. Perhaps the best known association is with Hodgkin disease, where a granulomatous hepatitis can precede a diagnosis of Hodgkin disease by months to years. The granulomas are typically small, epithelioid, and otherwise nondescript. Non-Hodgkin lymphomas can also rarely be associated with granulomas.[4,5] Other tumors that can occasionally have granulomas, either within the tumors or in the background liver, include conventional hepatocellular carcinoma,[4,6] fibrolamellar carcinoma, cholangiocarcinoma,[4] and metastatic tumors (Figure 7.30).[3]

IDIOPATHIC GRANULOMAS

Follow-up clinical and laboratory findings are important to determine the most likely cause of granulomas seen on biopsy; histology alone is insufficient. For example, one study reported that follow-up testing identified a likely cause in 17 of 24 biopsies with histologically idiopathic granulomas.[94] Nonetheless, approximately one-third of all biopsies with granulomas will remain idiopathic despite a full clinical workup (Figure 7.31). In many of these cases, repeat biopsies will continue to show granulomas. In most of these idiopathic cases, the granulomas are small, epithelioid, sparse, and without necrosis. The background liver

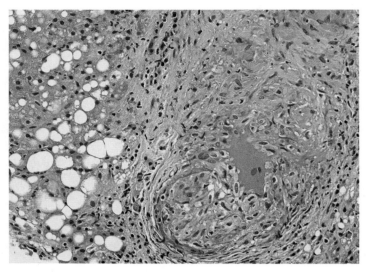

FIGURE 7.31 Incidental idiopathic granuloma. Several granulomas were seen in this liver biopsy performed to stage and grade nonalcoholic fatty liver disease. No cause was identified.

generally has no fibrosis, unless there is another chronic liver disease such as chronic hepatitis C, chronic hepatitis B, or NAFLD. At this point, all available data suggest these idiopathic granulomas are not a cause of clinically significant liver disease and most likely represent a nonspecific reactive change.

OTHER CAUSES

Other rare causes of granulomas include the following: Sjogren syndrome,[95] gout,[3] vasculitis,[6] polymyalgia rheumatic,[5] juvenile chronic arthritis,[5] graft-versus-host disease,[5] jejunoileal bypass surgery,[5] and resolving chronic biliary tract disease.[5] Autoimmune hepatitis with granulomas but without features of PBC has also been identified in several studies.[5-7] This list is extensive but not exhaustive and other rare causes of granulomas have been reported.

RHEUMATOID NODULES are not granulomas per se, but they can involve the liver,[96,97] where they can mimic a large necrotizing granuloma. Rheumatoid nodules have a central zone that is almost acellular, being composed of fibrin and varying degrees of necrosis, surrounded by an outer rim formed by palisading histiocytes, chronic inflammation, and fibrosis (Figure 7.32). In time, lesions can become mostly fibrotic.

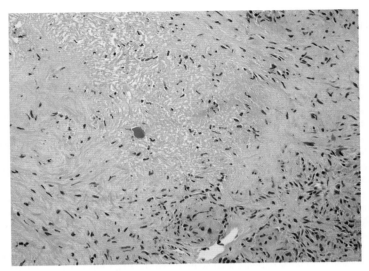

FIGURE 7.32 **Rheumatoid nodule.** This rheumatoid nodule shows an acellular center composed of fibrin and focal necrosis. In the lower right of the image, the outer rim of palisading histiocytes and chronic inflammation is seen.

REFERENCES

1. Drebber U, Kasper HU, Ratering J, et al. Hepatic granulomas: histological and molecular pathological approach to differential diagnosis—A study of 442 cases. *Liver Int.* 2008;28:828-834.

2. Lagana SM, Moreira RK, Lefkowitch JH. Hepatic granulomas: pathogenesis and differential diagnosis. *Clin Liver Dis.* 2010;14:605-617.

3. McCluggage WG, Sloan JM. Hepatic granulomas in Northern Ireland: a thirteen-year review. *Histopathology.* 1994;25:219-228.

4. Turhan N, Kurt M, Ozderin YO, et al. Hepatic granulomas: a clinicopathologic analysis of 86 cases. *Pathol Res Pract.* 2011;207:359-365.

5. Gaya DR, Thorburn D, Oien KA, et al. Hepatic granulomas: a 10-year single centre experience. *J Clin Pathol.* 2003;56:850-853.

6. Dourakis SP, Saramadou R, Alexopoulou A, et al. Hepatic granulomas: a 6-year experience in a single center in Greece. *Eur J Gastroenterol Hepatol.* 2007;19:101-104.

7. Geramizadeh B, Jahangiri R, Moradi E. Causes of hepatic granuloma: a 12-year single center experience from southern Iran. *Arch Iran Med.* 2011;14:288-289.

8. Moreno-Merlo F, Wanless IR, Shimamatsu K, et al. The role of granulomatous phlebitis and thrombosis in the pathogenesis of cirrhosis and portal hypertension in sarcoidosis. *Hepatology.* 1997;26:554-560.

9. Saito T, Harada K, Nakanuma Y. Granulomatous phlebitis of small hepatic vein. *J Gastroenterol Hepatol.* 2002;17:1334-1339.

10. Snyder N, Martinez JG, Xiao SY. Chronic hepatitis C is a common associated with hepatic granulomas. *World J Gastroenterol.* 2008;14:6366-6369.

11. Tahan V, Ozaras R, Lacevic N, et al. Prevalence of hepatic granulomas in chronic hepatitis B. *Dig Dis Sci.* 2004;49:1575-1577.

12. Carreno Hernandez MC, Garrido Paniagua S, Colomes Iess M, et al. Accelerated silicosis with bone marrow, hepatic and splenic involvement in a patient with lung transplantation. *BMJ Case Rep.* 2019;12.

13. Cortex Pimentel J, Peixoto Menezes A. Pulmonary and hepatic granulomatous disorders due to the inhalation of cement and mica dusts. *Thorax.* 1978;33:219-227.

14. Pimentel JC, Menezes AP. Liver granulomas containing copper in vineyard sprayer's lung. A new etiology of hepatic granulomatosis. *Am Rev Respir Dis.* 1975;111:189-195.

15. Yamamoto T, Ishii M, Nagura H, et al. Transient hepatic fibrin-ring granulomas in a patient with acute hepatitis A. *Liver.* 1995;15:276-279.

16. Ruel M, Sevestre H, Henry-Biabaud E, et al. Fibrin ring granulomas in hepatitis A. *Dig Dis Sci.* 1992;37:1915-1917.

17. Nenert M, Mavier P, Dubuc N, et al. Epstein-Barr virus infection and hepatic fibrin-ring granulomas. *Hum Pathol.* 1988;19:608-610.

18. Glazer E, Ejaz A, Coley CJ II, et al. Fibrin ring granuloma in chronic hepatitis C: virus-related vasculitis and/or immune complex disease? *Semin Liver Dis.* 2007;27:227-230.

19. Pellegrin M, Delsol G, Auvergnat JC, et al. Granulomatous hepatitis in Q fever. *Hum Pathol.* 1980;11:51-57.

20. Jang YR, Shin Y, Jin CE, et al. Molecular detection of *Coxiella burnetii* from the formalin-fixed tissues of Q fever patients with acute hepatitis. *PLoS One.* 2017;12:e0180237.

21. Marazuela M, Moreno A, Yebra M, et al. Hepatic fibrin-ring granulomas: a clinicopathologic study of 23 patients. *Hum Pathol.* 1991;22:607-613.

22. Moreno A, Marazuela M, Yebra M, et al. Hepatic fibrin-ring granulomas in visceral leishmaniasis. *Gastroenterology.* 1988;95:1123-1126.

23. Khanlari B, Bodmer M, Terracciano L, et al. Hepatitis with fibrin-ring granulomas. *Infection.* 2008;36:381-383.

24. Font J, Bruguera M, Perez-Villa F, et al. Hepatic fibrin-ring granulomas caused by *Staphylococcus epidermidis* generalized infection. *Gastroenterology.* 1987;93:1449-1451.

25. Vanderstigel M, Zafrani ES, Lejonc JL, et al. Allopurinol hypersensitivity syndrome as a cause of hepatic fibrin-ring granulomas. *Gastroenterology.* 1986;90:188-190.

26. Stricker BH, Blok AP, Babany G, et al. Fibrin ring granulomas and allopurinol. *Gastroenterology.* 1989;96:1199-1203.

27. Everett J, Srivastava A, Misdraji J. Fibrin ring granulomas in checkpoint inhibitor-induced hepatitis. *Am J Surg Pathol.* 2017;41:134-137.

28. de Bayser L, Roblot P, Ramassamy A, et al. Hepatic fibrin-ring granulomas in giant cell arteritis. *Gastroenterology.* 1993;105:272-273.

29. Murphy E, Griffiths MR, Hunter JA, et al. Fibrin-ring granulomas: a non-specific reaction to liver injury? *Histopathology.* 1991;19:91-93.

30. Roberts IS, Armstrong GR. Hepatic fibrin-ring granulomas. *Histopathology.* 1992;20:549.

31. Liu YC, Tomashefski J Jr, McMahon JT, et al. Mineral-associated hepatic injury: a report of seven cases with X-ray microanalysis. *Hum Pathol.* 1991;22:1120-1127.

32. Allaire GS, Goodman ZD, Ishak KG, et al. Talc in liver tissue of intravenous drug abusers with chronic hepatitis. A comparative study. *Am J Clin Pathol.* 1989;92:583-588.

33. Nihon-Yanagi Y, Ishiwatari T, Otsuka Y, et al. A case of postoperative hepatic granuloma presumptively caused by surgical staples/clipping materials. *Diagn Pathol.* 2015;10:90.

34. Peoc'h M, Moulin C, Pasquier B. Systemic granulomatous reaction to a foreign body after hip replacement. *N Engl J Med.* 1996;335:133-134.

35. Ballestri M, Baraldi A, Gatti AM, et al. Liver and kidney foreign bodies granulomatosis in a patient with malocclusion, bruxism, and worn dental prostheses. *Gastroenterology.* 2001;121:1234-1238.

36. Lavranos G, Kouma D, Deveros A, et al. Still's-like disease induced by breast implants in a middle-aged female Health professional. *Eur J Case Rep Intern Med.* 2017;4:000513.

37. Nowacki NB, Arnold MA, Frankel WL, et al. Gastrointestinal tract-derived pulse granulomata: clues to an underrecognized pseudotumor. *Am J Surg Pathol.* 2015;39:84-92.

38. Dincsoy HP, Weesner RE, MacGee J. Lipogranulomas in non-fatty human livers. A mineral oil induced environmental disease. *Am J Clin Pathol.* 1982;78:35-41.

39. Boitnott JK, Margolis S. Saturated hydrocarbons in human tissues. 3. Oil droplets in the liver and spleen. *Johns Hopkins Med J.* 1970;127:65-78.

40. Carlton WW, Boitnott JK, Dungworth DL, et al. Assessment of the morphology and significance of the lymph nodal and hepatic lesions produced in rats by the feeding of certain mineral oils and waxes. Proceedings of a pathology workshop held at the Fraunhofer Institute of Toxicology and Aerosol Research Hannover, Germany, May 7-9, 2001. *Exp Toxicol Pathol.* 2001;53:247-255.

41. Zhu H, Bodenheimer HC Jr, Clain DJ, et al. Hepatic lipogranulomas in patients with chronic liver disease: association with hepatitis C and fatty liver disease. *World J Gastroenterol.* 2010;16:5065-5069.

42. Delladetsima JK, Horn T, Poulsen H. Portal tract lipogranulomas in liver biopsies. *Liver.* 1987;7:9-17.

43. Kleiner DE, Brunt EM, Van Natta M, et al. Design and validation of a histological scoring system for nonalcoholic fatty liver disease. *Hepatology.* 2005;41:1313-1321.

44. Howard PF, Smith JW. Diagnosis of disseminated coccidioidomycosis by liver biopsy. *Arch Intern Med.* 1983;143:1335-1338.

45. Ragnaud JM, Dupon M, Echinard E, et al. Hepatic manifestations of psittacosis. Article in French. *Gastroenterol Clin Biol* 1986;10:234-237.

46. Singh S, Verma Y, Pandey P, et al. Granulomatous hepatitis by Nocardia species: an unusual case. *Int J Infect Dis.* 2019;81:97-99.

47. Cornog JL Jr, Hanson CW. Psittacosis as a cause of miliary infiltrates of the lung and hepatic granulomas. *Am Rev Respir Dis.* 1968;98:1033-1036.

48. Middelveen M, McClain S, Bandoski C, et al. *Granulomatous hepatitis associated with chronic Borrelia burgdorferi infection: a case report.* In: *Biology and Environmental Science Faculty Publications Volume Paper 33.* 2014.

49. Case records of the Massachusetts General Hospital. Weekly clinicopathological exercises. Case 27-1983. A 25-year-old homosexual man with persistent fever and liver disease. *N Engl J Med.* 1983;309:35-43.

50. Roberts-Thomson IC, Anders RF, Bhathal PS. Granulomatous hepatitis and cholangitis associated with giardiasis. *Gastroenterology.* 1982;83:480-483.

51. Brenner DJ, Hollis DG, Moss CW, et al. Proposal of Afipia gen. nov., with Afipia felis sp. nov. (formerly the cat scratch disease bacillus), Afipia clevelandensis sp. nov. (formerly the Cleveland Clinic Foundation strain), Afipia broomeae sp. nov., and three unnamed genospecies. *J Clin Microbiol.* 1991;29:2450-2460.

52. Debre R, Lamy M, Jammet M, et al. La maladie des griffes de chat. *Bull Mem Soc Med Hop Paris.* 1950;66:76-79.

53. Florin TA, Zaoutis TE, Zaoutis LB. Beyond cat scratch disease: widening spectrum of Bartonella henselae infection. *Pediatrics.* 2008;121:e1413-25.

54. Weinspach S, Tenenbaum T, Schonberger S, et al. Cat scratch disease – Heterogeneous in clinical presentation: five unusual cases of an infection caused by Bartonella henselae. *Klin Padiatr.* 2010;222:73-78.

55. Lamps LW, Gray GF, Scott MA. The histologic spectrum of hepatic cat scratch disease. A series of six cases with confirmed Bartonella henselae infection. *Am J Surg Pathol.* 1996;20:1253-1259.

56. Angelakis E, Raoult D. Pathogenicity and treatment of Bartonella infections. *Int J Antimicrob Agents*. 2014;44:16-25.

57. Wyatt HV. How Themistocles Zammit found Malta Fever (brucellosis) to be transmitted by the milk of goats. *J R Soc Med*. 2005;98:451-454.

58. Robichaud S, Libman M, Behr M, et al. Prevention of laboratory-acquired brucellosis. *Clin Infect Dis*. 2004;38:e119-22.

59. Young EJ, Hasanjani Roushan MR, Shafae S, et al. Liver histology of acute brucellosis caused by Brucella melitensis. *Hum Pathol*. 2014;45:2023-2028.

60. Akritidis N, Tzivras M, Delladetsima I, et al. The liver in brucellosis. *Clin Gastroenterol Hepatol*. 2007;5:1109-1112.

61. Young EJ. Brucella melitensis hepatitis: the absence of granulomas. *Ann Intern Med*. 1979;91:414-415.

62. Colmenero JD, Reguera JM, Martos F, et al. Complications associated with Brucella melitensis infection: a study of 530 cases. *Medicine (Baltimore)*. 1996;75:195-211.

63. Amarapurkar A, Agrawal V. Liver involvement in tuberculosis – An autopsy study. *Trop Gastroenterol*. 2006;27:69-74.

64. Xing X, Li H, Liu WG. Hepatic segmentectomy for treatment of hepatic tuberculous pseudotumor. *Hepatobiliary Pancreat Dis Int*. 2005;4:565-568.

65. Scriven JE, Scobie A, Verlander NQ, et al. Mycobacterium chimaera infection following cardiac surgery in the United Kingdom: clinical features and outcome of the first 30 cases. *Clin Microbiol Infect*. 2018;24(11):1164-1170.

66. Shafizadeh N, Hale G, Bhatnagar J, et al. Mycobacterium chimaera hepatitis: a new disease entity. *Am J Surg Pathol*. 2019;43:244-250.

67. Han XY, Seo YH, Sizer KC, et al. A new *Mycobacterium* species causing diffuse lepromatous leprosy. *Am J Clin Pathol*. 2008;130:856-864.

68. Norouzi S, Aghamohammadi A, Mamishi S, et al. Bacillus Calmette-Guerin (BCG) complications associated with primary immunodeficiency diseases. *J Infect*. 2012;64:543-554.

69. Perez-Jacoiste Asin MA, Fernandez-Ruiz M, Lopez-Medrano F, et al. Bacillus Calmette-Guerin (BCG) infection following intravesical BCG administration as adjunctive therapy for bladder cancer: incidence, risk factors, and outcome in a single-institution series and review of the literature. *Medicine (Baltimore)*. 2014;93:236-254.

70. Leebeek FW, Ouwendijk RJ, Kolk AH, et al. Granulomatous hepatitis caused by Bacillus Calmette-Guerin (BCG) infection after BCG bladder instillation. *Gut*. 1996;38:616-618.

71. McHugh J, Mackowiak PA. Death in the white house: president William Henry Harrison's atypical pneumonia. *Clin Infect Dis*. 2014;59:990-995.

72. Ahmed A, Ahmed B. Jaundice in typhoid patients: differentiation from other common causes of fever and jaundice in the tropics. *Ann Afr Med*. 2010;9:135-140.

73. Arif N, Khan AA, Iqbal Z. Hepatic involvement with typhoid fever: a report of nine patients. *J Pak Med Assoc*. 1990;40:4-9.

74. Ramachandran S, Godfrey JJ, Perera MV. Typhoid hepatitis. *J Am Med Assoc*. 1974;230:236-240.

75. Pramoolsinsap C, Viranuvatti V. Salmonella hepatitis. *J Gastroenterol Hepatol*. 1998;13:745-750.

76. Zanchi AC, Gingold AR, Theise ND, et al. Necrotizing granulomatous hepatitis as an unusual manifestation of Lyme disease. *Dig Dis Sci*. 2007;52:2629-2632.

77. Trevisanato SI. The 'Hittite plague', an epidemic of tularemia and the first record of biological warfare. *Med Hypotheses*. 2007;69:1371-1374.

78. Evans ME, Gregory DW, Schaffner W, et al. Tularemia: a 30-year experience with 88 cases. *Medicine (Baltimore)*. 1985;64:251-269.

79. Lamps LW, Havens JM, Sjostedt A, et al. Histologic and molecular diagnosis of tularemia: a potential bioterrorism agent endemic to North America. *Mod Pathol.* 2004;17:489-495.

80. Lamps LW, Molina CP, West AB, et al. The pathologic spectrum of gastrointestinal and hepatic histoplasmosis. *Am J Clin Pathol.* 2000;113:64-72.

81. Ozaras R, Tahan V, Mert A, et al. The prevalence of hepatic granulomas in chronic hepatitis C. *J Clin Gastroenterol.* 2004;38:449-452.

82. Arkema EV, Cozier YC. Epidemiology of sarcoidosis: current findings and future directions. *Ther Adv Chronic Dis.* 2018;9:227-240.

83. Devaney K, Goodman ZD, Epstein MS, et al. Hepatic sarcoidosis. Clinicopathologic features in 100 patients. *Am J Surg Pathol.* 1993;17:1272-1280.

84. Ferrell LD, Lee R, Brixko C, et al. Hepatic granulomas following liver transplantation. Clinicopathologic features in 42 patients. *Transplantation.* 1995;60:926-933.

85. van den Berg JM, van Koppen E, Ahlin A, et al. Chronic granulomatous disease: the European experience. *PLoS One.* 2009;4:e5234.

86. Hussain N, Feld JJ, Kleiner DE, et al. Hepatic abnormalities in patients with chronic granulomatous disease. *Hepatology.* 2007;45:675-683.

87. Szekely A, Peter M Jr, Erdos M, et al. Hepatic abscess as the single manifestation of X-linked chronic granulomatous disease. *Pediatr Blood Cancer.* 2012;58:828-829.

88. Daniels JA, Torbenson M, Vivekanandan P, et al. Hepatitis in common variable immunodeficiency. *Hum Pathol.* 2009;40:484-488.

89. Crotty R, Taylor MS, Farmer JR, et al. Spectrum of hepatic manifestations of common variable immunodeficiency. *Am J Surg Pathol.* 2020;44:617-625.

90. Fernandez-Ruiz M, Guerra-Vales JM, Francisco-Javier CF, et al. Fever of unknown origin in a patient with common variable immunodeficiency associated with multisystemic granulomatous disease. *Intern Med.* 2007;46:1197-1202.

91. Patedakis Litvinov BI, Pathak AP. Granulomatous hepatitis in a patient with Crohn's disease and cholestasis. *BMJ Case Rep.* 2017;2017:bcr2017220988.

92. Rojas-Feria M, Castro M, Suarez E, et al. Hepatobiliary manifestations in inflammatory bowel disease: the gut, the drugs and the liver. *World J Gastroenterol.* 2013;19:7327-7340.

93. Hilzenrat N, Lamoureux E, Sherker A, et al. Cholestasis in Crohn's disease: a diagnostic challenge. *Can J Gastroenterol.* 1997;11:35-37.

94. Cunnigham D, Mills PR, Quigley EM, et al. Hepatic granulomas: experience over a 10-year period in the West of Scotland. *Q J Med.* 1982;51:162-170.

95. Miller EB, Shichmanter R, Friedman JA, et al. Granulomatous hepatitis and Sjogren's syndrome: an association. *Semin Arthritis Rheum.* 2006;36:153-158.

96. Smits JG, Kooijman CD. Rheumatoid nodules in liver. *Histopathology.* 1986;10:1211-1213.

97. Campani C, Guido M, Colagrande S, et al. A large rheumatoid nodule mimicking hepatic malignancy. *Hepatology.* 2019;69:1345-1348.

8

DRUG-INDUCED LIVER INJURY

OVERALL APPROACH TO LIVER BIOPSY AND DRUG REACTION

Drug reactions affecting the liver are commonly called drug-induced liver injury (DILI), and the terms can be used interchangeably. DILI is an important cause of clinical hepatitis; in the USA, the most common categories of medications that have been linked to DILI are acetaminophen, antibiotics, central nervous system agents, antihypertensive agents, and antidiabetic agents.[1] Dietary supplements were identified as the cause of DILI in 9% of cases in one large registry-based paper.[1] In children, the most common agents are antibiotics and central nervous system agents.[2]

In most cases of DILI, the clinical findings strongly suggest the correct diagnosis, the medication is stopped, and the patient is followed until liver enzymes normalize, with no need for a biopsy. Thus, the cases of DILI seen in surgical pathology mostly fall into one of these three categories: (1) medications that are fairly new to the market (usually in the first 5 years), since the clinical team will have less experience with their toxicity profile; (2) patients with complicated clinical histories where multiple medications or other risk factors for liver disease are present, and the biopsy will (hopefully) help identify the most likely agent; (3) herbal remedies/nutrient supplements, both because patients often under-report their use to the clinical team and because the formulation of the remedies/supplements can change over time, even for the same product.

There are no pathognomonic findings that can be used to identify a drug reaction and the histological findings can vary substantially between different medications. Thus, it is important to have a high degree of suspicion and to routinely consider drug reactions in your differential. In addition, it is important to remember that any given drug can induce multiple patterns of injury. As an illustration, tamoxifen therapy has been associated with acute hepatitis, massive liver necrosis, peliosis hepatitis, steatosis, steatohepatitis, and cholestasis.[3] For this reason, if a patient has recently started a new medication, and then develops acute onset hepatitis, it certainly can be helpful if you find a reported pattern of injury on the liver biopsy, one that has been previously associated with the given drug, but this is not required to suggest the diagnosis of DILI.

In addition, because the list of drug reactions is long and constantly expanding, it is best not to rely solely on long tables of drugs reactions published in books or review articles when evaluating a specific case. Instead, it is better to check the literature through search engines such as PubMed or commercial databases, as new patterns of injury may have been reported for a given drug. For example, the LiverTox website is free and is an excellent source of information http://livertox.nih.gov/. Nonetheless, tables of drug reaction patterns can be a helpful starting point and several tables are included in this chapter. These tables were chosen to focus on specific patterns of injury, both by way of illustration and to provide some lists for specific patterns of injury that can be relatively harder to elicit from the literature.

BASIC MECHANISMS OF INJURY. There are three major mechanisms by which DILI causes liver injury: directly toxic drug reactions (also called intrinsic), idiosyncratic drug reactions, and allergic drug reactions (also called hypersensitivity). Each of these is discussed in more detail below, along with specific examples. Idiosyncratic drug reactions are the most common type of DILI seen in routine surgical pathology. Finally, there is a fourth pattern where medications are not necessarily the sole cause of a pattern of injury, but instead, lead to exacerbation of an injury pattern that was already present; this is seen almost exclusively with fatty liver disease.

Making a Diagnosis of DILI

- Acute onset liver enzyme elevations (most common)
- Temporal correlation that fits for both timing, and if it is an intrinsic drug reaction, for dose exposure
- For any histological pattern of injury, there is a differential and other etiologies for that given pattern of injury should be reasonably excluded by additional stains, clinical history, and/or serological tests
- For idiosyncratic DILI, the main differential diagnoses autoimmune hepatitis and viral hepatitis
- The biopsy findings should be compatible with DILI for the medication(s) the patient has been exposed to

MAKING THE DIAGNOSIS. Pathologists recognize that DILI can have a wide range of histological manifestations. In fact, essentially all of the different histological injury patterns seen on liver biopsy specimens have been associated with a medication effect at some point. This understanding of the many possible faces of DILI is very important but can tempt one into a somewhat nihilistic approach to the diagnosis of a drug reaction. As astutely put to me by one trainee, "If all histological patterns are possibly DILI, then it's not really a histological diagnosis anyway"; although I could not tell if he was unusually discerning or sarcastic, the truth is that the diagnosis of DILI is not made solely by the pathologist.

How, then, is a diagnosis made? The best approach is to have a high index of suspicion for a drug reaction when (1) there is a history of acute onset liver injury, (2) there is a temporal correlation with a medication, (3) other possibilities in the differential for a given pattern of injury are reasonably excluded, and the biopsy findings provide no better explanation for the active liver injury than DILI, (4) autoimmune hepatitis and viral hepatitis have been reasonably excluded by clinical and serological findings for hepatitic patterns of injury, and (5) the biopsy findings are consistent with the changes expected for medications to which the patient has been exposed.

In terms of the last point, as noted previously, it is important to not be overly dogmatic that the histological findings you see in the specimen are exactly the same as found in textbooks or internet images. Of course, some medications do have a "signature" pattern of injury, but this is not true in most cases of idiosyncratic DILI, where a given medication will have a "most common pattern," but also a much wider range of acceptable injury patterns. On the other hand, some patterns of injury would not be well-explained as DILI for a given medication. For example, an acute granulomatous hepatitis would not be a good fit for acetaminophen injury.

Several points can be considered when assessing whether a patient has a temporally compatible history of exposure. For direct toxins, such as acetaminophen, assessment includes evaluation of both a temporal association as well as the amount of exposure, as toxicity is associated with both. For idiosyncratic drug reactions, a compatible exposure history includes current usage of the medication or recent usage of the medication, but the dosage per se is not particularly relevant. Most idiosyncratic drug reactions occur within the first several weeks of exposure to a new medication. It is well accepted, however, that in rare cases a medication may have been in use for months to years before a drug reaction develops.

Finally, at the time of sign-out, most cases of DILI should be considered as being "most consistent with DILI given the currently available clinical and laboratory findings," and not as "biopsy-proven DILI." New clinical information or new laboratory results can sometimes lead to reclassification of biopsy findings on cases that were previously considered to be "most consistent with" a drug reaction. To illustrate this point, in one study, several cases of hepatitis that a panel of expert hepatologists determined by consensus were most likely to be DILI, were later reclassified as acute hepatitis E virus (HEV) infection when newly available HEV testing was retrospectively applied to these cases.[4] Acute HCV is also an important mimic of drug reactions and sometimes has to be excluded by RNA testing, as antibody testing can miss acute cases.[1]

HISTOLOGICAL CLUES TO A DRUG REACTION

Prominent eosinophils in the portal tracts and/or lobules can suggest an allergic-type drug reaction (Figure 8.1, eFig. 8.1). While this clue is useful, it is rarely seen in surgical pathology because most allergic drug reactions are evident clinically and biopsies are not necessary for diagnosis or management. Instead, most biopsied drug reactions are of the idiosyncratic type and show a hepatitic or cholestatic pattern of injury. For cases that do show eosinophilic-rich portal inflammation, the differential diagnosis also includes mast cell disease, Rosia Dorfman disease, Langerhans histiocytosis, and Hodgkin lymphoma.

Bland lobular cholestasis is another potential clue to a drug reaction (Figure 8.2). This pattern of injury shows lobular cholestasis but no evidence for biliary tract disease, no significant inflammation, and no fibrosis. This pattern is not specific but is most commonly seen as part of DILI, especially if it is associated with an acute onset of liver enzyme elevations and the patient is not septic or otherwise severely ill.

For biopsies with a hepatitic pattern of injury, an uncommon but important clue to the diagnosis of DILI can be inflammatory patterns that do not fit well for autoimmune hepatitis or viral hepatitis, the most common diseases in the differential for a hepatitic pattern of injury. For example, a biopsy may show a mild but definite lobular hepatitis as well as significant injury to the bile ducts, a pattern that would not be typical for either autoimmune hepatitis or viral hepatitis.

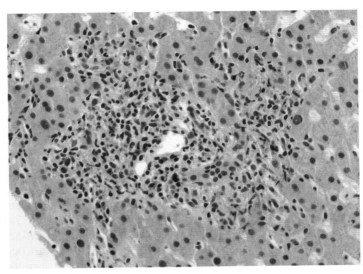

FIGURE 8.1 **Eosinophilic drug reaction.** This drug reaction from atorvastatin showed portal-based inflammation with lymphocytes, plasma cells, and numerous eosinophils.

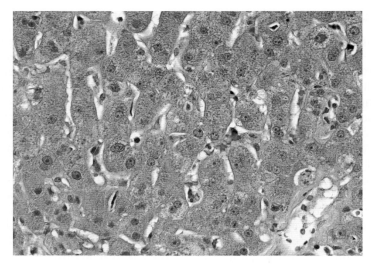

FIGURE 8.2 **Bland lobular cholestasis drug reaction.** This drug reaction shows a canalicular cholestasis pattern of injury, with no significant inflammation.

IDIOPATHIC PATTERNS OF INJURY

Idiosyncratic drug reactions by definition are not dose-related and cannot be predicted on an individual level. They most commonly have a hepatitic pattern of injury, showing predominately lymphocytic inflammation in the lobules and the portal tracts. The diagnosis requires exclusion of viral hepatitis (A, B, C, E) and autoimmune hepatitis. Several additional common patterns for DILI are described in more detail below. Also of note, the changes seen with any given drug often show a common pattern of injury, but there can be wide variations in the histological findings. Thus, finding a "typical pattern" for a given drug is helpful but is not necessary to diagnose a drug reaction. Most idiosyncratic drug reactions are not associated with significant fibrosis, so fibrosis in most cases suggests an alternative injury process.

Hepatic Pattern

Hepatitic patterns of DILI show lobular inflammation that is predominately lymphocytic and ranges from mild to marked in severity, often accompanied by varying degrees of lobular disarray and apoptotic hepatocytes (Figure 8.3). Some cases can show a zone 3 accentuation of the inflammation, including either subacute (Figure 8.4) or acute zone 3 necrosis (eFig. 8.2). Lobular cholestasis can also be seen. The portal inflammation can range from mild to severe and is mostly lymphocytic, but occasional plasma cells, neutrophils, and eosinophils are common and sometimes can be prominent. Interface activity can be present (Figure 8.5), in particular if there is moderate or greater portal inflammation.

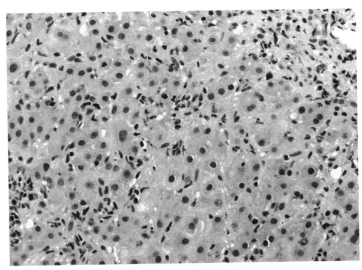

FIGURE 8.3 **Idiopathic drug reaction, lobular hepatitis.** This drug reaction was induced by an herbal remedy and shows a hepatitic pattern of injury.

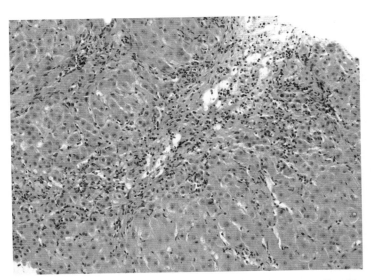

FIGURE 8.4 **Idiopathic drug reaction, lobular hepatitis with zone 3 pattern.** In this case of atorvastatin drug-induced liver injury (DILI), there is a zone 3 accentuation of the lobular inflammation with loss of zone 3 hepatocytes, indicating subacute necrosis.

The differential for a hepatitic pattern of injury is largely that of viral hepatitis and autoimmune hepatitis. Of note, the histological findings in viral hepatitis, autoimmune hepatitis, and hepatitic patterns of DILI have sufficient overlap that in most cases, a diagnosis cannot be confidently made based solely on the histology. Specifically, plasma cell–rich inflammation,

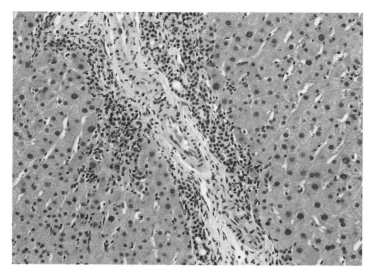

FIGURE 8.5 **Idiopathic drug reaction, interface activity.** This example of diclofenac-induced drug-induced liver injury (DILI) showed predominately portal-based inflammation with interface activity.

interface activity, and zone 3 predominant inflammation are not etiologically specific and can be seen in all three of these entities.

Importantly, several idiosyncratic drug reactions can have a plasma cell–rich hepatitic pattern that closely mimics autoimmune hepatitis (Figure 8.6, eFig. 8.3), and can be associated with elevated serum antinuclear (ANA) and/or antismooth muscle (ASMA) antibody titers. These drugs include minocycline (used to treat acne), methyldopa (used to treat hypertension), clometacin (anti-inflammatory drug), and nitrofurantoin (used to treat urinary tract infections) (Table 8.1). These drug reactions can start soon after beginning the medication or can take several years to develop. These cases are sometimes called drug-induced autoimmune hepatitis,[24] but they are not the same disease as autoimmune hepatitis and that distinction requires clinical follow-up, so is a term best avoided in surgical pathology reports.

Infliximab, a monoclonal antibody against tumour necrosis factor (TNF) alpha, can also lead to an autoimmune-like pattern of hepatitis; of note, infliximab, can also induce serum ANA and ASMA autoantibodies, so a diagnosis of autoimmune hepatitis should be approached with caution if a patient has a relevant history of these therapies.[25]

Resolving Pattern of Hepatitis

In some cases, a biopsy may be performed because a drug reaction was clinically suspected, but the medication was stopped prior to the biopsy. Biopsies in this setting often show a resolving hepatitis pattern, with absent

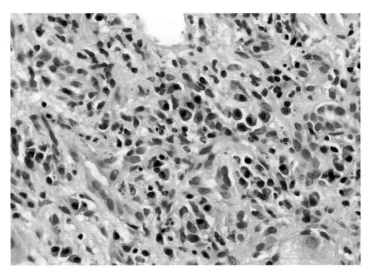

FIGURE 8.6 **Plasma cell–rich drug reaction.** Numerous portal plasma cells are seen in this drug reaction.

to minimal lobular lymphocytic inflammation and minimal to focally mild portal lymphocytic inflammation. The lobules and portal tracts commonly show small Kupffer cell aggregates (Figure 8.7), which may contain pigmented material in their cytoplasm and can be highlighted on periodic acid–Schiff with diastase (PASD) stain. The resolving hepatitis pattern can also be seen in patients after acute, self-limited viral hepatitis.

Prolonged Liver Enzyme Elevations After Stopping a Medication

In most cases of DILI, the liver injury resolves fairly promptly after stopping the drug, within 2 to 4 weeks, but occasionally, it may take a few months for the liver enzymes to completely normalize. In general, DILI that caused significant clinical cholestasis tends to resolve more slowly than DILI that is purely or primarily hepatitic. Uncommonly, patients may have prolonged elevations in liver enzymes or bilirubin levels after stopping the medication, leading to a biopsy to rule out underlying liver disease. The biopsies findings in this setting usually do not show evidence for an underlying liver disease but instead demonstrate only minimal inflammatory or cholestatic changes. Most of these cases represent the tail-end of the recovery curve; there currently is no compelling evidence for progression to ongoing chronic hepatitis, advanced fibrosis, or cirrhosis in these cases. For this reason, a biopsy that shows significant ongoing hepatitic or biliary injury after stopping the medication suggests the medication was not the cause of the liver injury, or there is an underlying liver disease.

TABLE 8.1 Drugs That Can Be Associated With Both an Autoimmune Hepatitis-Like Pattern of Injury on Biopsy as Well as Positive Autoantibody Serologies. A Representative Reference Is Provided

Drug	Comments
Strongest association	
Atorvastatin (Lipitor)[5]	Statin used to lower cholesterol
Clometacin[6]	Nonsteroidal anti-inflammatory drug (NSAID)
Diclofenac[7]	NSAID
Dihydralizine[8]	Antihypertensive
Halothane[9]	Inhalational general anesthetic
Infliximab[10,11]	Antibody against tumor necrosis factor alpha
Interferon[12,13]	Can be seen in the postliver transplant setting
Isoniazid[9]	Tuberculosis treatment
Methyldopa[14]	Antihypertensive
Minocycline[15]	Antibiotic
Nitrofurantoin[15]	Antibiotic
Oxyphenisatin[16]	Herbal laxative
Tienilic acid[17]	Diuretic
Propylthiouracil[18]	Treatment for hyperthyroid disease
Others	
Benzbromarone[19]	Inhibitor of xanthine oxidase used to treat gout
Cefaclor[19]	Antibiotic
Cephalexin[15]	Antibiotic
Loxoprofen sodium hydrate[19]	NSAID
Ofloxacin[19]	Antibiotic
Ornidazole[20]	Antiprotozoan
Prometrium[15]	Progesterone
Pemoline[21]	Simulant used to treat attention-deficit hyperactivity disorder (ADHD) and narcolepsy
Rosuvastatin (Crestor)[22]	Statin used to lower cholesterol
Simvastatin[5]	Statin used to lower cholesterol
Black Cohosh[23]	Herbal remedy

Granulomas

Granulomas in DILI are commonly associated with a granulomatous hepatitis pattern of injury, where the biopsy shows lymphocytic inflammation of the portal tracts and lobules accompanied by scattered, often poorly formed granulomas. The granulomas can be found in the lobules

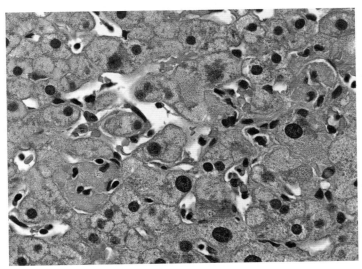

FIGURE 8.7 **Resolving hepatitis.** A biopsy was performed for an acute hepatitis caused by a drug reaction. The active injury was largely absent by the time the biopsy was performed, but numerous pigmented Kupffer cells are present in the lobules.

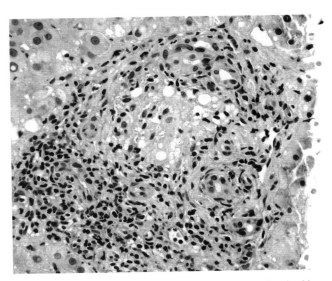

FIGURE 8.8 **Granulomas in drug reaction.** This drug reaction had loose, poorly formed granulomas in the portal tracts.

(Figure 8.8), the portal tracts, and rarely can involve bile ducts. Less often, granulomas with little or no inflammation are the main histological finding.

Granulomas in DILI can have a range of morphologies, but most are loose and poorly formed in the setting of a marked lobular hepatitis, or

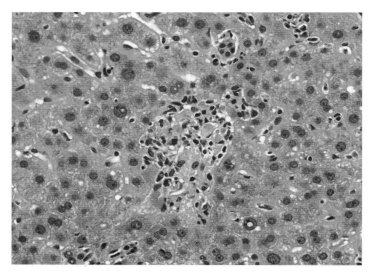

FIGURE 8.9 **Granulomas in drug reaction.** This case of lisinopril drug-induced liver injury (DILI) showed mild lobular hepatitis and scattered lobular epithelioid granulomas.

are well-formed epithelioid granulomas (Figure 8.9). Fibrin ring granulomas can also be seen. The differential for granulomas in the liver is broad and there are no immunohistochemical stains that can identify the etiology of granulomas, outside of organism stains. Most granulomas seen in liver biopsies are not drug-related but instead primary biliary cholangitis (PBC)–related, idiopathic, sarcoidosis-related, or infection-associated.[26] Granulomas in the setting of DILI are not fibrotic (as they often are in cases of sarcoidosis), and most often there is no fibrosis in the background liver, unless there is an underlying chronic liver disease with a superimposed DILI. Granulomas caused by DILI do not show central necrosis, a finding that would favor infection. Antimitochondrial antibodies (AMA) positivity and features of chronic cholestatic liver disease would favor PBC. Polarization can help identify foreign body granulomas, but foreign body granulomas would be an incidental finding if seen in the context of DILI. Stains to rule out fungal and acid-fast infections are important.

Cholangitic Pattern

The cholangitic pattern of injury is most commonly seen with antibiotics and shows active bile duct injury, with lymphocytosis of the bile duct epithelium, reactive epithelial changes, and apoptotic epithelial bodies. The amount of duct-centered inflammation can range from mild (Figure 8.10) to striking (Figure 8.11). The portal inflammation is often mixed, with lymphocytes and neutrophils. There also can be histiocyte-rich inflammation that is vaguely granulomatous, often associated with more severe bile duct injury.

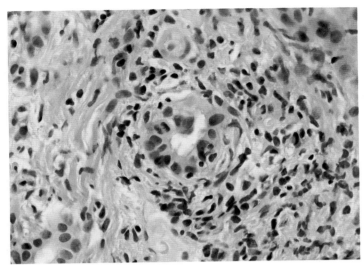

FIGURE 8.10 **Cholangitic pattern of drug reaction.** The inflammation is overall mild but there is clear bile duct lymphocytosis and injury in this case of Augmentin drug-induced liver injury (DILI).

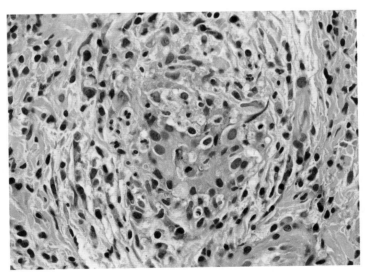

FIGURE 8.11 **Cholangitic pattern of drug reaction.** There is striking lymphocytic inflammation and severe bile duct injury in this case. Occasional eosinophils are also seen.

Bland Lobular Cholestasis Pattern

Varying degrees of cholestasis can be present in biopsies with a hepatitic pattern of injury or with a cholangitic pattern of injury, but this section is focused on the injury pattern that shows lobular cholestasis without

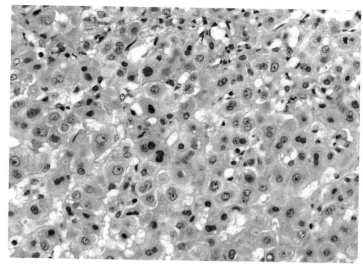

FIGURE 8.12 **Bland lobular cholestasis drug reaction.** This biopsy is from a young man who presented with cholestasis after using body-building supplements that contained androgens.

significant bile duct injury, bile duct loss, changes of obstruction, or significant lobular hepatitis (Figure 8.12). This pattern of injury is commonly seen with oral contraceptives or anabolic steroids but can also be seen with a wide range of other medications. The cholestasis often has a zone 3 predominance. Bile can be seen in the hepatocyte cytoplasm or in the bile canaliculi. Bile is not present in the bile ducts and there is no or minimal bile ductular reaction. Lobular cholestasis can persist for several months after discontinuing the offending drug.

The differential for bland lobular cholestasis includes sepsis, heart failure, hypothyroidism, and critically ill individuals, for example those in intensive care units. In most of these settings, however, biopsies are not performed because the clinical findings provide an explanation for the liver dysfunction. If biopsies are performed in this setting, they show a similar pattern of bland lobular cholestasis.

Ductopenic Pattern

Loss of intrahepatic bile ducts is a rare but important pattern of DILI (Figure 8.13 and Table 8.2). This pattern can be very subtle and cytokeratin immunostains are helpful to confirm and quantify bile duct loss; cytokeratin 7 (CK7) is best for this task, as it will also show zone 1 intermediate hepatocytes, which are invariably present in cases of true bile duct loss. When evaluating the biopsy for bile duct loss, the size of the portal tract should be taken into account, since loss of bile ducts in large or medium-sized portal tracts is essentially always abnormal. In contrast,

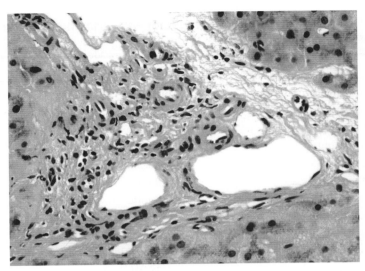

FIGURE 8.13 **Ductopenia.** No bile ducts were seen in most of the portal tracts in this biopsy.

approximately 50% of smaller portal tracts should have bile duct loss to confidently diagnosis ductopenia. Looking for unpaired hepatic arteries can improve the detection of bile duct loss.[50] In cases of drug-induced ductopenia, the remaining ducts often show atrophic changes, and the overall findings tend to be similar to that of chronic rejection in the liver allograft. There can be lobular cholestasis, especially in cases with prolonged ductopenia. The portal tracts often have minimal to mild nonspecific lymphocytic inflammation.

Cases of ductopenia resulting from DILI typically do not show bile ductular proliferation, bile duct duplication, onion-skin fibrosis, or fibroobliterative duct lesions. If any of these latter changes are present, then the ductopenia is unlikely to be drug-related. Likewise, significant fibrosis is typically not part of the drug-associated ductopenic pattern of injury and would favor an alternative form of chronic biliary tract disease. In all cases, imaging of the biliary tract should be performed to exclude bile duct loss secondary to chronic biliary obstruction.

Fatty Pattern

Drug reactions can cause both a macrovesicular and microvesicular pattern of injury. Overall, an estimated 2% of cases of nonalcoholic fatty liver disease are drug-related.[3] The diagnosis of a macrovesicular steatosis pattern of DILI requires exclusion of other diseases, including the metabolic syndrome, alcohol, Wilson disease, celiac disease, protein malnutrition, and cystic fibrosis. Steroids are one of the more commonly encountered drug-induced causes of steatosis, but there are many others

TABLE 8.2 **Drugs Associated With Ductopenia, Also Known as the Vanishing Bile Duct Syndrome**	
Drug	Comments
Amoxicillin/clavulanic acid[27]	Antibiotic
Anabolic steroids[28]	
Azithromycin[29]	Antibiotic
Carbamazepine[30]	Used to treat epilepsy
Chlorpromazine (Thorazine)[31]	Antipsychotic
Ciprofloxacin[32]	Antibiotic
Flucloxacillin[33]	Antibiotic
fluoroquinolone[34]	Antibiotic
Gold salt therapy[35]	
Ibuprofen[36]	Nonsteroidal anti-inflammatory drug (NSAID)
Interferon therapy[37]	
Itraconazole[38]	Antifungal
Meropenem[39]	Antibiotic
Moxifloxacin[40]	Antibiotic
Naproxen[41]	NSAID
Nevirapine[42]	Reverse transcriptase inhibitor
Tenoxicam[43]	NSAID
Terbinafine[44]	Antifungal
Thiabendazole[45]	Antifungal
Tibolone and St Johns Wort[46]	Synthetic hormone and Herbal remedy
Trimethoprim-sulfamethoxazole[47]	Antibiotic
Total parenteral nutrition[48]	Up to 25% of cases in one study
Valproic acid[49]	Used to treat epilepsy

(Table 8.3). Steatohepatitis, with ballooned hepatocytes and Mallory hyaline, is rarely seen as a drug effect, other than with amiodarone or irinotecan. Methotrexate can have a steatohepatitis pattern, often with fibrosis.

AMIODARONE. Overall, an estimated 1% to 4% of individuals on chronic amiodarone therapy will develop steatohepatitis.[53,54] The risk of steatohepatitis is associated more with the duration of therapy than with the dosage, with most cases having at least a year of exposure.[3] The total accumulated dose, however, also appears to be a risk factor. Amiodarone becomes very concentrated in the liver, where it can reach levels as high as 1% of the wet weight of the liver over time.[3] Amiodarone also has a very long half-life in the liver and can continue to cause liver injury after the medication is

TABLE 8.3 Drugs Associated With a Macrovesicular Steatosis Pattern of Injury

Drug	Comments
Amiodarone	One of the most common causes of drug-induced steatohepatitis
Cannabis	Limited data; reported in the setting of chronic hepatitis C[51]
Glucocorticoids	
Irinotecan	Chemotherapeutic, commonly used in colon cancer
Methotrexate	
Nucleoside reverse transcriptase inhibitors	HIV treatment
Oxaliplatin	Chemotherapeutic, commonly used in colon cancer
Perhexiline	Antianginal agent
Protease inhibitors	HIV treatment, can be associated with lipodystrophy
Tamoxifen	Estrogen receptor antagonist. 30%-40% of breast cancer patients under treatment will develop fatty liver disease in the first 2 y of therapy[52]

stopped. Amiodarone-induced injury can lead to macrovesicular steatosis with generally mild lobular inflammation. Despite the often mild fatty change, most cases show moderate to marked hepatocellular ballooning and abundant Mallory hyaline (Figure 8.14). This disproportionately severe ballooning, compared to the degree of steatosis, can closely mimic severe alcoholic liver disease.[55] In fact, balloon cells will predominate with only little fatty change in some cases. Cholestasis and granulomas have also been reported.[56,57]

Several drugs are thought to precipitate fatty liver disease, or exacerbate the disease activity in individuals with the metabolic syndrome or alcohol use. These drugs include estrogens, tamoxifen, and nifedipine. At a practical level, biopsies to rule out DILI in this setting are best approached by fully reporting the amount of fat, degree of ongoing injury, and fibrosis and noting that the biopsy findings do not reliably separate DILI from ordinary fatty liver disease but that certain drugs are thought to exacerbate fatty liver disease in patients with underlying risk factors. Furthermore, the relative contributions from DILI versus the metabolic syndrome/alcohol use is not reliably made by biopsy.

PHOSPHOLIPIDOSIS. Some drugs, such as amiodarone, perhexiline maleate, and diethylaminoethoxyhexestrol can cause steatohepatitis, with or

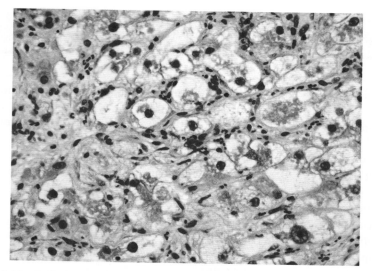

FIGURE 8.14 **Amiodarone drug-induced liver injury (DILI).** The biopsy shows severe ballooning with little steatosis.

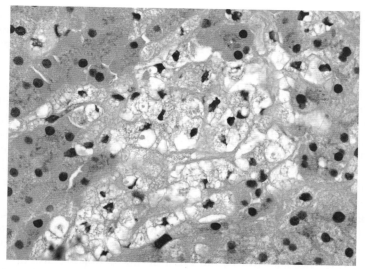

FIGURE 8.15 **Phospholipidosis.** The biopsy shows distinct clusters of enlarged Kupffer cells with foamy cytoplasm. This case is more striking than many.

without an additional finding called *phospholipidosis*. Phospholipidosis is characterized by enlarged Kupffer cells with foamy appearing cytoplasm (Figure 8.15). This finding can be difficult to reliably identify on hematoxylin and eosin (H&E) stains when mild, but when well developed, the changes are striking and can mimic a storage disorder, such as Niemann

Pick disease. On electron microscopy, the foamy Kupffer cells show lamellar inclusions in lysosomes.

Phospholipidosis can also be seen with a wide variety of medications that are not associated with fatty liver disease.[58] There continues to be uncertainty as to whether phospholipidosis represents a toxic effect or an adaptive response.

MICROVESICULAR STEATOSIS PATTERN. The microvesicular pattern of steatosis is rare but can be seen with Reye syndrome and with medications that impair mitochondrial function, including valproic acid, tetracycline, and zidovudine. With microvesicular steatosis, the hepatocytes have numerous tiny vacuoles that fill their cytoplasm (Figure 8.16). The microvesicular steatosis is typically diffuse, although there may be some zonal accentuation. The presence of occasional medium- or large-sized fat droplets is still consistent with the diagnosis.

Isolated Hyperammonemia

Rarely, patients can present with isolated elevations in serum ammonia, raising concern for advanced cirrhosis. The two most common medications that have been linked to this pattern of DILI are valproic acid[59] and infusion of high-dose 5-fluorouracil for chemotherapy.[60] The elevated ammonia levels typically lead to assessment by noninvasive markers of fibrosis and, if these are negative for advanced fibrosis, can sometimes lead to a biopsy to rule out advanced fibrosis or other parenchymal disease.

In cases that show no evidence for an underlying, undiagnosed liver disease, the biopsy findings generally fall into the almost normal liver

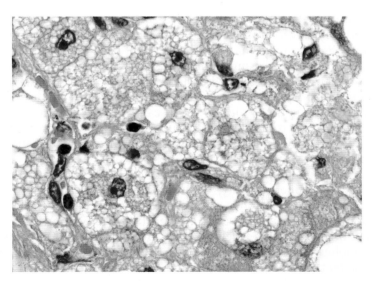

FIGURE 8.16 **Microvesicular steatosis.** The hepatocytes are swollen by numerous tiny droplets of fat.

pattern, although some cases can show minimal, nonspecific portal or lobular lymphocytic inflammation, or minimal macrovesicular steatosis. The differential for this pattern of injury (isolated elevations in serum ammonia; histology shows an almost normal liver biopsy) includes portosystemic shunts,[61] urea cycle defects,[62] and infections with urease producing bacteria—often originating in the urinary tract.[63,64]

Toxic Injury Patterns

Direct toxins cause liver injury in a reproducible and dose-dependent fashion. In most cases, the injury occurs in a few days after exposure. Examples include acetaminophen, mushroom poisoning, and miscellaneous household and industrial chemicals. For most of these agents, the basic pattern of injury is direct necrosis with relatively little inflammation. The surviving hepatocytes often show mild reactive fatty changes, with small- and medium-sized fat droplets, as well as cholestasis. In most cases, the necrosis has a zone 3 pattern. Toxicity from phosphorous, ferrous sulfate, and cocaine, however, have all been associated with a zone 1 pattern of necrosis.[65,66] With more severe injury, the necrosis is often panacinar and no zonation will be evident.

ACETAMINOPHEN TOXICITY. Acetaminophen toxicity is a classic example of a direct liver toxin, with the degree of injury predicted by the level of exposure. Acetaminophen toxicity is one of the most important causes of acute liver failure, representing up to 50% of cases in the USA and 75% of cases in the United Kingdom, although in other countries, such as Japan, the frequency is lower.

Acetaminophen toxicity occurs in individuals who intentionally take large quantities at single time points as suicide attempts (approximately 40%). An even larger proportion of individuals have unintentional overdoses that often occur in the setting of alcohol use, or in cases of chronic pain, where patients are using medications that contain both narcotics and acetaminophen. Hepatic injury is usually not seen unless there is greater than 7.5 g of exposure, with severe liver damage seen with 15 to 25 g of exposure. The toxic threshold, however, can be lower in individuals with fatty liver disease, chronic alcohol consumption, and use of drugs that stimulate the P-450 enzyme system, including carbamazepine, dimetidine, isoniazid, and phenytoin.

The median alanine aminotransferase (ALT) levels is 4300 IU/L with severe acetaminophen toxicity, while bilirubin levels are only modestly elevated, usually in the range of 4 mg/dL. By way of contrast, idiosyncratic DILI tends to have lower ALT levels (average of approximately 500 IU/L) but higher bilirubin levels (average around 20 mg/dL). Treatment of acetaminophen toxicity with N-acetylcysteine is very effective when given within the first 24 hours of presentation.

Histologically, the liver shows hepatocyte necrosis with relatively little inflammation in the lobules or portal tracts. In milder cases, the necrosis can have a zone 3 distribution (Figure 8.17), while severe cases can show panacinar necrosis (eFig. 8.4). In cases with very early hepatocellular necrosis, the Kupffer cells and endothelial cells are often still alive and in their normal locations. Remaining, viable hepatocytes are often cholestatic and commonly show mild microvesicular steatosis. If the specimen is from a later time point, there may be mild lobular inflammation in the areas of necrosis and the portal tracts can show a brisk bile ductular proliferation, one that can extend into areas of parenchymal collapse. At these later time points, the Kupffer cells may also show significant iron accumulation, as can the proliferating bile ductules. While special stains are generally not needed, occasionally a special stain can be useful to demonstrate the necrosis for diagnosis or presentations to clinical colleagues. Useful stains include a CD10 or polyclonal carcinoembryonic antigen (CEA), which will show loss of the canalicular staining pattern in the necrotic areas (Figure 8.18).

ALLERGIC INJURY PATTERN

Cases of allergic-type DILI are rarely biopsied because patients typically have other clinical findings that suggest the diagnosis, such as hives or wheezing or peripheral eosinophilia. Occasionally, however, the clinical findings can be diminished or obscured by other comorbid conditions, leading to liver biopsies as part of the investigation into the cause of new onset hepatitis. In most cases, the drug exposure will have been within the past few days or weeks.

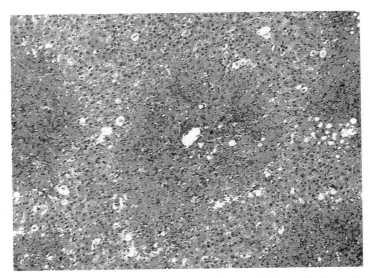

FIGURE 8.17 **Acetaminophen toxicity.** Necrosis is seen with a zonal pattern. The necrosis involves zones 3 and 2, with sparing of the zone 1, or perioportal, hepatocytes.

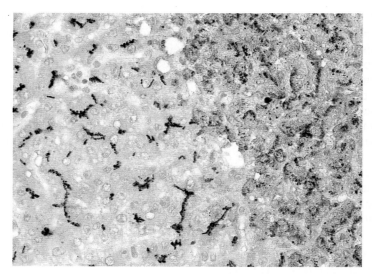

FIGURE 8.18 **Zone 3 necrosis, CD10 immunostain.** The area of necrosis shows loss of the normal canalicular staining pattern (right side of image), while the viable hepatocytes show a normal staining pattern (left side of image).

The biopsy shows increased eosinophils in the portal tracts and sinusoids. The portal tracts also typically show mild to moderate, patchy lymphocytic inflammation. The lobules can show mild lymphocytic inflammation and occasional apoptotic bodies.

Of note, cases of otherwise typical chronic viral hepatitis, autoimmune hepatitis, and PBC can sometimes have a focal, mild prominence in portal tract eosinophils, so the mere presence of eosinophils does not always indicate a drug reaction. Likewise, a prominence in sinusoidal eosinophils can be seen with peripheral eosinophilia from many different causes that are not a result of DILI; in these cases, there is minimal or absent lobular injury, as the eosinophils are simply passing through the liver sinusoids and their prominence in the biopsy reflects the increased numbers in the blood.

DRESS SYNDROME A severe type of allergic DILI is called the DRESS syndrome, which stands for Drug Reaction with Eosinophilia and Systemic Symptoms. This severe drug reaction, which has a mortality rate of up to 10%,[67] is unusual because it typically develops later than most allergic-type drug reactions, often starting 3 or more weeks after the triggering medication was begun. DRESS can even develop several weeks after cessation of the offending medication. The most common drugs that cause the DRESS syndrome are carbamazepine (27% of cases), allopurinol (11%), lamotrigine (6%), phenobarbital (6%), nevirapine (5%), phenytoin (4%), and abacavir (3%), but the full list is very long with many less common trigger medications.[68]

The liver is typically involved, but, in most cases, the diagnosis is made on clinical grounds (Table 8.4) and biopsies are not needed. When biopsied, the liver shows moderate to marked portal inflammation that has a striking enrichment for eosinophils (Figure 8.19), along with lobular inflammation that is also enriched for eosinophils. Additional findings may include noncaseating, epithelioid granulomas, and lymphocytic cholangitis.[69] Cases with severe lobular injury commonly show necrosis, which can range from zone 3 to panacinar. Rare examples of DRESS with zone 1 necrosis have also been reported.[69]

TABLE 8.4   Clinical Features of the DRESS Syndrome

• Fever, that is, greater than 38 °C
• Rash
• Lymphadenopathy in at least two locations
• Peripheral blood tests
  • Either lymphocytosis or lymphopenia. The lymphocytes often show cytological atypia.
  • Eosinophilia
  • Thrombocytopenia

DRESS, Drug reaction with eosinophilia and systemic symptoms.

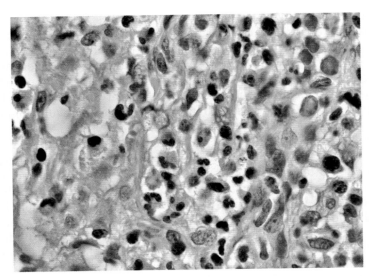

FIGURE 8.19   **DRESS syndrome.** The biopsy shows marked eosinophil infiltrates in the portal tracts.

OTHER PATTERNS

Medications Associated With Fibrosis

Fibrosis is an uncommon finding in cases of DILI but is well recognized for several medications. On the other hand, a wide variety of drugs have been associated with liver fibrosis in case reports and case series, but causality is often difficult to prove, or evenly strongly suggest, as many individuals have comorbidities that could adequately explain the fibrosis, such as the metabolic syndrome. Likewise, a number of drugs have been associated with the development of cirrhosis. For example, one large registry-based study identified cases of cirrhosis that were thought to be caused by idiosyncratic drug reactions from tamoxifen, ebrotidine, and amoxicillin–clavulanic acid.[70] A second registry-based study found cryptogenic cirrhosis in 0.7% of individuals after long term follow-up for a drug-induced hepatitis.[71] Causation, however, can be difficult to convincingly demonstrate. This is not meant to say that drug reactions cannot cause fibrosis or cirrhosis, as the ability to cause fibrosis has been demonstrated for a few specific drugs. On the other hand, the mere taking of a fibrogenic drug does not necessarily indicate it is the cause of fibrosis in a specific liver biopsy specimen. Instead, each biopsy has to be evaluated on its own merits and in its own unique clinical and laboratory context. Methotrexate is discussed next, as one example of a drug that has been strongly associated with fibrosis risk.

METHOTREXATE. Low-dose, chronic methotrexate use is a risk factor for the development of significant fibrosis.[72,73] Methotrexate is an important medication for the management of chronic diseases, such as psoriasis and rheumatoid arthritis, and remains a valuable therapeutic agent despite the fibrosis risk. Risk factors for fibrosis include the cumulative dose and the presence of other chronic liver disease, in particular fatty liver disease.[73] Historically, liver biopsies were often performed at baseline and periodically after the introduction of the medication to monitor for fibrosis development, but this role has diminished considerably with noninvasive markers of fibrosis.[74]

The fibrosis pattern can include both portal fibrosis and pericellular fibrosis (Figure 8.20). The medication is frequently stopped when there is moderate portal fibrosis or bridging fibrosis. In addition to the fibrosis, the liver can show fatty change (Figure 8.21), hepatocyte nuclear pleomorphism, and portal lymphocytic inflammation that is generally mild but can be focally moderate. Many patients will also have risk factors for fatty liver disease, such as the metabolic syndrome, and the histological findings do not clearly separate drug effect from ordinary fatty liver disease in these individuals. In fact, it is an open question to what extent methotrexate use causes significant fibrosis if the patient does not also have fatty liver disease.

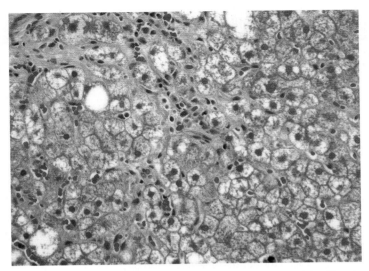

FIGURE 8.20 **Methotrexate injury.** A trichrome stain shows pericellular fibrosis.

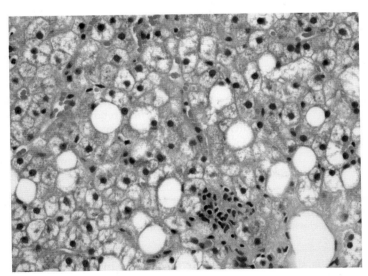

FIGURE 8.21 **Methotrexate injury.** Mild macrovesicular steatosis and mild lobular inflammation is present.

Despite having been largely replaced by noninvasive markers of fibrosis, biopsies are still performed in cases with discordant results between clinical findings and noninvasive markers of fibrosis, or when there are concerns for other disease processes. The fibrosis seen on biopsy is then helpful in determining whether to continue methotrexate therapy. A grading schema for methotrexate injury has long been available and the current,

TABLE 8.5	Grading Schema for Methotrexate Toxicity
Grade	**Histological Description**
1	Normal
	Mild steatosis
	Mild nuclear variability
	Mild portal inflammation
	Allowed fibrosis is not specified, typically none
2	Moderate to marked steatosis
	Moderate to marked nuclear variability
	Moderate to marked portal inflammation
	Allowed fibrosis is not specified, typically none or minimal portal fibrosis
3	3A: "mild" fibrosis.[1]
	3B: "moderate to severe" fibrosis.[1]
4	Cirrhosis
	Suggested Clinical Implications
1	Can continue to receive methotrexate therapy
2	Can continue to receive methotrexate therapy
3A	Can continue to receive methotrexate therapy but should have a repeat liver biopsy after approximately 6 mo of continued therapy.
3B	Should not be given further methotrexate therapy. However, exceptional circumstances may require continued methotrexate therapy with careful follow-up.
4	Should not be given further methotrexate therapy. However, exceptional circumstances may require continued methotrexate therapy with careful follow-up.

Original paper.[75] There is some ambiguity about what was precisely meant by mild fibrosis versus moderate to severe fibrosis in the published schema. In general practice, portal fibrosis is commonly classified as 3A, while bridging fibrosis is classified as 3B.

revised form[75] is shown in Table 8.5. There remain some questions on the structure of the schema (because it combines fat and inflammation in the same score as the fibrosis), so many pathologists choose not to use it for clinical care. Whatever approach you choose, important findings to convey in the pathology report are the amounts of fibrosis, steatosis, and active injury (balloon cells, lobular and portal inflammation).

Vascular Changes Associated With Drug Effects

Drug-induced vascular changes are most commonly seen in the setting of chemotherapy and include veno-occlusive disease, also known as sinusoidal obstructive syndrome, and nodular regenerative hyperplasia. Other examples of drug-induced vascular changes include peliosis hepatis and vascular thrombosis. These patterns of injury are discussed in Chapter 13.

Drug-Induced Cytoplasmic Changes and Inclusions

Drug effects can lead to abnormal endoplasmic reticulum (ER) proliferation in hepatocytes, leading to distinctive cytoplasmic changes. These changes can be associated with mild liver enzyme elevations but never with moderate or greater liver enzyme elevations and there is no risk of fibrosis; thus, these ER proliferations are often considered to be adaptive responses rather than true drug-induced liver injuries. The ER changes can be categorized into several different histological patterns.

First, the hepatocytes can show a diffuse, gray, homogenous change to their cytoplasm. For example, this change can be seen in individuals with HIV/HCV coinfection, usually as an incidental finding. Similar ER changes (Figure 8.22) can be seen with the use of phenobarbital or barbiturates.[76] The distribution of hepatocytes with the ER changes can vary from case to case, with milder cases showing zonation (often zone 3) and patchiness. Often this change is referred to as "induced" hepatocytes.

A second major pattern of ER proliferation has been described as "two-tone" hepatocytes, where hepatocytes have two distinct colors to their cytoplasm, with normal cytoplasmic eosinophilia in one half, while the other half of the cytoplasm has a distinctive homogenous gray color.

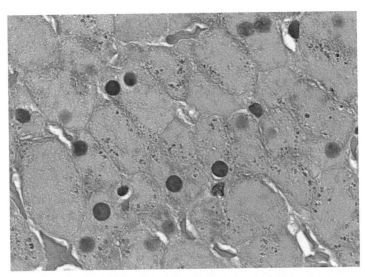

FIGURE 8.22 **Smooth endoplasmic reticulum proliferation.** The hepatocytes show an amphophilic change that fills the cytoplasm, displacing some of the lipofuscin (granular brown material) to the edge of the hepatocyte cytoplasm; this case is secondary to phenobarbital therapy.

The gray color of ER proliferation can be adjacent to the bile canaliculi (Figure 8.23) or can be perisinusoidal in location. The two-tone pattern can be highlighted nicely by PAS stains (Figure 8.24) and appears to be associated with a variety of drugs, often in individuals who are immunosuppressed and taking a number of different medications.

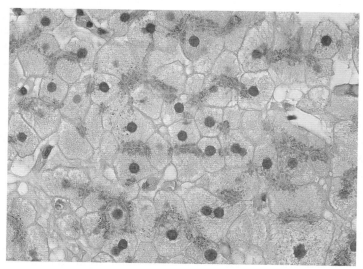

FIGURE 8.23 **Drug reaction with "two-tone hepatocytes."** The hepatocytes have two distinct colors to the cytoplasm, with the endoplasmic reticulum proliferation leading to light gray cytoplasm juxtaposed to more basophilic cytoplasm adjacent to the bile canaliculi.

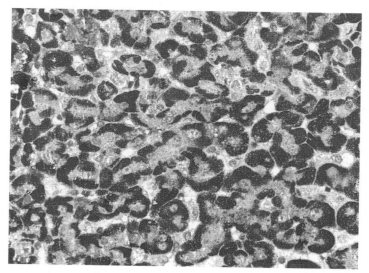

FIGURE 8.24 **Drug reaction with two tone hepatocytes.** A PAS stain highlights the cytoplasmic changes.

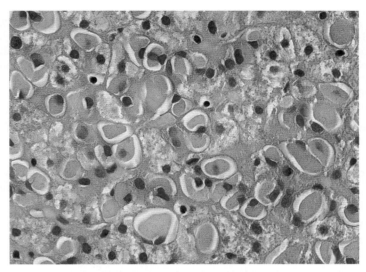

FIGURE 8.25 **Glycogen pseudoground glass.** This biopsy, from an immunosuppressed individual taking numerous medications, shows striking cytoplasmic changes, with large amphophilic inclusions in the hepatocytes.

In a third pattern, the ER proliferation can lead to distinctive hepatocyte inclusions (Figure 8.25, eFig. 8.5), a pattern termed "glycogen pseudoground glass" because it histologically closely resembles the ground glass changes that can be seen in cases of long-standing chronic hepatitis B virus (HBV) infection.[77] The inclusions are strongly PAS-positive, diastase sensitive, and electron microscopy suggests they are composed of glycogen with abnormal folding patterns.[77-79] The inclusions can be associated with mild liver enzyme elevations, but are not a cause of significant liver disease, with no evidence for causing fibrosis or other clinical problems. They can be present in follow-up biopsies.

There does not appear to be a single drug or class of drugs that can consistently cause the pseudoground glass change, and different drugs can lead to this same effect. The common denominator in most cases is immunosuppression combined with numerous medications. On the other hand, this same cytoplasmic change can occasionally be seen in individuals on single medications who are without obvious immunosuppression. The histological differential includes ground glass changes that can be seen in later stages of chronic HBV infection. Immunostains for HBV surface antigen are helpful in ruling out HBV infection. The differential also includes drug effects such as cyanamide, Lafora bodies, fibrinogen inclusions, and uremia (Table 8.6). Most types of inclusions are PAS-positive and PASD sensitive. PAS diastase sensitivity can be of help in this differential but should be interpreted cautiously because the degree of sensitivity or resistance to digestion can vary between laboratories. In most cases with inclusions, the distinctive clinical situations will clarify their etiology.

TABLE 8.6 Differential for Pseudo–Ground Glass–Type Inclusions in Hepatocytes

Type of Inclusion	Staining Properties	Electron Microscopy Findings
Glycogen pseudo-ground glass	PAS + diastase-sensitive colloidal iron-negative[a]	glycogen, occasional organelles[b]
Cyanamide	PAS + diastase-sensitive[c]	glycogen granules and dilated smooth endoplasmic reticulum
Fibrinogen	PAS– Fibrinogen + C3, C4 positive +/–	granular/fibrillar material within rough endoplasmic reticulum
Type IV glycogen storage disease	PAS + partially diastase-sensitive[d] colloidal iron-negative	nonmembrane-bound fibrillar and granular material
Lafora bodies	PAS + diastase-resistant colloidal iron-positive	fibril-like structures and electron-dense clumps
Uremia	PAS +	smooth endoplasmic reticulum

PAS, periodic acid–Schiff.

[a]Colloidal iron is generally negative in the inclusions, but depending on the quality of the stain, there can be areas where the hepatocytes all have a generalized blue color–in these overstained areas the inclusions will be positive.

[b]Additional details of the organelles was obscured by poor preservation.

[c]Cyanamide psuedoground glass has been described as both diastase-sensitive[80,81] and diastase-resistant.[82] Most cases in the literature appear to be diastase-sensitive.

[d]The inclusions in type IV glycogen storage disease is variably diastase-sensitive.[83,84]

Of note, fibrinogen-type inclusions are the only inclusions consistently PAS negative. Fibrinogen-type inclusions occur in two distinctly different clinical settings. The morphological findings, however, are about the same, so the clinical setting is important. Most often, they are nonspecific inclusions seen in the setting of other concomitant liver diseases.[85] Rarely, they are the histological manifestation of fibrinogen storage disease; in this setting, patients will have histories of either bleeding disorders or hypercoagulable disorders, depending on the specific site of the fibrinogen mutation.

Glycogenic Hepatopathy

Some drugs can lead to hepatic glycogenosis, with the biopsy showing enlarged pale hepatocytes, their cytoplasm filled with glycogen (Figure 8.26, eFig. 8.6). Corticosteroids are the most common drug association, which can be seen in a subset of patients after they receive a steroid bolus. With chronic use, corticosteroids can also cause steatosis.

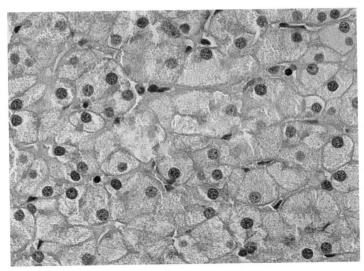

FIGURE 8.26 **Steroid-induced hepatic glycogenosis.** The hepatocytes are enlarged and pale appearing.

Excess Vitamin A

Excess intake of vitamin A has been a recognized cause of liver disease for over 50 years. Patients can have either acute or chronic presentations, although essentially all of the cases seen in surgical pathology specimens will be from chronic exposure. Patients with acute vitamin A toxicity can have severe headaches, vertigo, blurred vision, nausea, muscle pain, skin desquamation, and alopecia. Acute toxicity results from very high doses of vitamin A, usually >100 times the recommended dietary allowance (RDA).[86] In contrast, chronic toxicity typically develops in patients with at least 6 months of exposure to vitamin A doses that are >10 the RDA; most of these patients are asymptomatic and are picked up by mild persistent liver enzyme elevations.

The vast majority of chronic vitamin A toxicity occurs when patients consume too much preformed vitamin A, usually because of excess use of vitamins or dietary supplements. Rare cases of acute vitamin A toxicity have been reported after individuals ate too much liver of certain animals, such as seal or polar bear,[87] since these livers contain so much vitamin A. The liver of some fish, such as the grouper, can also have so much vitamin A that it causes acute toxicity when eaten by humans.[88]

In terms of chronic toxicity, topical Retin-A has been linked to stellate cell hyperplasia, suggesting chronic vitamin A toxicity.[89] On the other hand, vitamin A toxicity does not result from eating lots of vegetables, even those that are rich in beta-carotenes, the precursor to vitamin A, as the conversion of beta-carotenes to vitamin A is tightly regulated by the body, preventing excess.

The most common presentation with chronic exposure is mild but persistent aspartate aminotransferase (AST) and ALT elevations and a biopsy that at first review appears to be "almost normal." The histological correlate of vitamin A excess is enlarged and lipid-laden stellate cells, but these can be easily overlooked and the clinical information of excess vitamin A intake is almost always lacking. Thus, some very careful microscopy and a high degree of suspicion are usually necessary to make the diagnosis. An important point to remember: normal serum levels of vitamin A do not exclude vitamin A toxicity[90] because large proportions of vitamin A circulate as esters bound to plasma proteins and thus will not be evident in routinely used serum tests.[91] Measuring total serum retinyl esters may be a more reliable way to determine if there are excess total body vitamin A levels.[86]

Histologically, the main finding is stellate cell hyperplasia, with stellate cells that are enlarged (hypertrophy) and increased in number (hyperplasia). The stellate cell cytoplasm is filled with small lipid vacuoles giving the cytoplasm a bubbly appearance (Figure 8.27, eFig. 8.7). The presence of a true hyperplasia—a definite increase in numbers—is an important part of the making the diagnosis of vitamin A toxicity, as rare stellate cells can occasionally be seen in many diseases that have nothing to do with vitamin A toxicity. Nonetheless, even in a true hyperplasia, the lipid laden stellate cells remain relatively sparse in the biopsy, typically about 20 per 10 high-power fields (40× lens), with a range of about 10 to 60. In contrast, careful examination of biopsies in the setting of other liver diseases generally shows 0 to 2 stellate cells per 10 hpf.

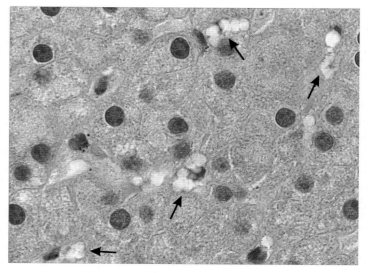

FIGURE 8.27 **Stellate cell hyperplasia.** Stellate cells (arrows) are enlarged by numerous small cytoplasmic vacuoles that indent the nuclei.

The sinusoidal location of the stellate cells and the shape of their nuclei usually permit one to distinguish stellate cell lipidosis from hepatocytes that have fat. On the other hand, many patients with fatty liver disease, especially those with marked steatosis plus mild to moderate lobular inflammation (ie, an "active steatohepatitis"), will have a Kupffer cell hyperplasia, and many of these Kupffer cells will have abundant smaller droplets of fat in their cytoplasm, which can closely mimic stellate cells. In addition, cholestatic liver disease can have Kupffer cell hyperplasia, where the Kupffer cells often showing vacuolated cytoplasm that can be misinterpreted as stellate cell hyperplasia. In fact, a fair number of images published in papers and sometimes textbooks appear to be reactive Kupffer cells and not really stellate cells. One useful clue to avoid this mistake is this: in cases where Kupffer cell hyperplasia is mimicking stellate cells, the vacuolated Kupffer cells tend to be much more frequent and prominent than true stellate cell hyperplasia caused by vitamin A excess. Nonetheless, because of the histological overlap, a diagnosis of stellate cell hyperplasia in the setting of significant fatty liver disease or cholestatic liver disease should be approached cautiously and is probably best avoided, especially if you see only a few stellate cells.

Other findings in vitamin A toxicity can include nodular regenerative hyperplasia and mild chronic inflammation.[92] Even relatively low levels of excess vitamin A intake can lead to liver disease, if taken long enough in susceptible individuals.[92] Fibrosis can be seen, but typically, only after years-to-decades of excess vitamin A intake.[92]

No immunostain is currently available that reliably highlights stellate cells in the setting of vitamin A excess: smooth muscle actin and fascin immunostains have not been helpful in my experience. CD68 can be helpful to exclude foamy Kupffer cells in select cases, but it can be very challenging to map the H&E findings to the immunostain findings on a cell-by-cell basis.

Chemotherapy-Related Changes

Sometimes, chemotherapy-associated liver injury is called CALI, instead of DILI. The most common patterns of injury are vascular disease, fatty liver disease, or a hepatitic pattern of injury.

Vascular injury most often results from damage to the sinusoidal endothelial cells, leading to a congestive pattern of injury called sinusoidal obstructive syndrome or veno-occlusive disease.[93] In surgical pathology specimens, the most common chemotherapy agent to lead to this pattern of injury is oxaliplatin. In general, biopsies are not performed to make a diagnosis of oxaliplatin DILI, but instead, these findings are usually incidental changes in the background liver parenchyma of specimens resected for metastatic colon adenocarcinoma.

The histological findings show moderate to marked sinusoidal dilatation and congestion (Figure 8.28). These changes are focused in zone 3 and can lead to a "bridging congestion" pattern, where areas of zone 3

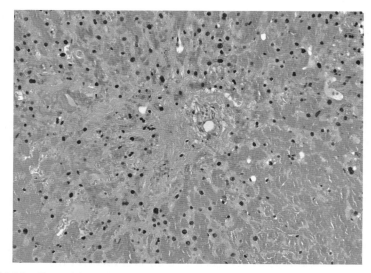

FIGURE 8.28 **Sinusoidal obstructive syndrome.** There is sclerosis of the central vein and marked sinusoidal congestion.

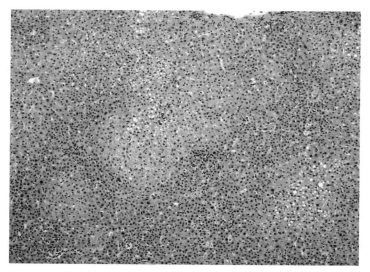

FIGURE 8.29 **Nodular regenerative hyperplasia.** The background liver shows nodularity without fibrosis in this resection specimen for treated colonic adenocarcinoma.

congestion extend from central veins to central veins. Changes of nodular regenerative hyperplasia are often present (Figure 8.29), and can range from subtle and equivocal (most often) to well-developed.[94-96] The central veins can also show fibrosis, with partial or complete occlusion by loose collagen. This finding is typically focal and is often best appreciated on trichrome stain. Zone 3 hepatocyte atrophy can also be seen. Unless there are additional disease processes affecting the liver, this pattern of chemotherapy-related injury does not have significant portal or lobular inflammation and does not have changes of downstream biliary obstruction.

Fatty liver disease is a second common pattern of DILI seen following chemotherapy. The changes include both steatosis, which can range from mild to marked, as well as steatohepatitis, with ballooned hepatocytes, mild lobular inflammation, and occasional Mallory hyaline. This pattern of injury is sometimes referred to as chemotherapy-associated steatosis or steatohepatitis or CAS/CASH[97] and is most often associated with irinotecan and to a lesser degree with oxaliplatin.[95] Essentially all individuals with CAS/CASH also have risk factors for the metabolic syndrome,[96] and this form of DILI appears to result from synergistic changes between the chemotherapy and other underlying risk factors of the metabolic syndrome.

CHECKPOINT INHIBITORS. Hepatitic patterns of injury following chemotherapy can occur in the setting of checkpoint inhibitors. For example, Ipilimumab is a monoclonal antibody that blocks the action of CTLA-4. CTLA-4 is a receptor that downregulates the immune system; when this receptor is blocked by antibodies, the immune system is more active against the tumor. The same basic mechanism of DILI is true for other checkpoint inhibitors, such as those targeting PD1 or PDL1.

In some patients, the immune system also becomes active against the nonneoplastic hepatocytes, leading to a hepatitic pattern of injury, with either a panlobular hepatitis or a zone 3 predominate hepatitis (Figure 8.30).[98-100] With more severe cases, the lobules can also show Kupffer cell

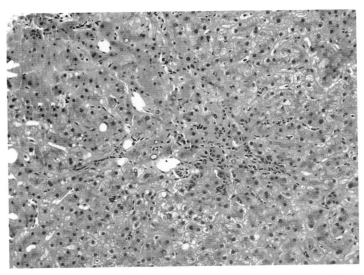

FIGURE 8.30 **Hepatitic pattern, Ipilimumab DILI**. The lobules show a mild hepatitis with a zone 3 accentuation.

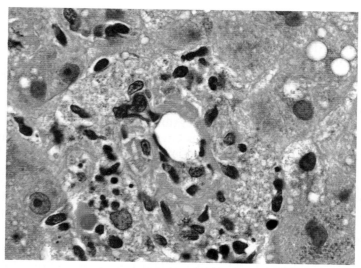

FIGURE 8.31 **Granuloma, Ipilimumab DILI.** In this case with a background of fatty liver disease, the lobules also showed fibrin ring-type granulomas.

hyperplasia with the formation of loose granulomas.[101] True epithelioid granulomas are occasionally present; fibrin ring granulomas can be seen too, mostly when the background liver shows fatty disease (Figure 8.31).[102] Overall, the hepatitis is morphologically nondescript and the broader differential includes autoimmune hepatitis and acute viral hepatitis. If the patient has a history of chronic HBV, reactivation of HBV is also in the histological differential and should be excluded.[103]

In some cases, the injury pattern can be more duct-centered, with active bile duct injury, including lymphocytic cholangitis that suggests PBC and/or changes that suggest biliary obstruction. In fact, some patients can develop primary sclerosing cholangitis (PSC)–like changes of the extrahepatic bile ducts that are evident on imaging.[101] Autoimmune conditions in other organs can also develop and most patients are treated by discontinuing the medication and/or steroid therapy.[104] Checkpoint inhibitors have also been associated with nodular regenerative hyperplasia.[105]

REFERENCES

1. Chalasani N, Fontana RJ, Bonkovsky HL, et al. Causes, clinical features, and outcomes from a prospective study of drug-induced liver injury in the United States. *Gastroenterology*. 2008;135:1924-1934.

2. Molleston JP, Fontana RJ, Lopez MJ, et al. Characteristics of idiosyncratic drug-induced liver injury in children: results from the DILIN prospective study. *J Pediatr Gastroenterol Nutr*. 2011;53:182-189.

3. Farrell GC. Drugs and steatohepatitis. *Semin Liver Dis*. 2002;22:185-194.

4. Davern TJ, Chalasani N, Fontana RJ, et al. Acute hepatitis E infection accounts for some cases of suspected drug-induced liver injury. *Gastroenterology*. 2011;141:1665-1672.

5. Alla V, Abraham J, Siddiqui J, et al. Autoimmune hepatitis triggered by statins. *J Clin Gastroenterol*. 2006;40:757-761.

6. Islam S, Mekhloufi F, Paul JM, et al. Characteristics of clometacin-induced hepatitis with special reference to the presence of anti-actin cable antibodies. *Autoimmunity*. 1989;2:213-221.

7. Scully LJ, Clarke D, Barr RJ. Diclofenac induced hepatitis. 3 cases with features of autoimmune chronic active hepatitis. *Dig Dis Sci*. 1993;38:744-751.

8. Bourdi M, Gautier JC, Mircheva J, et al. Anti-liver microsomes autoantibodies and dihydralazine-induced hepatitis: specificity of autoantibodies and inductive capacity of the drug. *Mol Pharmacol*. 1992;42:280-285.

9. Czaja AJ. Drug-induced autoimmune-like hepatitis. *Dig Dis Sci*. 2011;56:958-976.

10. Doyle A, Forbes G, Kontorinis N. Autoimmune hepatitis during infliximab therapy for Crohn's disease: a case report. *J Crohns Colitis*. 2011;5:253-255.

11. Efe C. Drug induced autoimmune hepatitis and TNF-α blocking agents: is there a real relationship? *Autoimmun Rev*. 2013;12:337-339.

12. Fiel MI, Agarwal K, Stanca C, et al. Posttransplant plasma cell hepatitis (de novo autoimmune hepatitis) is a variant of rejection and may lead to a negative outcome in patients with hepatitis C virus. *Liver Transplant*. 2008;14:861-871.

13. Fiel MI, Schiano TD. Plasma cell hepatitis (de-novo autoimmune hepatitis) developing post liver transplantation. *Curr Opin Organ Transplant*. 2012;17:287-292.

14. Shalev O, Mosseri M, Ariel I, et al. Methyldopa-induced immune hemolytic anemia and chronic active hepatitis. *Arch Intern Med*. 1983;143:592-593.

15. Bjornsson E, Talwalkar J, Treeprasertsuk S, et al. Drug-induced autoimmune hepatitis: clinical characteristics and prognosis. *Hepatology*. 2010;51:2040-2048.

16. Dietrichson O. Chronic active hepatitis. Aetiological considerations based on clinical and serological studies. *Scand J Gastroenterol*. 1975;10:617-624.

17. Lecoeur S, Andre C, Beaune PH. Tienilic acid-induced autoimmune hepatitis: anti-liver and-kidney microsomal type 2 autoantibodies recognize a three-site conformational epitope on cytochrome P4502C9. *Mol Pharmacol*. 1996;50:326-333.

18. Maggiore G, Larizza D, Lorini R, et al. Propylthiouracil hepatotoxicity mimicking autoimmune chronic active hepatitis in a girl. *J Pediatr Gastroenterol Nutr*. 1989;8:547-548.

19. Sugimoto K, Ito T, Yamamoto N, et al. Seven cases of autoimmune hepatitis that developed after drug-induced liver injury. *Hepatology*. 2011;54:1892-1893.

20. Ersoz G, Vardar R, Akarca US, et al. Ornidazole-induced autoimmune hepatitis. *Turk J Gastroenterol*. 2011;22:494-499.

21. Sterling MJ, Kane M, Grace ND. Pemoline-induced autoimmune hepatitis. *Am J Gastroenterol*. 1996;91:2233-2234.

22. Wolters LM, Van Buuren HR. Rosuvastatin-associated hepatitis with autoimmune features. *Eur J Gastroenterol Hepatol*. 2005;17:589-590.

23. Guzman G, Kallwitz ER, Wojewoda C, et al. Liver injury with features mimicking autoimmune hepatitis following the use of black cohosh. *Case Rep Med*. 2009;2009:918156.

24. European Association for the Study of the Liver Electronic address: easloffice@easloffice.eu; Clinical Practice Guideline Panel: Chair; Panel members; EASL Governing Board representative. EASL clinical practice guidelines: drug-induced liver injury. *J Hepatol*. 2019;70:1222-1261.

25. Germano V, Picchianti Diamanti A, Baccano G, et al. Autoimmune hepatitis associated with infliximab in a patient with psoriatic arthritis. *Ann Rheum Dis*. 2005;64:1519-1520.

26. Drebber U, Kasper HU, Ratering J, et al. Hepatic granulomas: histological and molecular pathological approach to differential diagnosis—A study of 442 cases. *Liver Int.* 2008;28:828-834.

27. Chawla A, Kahn E, Yunis EJ, et al. Rapidly progressive cholestasis: an unusual reaction to amoxicillin/clavulanic acid therapy in a child. *J Pediatr.* 2000;136:121-123.

28. Capra F, Nicolini N, Morana G, et al. Vanishing bile duct syndrome and inflammatory pseudotumor associated with a case of anabolic steroid abuse. *Dig Dis Sci.* 2005;50:1535-1537.

29. Juricic D, Hrstic I, Radic D, et al. Vanishing bile duct syndrome associated with azithromycin in a 62-year-old man. *Basic Clin Pharmacol Toxicol.* 2010;106:62-65.

30. Ramos AM, Gayotto LC, Clemente CM, et al. Reversible vanishing bile duct syndrome induced by carbamazepine. *Eur J Gastroenterol Hepatol.* 2002;14:1019-1022.

31. Chlumska A, Curik R, Boudova L, et al. Chlorpromazine-induced cholestatic liver disease with ductopenia. *Cesk Patol.* 2001;37:118-122.

32. Bataille L, Rahier J, Geubel A. Delayed and prolonged cholestatic hepatitis with ductopenia after long-term ciprofloxacin therapy for Crohn's disease. *J Hepatol.* 2002;37:696-699.

33. Eckstein RP, Dowsett JF, Lunzer MR. Flucloxacillin induced liver disease: histopathological findings at biopsy and autopsy. *Pathology.* 1993;25:223-228.

34. Orman ES, Conjeevaram HS, Vuppalanchi R, et al. Clinical and histopathologic features of fluoroquinolone-induced liver injury. *Clin Gastroenterol Hepatol.* 2011;9:517.e3-523.e3.

35. Basset C, Vadrot J, Denis J, et al. Prolonged cholestasis and ductopenia following gold salt therapy. *Liver Int.* 2003;23:89-93.

36. Alam I, Ferrell LD, Bass NM. Vanishing bile duct syndrome temporally associated with ibuprofen use. *Am J Gastroenterol.* 1996;91:1626-1630.

37. Dousset B, Conti F, Houssin D, et al. Acute vanishing bile duct syndrome after interferon therapy for recurrent HCV infection in liver-transplant recipients. *N Engl J Med.* 1994;330:1160-1161.

38. Adriaenssens B, Roskams T, Steger P, et al. Hepatotoxicity related to itraconazole: report of three cases. *Acta Clin Belg.* 2001;56:364-369.

39. Schumaker AL, Okulicz JF. Meropenem-induced vanishing bile duct syndrome. *Pharmacotherapy.* 2010;30:953.

40. Robinson W, Habr F, Manlolo J, et al. Moxifloxacin associated vanishing bile duct syndrome. *J Clin Gastroenterol.* 2010;44:72-73.

41. Ali S, Pimentel JD, Ma C. Naproxen-induced liver injury. *Hepatobiliary Pancreat Dis Int.* 2011;10:552-556.

42. Kochar R, Nevah MI, Lukens FJ, et al. Vanishing bile duct syndrome in human immunodeficiency virus: nevirapine hepatotoxicity revisited. *World J Gastroenterol.* 2010;16:3335-3338.

43. Trak-Smayra V, Cazals-Hatem D, Asselah T, et al. Prolonged cholestasis and ductopenia associated with tenoxicam. *J Hepatol.* 2003;39:125-128.

44. Anania FA, Rabin L. Terbinafine hepatotoxicity resulting in chronic biliary ductopenia and portal fibrosis. *Am J Med.* 2002;112:741-742.

45. Groh M, Blanche P, Calmus Y, et al. Thiabendazole-induced acute liver failure requiring transplantation and subsequent diagnosis of polyarteritis nodosa. *Clin Exp Rheumatol.* 2012;30:S107-S109.

46. Etogo-Asse F, Boemer F, Sempoux C, et al. Acute hepatitis with prolonged cholestasis and disappearance of interlobular bile ducts following tibolone and *Hypericum perforatum* (St. John's wort). Case of drug interaction? *Acta Gastroenterol Belg.* 2008;71:36-38.

47. Yao F, Behling CA, Saab S, et al. Trimethoprim-sulfamethoxazole-induced vanishing bile duct syndrome. *Am J Gastroenterol.* 1997;92:167-169.

48. Naini BV, Lassman CR. Total parenteral nutrition therapy and liver injury: a histopathologic study with clinical correlation. *Hum Pathol.* 2012;43:826-833.

49. Gokce S, Durmaz O, Celtik C, et al. Valproic acid-associated vanishing bile duct syndrome. *J Child Neurol.* 2010;25:909-911.

50. Moreira RK, Chopp W, Washington MK. The concept of hepatic artery-bile duct parallelism in the diagnosis of ductopenia in liver biopsy samples. *Am J Surg Pathol.* 2011;35:392-403.

51. Hezode C, Zafrani ES, Roudot-Thoraval F, et al. Daily cannabis use: a novel risk factor of steatosis severity in patients with chronic hepatitis C. *Gastroenterology.* 2008;134:432-439.

52. Larrain S, Rinella ME. A myriad of pathways to NASH. *Clin Liver Dis.* 2012;16:525-548.

53. Lewis JH, Ranard RC, Caruso A, et al. Amiodarone hepatotoxicity: prevalence and clinicopathologic correlations among 104 patients. *Hepatology.* 1989;9:679-685.

54. Kum LC, Chan WW, Hui HH, et al. Prevalence of amiodarone-related hepatotoxicity in 720 Chinese patients with or without baseline liver dysfunction. *Clin Cardiol.* 2006;29:295-299.

55. Lewis JH, Mullick F, Ishak KG, et al. Histopathologic analysis of suspected amiodarone hepatotoxicity. *Hum Pathol.* 1990;21:59-67.

56. Rigas B, Rosenfeld LE, Barwick KW, et al. Amiodarone hepatotoxicity. A clinicopathologic study of five patients. *Ann Intern Med.* 1986;104:348-351.

57. Chang CC, Petrelli M, Tomashefski JF Jr, et al. Severe intrahepatic cholestasis caused by amiodarone toxicity after withdrawal of the drug: a case report and review of the literature. *Arch Pathol Lab Med.* 1999;123:251-256.

58. Reasor MJ, Hastings KL, Ulrich RG. Drug-induced phospholipidosis: issues and future directions. *Expert Opin Drug Saf.* 2006;5:567-583.

59. Wadzinski J, Franks R, Roane D, et al. Valproate-associated hyperammonemic encephalopathy. *J Am Board Fam Med.* 2007;20:499-502.

60. Nott L, Price TJ, Pittman K, et al. Hyperammonemia encephalopathy: an important cause of neurological deterioration following chemotherapy. *Leuk Lymphoma.* 2007;48:1702-1711.

61. Belenky A, Igov I, Konstantino Y, et al. Endovascular diagnosis and intervention in patients with isolated hyperammonemia, with or without ascites, after liver transplantation. *J Vasc Intervent Radiol.* 2009;20:259-263.

62. Acikalin A, Disel NR, Direk EC, et al. A rare cause of postpartum coma: isolated hyperammonemia due to urea cycle disorder. *Am J Emerg Med.* 2016;34(7):1324.e3-1324.e4.

63. Cordano C, Traverso E, Calabro V, et al. Recurring hyperammonemic encephalopathy induced by bacteria usually not producing urease. *BMC Res Notes.* 2014;7:324.

64. Albersen M, Joniau S, Van Poppel H, et al. Urea-splitting urinary tract infection contributing to hyperammonemic encephalopathy. *Nat Clin Pract Urol.* 2007;4:455-458.

65. Pestaner JP, Ishak KG, Mullick FG, et al. Ferrous sulfate toxicity: a review of autopsy findings. *Biol Trace Elem Res.* 1999;69:191-198.

66. Ramachandran R, Kakar S. Histological patterns in drug-induced liver disease. *J Clin Pathol.* 2009;62:481-492.

67. Lopez-Rocha E, Blancas L, Rodriguez-Mireles K, et al. Prevalence of DRESS syndrome. *Rev Alerg Mex.* 2014;61:14-23.

68. Cacoub P, Musette P, Descamps V, et al. The DRESS syndrome: a literature review. *Am J Med.* 2011;124:588-597.

69. Ichai P, Laurent-Bellue A, Saliba F, et al. Acute liver failure/injury related to drug reaction with eosinophilia and systemic symptoms: outcomes and prognostic factors. *Transplantation*. 2017;101:1830-1837.

70. Andrade RJ, Lucena MI, Kaplowitz N, et al. Outcome of acute idiosyncratic drug-induced liver injury: long-term follow-up in a hepatotoxicity registry. *Hepatology*. 2006;44:1581-1588.

71. Bjornsson E, Davidsdottir L. The long-term follow-up after idiosyncratic drug-induced liver injury with jaundice. *J Hepatol*. 2009;50:511-517.

72. Whiting-O'Keefe QE, Fye KH, Sack KD. Methotrexate and histologic hepatic abnormalities: a meta-analysis. *Am J Med*. 1991;90:711-716.

73. Lertnawapan R, Chonprasertsuk S, Siramolpiwat S. Association between cumulative methotrexate dose, non-invasive scoring system and hepatic fibrosis detected by Fibroscan in rheumatoid arthritis patients receiving methotrexate. *Int J Rheum Dis*. 2019;22:214-221.

74. Wang Z, Huang Y, Nossent H, et al. Hepascore predicts liver outcomes and all-cause mortality in long-term methotrexate users: a retrospective cohort study. *JGH Open*. 2020;4:1211-1216.

75. Roenigk HH Jr, Auerbach R, Maibach HI, et al. Methotrexate in psoriasis: revised guidelines. *J Am Acad Dermatol*. 1988;19:145-156.

76. Jezequel AM, Librari ML, Mosca P, et al. Changes induced in human liver by long-term anticonvulsant therapy Functional and ultrastructural data. *Liver*. 1984;4:307-317.

77. Wisell J, Boitnott J, Haas M, et al. Glycogen pseudoground glass change in hepatocytes. *Am J Surg Pathol*. 2006;30:1085-1090.

78. O'Shea AM, Wilson GJ, Ling SC, et al. Lafora-like ground-glass inclusions in hepatocytes of pediatric patients: a report of two cases. *Pediatr Dev Pathol*. 2007;10:351-357.

79. Bejarano PA, Garcia MT, Rodriguez MM, et al. Liver glycogen bodies: ground-glass hepatocytes in transplanted patients. *Virchows Arch*. 2006;449:539-545.

80. Bruguera M, Lamar C, Bernet M, et al. Hepatic disease associated with ground-glass inclusions in hepatocytes after cyanamide therapy. *Arch Pathol Lab Med*. 1986;110:906-910.

81. Hashimoto K, Hoshii Y, Takahashi M, et al. Use of a monoclonal antibody against Lafora bodies for the immunocytochemical study of ground-glass inclusions in hepatocytes due to cyanamide. *Histopathology*. 2001;39:60-65.

82. Zimmerman HJ, Ishak KG. Hepatic injury due to drugs and toxins. In: BC P, ed. *Pathology of the Liver*. Churchill-Livingstone; 1995:563-634.

83. Sahoo S, Blumberg AK, Sengupta E, et al. Type IV glycogen storage disease. *Arch Pathol Lab Med*. 2002;126:630-631.

84. Vazquez JJ. Ground-glass hepatocytes: light and electron microscopy. Characterization of the different types. *Histol Histopathol*. 1990;5:379-386.

85. Zen Y, Nishigami T. Rethinking fibrinogen storage disease of the liver: ground glass and globular inclusions do not represent a congenital metabolic disorder but acquired collective retention of proteins. *Hum Pathol*. 2020;100:1-9.

86. Penniston KL, Tanumihardjo SA. The acute and chronic toxic effects of vitamin A. *Am J Clin Nutr*. 2006;83:191-201.

87. Rodahl K, Moore T. The vitamin A content and toxicity of bear and seal liver. *Biochem J*. 1943;37:166-168.

88. Chiu YK, Lai MS, Ho JC, et al. Acute fish liver intoxication: report of three cases. *Changgeng Yi Xue Za Zhi*. 1999;22:468-473.

89. Levine PH, Delgado Y, Theise ND, et al. Stellate-cell lipidosis in liver biopsy specimens. Recognition and significance. *Am J Clin Pathol*. 2003;119:254-258.

90. Bucciol G, Cassiman D, Roskams T, et al. Liver transplantation for very severe hepatopulmonary syndrome due to vitamin A-induced chronic liver disease in a patient with Shwachman-Diamond syndrome. *Orphanet J Rare Dis*. 2018;13:69.

91. Miksad R, de Ledinghen V, McDougall C, et al. Hepatic hydrothorax associated with vitamin a toxicity. *J Clin Gastroenterol*. 2002;34:275-279.

92. Geubel AP, De Galocsy C, Alves N, et al. Liver damage caused by therapeutic vitamin A administration: estimate of dose-related toxicity in 41 cases. *Gastroenterology*. 1991;100:1701-1709.

93. Vigano L, De Rosa G, Toso C, et al. Reversibility of chemotherapy-related liver injury. *J Hepatol*. 2017;67:84-91.

94. Morris-Stiff G, White AD, Gomez D, et al. Nodular regenerative hyperplasia (NRH) complicating oxaliplatin chemotherapy in patients undergoing resection of colorectal liver metastases. *Eur J Surg Oncol*. 2014;40:1016-1020.

95. Vauthey JN, Pawlik TM, Ribero D, et al. Chemotherapy regimen predicts steatohepatitis and an increase in 90-day mortality after surgery for hepatic colorectal metastases. *J Clin Oncol*. 2006;24:2065-2072.

96. Ryan P, Nanji S, Pollett A, et al. Chemotherapy-induced liver injury in metastatic colorectal cancer: semiquantitative histologic analysis of 334 resected liver specimens shows that vascular injury but not steatohepatitis is associated with preoperative chemotherapy. *Am J Surg Pathol*. 2010;34:784-791.

97. Doherty DT, Coe PO, Rimmer L, et al. Hepatic steatosis in patients undergoing resection of colorectal liver metastases: a target for prehabilitation? A narrative review. *Surg Oncol*. 2019;30:147-158.

98. Johncilla M, Misdraji J, Pratt DS, et al. Ipilimumab-associated hepatitis: clinicopathologic characterization in a series of 11 cases. *Am J Surg Pathol*. 2015;39:1075-1084.

99. Kleiner DE, Berman D. Pathologic changes in ipilimumab-related hepatitis in patients with metastatic melanoma. *Dig Dis Sci*. 2012;57:2233-2240.

100. Zen Y, Yeh MM. Hepatotoxicity of immune checkpoint inhibitors: a histology study of seven cases in comparison with autoimmune hepatitis and idiosyncratic drug-induced liver injury. *Mod Pathol*. 2018;31:965-973.

101. Zen Y, Chen YY, Jeng YM, et al. Immune-related adverse reactions in the hepatobiliary system: second-generation checkpoint inhibitors highlight diverse histological changes. *Histopathology*. 2020;76:470-480.

102. Meyerson C, Naini BV. Something old, something new: liver injury associated with total parenteral nutrition therapy and immune checkpoint inhibitors. *Hum Pathol*. 2020;96:39-47.

103. Godbert B, Petitpain N, Lopez A, et al. Hepatitis B reactivation and immune check point inhibitors. *Dig Liver Dis*. 2020;53(4):452-455.

104. Chan KK, Bass AR. Autoimmune complications of immunotherapy: pathophysiology and management. *Br Med J*. 2020;369:m736.

105. LoPiccolo J, Brener MI, Oshima K, et al. Nodular regenerative hyperplasia associated with immune checkpoint blockade. *Hepatology*. 2018;68:2431-2433.

9

FATTY LIVER DISEASE

NONALCOHOLIC FATTY LIVER DISEASE

Nonalcoholic fatty liver disease (NAFLD) is the most common type of fatty liver disease seen in biopsy specimens. For the most part, the histological findings are relatively straightforward. The most common questions that arise for pathologists are these: (1) How do I make a diagnosis of steatosis versus steatohepatitis? (2) The patient has low-titer anti-nuclear antibody (ANA) positivity and some portal chronic inflammation. How do I tell if there is an element of autoimmune hepatitis? (3) What scoring system should I use? (4) The liver shows NAFLD, but the patient does not have the metabolic syndrome—what, then, is the differential? Each of these questions is addressed in the sections below, along with the clinical and histological findings and the differential diagnosis for fatty liver disease.

TERMINOLOGY

Fatty liver disease is a very broad term that includes any pattern of injury that has steatosis as a core part of the findings. For diagnostic purposes, steatosis (or fat) in the liver is further classified into macrovesicular and microvesicular patterns. For those cases with the macrovesicular pattern, the histological changes are further subclassified as *steatosis* versus *steatohepatitis*, with cases called steatohepatitis if there is fat plus histologically recognizable active lobular injury; this distinction is made to stratify for the risk of fibrosis progression. If there is insufficient evidence for steatohepatitis, common terms used for the diagnosis in the pathology report include *steatosis*, *simple steatosis*, or *nonalcoholic fatty liver*. In contrast to the macrovesicular pattern of injury, which by and large is a chronic pattern of injury that carries a risk for fibrosis/cirrhosis, microvesicular steatosis is typically an acute injury pattern that has no risk for fibrosis progression, so there is no need to divide it into steatosis versus steatohepatitis.

NONALCOHOLIC FATTY LIVER DISEASE (NAFLD). This is an umbrella term that includes all nonalcohol causes of macrovesicular steatosis. Since the overwhelming majority of these cases are caused by the metabolic syndrome, most people generally assume that you are referring to metabolic syndrome–related disease when you use the term NAFLD, unless you state otherwise. As a fore-warning, some people are unhappy with the term NAFLD and want to change it to *metabolic dysfunction–associated fatty liver disease* or MAFLD[1]; person-ally, I would vote for MetDysAssFatLivDisPrevKnownAsNonAlcFaLivDis—it is very comprehensive and has a nice ring to it.

METABOLIC SYNDROME, DEFINITION

The metabolic syndrome is the most common cause of fatty liver disease in the Western world. It is not necessary to know the clinical findings in order to diagnose fatty liver disease on the biopsy, but knowing the clinical features of the metabolic syndrome can be useful when you are looking at a specific case, discussing cases with your colleagues, or reading the literature. There are several competing definitions for the metabolic syndrome proposed by various professional organizations, but overall, these definitions are more alike than different, with the differences focusing on how to specifically mea-sure 4 widely accepted core features of the metabolic syndrome: (1) obesity (obesity is commonly defined as body mass index [BMI] > 30), (2) dyslipid-emia, (3) raised blood pressure, and (4) elevated fasting serum glucose levels and/or insulin resistance. Keep in mind, however, that not everyone with the metabolic syndrome will have fatty liver disease and not everyone with bone fide nonalcoholic fatty liver disease will meet the full definition of the metabolic syndrome. In fact, there is growing information about a group of patients called *metabolic obesity but normal weight*, where patients are normoweight or lean, as defined by their BMI, yet meet several or all of the other criteria for the metabolic syndrome, and can have fatty liver disease.[2]

CLINICAL ASSOCIATIONS

Most cases of NAFLD occur in middle-aged adults, but fatty liver disease can also be seen in children and teenagers. Aspartate aminotransferase (AST) and alanine aminotransferase (ALT) serum levels are mildly ele-vated, usually in the 40s and 50s IU/L, but about 20% of cases may have normal enzyme levels.[3,4] In addition, up to 5% of patients may have iso-lated alkaline phosphatase elevations but normal ALT and AST levels.[5] The metabolic syndrome is overall the most important risk factor for fatty liver disease, but there are many others (Table 9.1). For example, the metabolic syndrome can also develop in individuals with specific genetic diseases, including the Prader-Willi syndrome[30] and Turner syndrome.[24]

NATURAL HISTORY

In a subset of patients, fatty liver disease can lead to fibrosis and cirrhosis. This is important because advanced fibrosis represents one of the stron-gest risks for long-term morbidity and mortality in patients with the meta-bolic syndrome.[31,32] The biopsy can provide important information on the

TABLE 9.1 Differential for Macrovesicular Steatosis, After Excluding the Metabolic Syndrome, Alcoholic Liver Disease, and Drug Effect

Cause	Comment and or Reference
Metabolic conditions	
Elevated cortisol	
Diabetes mellitus	Can be seen in both type I and type II diabetic patients who do not have features of the metabolic syndrome
Growth hormone deficiency	[6]
Hypothyroid disease	[7]
Polycystic ovarian syndrome	[8]
Sepsis	[9]
Genetic disease	
Ataxia telangiectasia	[10]
Bardet-Biedl syndrome	
Citrullinemia	[11]
Congenital disorders of glycosylation	Small to intermediate-sized droplets of fat[12]
Congenital hypobetalipoproteinemia	Large droplet of fat[13]
Cystic fibrosis	Pediatric patients can be normoweight (fat possibly from malabsorption). In contrast, most adults with cystic fibrosis and fatty liver also have the metabolic syndrome[14-16]
Fatty acid oxidation disorders	[17]
Glycogen storage disease	Usually admixed with glycogenosis, except for glycogen storage disease type 0, which shows pure steatosis
Lipodystrophies	[18,19]
PFIC1 mutations	Steatosis also can be seen after transplantation in the liver allograft[20]
Porphyria cutanea tarda	[21]
Prader-Willi syndrome	[22]
Tyrosinemia	[23]
Turner syndrome	[24]
Urea cycle defects	For example, ornithine transcarbamylase deficiency. Most cases are dominated by glycogenosis or microvesicular steatosis, but macrovesicular steatosis can be seen[17]

TABLE 9.1 **Differential for Macrovesicular Steatosis, After Excluding the Metabolic Syndrome, Alcoholic Liver Disease, and Drug Effect** **(Continued)**

Cause	Comment and or Reference
Weber-Christian disease	25,26
Wilson disease	Biopsy can also have glycogenated nuclei and Mallory hyaline in periportal hepatocytes
Malnutrition and related	
Inflammatory diseases affecting the small bowel	Crohn disease, celiac disease, bacterial overgrowth
Gastrointestinal surgery	After jejunoileal bypass surgery or extensive small bowel resection
Malnutrition	Both marasmus and kwashiorkor can have fatty liver
Portal vein thrombosis	27,28
Anorexia	
Miscellaneous	
Volatile petrochemical products	29

current fibrosis stage as well as information on future fibrosis risk. The most important histological risk factors for fibrosis progression are steatohepatitis (vs steatosis), the degree of fibrosis on the current biopsy (more fibrosis, more risk for fibrosis progression), and concomitant liver diseases such as genetic hemochromatosis.

Fibrosis progression occurs in both steatosis (~40% of cases) and steatohepatitis (~40% of cases), but there is much slower progression with steatosis versus steatohepatitis; one study found an average progression of 1 fibrosis stage in 14 years for steatosis versus 1 fibrosis stage in 7 years for steatohepatitis.[33]

Studies have demonstrated that the fat in NAFLD can diminish as fibrosis progresses, and even disappear with cirrhosis. Thus, many cases of cryptogenic cirrhosis are associated with clinical findings of the metabolic syndrome and presumably represent fatty liver disease that has progressed to cirrhosis and lost the fatty change.[34]

Fatty liver disease is also a risk factor for inflammatory hepatic adenomas and for hepatocellular carcinoma.

TREATMENT

The most effective treatments for fatty liver disease are weight loss (if overweight or obese), increased exercise, control of blood sugar, and a balanced diet. Alcohol avoidance is commonly recommended. In terms of medication, there is no US Food and Drug Administration–approved drug treatment for fatty liver disease, so patients are generally treated "off-label" and there is no well-established, standard treatment algorithm. Nonetheless, patients are often treated with various insulin-sensitizing agents or drugs that modify various aspects of lipid metabolism if they have advanced fibrosis.

AUTOANTIBODIES

Many biopsies are received with information that the patient has mildly elevated autoantibodies in the setting of the metabolic syndrome, with the clinical question of whether there is an additional component of autoimmune hepatitis. Multiple studies have shown that autoantibodies are seen in 20% to 30% of individuals with fatty liver disease.[35-37] The most common autoantibodies are ANA and/or anti-smooth muscle antibody (ASMA). They are typically low titer. Some studies, but not all,[35] have found an association with more advanced liver fibrosis or more active liver disease.[36] These frequent, but low-titer autoantibodies do not indicate autoimmune hepatitis in isolation. Overall, about 8% of patients with the metabolic syndrome plus elevated serum autoantibodies have histological findings that indicate an additional component of autoimmune hepatitis, which is why biopsies are commonly performed.[36] In these cases, the diagnosis of autoimmune hepatitis should be made in the usual fashion, based on the presence of typical clinical, serological, and histological findings. Anti-mitochondrial antibody is positive less frequently, in about 2% of patients with fatty liver disease, and most of these patients will also lack histological findings of primary biliary cirrhosis/cholangitis.[38,39]

HISTOLOGICAL FINDINGS

Historical Overview

The core histological findings of NAFLD include varying degrees of fat, balloon cells, inflammation, and fibrosis. These were first systematically described in a seminal paper from Mayo Clinic in 1980.[40] This was followed by a large body of literature that more fully fleshed out the range of histological findings in NAFLD and proposed varying grading and staging systems. A subsequent, large National Institutes of Health–funded clinical trial, called the nonalcoholic steatohepatitis research network (NASH-CRN), has generated important data on the natural history, treatment, and pathology of fatty liver disease, including developing a scoring system and publishing many key papers on the histological and clinical findings in NASH. Currently, the two most commonly used grading and staging systems for steatohepatitis are the NASH-CRN[41] and the FAS system.[42]

Differentiating Steatosis From Steatohepatitis

For clinical care, there is a lot of emphasis on differentiating steatosis from steatohepatitis, because fibrosis progression in steatosis is generally slow, whereas steatohepatitis has approximately a 30% risk for developing significant fibrosis and 15% risk for cirrhosis.[43] Historically, it was thought that steatosis and steatohepatitis were essentially two separate diseases and that steatohepatitis was relatively permanent once it developed.[44] Subsequent research, however, has shown that this is not quite true. Instead, patients routinely shift back and forth between steatosis and steatohepatitis throughout their clinical course.[45-48] Thus, the current model is that NAFLD is a single disease pattern with a range in the degree of active injury; the lowest grade of injury is called steatosis and higher grades of injury are called steatohepatitis. This makes good sense and NAFLD is now brought into the fold of other major patterns of chronic liver disease, such as chronic viral hepatitis and autoimmune hepatitis, all of which are single diseases with varying degrees of active injury and fibrosis. Thus, the distinction between steatosis and steatohepatitis is important for clinical care purposes, but we as pathologists are essentially dividing cases into those with no or minimal lobular injury (steatosis) versus those with more than minimal active lobular injury (steatohepatitis).

The core notion of separating steatosis from steatohepatitis is as follows: both should show at least mild fat (at least 5% macrovesicular steatosis), but steatohepatitis should also have evidence for "active" or "ongoing" injury. Both steatosis and steatohepatitis may or may not have fibrosis; fibrosis is an indicator of chronic injury and not of active injury, so it is not used to differentiate steatosis from steatohepatitis. Portal inflammation is often present, especially with more advanced fibrosis but is not used to distinguish steatosis from steatohepatitis. It is generally agreed that the active injury can have elements of balloon cells (plus or minus Mallory hyaline), lobular hepatitis, and apoptosis,[49] with the first two elements being the most important.[41]

There are different opinions among expert pathologists over the exact minimal features needed for the "active injury" that differentiates steatosis from steatohepatitis, which have led to two major approaches. The first approach requires only ballooned hepatocytes,[41] whereas the second approach requires at least mild lobular inflammation plus ballooned hepatocytes.[42] In the vast majority of cases, either approach leads to the same answer, since biopsies with readily identified balloon cells will typically also have at least mild patchy lobular hepatitis and occasionally rare apoptotic bodies. Both approaches agree that biopsies with no hepatocyte ballooning and no or minimal lobular inflammation do not qualify for steatohepatitis. Additional areas of generally uniform agreement and disagreement for distinguishing steatosis versus steatohepatitis are summarized in Table 9.2.

Of note, most borderline cases are more concerning to pathologists (who often spend more time perseverating over them than is warranted) than clinicians, since the disease in these cases is very mild anyway. Overall, these "tweener" cases are best approached by accurately conveying the amount of fat, the degree of active lobular injury, and the fibrosis stage. For the diagnostic line in the pathology report, reasonable terms include

TABLE 9.2 Areas of Diagnostic Consensus and Nonconsensus in Fatty Liver Disease

Fat	Balloon Cells	Lobular Inflammation	Diagnostic Category
Minimal (<5%)	None	Minimal or mild	Consensus: not steatohepatitis
Minimal (<5%)	Possibly; equivocal balloon cells only	Minimal or mild	*No consensus*: I call these steatosis
Minimal (<5%)	Yes, classic	Minimal or greater	*No consensus*: I call these steatohepatitis
Mild or greater	None	Minimal or mild	Consensus: not steatohepatitis
Mild or greater	None	Greater than mild	*No consensus*: I call these steatohepatitis
Mild or greater	Possibly; equivocal balloon cells only	Minimal or mild	*No consensus*: I call these steatosis
Mild or greater	Possibly; equivocal balloon cells only	Greater than mild	*No consensus*: I call these steatohepatitis
Mild or greater	Yes, classic	Absent or minimal	*No consensus*: NASH-CRN calls these steatohepatitis; SAF does not
Mild or greater	Yes, classic	Mild or greater	Consensus: steatohepatitis

minimally active steatohepatitis (my preference) or *borderline steatohepatitis*. Most of these cases generally fall into one of the following categories.

1. *No ballooned hepatocytes, more than minimal lobular inflammation.* Rare biopsies have no balloon cells but have sufficient lobular hepatitis, and perhaps occasional apoptotic bodies, sufficient to make a reasonable pathologist uncomfortable with a diagnosis of only steatosis.

2. *Discrepancies in identifying ballooned hepatocytes.* There can be disagreement on whether balloon cells are present, especially when they are rare or when the liver also shows areas of glycogenosis. In these cases, one expert pathologist may believe a given cell has definite ballooning, whereas another expert pathologist will find that exact same cell to decidedly not show ballooning. This challenge is not a practical problem in most cases, as most biopsies with steatohepatitis will show

at least a few uniformly convincing balloon cells. However, if a biopsy shows a single balloon cell candidate, not all pathologists may come to the same diagnosis, even if some pathologists are quite certain about it.

3. *Only equivocal ballooned cells present.* Some biopsies have only equivocal ballooned hepatocytes, where most pathologists will agree that a few cells "look funny" but lack the definite features of ballooned hepatocytes. Some authors have suggested calling these cells *nonclassic ballooned hepatocytes* and some have recommended their use in diagnosing steatohepatitis. This may work OK in research studies, where biopsies undergo central review by expert pathologists, but enthusiasm for using nonclassic ballooned hepatocytes for general clinical purposes has been muted because of concerns this approach leads to further degradation of reproducibly identifying balloon cells. At a practical level, if you have a possible balloon cell, but are not sure about it (and feel you might be embarrassed by showing it to your colleague, who is likely to disagree with you anyway), then keep looking at the rest of the biopsy, as a true steatohepatitis, the ones that are clinically important because of their higher risk for fibrosis, will typically have more than a single equivocal balloon cell per specimen.

In sum, there is no experimental evidence that satisfactorily resolves the question of how to best classify cases that straddle the line between steatosis and steatohepatitis, so I believe the most prudent course is to use a constellation of findings for active injury: if there are classic balloon cells present, then diagnose steatohepatitis; if there are no classic balloon cells, but there is more than the usual minimal lobular hepatitis of steatosis, then also diagnose steatohepatitis. If a biopsy has less than 5% fat, but definite balloon cells, then it is also reasonable to classify the case as minimally active steatohepatitis. If there are no balloon cells and only minimal to patchy mild lobular inflammation, then diagnose steatosis.

Steatosis

Key Points for Evaluating Macrovesicular Steatosis

- Score the macrovesicular component only
- Estimate the percent of fat at low power (for example 4× or 10×)
- Classify steatosis as minimal (<5%), mild (5%-33%), moderate (34%-66%), or severe (>66%)
- At least 5% macrovesicular steatosis is typically required in order to diagnose steatohepatitis

TERMINOLOGY. In cases of macrovesicular steatosis, the fat vacuoles are large, typically one per cytoplasm, and often push the nucleus to the side (Figure 9.1). Nonetheless, there will be many areas where hepatocytes have fat droplets of intermediate size (Figure 9.2) and some areas where the fat

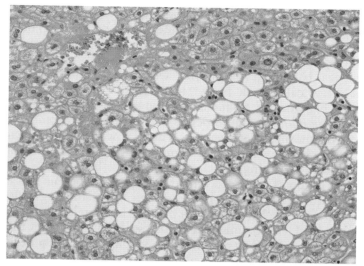

FIGURE 9.1 **Macrovesiclar steatosis.** The lobules show a macrovesicular pattern of steatosis.

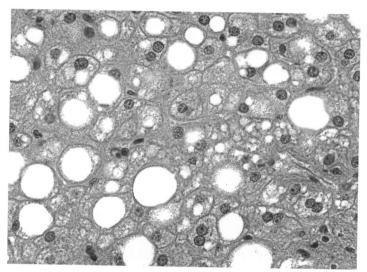

FIGURE 9.2 **Steatosis with intermediate-sized fat droplets.** Most cases of macrovesicular steatosis will also have hepatocytes that have small and intermediate-sized fat droplets.

droplets are tiny. These latter findings should not worry you when using the term "macrovesicular steatosis"—the big fat droplets have to start from somewhere. Some pathologists use the term *mixed micro and macrovesicular steatosis* in their pathology reports, since they see the smaller droplets of fat along with the large droplets of fat, but this terminology is not necessary, as all cases of macrovesicular steatosis are fully understood to have smaller droplets of fat. In fact, although it is not the weightiest of matters, it is best to avoid the terminology of mixed micro and macrovesicular steatosis because it misapplies well-established histological terminology.

HOW TO ESTIMATE THE PERCENT FAT? The amount of fat is estimated by examining the entire specimen at a 4× or 10× lens and assessing the average proportion of hepatocytes with macrovesicular steatosis. You can choose whether you like to estimate the percent of the lobular area that has steatosis or whether you prefer to estimate the percent of hepatocytes with steatosis; it all works out about the same, since hepatocytes have a fairly constant size in all people.

The amount of fat is generally scored as minimal (less than 5%), mild (5%-33%), moderate (34%-66%), or marked (greater than 66%). The general consensus is that only the macrovesicular component should be scored. Some cases can have relatively more abundant intermediate-sized fat droplets and may be more challenging to score. If you use too high of a magnification, it makes scoring even more difficult, so stay around a 10× to make your estimate. Another common error is to overthink this process. If you try to decide between 33% fat and 34% fat (which differentiates mild from moderate steatosis), you are likely to feel a little uncertain about your final fat estimate—instead, use a low-power lens and think in terms of minimal, mild, moderate, and marked. This works well because the human eye is much better at global classification than it is at determining precise percentages; the percentages that accompany the categories of minimal, mild, moderate, and marked steatosis are for reference in the hopes of uniform categories across the literature. When there is a lot of fat, a useful approach for distinguishing between moderate and severe steatosis is to consider what proportion of hepatocytes *do not* have steatosis.

In the midst of all of the complexities that could affect the accuracy of scoring the amount of fat, do not forget this key guiding principle: histological fat grade is a skilled estimate that provides necessary and sufficient information for patient care; there is no need for greater precision than that. Clinicians in your hospital, on the other hand, may prefer a semiquantitative estimate of the percent of fat, in addition to the commonly used grades of minimal/mild/moderate/severe. If so, a reasonable approach is to estimate the amount of steatosis to the nearest 10%. There is certainly no clinical need to estimate the fat any more precisely, and the human eye cannot reliably do much better anyway.

CASES WITH BORDERLINE STEATOSIS. A minimum of 5% macrovesicular steatosis is the official cut-off needed to diagnosis steatosis and steatohepatitis. Of course, this cut-off is arbitrary and is intended to by a rough guide, one written in sand and not stone. For example, if the fat looks to be less than 5%, but has a zone 3 pattern and shows ballooned hepatocytes, then those cases are reasonably called steatohepatitis.

FAT DISTRIBUTION. The fat can be distributed in different patterns within the hepatic lobules. With a zone 3 distribution (Figure 9.3), the fat clusters around the central veins, whereas with a zone 1 pattern the fat clusters around the portal tracts (Figure 9.4, eFig. 9.1). In cases with moderate or greater fat, it can be easier to look for what zone is spared from the fat when making this distinction. For example, a zone 3 pattern

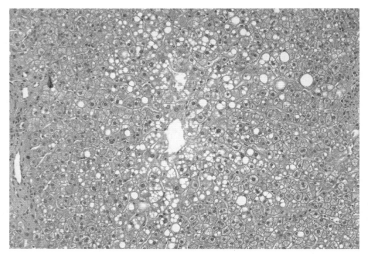

FIGURE 9.3 **Steatosis in a zone 3 pattern.** The lobules show macrovesicular steatosis around the central vein (ie, zone 3 pattern).

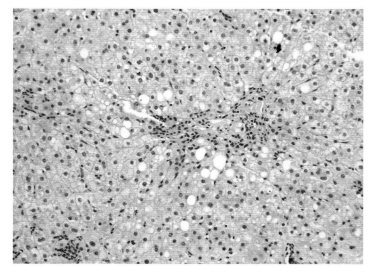

FIGURE 9.4 **Steatosis in a zone 1 pattern.** There is mild macrovesicular steatosis in zone 1. The pattern is most commonly seen in children and teenaged patients.

of fat will have little or no fat around the portal tracts. With a panacinar distribution, the fat is typically moderate to marked and no strong zonal distribution patterns are evident (Figure 9.5). In cases with an azonal fat distribution, the steatosis is typically mild but no strong zonal distribution patterns are evident (Figure 9.6). Currently, the zonal patterns

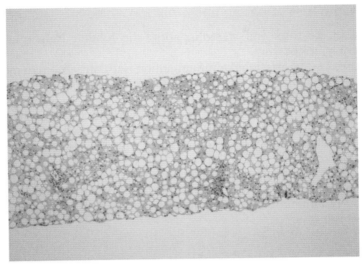

FIGURE 9.5 **Fat, panacinar pattern.** There is severe macrovesicular steatosis with no clear zonation.

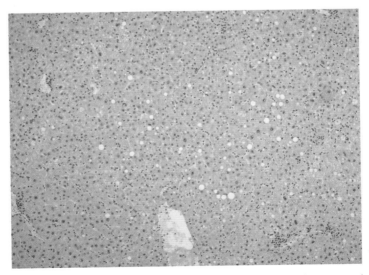

FIGURE 9.6 **Fat, azonal pattern.** The macrovesicular steatosis shows no clear zonal pattern.

do not have any diagnostic significance/clinical management relevance. Nonetheless, the zone 1 pattern of steatosis is more common in children and teenagers,[50] although it can also be seen in adults.

Inflammation

Key Points for Evaluating Inflammation

- In both steatosis and steatohepatitis, the lobular inflammation is mostly lymphocytic.
- In cases of steatosis, lobular inflammation is usually absent to minimal.
- In cases of steatohepatitis, lobular inflammation is usually patchy mild to patchy moderate.
- Higher grades of lobular hepatitis (diffuse moderate or greater hepatitis) suggest an additional or superimposed disease process.
- Portal inflammation is predominately lymphocytic and generally minimal to mild.
- Portal inflammation can be patchy moderate, especially if there is advanced fibrosis.
- Portal inflammation is not included when determining the grade of active injury.

PORTAL INFLAMMATION. The portal tracts have inflammation that ranges from mild to focally moderate and is composed predominately of lymphocytes, with only rare and inconspicuous plasma cells (Figure 9.7). In general, biopsies with fibrosis tend to have more portal chronic inflammation than biopsies without fibrosis. Although the inflammation can be focally moderate with more advanced fibrosis, it is generally on the low end of moderate, and biopsies with moderate diffuse portal chronic inflammation or marked portal chronic inflammation should raise your suspicion for another disease process. I have seen several cases of clinically unknown chronic hepatitis C picked up this way, ie, the patient had fatty liver disease histologically, plus more than the expected chronic portal inflammation, and additional testing revealed previously unknown chronic hepatitis C (Figure 9.8).

LOBULAR INFLAMMATION. The lobular inflammation is generally mild in fatty liver disease (Figure 9.9), including both steatosis and steatohepatitis, ranging from minimal to focally moderate. A biopsy with either diffuse moderate lobular inflammation or with marked lobular hepatitis would be unusual for steatohepatitis and suggests a concomitant, separate disease process (Figure 9.10); this is particularly true if the patient presented with a recent increase in serum AST or ALT levels. The lobular inflammation in fatty liver disease is mostly lymphocytic. Neutrophils in

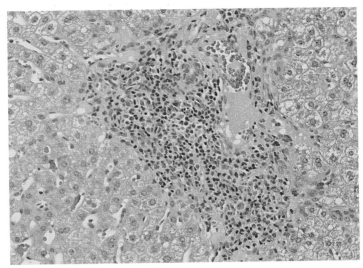

FIGURE 9.7 **NAFLD, portal inflammation.** This wedge biopsy showed focally moderate portal chronic inflammation.

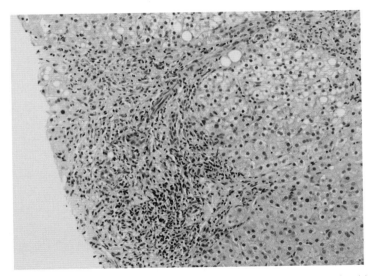

FIGURE 9.8 **NAFLD, too much portal inflammation.** In this case, a wedge biopsy was obtained at the time of bariatric surgery for grading and staging NAFLD in the setting of the metabolic syndrome. There was diffuse moderate to marked portal chronic inflammation, which suggested an additional disease process such as chronic hepatitis C; subsequent testing showed the patient was hepatitis C positive. Focal portal tracts can show moderate portal chronic inflammation in fatty liver disease, but there should not be diffusely moderate, or greater, portal chronic inflammation.

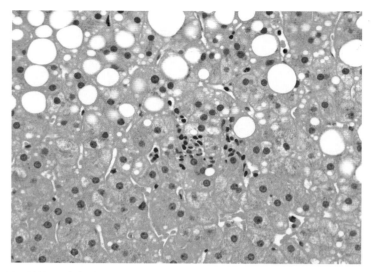

FIGURE 9.9 **NAFLD, lobular inflammation.** This biopsy shows mild patchy lobular hepatitis composed of lymphocytes.

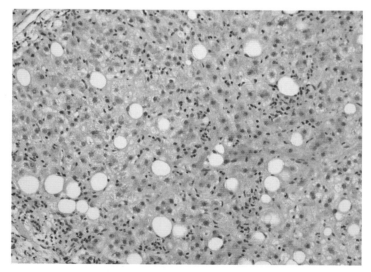

FIGURE 9.10 **NAFLD, lobular inflammation.** This biopsy shows moderate, diffuse lobular hepatitis, which is more than is typical for NAFLD.

the lobules are relatively rare in NAFLD, except for when there is markedly active disease with numerous balloon cells and abundant Mallory hyaline, where focal neutrophils may be seen around a balloon cell, a finding called *satellitosis* (eFig. 9.2). Neutrophils in the lobules are more common in cases of alcoholic-related steatohepatitis, as discussed further

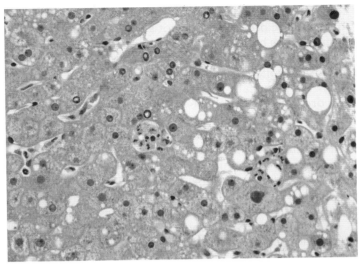

FIGURE 9.11 **Surgical hepatitis.** This resection specimen shows mild macrovesicular steatosis without steatohepatitis. The small aggregates of neutrophils in the sinusoids represent surgical hepatitis.

below. As a diagnostic pitfall, beware that wedge biopsies or resections can show surgical hepatitis (Figure 9.11, eFigs. 9.3 and 9.4). When the background liver also shows fatty change, the surgical hepatitis can sometimes be misinterpreted as steatohepatitis. Surgical hepatitis, however, shows small clusters or aggregates of neutrophils in the sinusoids, often with a zone 3 distribution that may include the central veins themselves. These small sinusoidal neutrophilic aggregates will not be associated with ballooned hepatocytes. The cause of surgical hepatitis is not entirely clear, but it is an incidental finding.

Ballooned Hepatocytes (Also Called Ballooned Cells)

Key Points for Ballooned Hepatocytes

- Ballooned hepatocytes are defined by hematoxylin and eosin (H&E) findings.
- They are essentially always larger than adjacent hepatocytes.
- They have rarified cytoplasm with thin wisps of pink cytoplasm.
- They may or may not have Mallory hyaline.
- They generally do not have fat.

Balloon cells are hepatocytes that are injured but not yet dead. The precise molecular reason(s) for their distinctive appearance is not clear.

Balloon cells can also be seen in other diseases, such as cholestatic liver disease, so their mere presence does not always indicate steatohepatitis.

Balloon cells are big, typically 1.5× or greater in size than their neighbors, and have large amounts of clear, rarified cytoplasm, often with scattered small eosinophilic clumps of condensed proteins (Mallory hyaline) (Figure 9.12). They typically lack fat droplets or have only small inconspicuous fat droplets. Balloon cells can be found anywhere but are most commonly located in zone 3. When there is advanced fibrosis, the balloon cells are often located near the fibrous bands. They should stand out from the adjacent hepatocytes when scanning on a low-power lens (Figure 9.13, eFigs. 9.5 and 9.6). If you spend too much time with your 40X lens, lots of hepatocytes may soon start to look like balloon cells, even when they are not. This is especially true if the biopsy also shows areas of glycogenosis, which is common in fatty liver disease, as these glycogen-laden hepatocytes can be slightly enlarged, have clear cytoplasm, and closely mimic balloon cells. One useful clue is that glycogen-laden hepatocytes tend to be found in contiguous patches that contain many affected hepatocytes, not as individual cells that pop out of the background at low power examination, like balloon cells do.

Balloon cells often contain Mallory hyaline, and almost all Mallory hyaline will be seen within balloon cells. Mallory hyaline is also referred to as Mallory-Denk bodies. Mallory hyaline is an eosinophilic material in the hepatocyte cytoplasm that can be either clumpy or ropy (Figure 9.14). Mallory hyaline is composed of damaged and ubiquitinated cytoskeleton proteins. Although immunostains are not necessary, you can stain the Mallory hyaline with ubiquitin, p62, or cytokeratins 8 and 18.

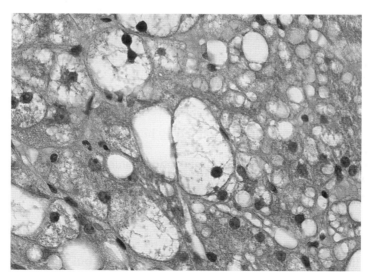

FIGURE 9.12 **Balloon cells, high power.** Several balloon cells can be seen in this image.

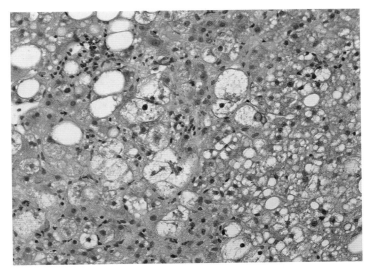

FIGURE 9.13 **Balloon cells, low power.** These balloon cells stand out with their abundant rarified cytoplasm that has small clumps of eosinophilic material.

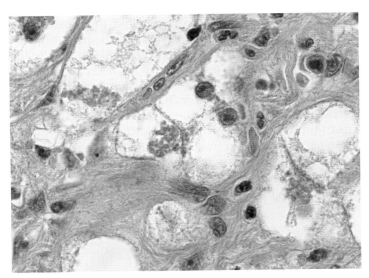

FIGURE 9.14 **Mallory hyaline.** Mallory hyaline is seen as pink cytoplasmic aggregates in these ballooned hepatocytes.

There are many balloon cells that all pathologists will agree on; these have been called *classic balloon cells*. In addition, there are many possible balloon cells that are in the "eye of the beholder" (Figure 9.15); these tend to have clear-ish and sometimes clumpy cytoplasm but are not truly ballooned in size, compared with adjacent hepatocytes; they also lack Mallory hyaline. These cells are sometimes called *nonclassic*

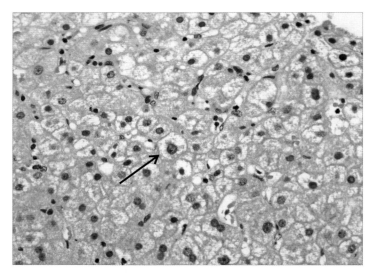

FIGURE 9.15   **Equivocal balloon cell.** Is there a balloon cell at the arrow? Some will say yes and some will say no and some will say they do not know.

balloon cells, a term that seems to imply that they are actual balloon cells but with an unusual morphology; the real question, however, is whether they should be considered balloon cells at all. Reliably identifying possible ballooned hepatocytes is not easy, and definitely not widely reproducible! Thus, their clinical/diagnostic relevance is unclear and it is best not to perseverate over these types of cells and move on to the rest of the biopsy, looking for classic balloon cells; if classic balloon cells are not found, then the histological differential is typically that of steatosis versus minimally active steatohepatitis, a differential that, at least at this point, is intriguing mostly to academic pathologists.

OTHER FINDINGS IN FATTY LIVER DISEASE

Common Additional Findings

- Lipogranulomas
- Megamitochondria
- Patches of microvesicular steatosis
- Glycogenated hepatocytes
- Glycogenotic nuclei
- Aberrant lobular arteries

Note: None of these findings are useful for distinguishing steatosis from steatohepatitis, nor are they used for any other diagnostic purpose. Thus, they do not need to be included in pathology reports.

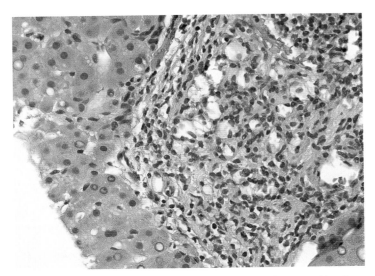

FIGURE 9.16   **Lipogranuloma.** A large lipogranuloma is seen in a portal tract.

LIPOGRANULOMAS are most commonly seen in portal tracts or in the central vein areas. They are composed of aggregates of histiocytes with medium-sized and large lipid droplets (Figure 9.16). Admixed lymphocytes are common, and occasional eosinophils may be present. Many of them will be associated with focal fibrosis,[51] but they are not associated with fibrosis progression per se.

MEGAMITOCHONDRIA. Hepatocytes in fatty liver disease often have megamitochondria, small eosinophilic structures in the cytoplasm that can range in size from 1 to 6 μm. They can be single or multiple, and their shape varies from round, to oval, to needle shaped (Figure 9.17). Their frequency in biopsy material tends to correlate with how hard you look for them, but they are easily found without much looking in about 15% of NAFLD cases.[41] They are not specific for fatty liver disease and are seen in a wider variety of liver diseases. Overall, they are more common in steatohepatitis and in older-aged patients,[52] but are neither necessary nor specific for the diagnosis of steatohepatitis.

PATCHES OF MICROVESICULAR STEATOSIS. About 10% of biopsies showing typical nonalcoholic fatty liver disease will have small, circumscribed patches of microvesicular steatosis (Figures 9.18 and 9.19). These small patches are more frequent when there is marked steatosis and active steatohepatitis in the rest of the biopsy.[53] They are also more common in biopsy specimens with advanced fibrosis.[53] Outside of these correlates, their pathogenesis is unclear, but there is no clinical significance. Their greatest importance, at least currently, is to not overinterpret them as indicating a true microvesicular steatosis pattern of injury.

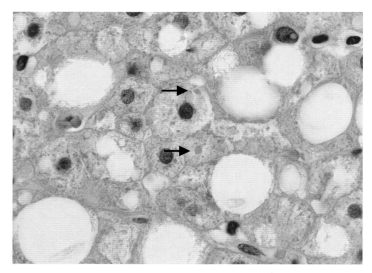

FIGURE 9.17 **Megamitochondria.** Several megamitochondria are seen in this case of fatty liver disease (arrows).

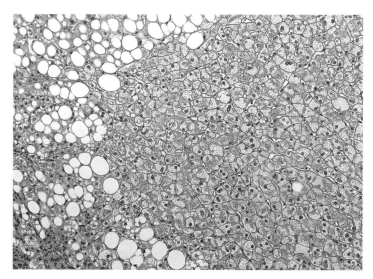

FIGURE 9.18 **Patch of microvesicular steatosis.** A small round patch of microvesicular steatosis stands out in a background of macrovesicular steatosis.

HEPATIC GLYCOGENOSIS. Contiguous patches of hepatocytes can show cytoplasmic rarefication owing to glycogen accumulation. Overall, focal glycogenosis is seen in nearly 50% of cases of nonalcoholic steatohepatitis and is more common in patients with higher serum glucose levels and patients who use insulin.[54] The most important point is to not interpret this finding as glycogenic hepatopathy, which has similar findings at the

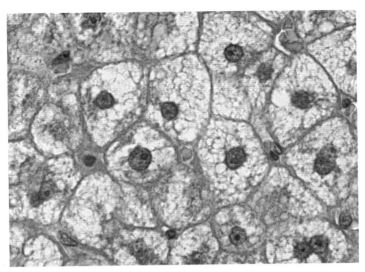

FIGURE 9.19 **Microvesicular steatosis, high power.** The cells contain small droplets of fat that fill the cytoplasm. Same case preceding image.

individual cell level but is a diffuse process associated with poorly controlled (typically) type 1 diabetes. In fatty liver disease, hepatocytes with glycogen accumulation can also sometimes mimic balloon cells.

GLYCOGENATED NUCLEI are found in approximately 45% to 65% of biopsies with NAFLD.[27,41] Hepatocytes with glycogenated nuclei tend to cluster (Figure 9.20), but single, scattered hepatocytes with glycogenated nuclei can also be seen. Overall, glycogenated nuclei correlate with diabetes mellitus[55] but have no diagnostic relevance.

ABERRANT CENTRAL ARTERIES. In livers with advanced fibrosis, scarred central veins/zone 3 regions can have in-growth of branches of the hepatic artery.[56] These scared and arterialized central veins can mimic portal tracts with ductopenia, because there are discrete areas of fibrosis with both an artery and vein (Figure 9.21), but careful evaluation of the overall biopsy typically resolves this issue. These abnormal branches of the hepatic artery can be seen in both alcoholic and nonalcoholic steatohepatitis with advanced fibrosis.

METABOLIC SYNDROME WITHOUT FAT. Based on liver biopsies obtained during bariatric surgery, approximately 10% of patients with the metabolic syndrome will have no fat in the liver, despite evaluation of a large wedge biopsy specimen.[27,57,58] This subgroup of patients has not been well characterized, but there is no clear difference in age or gender compared with those individuals with fat in their biopsies. In cases that lack fat, the biopsies generally show mild portal chronic inflammation with rare portal tracts that may approach moderate chronic inflammation. The lobules show no or minimal chronic inflammation, and fibrosis is generally absent.

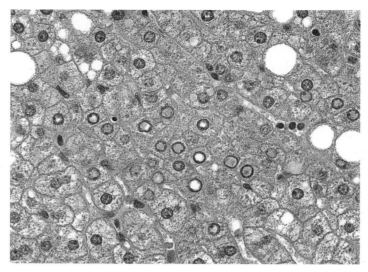

FIGURE 9.20 **Glycogenated nuclei.** Some of the hepatocytes have round clear nuclear inclusions.

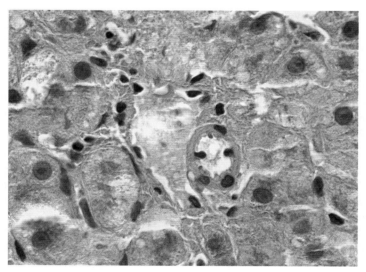

FIGURE 9.21 **Aberrant central artery.** A hepatic artery has grown into the lobules and is adjacent to a small central vein in this case of alcoholic liver disease.

ALCOHOL-ASSOCIATED LIVER DISEASE

The histology of alcohol-related fatty liver disease can range from simple steatosis to markedly active steatohepatitis. Alcohol-associated fatty liver disease shares many histological similarities with nonalcohol fatty liver disease. In most cases, there is no reliable way to distinguish between these two causes of fatty liver based on solely histological findings. There are, however, a few findings that favor alcohol-related liver disease. First, if there is diffuse sclerosis of the central veins (Figure 9.22), this tends to favor alcohol-related liver disease, a finding called *central hyaline sclerosis* or *sclerosing hyaline necrosis* in the older literature.[59]

Second, if the balloon cells and Mallory hyaline are striking and diffuse (Figure 9.23), this favors alcohol-related liver disease; in many of

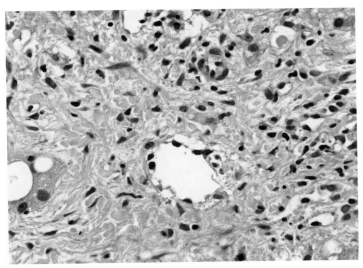

FIGURE 9.22 **Alcohol liver disease, central vein sclerosis.** In this case of alcoholic liver cirrhosis, the central vein lumen is narrowed from scarring. A small artery can also be seen in the upper middle of this image.

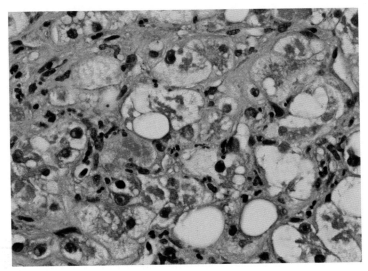

FIGURE 9.23 **Alcohol liver disease.** Numerous ballooned hepatocytes are seen with abundant Mallory hyaline.

these cases, the lobules also show somewhat prominent neutrophil infil-trates (Figure 9.24). Third, lobular cholestasis can be present and, when it is, both favors alcoholic steatohepatitis and is an adverse prognostic finding.[60] Fourth, in some cases, the trichrome will demonstrate strong and diffuse pericellular fibrosis throughout the lobules (Figure 9.25). In fact, in

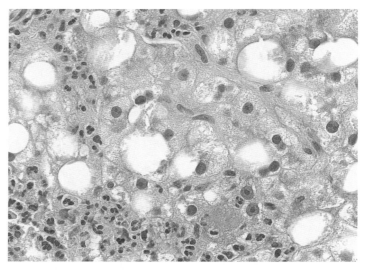

FIGURE 9.24 **Alcohol liver disease.** The lobules show cholestasis and numerous neutro-phils in this case of markedly active alcoholic hepatitis.

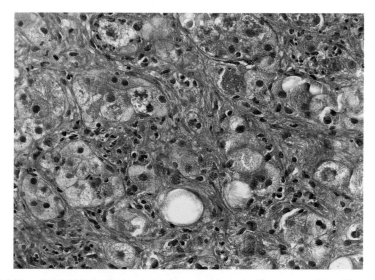

FIGURE 9.25 **Alcohol liver disease, trichrome.** Marked diffuse pericellular fibrosis is seen in this case of alcoholic cirrhosis.

some patients with active, heavy alcohol use and cirrhosis, there can be diffuse lobular fibrosis without well-formed nodules, with nodules forming only after the patient has reduced alcohol consumption and the liver can begin to regenerate.

If you want to use a formal grading/staging system for clinical care, both the nonalcoholic steatohepatitis (NAS) and steatosis, activity, fibrosis (SAF) work fine for alcoholic liver disease, even though they were designed for NAFLD. Alcohol-specific grading and staging systems have been created, such as the Alcoholic Hepatitis Histologic Score,[61] and they work well too; these systems commonly incorporate features that are more frequent in alcoholic liver disease, such as lobular cholestasis.

SCORING SYSTEMS

There are many fine scoring systems for research and/or clinical purposes, such as the NAS score (Tables 9.3 and 9.4) developed by the NASH-CRN.[41] In the NAS system, fat is scored from 0 to 3, lobular inflammation is scored from 0 to 3, and balloon cells are scored from 0 to 2; the sum of these 3 scores then gives the final NAS score. Lobular inflammation is scored using a 20× lens (Table 9.3), usually by averaging the counts for five different fields. Balloon cells are scored as 1 if there are only a few classic balloon cells in the entire biopsy, with a score of 2 given if they are easily found and present and in at least several 20× fields. Biopsies with a total NAS score of 0 to 2 often correlate with a diagnosis of steatosis, whereas cases with a NAS grade of 5 or greater almost always correlates with a diagnosis of steatohepatitis. On the other hand, biopsies with activity scores of 3 or 4 can be either steatosis or steatohepatitis.

The SAF is another excellent scoring system (Tables 9.5 and 9.6 show the grading system; the fibrosis staging system is the same as in NASH-CRN) and has the added feature of a clear separation of the fat from the ongoing hepatic injury (inflammation, balloon cells).

The use of scoring systems should not be a substitute for the diagnosis but instead is designed to convey the degree of active injury. In fact, the NAS scoring system, as well as most others, was designed for research purposes and was not originally intended for routine diagnostic use.[62] Nonetheless, there seems to be certain inevitability to including a scoring system in pathology reports, as pathologists and clinicians often have strong desires for them. Occasionally, the desire for scoring systems is built, at least to some degree, on the belief that a scoring system makes the report less descriptive and more scientific: it does not, as numbers are simply being substituted for adjectives. Other potential misunderstandings about scoring systems are discussed in Chapter 1.

If you or your clinical colleagues want to use a formal scoring system, there is nothing wrong with that approach and they have some useful

TABLE 9.3 NAS Scoring System for NAFLD

Component	Score	Degree of Injury	Notes
Macrovesicular steatosis			Use a 4× or 10× lens
	0	Less than 5%	
	1	5%-33%	
	2	34%-66%	
	3	67%-100%	
Lobular inflammation			Score with a 20× lens, averaging at least five fields
			Acidophils are also included in the score
	0	None	
	1	<2 Foci	
	2	2-4 Foci	
	3	>4 Foci	
Ballooned hepatocytes			Only convincing balloon cells should be counted
	0	None	
	1	Few	One to a few per entire biopsy
	2	Many	Easily found, present in at least several fields
Total NAS grade	Add together all components for total, out of 8		

The scores are summed for a maximum of 8 points.[41]
From the NASH-CRN Study Group.[41]

TABLE 9.4 NASH CRN Fibrosis Staging System

Fibrosis Stage	Histological Findings
1a	Mild pericellular fibrosis; only seen on trichrome stain
1b	Moderate pericellular fibrosis; readily seen on H&E stain
1c	Only portal fibrosis with no pericellular fibrosis
2	Portal fibrosis (any) and pericellular fibrosis (any)
3	Bridging fibrosis
4	Cirrhosis

TABLE 9.5 SAF Scoring System

Score	Fat	Balloon Cells	Lobular Inflammation
0	Minimal (<5%)	None	None
1	6%-33%	Balloon cells have rounded contours with clear reticular cytoplasm. Size is similar to normal hepatocytes. Typically few in number	<2 Foci per 20× field
2	34%-66%	Cells are rounded with clear cytoplasm and twice as large as normal hepatocytes. Typically many in number	>2 Foci per 20× field
3	67%-100%		

The scores are not summed but instead reported out separately.
Note 1: Original paper.[42]
Note 2: Fibrosis staging uses the same schema as the NASH CRN system shown in Table 9.4.
Note 3: Reported out as steatosis, activity, fibrosis. For example, a case with 20% steatosis, <2 foci of inflammation per 20× field, and bridging fibrosis would be reported as S1 A1 F3.

TABLE 9.6 FLIP Algorithm,[63] Which Is Used to Interpret the Results of the SAF Scoring System Shown in Table 9.5

Steatosis	Ballooning	Lobular Inflammation	Diagnosis
1 or greater	0	Any	Steatosis
1 or greater	1	0	Steatosis
1 or greater	1	1	NASH
1 or greater	1	2	NASH
1 or greater	2	0	Steatosis
1 or greater	2	1	NASH
1 or greater	2	2	NASH

features. For example, they have the advantage of ensuring that all of the key features of steatohepatitis are addressed, at least to a reasonable degree. They certainly make research studies easier too. If a system is used, it is important that you and your clinical colleagues understand the system, including the strengths and weakness of scoring systems in general, as well as any weaknesses unique to that system. In terms of patient care, it remains best practice to make your diagnosis based on the patterns discussed above and then, if desired, provide the scoring for fat, active injury, and fibrosis separately.

Finally, the best way to compare paired biopsy specimens from a patient, in order to compare disease activities or to look for fibrosis progression, is to pull out the old case and directly compare the old and the new biopsy together, even if that delays the full report for a while; this side-by-side comparison can also be handled using an addendum. In most cases, comparing scores alone is a poor substitute and one not to be eagerly embraced.

Fibrosis Staging

The NASH-CRN fibrosis staging system is currently the most widely used and was based on earlier publications by Brunt and colleagues. The SAF system for grading also uses the NASH-CRN schema for fibrosis staging. New fibrosis staging systems are being developed around clinical trials, which add additional stages of fibrosis and/or tweak the currently defined fibrosis stages, but these have not yet been fully validated or published.

Fibrosis in fatty liver disease usually begins as pericellular fibrosis, also called perisinusoidal fibrosis, or sinusoidal fibrosis (Figure 9.26, eFig. 9.7). This pattern of fibrosis typically begins in the zone 3 regions and can be very focal or have a more diffuse distribution in severe cases. As fibrosis progresses, the liver will develop portal fibrosis, although some biopsies can also show isolated portal fibrosis, without pericellular fibrosis. In any case, the portal fibrosis can subsequently progress through bridging fibrosis and cirrhosis (Table 9.2). Also, of note, early fibrosis can have a portal-based pattern in children with fatty liver disease, since they are more likely to have a zone 1 pattern of fat.

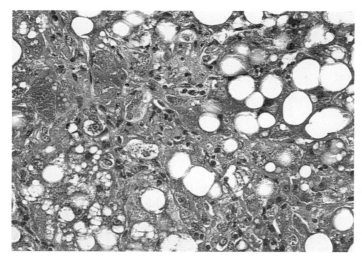

FIGURE 9.26 **Pericellular fibrosis, trichrome stain.** Zone 3 pericellular fibrosis is present.

OTHER CAUSES OF MACROVESICULAR STEATOSIS

After excluding NAFLD, drug effects, and alcohol as causes of fatty liver disease, there are still many possibilities in the differential (Table 9.1). Although each of these are rare, they are common enough as a group that you are likely to experience cases of fatty liver disease without evidence of the metabolic syndrome, alcohol, or drug effects during your career. Some of the more common of these entities are discussed in additional detail below, whereas other entities are discussed in other sections of this book.

DRUG-INDUCED LIVER INJURY (DILI) can manifest as fatty liver disease. In most of these cases, however, medications are likely exerting a synergistic effect, as most patients will also have the metabolic syndrome or several of its key features. As one example, most patients who develop fatty liver disease while taking methotrexate also have features of the metabolic syndrome.[64] As a second example, patients with colonic adenocarcinoma may develop fatty liver disease after treatment with irinotecan and oxaliplatin[65]; most of these patients will also have the metabolic syndrome.[66]

In general, fatty liver disease that is associated with medications has essentially identical histological findings to those of conventional NAFLD from the metabolic syndrome, ranging from steatosis to steatohepatitis. In fact, there is no reliable way to determine by histology the relative contributions of DILI versus the metabolic syndrome to the degree of fat, active injury, or steatosis. As an exception, the findings in amiodarone-related DILI do not look like ordinary NAFLD, as the hepatocytes often show relatively little fat but severe hepatocyte ballooning and abundant Mallory hyaline.

MALNUTRITION is a well-known but rare cause of a fatty liver disease. Malnutrition from food insufficiency is commonly categorized as either marasmus or kwashiorkor. Although both are rare in the developed world, they can be seen in cases of child abuse by starvation[67] or in cases where infants and toddlers are kept on nonstandard diets. Kwashiorkor develops when there is enough total caloric intake but insufficient protein intake and is associated with pedal edema, an enlarged abdomen, hepatic steatosis, and an increased risk for infections. Kwashiorkor is most commonly seen in infants when they are weaned from breast-feeding and moved to diets high in carbohydrates but low in proteins. Fatty liver is seen in greater than 90% of individuals with kwashiorkor and is typically severe.[68]

In contrast, marasmus results from total caloric insufficiency and individuals are typically emaciated with loose, dry skin and lack the edema and enlarged abdomen of kwashiorkor. Although fatty liver is almost always associated with kwashiorkor, it is also commonly present in marasmus.[68] In addition, anorexia nervosa can also cause severe fatty liver disease.[69]

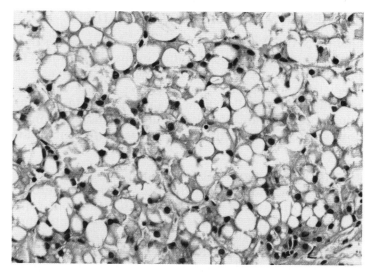

FIGURE 9.27 **Fatty liver disease after small bowel surgery.** This patient developed marked fatty liver disease after Roux-en-Y gastric bypass.

Finally, medication-induced injury to the small bowel can rarely lead to fatty liver disease because of malabsorption, one example being olmesartan enteropathy.[70]

ABDOMINAL SURGERY functions in many ways like malnutrition when large segments of the small bowel are removed and the remainder is insufficient for proper nutrient absorption (Figure 9.27). Malnutrition-associated fatty liver disease can also result from pyloric obstruction following liver transplant.[71] Steatosis or steatohepatitis also develops following pancreatic resection (Whipple) in about 50% of patients from malnutrition due to bowel loss and from exocrine insufficiency.[72] The pathology findings can range from steatosis to severe steatohepatitis.[71,73]

PORTAL VEIN THROMBOSIS. Acute portal vein thrombosis can also lead to fatty liver disease (Figure 9.28). In one study, fatty liver disease was present in 80% of 138 individuals with idiopathic portal vein thrombosis.[28] In addition, macrovesicular steatosis has been reported following portal vein or hepatic artery thrombosis in transplanted livers.[27] Some individuals can also have the metabolic syndrome, but some persons do not and the mechanism is unclear; it may be that obstruction of the portal vein prevents adequate nutrition from reaching the liver through the portal circulation.

WILSON DISEASE. In approximately 5% to 10% of children with Wilson disease,[74] biopsies show a rather nondescript pattern of fatty liver disease on liver biopsy (Figure 9.29). In some cases, particularly in older children or young adults, the fat can also be associated with Mallory hyaline in the periportal hepatocytes. These cases can mimic NAFLD, and the best approach is to have a high degree of suspicion, especially with cases of NAFLD in teenagers and young adults who do not have risk factors for the metabolic syndrome.

The fat in Wilson disease is often not associated with obesity or the metabolic syndrome and in these cases appears to be a direct consequence of the copper deposition, at least in part.[75] In fact, the amount

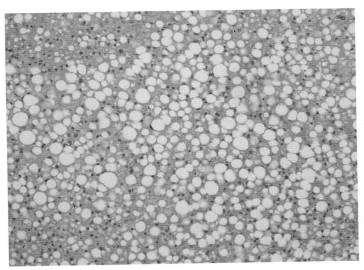

FIGURE 9.28   **Fatty liver disease after portal vein thrombosis.** Acute portal vein thrombosis led to fatty liver in this allograft liver biopsy.

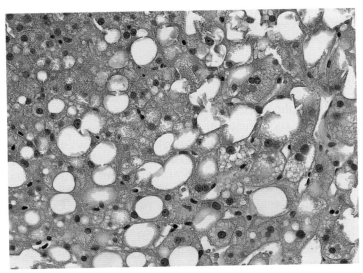

FIGURE 9.29   **Wilson disease.** Moderate macrovesicular steatosis is the main histological finding in this case of Wilson disease.

of fat correlates with the amount of tissue copper.[75] Nonetheless, the amount of fat is considerably more than the amount of copper visible on copper stain.

MICROVESICULAR STEATOSIS

Microvesicular steatosis is a distinctive pattern of injury where the hepatocyte cytoplasm is filled with numerous small droplets of fat that give the hepatocytes a "bubbly" appearance. The diagnosis is made based on H&E findings; Oil red O stains are neither necessary nor desirable. This injury pattern is very rare and is associated with mitochondrial injury from various causes, most commonly drug reactions, alcoholic foamy degeneration, or acute fatty liver of pregnancy. The differential is much longer and includes many disease processes that are of equal or greater rarity (Table 2.2, Chapter 2). Alcoholic foamy degeneration is further discussed as one example of this disease pattern. Acute fatty liver of pregnancy is discussed in Chapter 17.

To make a diagnosis of a microvesicular steatosis pattern of injury, these two features must be met, the first reflecting the morphology of the individual cell and the second the distribution of the microvesicular steatosis: (1) individual hepatocytes should have their entire cytoplasm filled with tiny vacuoles of fat, leading to a bubbly appearance and (2) the cells with microvesicular steatosis should be diffuse throughout the liver. The second criterion distinguishes this pattern from the focal patches of microvesicular steatosis that are common in ordinary steatohepatitis. This does not mean, however, that every hepatocyte needs to show microvesicular steatosis, as some milder cases may show the change in all zone 3 hepatocytes but with relatively normal-appearing zone 1 hepatocytes. In addition, a few scattered foci of macrovesicular steatosis are acceptable, but the main pattern should be microvesicular steatosis.

ALCOHOLIC FOAMY LIVER DEGENERATION. There are only limited data on the prevalence of alcoholic foamy degeneration, but one study from Spain reported a frequency of 2.3% in a study of nearly 400 sequential liver biopsies in alcoholic patients.[76] This unique pattern of alcohol-related liver injury leads to diffuse microvesicular steatosis (Figure 9.30). In milder cases, the microvesicular steatosis may have a zone 3 distribution with relative sparing of the zone 1 hepatocytes. In the spared hepatocytes, megamitochondria can be prominent. There is usually some degree of concomitant macrovesicular steatosis too.[77] The differential primarily includes drug effect. Although many other rare diseases can have a microvesicular steatosis pattern, the alcohol history quickly narrows the differential diagnosis.

The precise trigger for alcoholic foamy liver degeneration is unknown, but the injury pattern can be associated with increased alcohol consumption in patients with known but stable alcoholic liver disease; in some cases, patients feel sufficiently ill that they stop drinking days or weeks

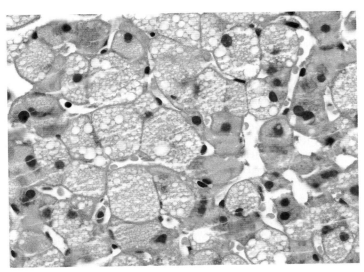

FIGURE 9.30 **Alcoholic foamy degeneration.** The hepatocyte shows diffuse microvesicular steatosis with no significant lobular inflammation.

before the biopsy. Clinically, the AST and ALT levels can be high, often over 500 IU/L and sometimes over 1000 IU/L,[77] but the biopsies show little or no lobular inflammation. Mild nonspecific portal chronic inflammation can be present. The classic AST:ALT ratio of greater than 2 (normal less than 1), which is not specific but is commonly seen in alcohol-related liver disease, may be closer to 1.[78]

REFERENCES

1. Eslam M, Newsome PN, Sarin SK, et al. A new definition for metabolic dysfunction-associated fatty liver disease: an international expert consensus statement. *J Hepatol.* 2020;73:202-209.
2. Kim D, Kim WR. Nonobese fatty liver disease. *Clin Gastroenterol Hepatol.* 2017;15:474-485.
3. Neuschwander-Tetri BA, Clark JM, Bass NM, et al. Clinical, laboratory and histological associations in adults with nonalcoholic fatty liver disease. *Hepatology.* 2010;52:913-924.
4. Verma S, Jensen D, Hart J, et al. Predictive value of ALT levels for non-alcoholic steatohepatitis (NASH) and advanced fibrosis in non-alcoholic fatty liver disease (NAFLD). *Liver Int.* 2013;33:1398-1405.
5. Pantsari MW, Harrison SA. Nonalcoholic fatty liver disease presenting with an isolated elevated alkaline phosphatase. *J Clin Gastroenterol.* 2006;40:633-635.
6. Johannsson G, Bengtsson BA. Growth hormone and the metabolic syndrome. *J Endocrinol Invest.* 1999;22:41-46.
7. Chung GE, Kim D, Kim W, et al. Non-alcoholic fatty liver disease across the spectrum of hypothyroidism. *J Hepatol.* 2012;57:150-156.
8. Kumarendran B, O'Reilly MW, Manolopoulos KN, et al. Polycystic ovary syndrome, androgen excess, and the risk of nonalcoholic fatty liver disease in women: a longitudinal study based on a United Kingdom primary care database. *PLoS Med.* 2018;15:e1002542.

9. Koskinas J, Gomatos IP, Tiniakos DG, et al. Liver histology in ICU patients dying from sepsis: a clinico-pathological study. *World J Gastroenterol.* 2008;14:1389-1393.

10. Weiss B, Krauthammer A, Soudack M, et al. Liver disease in pediatric patients with Ataxia Telangiectasia: a novel report. *J Pediatr Gastroenterol Nutr.* 2016;62:550-555.

11. Takagi H, Hagiwara S, Hashizume H, et al. Adult onset type II citrullinemia as a cause of non-alcoholic steatohepatitis. *J Hepatol.* 2006;44:236-239.

12. Damen G, de Klerk H, Huijmans J, et al. Gastrointestinal and other clinical manifestations in 17 children with congenital disorders of glycosylation type Ia, Ib, and Ic. *J Pediatr Gastroenterol Nutr.* 2004;38:282-287.

13. Black DD, Hay RV, Rohwer-Nutter PL, et al. Intestinal and hepatic apolipoprotein B gene expression in abetalipoproteinemia. *Gastroenterology.* 1991;101:520-528.

14. Yap JY, O'Connor C, Mager DR, et al. Diagnostic challenges of nonalcoholic fatty liver disease (NAFLD) in children of normal weight. *Clin Res Hepatol Gastroenterol.* 2011;35:500-505.

15. Collardeau-Frachon S, Bouvier R, Le Gall C, et al. Unexpected diagnosis of cystic fibrosis at liver biopsy: a report of four pediatric cases. *Virchows Arch.* 2007;451:57-64.

16. Ayoub F, Trillo-Alvarez C, Morelli G, et al. Risk factors for hepatic steatosis in adults with cystic fibrosis: similarities to non-alcoholic fatty liver disease. *World J Hepatol.* 2018;10:34-40.

17. Hourigan SK, Torbenson M, Tibesar E, et al. The full spectrum of hepatic steatosis in children. *Clin Pediatr (Phila).* 2015;54:635-642.

18. Powell EE, Searle J, Mortimer R. Steatohepatitis associated with limb lipodystrophy. *Gastroenterology.* 1989;97:1022-1024.

19. Africa JA, Behling CA, Brunt EM, et al. In children with nonalcoholic fatty liver disease, zone 1 steatosis is associated with advanced fibrosis. *Clin Gastroenterol Hepatol.* 2018;16:438-446.e1.

20. Miyagawa-Hayashino A, Egawa H, Yorifuji T, et al. Allograft steatohepatitis in progressive familial intrahepatic cholestasis type 1 after living donor liver transplantation. *Liver Transpl.* 2009;15:610-618.

21. Lefkowitch JH, Grossman ME. Hepatic pathology in porphyria cutanea tarda. *Liver.* 1983;3:19-29.

22. Fintini D, Inzaghi E, Colajacomo M, et al. Non-alcoholic fatty liver disease (NAFLD) in children and adolescents with Prader-Willi syndrome (PWS). *Pediatr Obes.* 2016;11:235-238.

23. Fernandez-Lainez C, Ibarra-Gonzalez I, Belmont-Martinez L, et al. Tyrosinemia type I: clinical and biochemical analysis of patients in Mexico. *Ann Hepatol.* 2014;13:265-272.

24. Roulot D. Liver involvement in Turner syndrome. *Liver Int.* 2013;33:24-30.

25. Kimura H, Kako M, Yo K, et al. Alcoholic hyalins (Mallory bodies) in a case of Weber-Christian disease: electron microscopic observations of liver involvement. *Gastroenterology.* 1980;78:807-812.

26. Wasserman JM, Thung SN, Berman R, et al. Hepatic Weber-Christian disease. *Semin Liver Dis.* 2001;21:115-118.

27. Silverman JF, O'Brien KF, Long S, et al. Liver pathology in morbidly obese patients with and without diabetes. *Am J Gastroenterol.* 1990;85:1349-1355.

28. Di Minno MN, Tufano A, Rusolillo A, et al. High prevalence of nonalcoholic fatty liver in patients with idiopathic venous thromboembolism. *World J Gastroenterol.* 2010;16:6119-6122.

29. Cotrim HP, Andrade ZA, Parana R, et al. Nonalcoholic steatohepatitis: a toxic liver disease in industrial workers. *Liver.* 1999;19:299-304.

30. Brambilla P, Crino A, Bedogni G, et al. Metabolic syndrome in children with Prader-Willi syndrome: the effect of obesity. *Nutr Metab Cardiovasc Dis.* 2011;21:269-276.

31. Angulo P, Kleiner DE, Dam-Larsen S, et al. Liver fibrosis, but No other histologic features, is associated with long-term outcomes of patients with nonalcoholic fatty liver disease. *Gastroenterology*. 2015;149:389-397.e10.

32. Ekstedt M, Hagstrom H, Nasr P, et al. Fibrosis stage is the strongest predictor for disease-specific mortality in NAFLD after up to 33 years of follow-up. *Hepatology*. 2015;61:1547-1554.

33. Singh S, Allen AM, Wang Z, et al. Fibrosis progression in nonalcoholic fatty liver vs nonalcoholic steatohepatitis: a systematic review and meta-analysis of paired-biopsy studies. *Clin Gastroenterol Hepatol*. 2015;13:643-654.e1-e9; quiz e39-40.

34. Maheshwari A, Thuluvath PJ. Cryptogenic cirrhosis and NAFLD: are they related? *Am J Gastroenterol*. 2006;101:664-668.

35. Vuppalanchi R, Gould RJ, Wilson LA, et al. Clinical significance of serum autoantibodies in patients with NAFLD: results from the nonalcoholic steatohepatitis clinical research network. *Hepatol Int*. 2012;6:379-385.

36. Adams LA, Lindor KD, Angulo P. The prevalence of autoantibodies and autoimmune hepatitis in patients with nonalcoholic Fatty liver disease. *Am J Gastroenterol*. 2004;99:1316-1320.

37. Cotler SJ, Kanji K, Keshavarzian A, et al. Prevalence and significance of autoantibodies in patients with non-alcoholic steatohepatitis. *J Clin Gastroenterol*. 2004;38:801-804.

38. Loria P, Lonardo A, Leonardi F, et al. Non-organ-specific autoantibodies in nonalcoholic fatty liver disease: prevalence and correlates. *Dig Dis Sci*. 2003;48:2173-2181.

39. Ravi S, Shoreibah M, Raff E, et al. Autoimmune markers do not impact clinical presentation or natural history of steatohepatitis-related liver disease. *Dig Dis Sci*. 2015;60:3788-3793.

40. Ludwig J, Viggiano TR, McGill DB, et al. Nonalcoholic steatohepatitis: Mayo Clinic experiences with a hitherto unnamed disease. *Mayo Clin Proc*. 1980;55:434-438.

41. Kleiner DE, Brunt EM, Van Natta M, et al. Design and validation of a histological scoring system for nonalcoholic fatty liver disease. *Hepatology*. 2005;41:1313-1321.

42. Bedossa P, Poitou C, Veyrie N, et al. Histopathological algorithm and scoring system for evaluation of liver lesions in morbidly obese patients. *Hepatology*. 2012;56:1751-1759.

43. Ong JP, Younossi ZM. Epidemiology and natural history of NAFLD and NASH. *Clin Liver Dis*. 2007;11:1-16, vii.

44. Fielding CM, Angulo P. Hepatic steatosis and steatohepatitis: are they really two distinct entities? *Curr Hepatol Rep*. 2014;13:151-158.

45. McPherson S, Hardy T, Henderson E, et al. Evidence of NAFLD progression from steatosis to fibrosing-steatohepatitis using paired biopsies: implications for prognosis and clinical management. *J Hepatol*. 2015;62:1148-1155.

46. Pais R, Charlotte F, Fedchuk L, et al. A systematic review of follow-up biopsies reveals disease progression in patients with non-alcoholic fatty liver. *J Hepatol*. 2013;59:550-556.

47. Hagstrom H, Elfwen O, Hultcrantz R, et al. Steatohepatitis is not associated with an increased risk for fibrosis progression in nonalcoholic fatty liver disease. *Gastroenterol Res Pract*. 2018;2018:1942648.

48. Wong VW, Wong GL, Choi PC, et al. Disease progression of non-alcoholic fatty liver disease: a prospective study with paired liver biopsies at 3 years. *Gut*. 2010;59:969-974.

49. Yeh MM, Belt P, Brunt EM, et al. Acidophil bodies in nonalcoholic steatohepatitis. *Hum Pathol*. 2016;52:28-37.

50. Brunt EM, Kleiner DE, Carpenter DH, et al. Nonalcoholic fatty liver disease: reporting histologic findings in clinical practice. *Hepatology*. 2021;73:2028-2038.

51. Zhu H, Bodenheimer HC Jr, Clain DJ, et al. Hepatic lipogranulomas in patients with chronic liver disease: association with hepatitis C and fatty liver disease. *World J Gastroenterol*. 2010;16:5065-5069.

52. Noureddin M, Yates KP, Vaughn IA, et al. Clinical and histological determinants of nonalcoholic steatohepatitis and advanced fibrosis in elderly patients. *Hepatology.* 2013;58:1644-1654.

53. Tandra S, Yeh MM, Brunt EM, et al. Presence and significance of microvesicular steatosis in nonalcoholic fatty liver disease. *J Hepatol.* 2011;55:654-659.

54. Allende DS, Gawrieh S, Cummings OW, et al. Glycogenosis is common in nonalcoholic fatty liver disease and is independently associated with ballooning, but lower steatosis and lower fibrosis. *Liver Int.* 2021;41:996-1011.

55. Abraham S, Furth EE. Receiver operating characteristic analysis of glycogenated nuclei in liver biopsy specimens: quantitative evaluation of their relationship with diabetes and obesity. *Hum Pathol.* 1994;25:1063-1068.

56. Gill RM, Belt P, Wilson L, et al. Centrizonal arteries and microvessels in nonalcoholic steatohepatitis. *Am J Surg Pathol.* 2011;35:1400-1404.

57. Xanthakos S, Miles L, Bucuvalas J, et al. Histologic spectrum of nonalcoholic fatty liver disease in morbidly obese adolescents. *Clin Gastroenterol Hepatol.* 2006;4:226-232.

58. Reha JL, Lee S, Hofmann LJ. Prevalence and predictors of nonalcoholic steatohepatitis in obese patients undergoing bariatric surgery: a Department of Defense experience. *Am Surg.* 2014;80:595-599.

59. Alcoholic liver disease: morphological manifestations. Review by an international group. *Lancet.* 1981;1:707-711.

60. Spahr L, Rubbia-Brandt L, Genevay M, et al. Early liver biopsy, intraparenchymal cholestasis, and prognosis in patients with alcoholic steatohepatitis. *BMC Gastroenterol.* 2011;11:115.

61. Altamirano J, Miquel R, Katoonizadeh A, et al. A histologic scoring system for prognosis of patients with alcoholic hepatitis. *Gastroenterology.* 2014;146:1231-1239.e1-e6.

62. Brunt EM, Kleiner DE, Behling C, et al. Misuse of scoring systems. *Hepatology.* 2011;54:369-370; author reply 70-71.

63. Bedossa P, Consortium FP. Utility and appropriateness of the fatty liver inhibition of progression (FLIP) algorithm and steatosis, activity, and fibrosis (SAF) score in the evaluation of biopsies of nonalcoholic fatty liver disease. *Hepatology.* 2014;60:565-575.

64. Shetty A, Cho W, Alazawi W, et al. Methotrexate hepatotoxicity and the impact of nonalcoholic fatty liver disease. *Am J Med Sci.* 2017;354:172-181.

65. Vauthey JN, Pawlik TM, Ribero D, et al. Chemotherapy regimen predicts steatohepatitis and an increase in 90-day mortality after surgery for hepatic colorectal metastases. *J Clin Oncol.* 2006;24:2065-2072.

66. Ryan P, Nanji S, Pollett A, et al. Chemotherapy-induced liver injury in metastatic colorectal cancer: semiquantitative histologic analysis of 334 resected liver specimens shows that vascular injury but not steatohepatitis is associated with preoperative chemotherapy. *Am J Surg Pathol.* 2010;34:784-791.

67. Solarino B, Grattagliano I, Catanesi R, et al. Child starvation and neglect: a report of two fatal cases. *J Forensic Leg Med.* 2012;19:171-174.

68. Doherty JF, Adam EJ, Griffin GE, et al. Ultrasonographic assessment of the extent of hepatic steatosis in severe malnutrition. *Arch Dis Child.* 1992;67:1348-1352.

69. Sakada M, Tanaka A, Ohta D, et al. Severe steatosis resulted from anorexia nervosa leading to fatal hepatic failure. *J Gastroenterol.* 2006;41:714-715.

70. Non-Alcoholic Fatty Liver Disease Study G; Dolci M, Nascimbeni F, et al. Nonalcoholic steatohepatitis heralding olmesartan-induced sprue-like enteropathy. *Dig Liver Dis.* 2016;48:1399-1401.

71. Sanada Y, Urahashi T, Wakiya T, et al. Non-alcoholic steatohepatitis caused by malnutrition after pediatric liver transplantation. *Pediatr Int.* 2011;53:1077-1081.

72. Okabe H, Yamashita YI, Inoue R, et al. Postoperative nonalcoholic fatty liver disease is correlated with malnutrition leading to an unpreferable clinical course for pancreatic cancer patients undergoing pancreaticoduodenectomy. *Surg Today*. 2020;50:193-199.

73. Sim EH, Kwon JH, Kim SY, et al. Severe steatohepatitis with hepatic decompensation resulting from malnutrition after pancreaticoduodenectomy. *Clin Mol Hepatol*. 2012;18:404-410.

74. Kleine RT, Mendes R, Pugliese R, et al. Wilson's disease: an analysis of 28 Brazilian children. *Clinics*. 2012;67:231-235.

75. Liggi M, Murgia D, Civolani A, et al. The relationship between copper and steatosis in Wilson's disease. *Clin Res Hepatol Gastroenterol*. 2013;37:36-40.

76. Montull S, Pares A, Bruguera M, et al. Alcoholic foamy degeneration in Spain. Prevalence and clinico-pathological features. *Liver*. 1989;9:79-85.

77. Roth N, Kanel G, Kaplowitz N. Alcoholic foamy degeneration and alcoholic fatty liver with jaundice: often overlooked causes of jaundice and hepatic decompensation that can mimic alcoholic hepatitis. *Clin Liver Dis*. 2015;6:145-148.

78. Ruiz P, Michelena J, Altamirano J, et al. Hepatic hemodynamics and transient elastography in alcoholic foamy degeneration: report of 2 cases. *Ann Hepatol*. 2012;11:399-403.

10

AUTOIMMUNE HEPATITIS

DEFENITION AND KEY CLINICAL FINDINGS

Autoimmune hepatitis (AIH) is a self-perpetuating, immune-mediated injury of the liver. The degree of disease activity can wax and wane over time and can lead to cirrhosis, especially in untreated patients. AIH, by definition, requires exclusion of known causes of viral hepatitis as well as drug-induced liver injury (DILI). A definite diagnosis also requires compatible histological findings on liver biopsy.[1]

DIAGNOSTIC APPROACH

Key Elements in the Diagnosis of AIH

- Clinical findings
  - Most commonly young to middle-aged women
  - DILI should be excluded
  - In selected populations, diseases such as Wilsons should be excluded
- Laboratory findings
  - Exclusion of viral hepatitis
  - Hepatitic pattern of liver enzyme elevations
  - Elevated serum IgG levels
  - Positive serum autoantibodies: Antinuclear antibody (ANA), antismooth muscle antibodies (ASMA), liver kidney microsomal antibodies (LKM) 1, or liver cytosol antibodies (LC1)
- Histology findings
  - A hepatitic pattern of injury, typically with plasma cell–rich inflammation
  - The amount of active inflammation, necrosis, and fibrosis can vary.

The diagnosis of AIH can be fully established only after a systematic evaluation of clinical, laboratory, and histological findings; there is no single pathognomonic finding and the diagnosis is based on a combination of negative and positive findings. As part of making the diagnosis, a liver biopsy is required, but the diagnosis is never made solely by histological findings.

Liver biopsies have several important roles in AIH; they establish that a histological injury pattern is consistent with AIH, they assess the degree of active injury, they determine the stage of fibrosis, and they evaluate for other potential concomitant diseases. In many cases, there is, in fact, another known disease, such as fatty liver disease or primary biliary cirrhosis/cholangitis (PBC), but patients also have elevated serum autoantibodies, leading to liver biopsies in order to determine if there is an additional element of AIH.

CLINICAL FINDINGS

AIH has a strong female predominance (80% overall), but males are equally affected prior to puberty and in the elderly.[2,3] AIH has a bimodal distribution for age at first diagnosis, with a first peak at 10 to 20 years of age and the second around 40 years of age. It is important to remember, however, that approximately 20% of AIH cases present after the age 60 years.[3]

A genetic predisposition has been identified in many studies, with strong links to HLA DR3 and DR4 for type I AIH. Much of the molecular mechanisms that underlie this genetic predisposition, however, remain unclear. Likewise, the factors that initiate or trigger AIH have not been resolved. The overall trend appears to be that acute hepatitis can cause the immune system to newly recognize self-antigens as foreign in susceptible individuals, even if the hepatitis was not clinically apparent (for example, mild subclinical cases of acute Hepatitis A or drug reactions).

Rarely, in less than 1% of cases, patients will have parents or siblings with a history of AIH.[4] In a study of 64 patients who had AIH and were twins, only a single twin (monozygotic) developed AIH in over 1110 patient-years of follow-up.[4]

Presentation

In about 25% of cases, AIH presents as an acute unexplained hepatitis; this can include fulminant hepatitis in about 5% of overall cases. The most common clinical presentation, seen in about 50% of patients, is nonspecific complaints such as fatigue, malaise, abdominal pain, or anorexia. Finally, approximately 25% of individuals are identified during laboratory testing for other clinical indications and have largely asymptomatic liver disease at initial diagnosis.

The International Autoimmune Hepatitis Group (IAHG) has published a series of papers, including an early scoring system that was designed for research purposes,[5,6] but, perhaps inevitably, became used

TABLE 10.1   International Autoimmune Hepatitis Group Criteria for the Diagnosis of Autoimmune Hepatitis[7]

Variable	Cut-Off	Points
ANA or ASMA	≥1:40	1
ANA or ASMA	≥1:80	2[a]
or LKM	≥1:40	2[a]
or SLA	Positive	2[a]
IgG	>Upper normal limit	1
	>1.10 times upper normal limit	2
Liver histology (evidence of hepatitis is necessary)	Compatible with AIH	1
	Typical of AIH	2
Absence of viral hepatitis	Yes	2
Interpretation	**≥7: definite AIH**	
	≥6: probable AIH	

ANA, antinuclear antibody; ASMA, antismooth muscle antibodies; LKM, kidney microsomal antibodies; SLA, soluble liver antigen; AIH, autoimmune hepatitis.
[a]The maximum total points for all autoantibodies is 2 points, even if the patient scores more than 2.

for clinical diagnosis by some clinical groups. The IAHG subsequently revised the scoring system in the hope of making it more useful for routine clinical practice.[7] A working familiarity with the system is worthwhile (Table 10.1), but this system is still primarily used for research and teaching purposes and is not consistently used at most medical centers for clinical care.

In regards to the scoring system, your contribution is to determine whether the biopsy is "compatible with AIH," "typical of AIH," or neither of these. The paper defines "typical" AIH as having the following three features: (1) interface hepatitis accompanied by lymphocytic/lymphoplasmocytic infiltrates in the portal tracts; (2) emperipolesis—defined as active penetration by 1 cell into and through a larger cell; and (3) hepatic rosette formation. The scoring system defines any chronic lymphocytic hepatitis as sufficient for meeting the criteria of "compatible with AIH."

These criteria will undoubtedly be updated and modified, as several of them are not particularly helpful and others are ambiguous, but this is unlikely to influence how the pathologist approaches this entity for clinical care; instead, the primary goal of liver pathology will remain the same, to identify a hepatitic pattern of injury, most often with plasma cell–rich inflammation. Also, of note, this system is not recommended for use in research studying the AIH overlap syndromes.[1]

Caveat to the Simplified Criteria From the IAHG

The criteria in this paper are not laid out with complete clarity. The paper actually lists four criteria:
1. interface activity
2. lymphocytic/lymphoplasmocytic inflammation extending into the lobules
3. emperipolesis
4. rosette formation

The interpretation of criterion 2 has been inconsistent because it is ambiguous, sometimes being interpreted as restatement of criterion 1, sometimes as indicating a need for portal inflammation, and sometimes as a need for both portal and lobular inflammation.

Treatment

Individuals with AIH are treated by immunosuppression. Steroids, with or without azathioprine, are most often used as first-line therapy and remission can be achieved in up to 80% of persons. Individuals who do not respond to glucocorticoids and azathioprine may be given other immunosuppressive agents such as mycophenolate, cyclosporin, tacrolimus, or methotrexate. A large proportion of individuals, up to 85%, will have disease relapse as steroids are tapered and so require additional therapy.[8] The overall clinical course can be influenced by gender (males do worse), ethnicity (non-Caucasians do worse), and the amount of fibrosis at presentation (more fibrosis does worse).[9]

SEROLOGICAL FINDINGS AND SUBTYPES

Serum IgG levels are typically elevated in AIH. In addition, serum autoantibodies are positive in most cases, including ANA, ASMA, LKM, LC-1, and soluble liver antigen (SLA). These autoantibodies are used to define two subtypes of AIH (Table 10.2). In the pediatric population, AIH type 1 tends to be more common after puberty, while type 2 can be seen in younger children as well. In the pediatric population, antibody titers also tend to be lower than in adults. Overall, the histological findings do not correlate strongly with autoantibody patterns, at least not that has been recognized to date. Both types 1 and 2 AIH have similar responses to modern treatment algorithms,[14] but type 2 AIH tends to have more flares and a greater risk for fibrosis progression. Patients only rarely are positive for antibodies of both type 1 and type 2 AIH, but when this is the case, the clinical course tends to be more similar to type 2 AIH. Type 2 AIH can also be associated with IgA deficiency.

The specific self-antigens have been defined in most cases for the various autoantibodies used to support a diagnosis of AIH.[10] Multiple

TABLE 10.2 **Autoimmune Hepatitis Subtypes**		
Feature	Type 1	Type 2
Approximate frequency	95%	5%
Autoantibodies[10]	ANA alone 5%-10%	Anti-liver/kidney microsomal antibody (LKM type 1)
	ASMA alone, 35%	
	Both positive, 50%	
	Both negative, 5%-10%	Anti-liver cytosol (LC1)
Elevated serum IgG levels	>2× upper limit of normal in ~80%	>2× upper limit of normal in ~80%
Most common affected age group	Teens to adults (10 to elderly)	Pediatrics (2-18)
Other associated diseases	Various autoimmune conditions in 20%-40%[11,a]	IgA deficiency in up to 45%[12,13]
Histological findings	Hepatitis with prominent plasma cells	Hepatitis with prominent plasma cells
Progression to cirrhosis (approximate %)	45	80

ANA, antinuclear antibody; ASMA, antismooth muscle antibodies.
[a]Can be diagnosed either at the time of autoimmune hepatitis or subsequently.

self-antigens appear to be the target for ANA, including double-stranded DNA, chromatin, and ribonucleoprotein. For ASMA, the self-antigens include filamentous actin (F-actin), vimentin, and desmin; of these, F-actin ASMA is the most specific for AIH.[15] In type 2 AIH, LKM1 antibodies recognize cytochrome P450 CYP2D6, while the LC1 antibodies recognize formiminotransferase cyclodeaminase. Anti-SLA is now thought to be the same antibody as anti-LP-1 and recognizes selenocysteine synthase. Anti-SLA/LP can be positive in both type 1 and type 2 AIH, but, of note, can be the only positive autoantibody in a subset of patients. Thus, it can be helpful to test for this autoantibody when ANA, ASMA, and LKM1 antibodies are negative.

When interpreting antibody findings, the overall level of positivity is important. For example, low-titer antibodies are common in a wide variety of inflammatory conditions, and even in the general "healthy" adult population. Thus, low-titer autoantibodies do not provide strong support for a diagnosis of AIH in isolation. Likewise, high-titer autoantibodies can be found in some individuals with systemic autoimmune diseases, some of who also have very mild liver enzyme elevations, but whose biopsies show no evidence for AIH; in these cases, the high-titer autoantibodies are also insufficient evidence in isolation to make a diagnosis of AIH.

A diagnosis of AIH is most commonly based on both the presence of significant elevations of autoantibodies (variably defined, but the IAHG suggests a minimum of 1:40 or greater) and an otherwise unexplained hepatitis on biopsy (eg, viral hepatitis, DILI, etc, have been excluded). In most AIH cases, the titers will be 1:160 or higher. In otherwise healthy children, autoantibodies are rare and low-titer ANA and ASMA, such as 1:20, can also be significant.[3] ELISA methods have replaced traditional antibody titer evaluation in many medical centers. With ELISA testing, positive results are not reported with titers but with a numerical value; most individuals with AIH will have values significantly outside the normal range (more than just a point or two). The normal ranges will vary depending on the assay.

SERONEGATIVE AIH

All serologies are negative in about 10% to 20% of patients who are eventually classified as having AIH based on clinical and histological findings; this group is called seronegative AIH. These patients resemble typical AIH patients in their overall clinical findings, histological changes seen on liver biopsy, response to therapy, and overall clinical outcomes. Some patients who are initially seronegative, may develop autoantibodies during follow-up.[16]

HISTOLOGICAL FINDINGS

Most Common Histological Patterns in AIH

Patients Who Present With Clinical Findings

- Acute hepatitis pattern, with moderate to marked lobular inflammation ± necrosis
- Fulminant hepatitis
- Zone 3 accentuated lobular hepatitis

Patients Identified by Incidental Elevations of Liver Enzymes or by Clinical Findings Associated With Cirrhosis

- Nonspecific findings, mildly active chronic hepatitis pattern, with mild portal and lobular inflammation and fibrosis
- End-stage cirrhosis, usually with mild nonspecific inflammation

The histological findings in AIH tend to correlate with the clinical presentation. The classic findings, such as a plasma cell–rich hepatitis that demonstrates interface activity, hepatitic rosettes, and emperipolesis, are seen primarily in cases of acute hepatitis or fulminant hepatitis presentations. In contrast, a large group of patients come to clinical attention when elevated liver enzymes are identified incidentally, and this group of patients typically have milder inflammation, with or without advanced fibrosis.

Fulminant Hepatitis

In cases of fulminant hepatitis, the biopsy shows marked inflammation and there can be extensive hepatocyte necrosis. The inflammation is typically plasma cell–rich, with plasma cell clusters evident in both the portal tracts and the lobules. The degree of inflammation, however, can change quickly and be substantially reduced following steroid therapy, which is can be started prior to the biopsy. Of course, plasma cell–rich fulminant hepatitis is not specific for AIH, and viral hepatitis and DILI in particular need to be excluded.

The necrosis is often panacinar, but can be quite patchy, with one core or portion of a core showing panacinar necrosis, while another core shows milder inflammatory changes with no significant necrosis (Figure 10.1). Fibrosis staging in the presence of marked necrosis is often problematic, as the areas of necrosis can be blue on trichrome stain, mimicking fibrosis. A reticulin stain can sometimes help by demonstrating areas of compressed reticulin that represent areas of necrosis. Of note, the vast majority of cases of fulminant hepatitis have no or mild fibrosis at presentation.

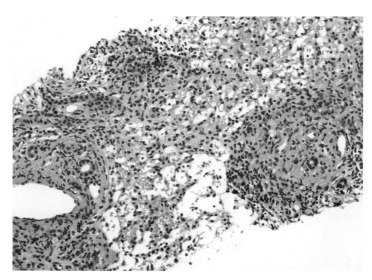

FIGURE 10.1 **Autoimmune hepatitis, patchy panacinar necrosis.** In this core, there is extensive panacinar necrosis, with loss of all hepatocytes and only residual portal tracts.

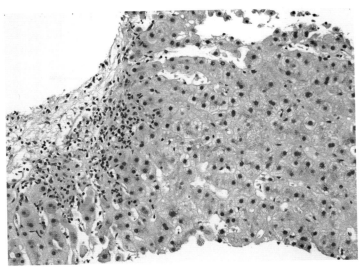

FIGURE 10.2 **Autoimmune hepatitis, patchy panacinar necrosis.** Same case as shown in Figure 10.1. A second biopsy core from the same procedure shows only focal zone 3 inflammation.

As livers with marked necrosis undergo recovery, usually following immunosuppressive therapy and a time interval of several weeks to months, they can develop striking regenerative nodules, nodules that can mimic tumors on imaging studies or on gross examination (Figure 10.2). These nodules can be several centimeters in diameter and can be haphazardly distributed, with the background liver showing extensive parenchymal collapse. In time, these areas of collapse can scar down, giving a very heterogeneous pattern of fibrosis, with areas of advanced fibrosis in one core (Figure 10.3), while other cores show only mild or no fibrosis (Figures 10.4 and 10.5).

Acute Hepatitis Presentation

Typical Features of Untreated AIH Presenting With Acute Liver Disease (Tends to Be a Continuum With Fulminant Hepatitis)

- Hepatitic pattern, usually with moderate or greater lobular and portal inflammation
  - Lobules may show regenerative rosettes
  - Emperipolesis may be present
  - Interface activity is usually moderate or greater
  - Plasma cell–rich inflammation in portal tracts and lobules
- Note: Incidentally identified cases, or those presenting with cirrhosis, usually have less inflammation, and plasma cells may be less prominent

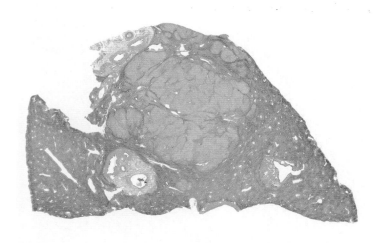

FIGURE 10.3 **Autoimmune hepatitis, regenerative nodule.** Varying-sized regenerative nodules were present in this liver transplanted for fulminant autoimmune hepatitis.

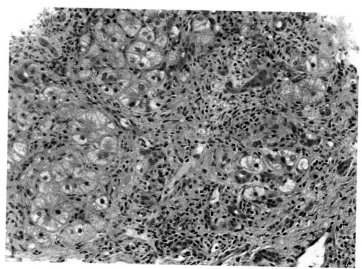

FIGURE 10.4 **Autoimmune hepatitis, patchy cirrhosis.** Multiple passes were obtained and several cores showed changes consistent with cirrhosis, while several other large cores showed no significant fibrosis (see next image).

The typical histological findings in acute AIH include moderate to marked portal inflammation with prominent plasma cells, interface activity, and moderate to marked lobular hepatitis. The lobules will also show scattered acidophil bodies, variable hepatocyte ballooning, and lobular disarray. The more severe hepatitic cases also commonly have lobular cholestasis

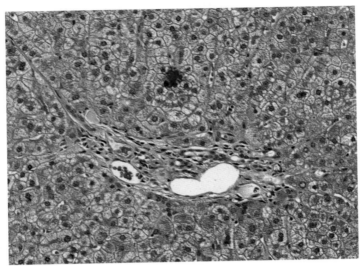

FIGURE 10.5 **Autoimmune hepatitis, patchy cirrhosis.** Multiple passes were obtained and several cores showed no significant fibrosis while others showed changes consistent with cirrhosis (see prior image).

and zone 3 necrosis. This "typical" pattern for AIH is important and helpful to recognize, but remember that (1) there are many variations to this pattern, (2) plasma cell–rich infiltrates can be seen in both drug reactions and acute viral hepatitis, and (3) interface activity is a reflection of the amount of active inflammation and not a very good indicator of etiology. Also, of note, neither emperipolesis nor hepatitic rosettes are specific for AIH, both instead being general findings in acute hepatitis from any etiology when there is moderate or marked activity.[17-19]

Portal Tracts

The portal tracts show lymphocytic inflammation that is typically moderate to marked (Figure 10.6), especially at first presentation of an acute hepatitis. The amount of plasma cells will vary, but plasma cells are evident and typically prominent (Figure 10.7; eFig. 10.1). The plasma cells can be immunostained and will show mostly IgG-positive plasma cells,[20] paralleling the increased serum immunoglobulin levels; this finding of predominantly IgG plasma cells, however, is not specific for AIH.[21] About 10% of cases can have few or no plasma cells, so their absence does not preclude a diagnosis of AIH.[17]

When it comes to identifying AIH on biopsy, interface activity is just as famous as plasma cells as a key feature of AIH (Figure 10.8; eFig. 10.2). Of note, however, interface activity is entirely nonspecific for AIH and is found in many other disease processes, including drug reactions, acute viral hepatitis, and chronic viral hepatitis. In fact, it is a common component of

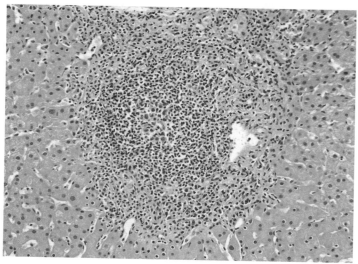

FIGURE 10.6 **Autoimmune hepatitis, portal tract.** The portal tract shows marked inflammation.

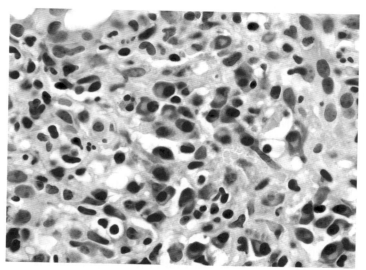

FIGURE 10.7 **Autoimmune hepatitis, portal tract.** Numerous plasma cells are seen.

most scoring systems for chronic viral hepatitis of any etiology. In addition, the sensitivity of interface activity for identifying AIH as a likely etiology, for example over that of portal or lobular plasma cell–rich inflammation, is not clear. Instead, interface activity seems to be best understood as a correlate of the degree of inflammatory activity for hepatitic patterns of injury resulting from any cause.

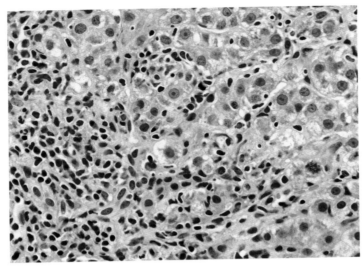

FIGURE 10.8 **Autoimmune hepatitis, interface activity.** The interface activity can have prominent plasma cells.

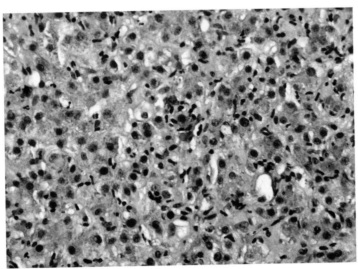

FIGURE 10.9 **Autoimmune hepatitis, lobular inflammation.** This case of autoimmune hepatitis shows moderate lobular inflammation.

Lobules

The lobules show varying amounts of lymphocytic inflammation, often with occasional single or small clusters of plasma cells (Figures 10.9 and 10.10; eFigs. 10.3 and 10.4). In some cases, the lobular inflammation can have a zone 3 predominant pattern. With marked hepatitis, zone 3

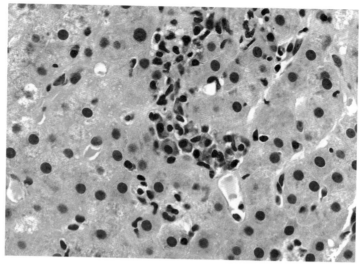

FIGURE 10.10 Autoimmune hepatitis, lobular plasma cells. An immunostain for IgG highlights numerous lobular plasma cells.

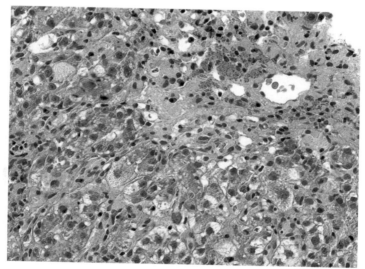

FIGURE 10.11 Autoimmune hepatitis, zone 3 necrosis. The central vein in the upper right of the image is surrounded by a rim of loose connective tissue with loss of hepatocytes.

necrosis is commonly present (Figure 10.11) and in severe cases, there can be bridging necrosis. With moderate to marked inflammation, the lobules often show cholestasis as well as hepatocyte rosettes (Figure 10.12). The hepatocyte rosettes are not specific for AIH and can be seen in zone 3, where they tend to be cholestatic rosettes, or in zone 1, where they are commonly called *regenerative rosettes*. Lobular neutrophils are unusual

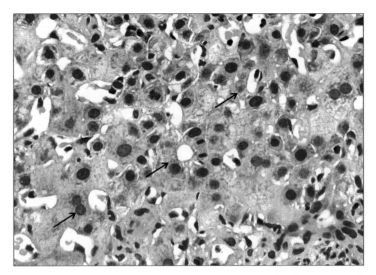

FIGURE 10.12 **Autoimmune hepatitis, hepatitic rosettes.** Circular regenerative rosettes can be seen (arrows).

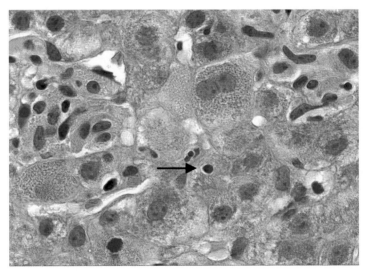

FIGURE 10.13 **Autoimmune hepatitis, emperipolesis.** The hepatocytes in autoimmune hepatitis will occasionally appear to have lymphocytes within their cytoplasm (arrow).

and suggest a drug reaction or acute viral hepatitis. Emperipolesis (Figure 10.13) is another feature identified by some authors as being useful, but in my experience this finding is difficult to reproducibly identify—ie, emperipolesis is often in the "eye of the beholder," with some pathologists having an easier time recognizing it than others (I find it hard).

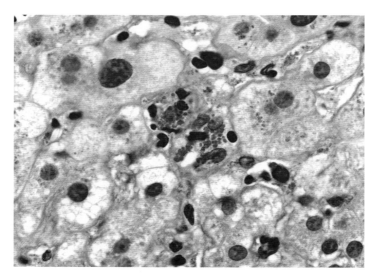

FIGURE 10.14 **Autoimmune hepatitis, Kupffer cell globules, periodic acid-Schiff with diastase (PASD) stain**. The PASD stain highlights globules in the Kupffer cells.

Periodic acid-Schiff with diastase (PASD) stains will highlight small round inclusions in the Kupffer cells in many cases (Figure 10.14). These small globules result from phagocytosis of immunoglobulins and will also stain with IgG; they are not, however, specific for AIH, being present in many diseases with elevated gamma globulins.

Zone 3 Pattern of Hepatitis

In some biopsies, the lobular hepatitis has a clear zone 3 accentuation. The zone 3 inflammation can range from mild to severe and is often accompanied by zone 3 necrosis in more severe cases. This pattern can be further subdivided into those with an isolated zone 3 hepatitis pattern and those that have zone 3 hepatitis plus the typical portal inflammation seen in conventual patterns of acute onset AIH. The isolated zone 3 pattern is seen in about 3% of patients (Figure 10.15; eFig. 10.5).[22-24] While this pattern is histologically distinct, the overall clinical presentation, laboratory findings, and clinical outcomes are broadly similar to conventional AIH. A zone 3 predominant pattern of hepatitis can also be seen with DILI and acute viral hepatitis, so is not specific for AIH.

AIH Undergoing Treatment

In patients with already established diagnoses of AIH, biopsies may be performed if there is concern for an additional, new liver injury, or if a patient is undergoing treatment and the clinical team wants to evaluate ongoing disease activity and/or to stage fibrosis. In this latter setting, residual inflammatory activity is present in 46% of follow-up biopsies and is

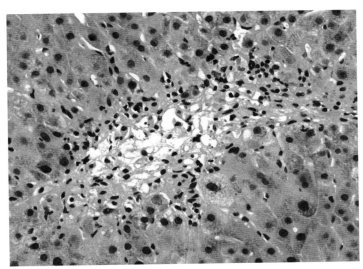

FIGURE 10.15 **Autoimmune hepatitis, zone 3 pattern.** The lobular inflammation in this case has a striking zone 3 accentuation.

associated with less interval improvement in fibrosis compared to those with no residual active AIH. Residual changes of active AIH is also associated with an increased risk of death or liver transplantation.[25] For cases with residual inflammation, however, the inflammatory changes are still milder than seen in baseline biopsies; as part of this, plasma cells are generally sparse or, when present, not as prominent as in the untreated baseline biopsy.

Cryptogenic Cirrhosis Pattern

Cryptogenic Cirrhosis Pattern

Diagnostic Approach: Reasonable to Suggest AIH When There Is

1. A known history of AIH plus no histological findings to indicate an alternative etiology.
2. AIH serologies are positive AND other common causes of cirrhosis have been excluded (fatty liver disease, viral hepatitis, etc) AND there are no findings that would suggest an alternative etiology.

Histological Findings

- Cirrhosis with mild nonspecific portal and septal chronic inflammation.
- Plasma cells, interface activity, and lobular hepatitis can be absent to mild.

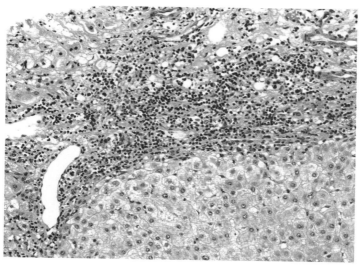

FIGURE 10.16 **Autoimmune hepatitis, cryptogenic cirrhosis.** This patient had a history of autoimmune hepatitis. The biopsy shows cirrhosis with nonspecific portal/septal inflammation.

Over time, AIH can "burn-out," in many patients, leading to a cirrhotic liver that has only nonspecific portal and septal lymphocytic inflammation (Figure 10.16).[26] Plasma cells are typically sparse but occasionally may still be mildly prominent. Portal inflammation is usually mild and interface activity and lobular hepatitis are either absent or minimal. Because these histological findings are nonspecific, the main role for pathology in this setting is to indicate that there are no findings inconsistent with a diagnosis of burned-out AIH. The final clinical diagnosis, then, is based on positive serologies, clinical and laboratory exclusion of other causes, and histology that is nonspecific but compatible with prior AIH.

Immunostain Findings

Immunostains can be helpful when the differential is between AIH and PBC (Figures 10.17 and 10.18). In AIH, IgG-positive plasma cells will predominate, while in PBC, IgM-positive plasma cells will be equal or greater in number than IgG-positive plasma cells in most cases, particularly in the medium-sized portal tracts.[20]

Fibrosis

The presence or absence of fibrosis is important information to convey in the biopsy report but does not specifically support or refute the diagnosis of AIH. There is sometimes a notion, particularly among clinical colleagues, that the presence of fibrosis in a liver biopsy of a patient with an acute hepatitis favors a diagnosis of AIH. This may be true in a very broad

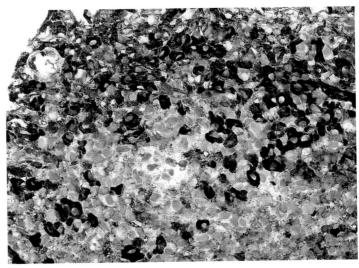

FIGURE 10.17 **Autoimmune hepatitis, immunostain for IgG.** Numerous IgG-positive plasma cells are seen in this case of autoimmune hepatitis.

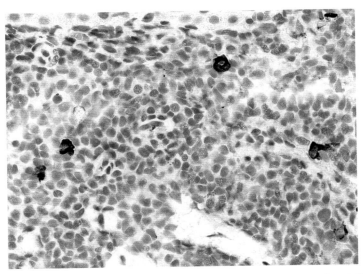

FIGURE 10.18 **Autoimmune hepatitis, immunostain for IgM.** Only a few IgM-positive plasma cells are seen (same portal tract as shown in preceding image).

sense, for example in large studies, but, at the individual patient level, the association is not sufficiently strong that it should change the usual diagnostic algorithm: the diagnosis of AIH is made in the setting of compatible clinical findings, laboratory findings, and histology findings, after other causes have been excluded. As can be seen, the presence or absence of fibrosis does not really enter in.

The presence of fibrosis in an acute hepatitis pattern does indicate an acute on chronic hepatitis, for which the differential includes AIH and hepatitis B virus (HBV) as well as DILI or acute viral hepatitis superimposed on other chronic liver diseases such as fatty liver disease. As a caveat, fibrosis staging can sometimes be challenging in the presence of marked inflammation or extensive necrosis. In general, fibrosis staging should be approached conservatively in this setting and it can be worthwhile to indicate this caveat when providing the fibrosis stage in the pathology report.

ASSOCIATIONS WITH OTHER DISEASES

AIH is associated with a wide range of other autoimmune conditions, the most common being autoimmune thyroiditis, rheumatoid arthritis, Sjogren syndrome, inflammatory bowel disease, and celiac disease.[11] Interestingly, first- and second-degree relatives of patients with AIH do not share this same increased risk for autoimmune diseases.[27]

On the other hand, individuals with systemic autoimmune conditions often have elevated serum autoantibodies and minimal or mild alanine aminotransferase (ALT) or aspartate aminotransferase (AST) elevations; some of these patients will undergo biopsies to rule out AIH. Most of these biopsy specimens will show minimal inflammatory changes with no fibrosis (Figure 10.19) and many will appear essentially normal: such cases behave differently than AIH and the term "autoimmune hepatitis" is best avoided in the pathology diagnosis (despite the elevated serum autoantibodies and

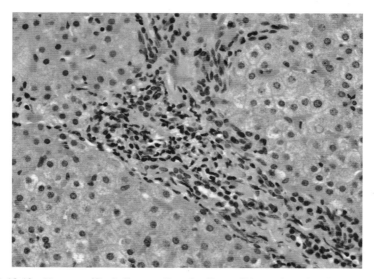

FIGURE 10.19 **Nonspecific inflammation in the setting of systemic autoimmune disease.** This patient had a connective tissue disorder and a high-titer antinuclear antibody (ANA). The biopsy shows minimal nonspecific portal inflammation, with no evidence for autoimmune hepatitis.

the minimal inflammatory changes in some cases). It is also best to avoid an older term that was sometimes applied to such cases, *nonspecific reactive hepatitis*, or to clearly indicate in your note what you intend the term to mean, since the term suffers from significant inconsistency in usage.

DIFFERENTATIAL DIAGNOSIS

Acute viral hepatitis can be plasma cell–rich, in particular hepatitis A virus (HAV) and HBV, and acute viral hepatitis should be excluded in all cases with an acute clinical presentation. DILI can also cause an acute onset hepatitis that closely mimics AIH, both serologically and histologically. Of these, minocycline and nitrofurantoin drug reactions currently make up the majority of cases.[28] A strong temporal association between the start of the hepatitis and the start of medication use may not be present, as these drugs may be in use for several years before the onset of clinical hepatitis. There are many other drugs that can also cause a hepatitis that mimics AIH[28] and it seems likely this list will continue to grow. Thus, a drug reaction has to be carefully excluded in every case. Wilson disease can also rarely present with histological findings that are indistinguishable from acute AIH.[29,30] For that reason, Wilson disease should be excluded in younger individuals who present with clinical and histological findings that suggest AIH.

AIH can also present as a result of incidentally discovered liver enzyme elevations. These cases typically have milder degrees of portal and lobular hepatitis, with or without fibrosis. In this setting, the differential is primarily that of chronic viral hepatitis and DILI. As discussed above, cirrhotic livers with nonspecific inflammatory changes can be linked to AIH, but only when supported by clinical and laboratory findings. Another common cause of cryptogenic cirrhosis is burned-out fatty liver disease, which should be excluded based on clinical findings. In some cases of cryptogenic cirrhosis, a firm diagnosis cannot be provided and the best approach is a prioritized differential, even after incorporating all histological, laboratory, and clinical findings.

ADULT SYNCYTIAL GIANT CELL HEPATITIS

Syncytial giant cell hepatitis is an uncommon pattern of liver injury defined by giant cell transformation of hepatocytes (Figure 10.20).[31,32] While this pattern does not represent a subtype of AIH, it is discussed here briefly because historically it was thought to represent a subtype of AIH, at least in many cases.

Conceptually, the term syncytial giant cell hepatitis is used when giant cell transformation is a dominant part of the histological findings, in contrast to the notion of giant cell transformation, which is a focal finding usually identified in the context of another recognizable disease process.

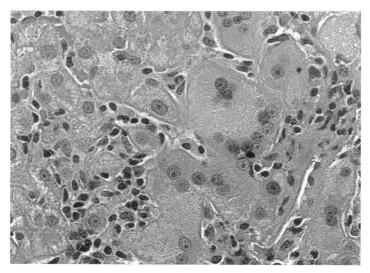

FIGURE 10.20 **Adult giant cell hepatitis.** The hepatocytes show giant cell transformation and there is a mild lobular hepatitis.

At the purely descriptive level—of how many hepatocytes are affected by giant cell change—there can be overlap between the notions of syncytial giant cell hepatitis as an independent pattern of injury and focal giant cell transformation that accompanies other patterns of injury, but the key difference remains that syncytial giant cell hepatitis is very rare and in most cases is an idiopathic pattern of injury, while giant cell transformation is much more common and is typically seen in the context of another recognizable disease process. Neither of these two important concepts have any particular link to AIH. For example, occasional cases of AIH will have focal giant cell transformation, but these same cases will have the ordinary clinical, laboratory, and histological findings of conventional AIH, and the giant cell transformation appears to be a mild nonspecific reactive change. On the other hand, the vast majority of cases with giant cell transformation lack the clinical, laboratory, and histological features of AIH.

In cases with the idiopathic syncytial giant cell hepatitis pattern of injury, the histological findings are dominated by giant cell transformation of hepatocytes. There can be portal and lobular lymphocytic inflammation, but this is usually on the milder side. A subset of cases is associated with autoimmune hemolytic anemia.[31,33-35] Giant cell hepatitis can recur after liver transplantation.[36,37]

Giant transformation of hepatocytes, on the other hand, can be seen in a larger number of known hepatitic and cholestatic patterns of liver injury, including hepatitis E,[38] hepatitis C,[31] and drug effects.[39] Other less common settings include Wilson disease[40] and HIV.[41] Cholestatic livers from many different causes can show focal giant cell transformation, especially in the pediatric population. Additional causes can be found in Table 2.5, Chapter 2. In all of these settings, the giant cells can be noted in the pathology report, if you wish, but in these cases the giant cell transformation is a mild, often focal, and incidental finding that should not be equated with the syncytial giant cell hepatitis pattern of injury, the latter being an idiopathic pattern of injury and not a focal finding that is seen in another pattern of injury.

OVERLAP SYNDROMES

In general, the most common overlap syndromes are between AIH and PBC or between AIH and primary sclerosing cholangitis (PSC). Overlap between PBC and PSC is exceedingly rare, although it has been reported.[42,43] The frequency of overlap syndromes varies considerably in the literature because the criteria for diagnosing overlap syndromes varies considerably. Nonetheless, it is likely in the 1% to 5% range at most.[1] Even within the "overlap" group, in most patients, one of the disease patterns will dominate the clinical, biochemical, and histological findings, suggesting that the overlap category is really a manifestation of a single primary disease process with some nonspecific histological findings that overlap with another disease. In this regard, the number of cases that truly have two distinct co-occurring diseases is probably much less than 1%. At a practical level, the autoimmune component of an overlap syndrome will be treated with oral corticosteroids, while the biliary component (if evident clinically by elevated alkaline phosphatase or bilirubin) is often treated with ursodeoxycholic acid (UDCA).[1] If you make a diagnosis of overlap syndrome, it is helpful to the clinical team to clearly indicate which is the predominate pattern of injury.

PBC and AIH Overlap

In general, a diagnosis of overlap syndrome should be considered when there are sufficient clinical, serological, and histological findings to support the presence of two distinct and different diseases. This approach sounds very reasonable but is often challenging to apply in practice. For example, elevated ANA titers are seen in up to a third of individuals with PBC. In addition, AMA titers can be positive in rare cases of otherwise typical AIH. Likewise, at the histological level, many cases of otherwise typical AIH will have some histological features that overlap with either PBC or PSC, such as mild patchy bile duct lymphocytosis or bile duct injury. As a second example, many cases of PBC have some interface activity. Thus, the mere presence of a histological finding that is recognized as being present in both conditions should not be the basis for a diagnosis of overlap syndrome.

When should the possibility of an overlap syndrome, then, be suggested by the pathologist? The histological findings of an overlap syndrome are essentially a composite of the findings in the two different diseases. For

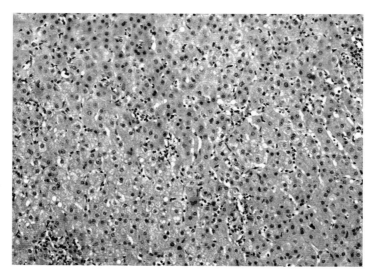

FIGURE 10.21 **Autoimmune hepatitis, primary biliary cirrhosis/cholangitis (PBC) overlap.** There was diffuse mild hepatitis in this case, too much lobular inflammation for PBC alone.

example, a biopsy might show a florid duct lesion plus a brisk lobular hepatitis (Figure 10.21), suggesting an AIH-PBC overlap. The most useful and practical approach is to first determine the major pattern of injury using the clinical, laboratory, and histological findings. If the major pattern of injury is AIH, then consider an overlap syndrome with PBC when there is a positive AMA, alkaline phosphatase levels >2× normal, *plus* florid duct lesions or other definite bile duct lymphocytic injury, chronic cholestatic injury, or bile duct loss. When the liver does not have advanced fibrosis, CK7 and Rhodanine stains can be very useful to look for early changes of cholate stasis. There are two important pitfalls to note. First, focal mild bile duct lymphocytosis is insufficient in isolation to indicate a component of PBC, being fairly common in AIH when there is moderate or marked portal inflammation. Secondly, portal or lobular granulomas have been reported in up to 10% of AIH cases[44] and do not indicate overlap syndrome if there is no other convincing evidence for biliary tract disease.

On the other hand, if you determine that the predominant injury pattern is PBC, then consider a diagnosis of overlap with AIH if the relevant serologies are positive and if there is mild and diffuse, or greater, degrees of lobular hepatitis; AST and ALT levels are typically (but not always) greater than 5× the upper limit of normal. Here too, there are several important diagnostic pitfalls. First, mild but patchy lobular inflammation can be seen with PBC alone, without an overlap syndrome, and can have a zone 3 accentuation. Secondly, interface activity is not particularly helpful for identifying an overlap syndrome; instead, it tends to parallel the degree of portal inflammation.

TABLE 10.3 Paris Criteria for Primary Biliary Cirrhosis-Autoimmune Hepatitis Overlap Syndrome[45]

Feature	Autoimmune Hepatitis Features (Two of Three are Needed)	PBC (Two of Three are Needed)
Liver enzymes	ALT ≥ 5 ULN	Alkaline phosotase ≥2 ULN or GGT ≥5 ULN
Serology	IgG ≥2 ULN or positive ASMA	AMA-positive
Histology	Interface hepatitis	Florid duct lesion

ALT, alanine aminotransferase; AMA, antimitochondrial antibodies; ASMA, antismooth muscle antibodies; GGT, gamma-glutamyl transpeptidase; PBC, primary biliary cirrhosis/cholangitis; ULN, upper limit of normal.

The Paris criteria are mostly a research tool used to help identify AIH-PBC overlap cases (Table 10.3). As a general observation, the Paris criteria are more sensitive but less specific than histological findings for the diagnosis of overlap syndrome, at least when the histology is evaluated with common sense. Thus, the Paris criteria are positive in most cases where the histological findings suggest AIH-PBC overlap using the approach above. On the other hand, there are a fair number of cases that meet the Paris criteria but do not have convincing histological findings of an overlap syndrome. Not surprisingly, using looser histological criteria lessens specificity. For example, specificity is diminished when using interface activity to suggest overlap with AIH in cases with PBC predominant patterns (which in 2009 was encouraged by The American Association for the Study of Liver Diseases [AASLD] guidelines). In discordant cases, where the histology does not suggest overlap while the Paris criteria do, or vice versa, there currently is no robust set of data to indicate "who is right", a particularly difficult knot to untie given the current challenges in diagnosing AIH and PBC in their own right. Anecdotally, following these patients over time can be helpful, as their liver enzyme profiles typically clarify the best diagnosis, when seen longitudinally over a sufficient length of time.

Autoimmune Sclerosing Cholangitis

Autoimmune sclerosing cholangitis is essentially an overlap syndrome between AIH and PSC. Unfortunately, there is some confusing language in this area, as the term "autoimmune cholangitis" (without the word "sclerosing") has also been used in the setting of AMA-negative PBC.

Autoimmune sclerosing cholangitis is more common in children and young adults and can be initially missed, as the biopsy may show changes of AIH with no features to strongly suggest biliary tract disease. Furthermore, the serum alkaline phosphatase and gamma-glutamyl transpeptidase (GGT) levels can be normal or only mildly increased in early stages of disease.

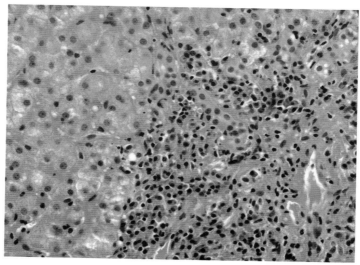

FIGURE 10.22 **Autoimmune sclerosing cholangitis.** The major pattern of injury in this biopsy was autoimmune hepatitis, but there was mild bile ductular proliferation in this and a few other portal tracts, a few intermediate hepatocytes, and imaging showed changes consistent with mild primary sclerosing cholangitis (PSC).

In other cases, the biopsy will show changes of AIH as well as changes that suggest obstructive biliary tract disease, so the diagnosis of an overlap syndrome can be suggested by histology on the index biopsy. In other cases, the biopsy findings will lack biliary features and the diagnosis of an AIH-PSC overlap syndrome is suggested during clinical follow-up when serum alkaline phosphatase and GGT levels become disproportionally elevated, despite treatment for the AIH. This pattern should prompt a cholangiogram to rule out an overlap syndrome.

In general, autoimmune sclerosing cholangitis is characterized by typical clinical and histological features of AIH, with positive ANA and or ASMA serologies, elevated serum IgG levels, and inflammatory changes consistent with AIH on the biopsy—along with imaging studies typical of PSC.[46] Histological changes of biliary obstruction may or may not be seen (Figure 10.22). Ulcerative colitis is strongly linked to both autoimmune sclerosing cholangitis and to PSC but is not linked to AIH. In fact, autoimmune sclerosing cholangitis should be ruled out by cholangiogram whenever making a diagnosis of AIH in a patient with a history of ulcerative colitis.

REFERENCES

1. Boberg KM, Chapman RW, Hirschfield GM, et al. Overlap syndromes: the International Autoimmune Hepatitis Group (IAIHG) position statement on a controversial issue. *J Hepatol.* 2011;54:374-385.
2. Roberts EA. Autoimmune hepatitis from the paediatric perspective. *Liver Int.* 2011;31:1424-1431.

3. Mieli-Vergani G, Vergani D. Autoimmune hepatitis. *Nat Rev Gastroenterol Hepatol.* 2011;8:320-329.

4. Gronbaek L, Vilstrup H, Pedersen L, et al. Family occurrence of autoimmune hepatitis: a Danish nationwide registry-based cohort study. *J Hepatol.* 2018;69:873-877.

5. Johnson PJ, McFarlane IG. Meeting report: International Autoimmune Hepatitis Group. *Hepatology.* 1993;18:998-1005.

6. Alvarez F, Berg PA, Bianchi FB, et al. International Autoimmune Hepatitis Group Report: review of criteria for diagnosis of autoimmune hepatitis. *J Hepatol.* 1999;31:929-938.

7. Hennes EM, Zeniya M, Czaja AJ, et al. Simplified criteria for the diagnosis of autoimmune hepatitis. *Hepatology.* 2008;48:169-176.

8. Czaja AJ. Advances in the current treatment of autoimmune hepatitis. *Dig Dis Sci.* 2012;57:1996-2010.

9. Verma S, Torbenson M, Thuluvath PJ. The impact of ethnicity on the natural history of autoimmune hepatitis. *Hepatology.* 2007;46:1828-1835.

10. Bogdanos DP, Mieli-Vergani G, Vergani D. Autoantibodies and their antigens in autoimmune hepatitis. *Semin Liver Dis.* 2009;29:241-253.

11. Teufel A, Weinmann A, Kahaly GJ, et al. Concurrent autoimmune diseases in patients with autoimmune hepatitis. *J Clin Gastroenterol.* 2010;44:208-213.

12. Mieli-Vergani G, Vergani D. Autoimmune hepatitis in children: what is different from adult AIH?. *Semin Liver Dis.* 2009;29:297-306.

13. Floreani A, Liberal R, Vergani D, et al. Autoimmune hepatitis: contrasts and comparisons in children and adults – a comprehensive review. *J Autoimmun.* 2013;46:7-16.

14. Czaja AJ. Diagnosis and management of autoimmune hepatitis: current status and future directions. *Gut Liver.* 2016;10:177-203.

15. Soares A, Cunha R, Rodrigues F, et al. Smooth muscle autoantibodies with F-actin specificity. *Autoimmun Rev.* 2009;8:713-716.

16. Miyake Y, Iwasaki Y, Kobashi H, et al. Clinical features of antinuclear antibodies-negative type 1 autoimmune hepatitis. *Hepatol Res.* 2009;39:241-246.

17. Suzuki A, Brunt EM, Kleiner DE, et al. The use of liver biopsy evaluation in discrimination of idiopathic autoimmune hepatitis versus drug-induced liver injury. *Hepatology.* 2011;54:931-939.

18. Gurung A, Assis DN, McCarty TR, et al. Histologic features of autoimmune hepatitis: a critical appraisal. *Hum Pathol.* 2018;82:51-60.

19. Balitzer D, Shafizadeh N, Peters MG, et al. Autoimmune hepatitis: review of histologic features included in the simplified criteria proposed by the international autoimmune hepatitis group and proposal for new histologic criteria. *Mod Pathol.* 2017;30:773-783.

20. Daniels JA, Torbenson M, Anders RA, et al. Immunostaining of plasma cells in primary biliary cirrhosis. *Am J Clin Pathol.* 2009;131:243-249.

21. Cabibi D, Tarantino G, Barbaria F, et al. Intrahepatic IgG/IgM plasma cells ratio helps in classifying autoimmune liver diseases. *Dig Liver Dis.* 2010;42:585-592.

22. Pratt DS, Fawaz KA, Rabson A, et al. A novel histological lesion in glucocorticoid-responsive chronic hepatitis. *Gastroenterology.* 1997;113:664-668.

23. Misdraji J, Thiim M, Graeme-Cook FM. Autoimmune hepatitis with centrilobular necrosis. *Am J Surg Pathol.* 2004;28:471-478.

24. Hofer H, Oesterreicher C, Wrba F, et al. Centrilobular necrosis in autoimmune hepatitis: a histological feature associated with acute clinical presentation. *J Clin Pathol.* 2006;59:246-249.

25. Dhaliwal HK, Hoeroldt BS, Dube AK, et al. Long-term prognostic significance of persisting histological activity despite biochemical remission in autoimmune hepatitis. *Am J Gastroenterol.* 2015;110:993-999.

26. Feld JJ, Dinh H, Arenovich T, et al. Autoimmune hepatitis: effect of symptoms and cirrhosis on natural history and outcome. *Hepatology.* 2005;42:53-62.

27. Gronbaek L, Vilstrup H, Pedersen L, et al. Extrahepatic autoimmune diseases in patients with autoimmune hepatitis and their relatives: a Danish nationwide cohort study. *Liver Int.* 2019;39:205-214.

28. Czaja AJ. Drug-induced autoimmune-like hepatitis. *Dig Dis Sci.* 2011;56:958-976.

29. Milkiewicz P, Saksena S, Hubscher SG, et al. Wilson's disease with superimposed autoimmune features: report of two cases and review. *J Gastroenterol Hepatol.* 2000;15:570-574.

30. Santos RG, Alissa F, Reyes J, et al. Fulminant hepatic failure: wilson's disease or autoimmune hepatitis? Implications for transplantation. *Pediatr Transplant.* 2005;9:112-116.

31. Devaney K, Goodman ZD, Ishak KG. Postinfantile giant-cell transformation in hepatitis. *Hepatology.* 1992;16:327-333.

32. Rabinovitz M, Demetris AJ. Postinfantile giant cell hepatitis associated with anti-M2 mitochondrial antibodies. *Gastroenterology.* 1994;107:1162-1164.

33. Maggiore G, Sciveres M, Fabre M, et al. Giant cell hepatitis with autoimmune hemolytic anemia in early childhood: long-term outcome in 16 children. *J Pediatr.* 2011;159:127-132 e1.

34. Akyildiz M, Karasu Z, Arikan C, et al. Successful liver transplantation for giant cell hepatitis and Coombs-positive hemolytic anemia: a case report. *Pediatr Transplant.* 2005;9:630-633.

35. Perez-Atayde AR, Sirlin SM, Jonas M. Coombs-positive autoimmune hemolytic anemia and postinfantile giant cell hepatitis in children. *Pediatr Pathol.* 1994;14:69-77.

36. Lerut JP, Claeys N, Ciccarelli O, et al. Recurrent postinfantile syncytial giant cell hepatitis after orthotopic liver transplantation. *Transpl Int.* 1998;11:320-322.

37. Pappo O, Yunis E, Jordan JA, et al. Recurrent and de novo giant cell hepatitis after orthotopic liver transplantation. *Am J Surg Pathol.* 1994;18:804-813.

38. Harmanci O, Onal IK, Ersoy O, et al. Postinfantile giant cell hepatitis due to hepatitis E virus along with the presence of autoantibodies. *Dig Dis Sci.* 2007;52:3521-3523.

39. Moreno-Otero R, Trapero-Marugan M, Garcia-Buey L, et al. Drug-induced postinfantile giant cell hepatitis. *Hepatology.* 2010;52:2245-2246.

40. Welte S, Gagesch M, Weber A, et al. Fulminant liver failure in Wilson's disease with histologic features of postinfantile giant cell hepatitis; cytomegalovirus as the trigger for both? *Eur J Gastroenterol Hepatol.* 2012;24:328-331.

41. Falasca L, Nonno FD, Palmieri F, et al. Two cases of giant cell hepatitis in HIV-infected patients. *Int J STD AIDS.* 2012;23:e3-e4.

42. Jeevagan A. Overlap of primary biliary cirrhosis and primary sclerosing cholangitis – a rare coincidence or a new syndrome. *Int J Gen Med.* 2010;3:143-146.

43. Kingham JG, Abbasi A. Co-existence of primary biliary cirrhosis and primary sclerosing cholangitis: a rare overlap syndrome put in perspective. *Eur J Gastroenterol Hepatol.* 2005;17:1077-1080.

44. de Boer YS, van Nieuwkerk CM, Witte BI, et al. Assessment of the histopathological key features in autoimmune hepatitis. *Histopathology.* 2015;66:351-362.

45. Chazouilleres O, Wendum D, Serfaty L, et al. Primary biliary cirrhosis-autoimmune hepatitis overlap syndrome: clinical features and response to therapy. *Hepatology.* 1998;28:296-301.

46. Gregorio GV, Portmann B, Karani J, et al. Autoimmune hepatitis/sclerosing cholangitis overlap syndrome in childhood: a 16-year prospective study. *Hepatology.* 2001;33:544-553.

11

BILIARY TRACT DISEASE AND CHOLESTATIC LIVER DISEASE

BLAND LOBULAR CHOLESTASIS PATTERN

The *bland lobular cholestasis* pattern of injury is characterized by lobular cholestasis as the main pattern of injury. The lobular cholestasis is usually mild to moderate and can show a hepatocellular, or canalicular, or mixed pattern (Figure 11.1). By definition, this pattern is not associated with significant inflammation, parenchymal necrosis, bile duct injury, bile duct loss, or changes of biliary obstruction. Ductopenia should be excluded using cytokeratin stains as needed, and correlation with imaging is needed to rule out biliary tract obstruction. In biopsy specimens, this pattern of injury is most commonly associated with drug-induced liver injury (DILI), but it can be seen with other rare conditions too (Table 11.1).

ACUTE BILIARY OBSTRUCTION

Acute Biliary Obstruction Pattern

Liver Enzymes
- Alkaline phosphatase ($\geq 2\times$ upper limit of normal [ULN]) or GGT elevations ($\geq 5\times$ ULN) predominate; aspartate transaminase (AST) and alanine transaminase (ALT) levels can be mildly elevated.
- Bilirubin levels can be elevated.

Histology
- Bile ductular proliferation is the predominant pattern.
- Portal inflammation is mild with mixed lymphocytes and neutrophils.
- Portal edema is uncommon but may be seen with acute, severe obstruction.
- Bile infarcts are very rare but can be seen with acute, severe obstruction.

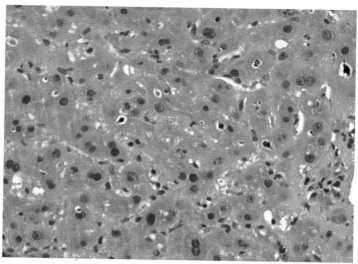

FIGURE 11.1 **Bland lobular cholestasis.** There is lobular cholestasis with no significant inflammation. The portal tracts (not seen in the image) showed no evidence for biliary obstruction.

TABLE 11.1 Differential for the Bland Lobular Cholestasis Pattern of Injury	
Common Causes in Surgical Pathology	**Notes**
Drug-induced liver injury	Most common cause seen in liver biopsy specimens.
Decompensated cirrhosis	Common in explanted livers. The cause for the clinical decompensation is often not evident on histology, but known precipitating factors include systemic infections and medication effect.
Uncommon Causes in Surgical Pathology	**Notes**
Bile salt deficiency diseases	FIC, BSEP, or MDR3 deficiency.
Intrahepatic cholestasis of pregnancy	Patients are commonly heterozygous for a bile salt deficiency mutation.
Multiorgan failure	Mostly seen in autopsy specimens.
Paraneoplastic syndromes	Example: Stauffer syndrome, from renal cell carcinoma.
	Not uncommon clinically, but rarely biopsied.
Sepsis	Mostly seen in autopsy specimens.
Thyroid disease	Not biopsied since the association is known clinically; it can be hypothyroid or hyperthyroid disease.

BSEP, bile salt export protein; FIC, familial intrahepatic cholestasis; MDR3, multidrug resistance protein type 3.

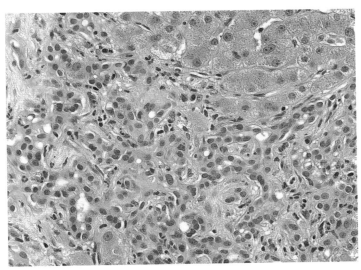

FIGURE 11.2 **Portal tract changes with obstruction.** This portal tract shows a brisk bile ductular proliferation.

Clinical Findings

The clinical findings for acute biliary tract obstruction include episodic right upper quadrant pain that is intense and radiates to the back. The pain can be associated with consuming fatty foods, but this association is neither sensitive nor specific. The clinical and imaging findings of acute biliary obstruction are typically characteristic enough to render a presumptive diagnosis, with imaging studies, showing dilatation of the extrahepatic biliary tree. Serum levels of alkaline phosphatase, γ-glutamyltransferase (GGT), and bilirubin are typically elevated. Biopsies of the liver are only rarely performed.

Histologic Findings

Biopsies in the setting of acute biliary obstruction predominately show portal tract changes (Figure 11.2), with a combination of bile ductular proliferation and portal tract inflammation that is composed of mixed neutrophils and lymphocytes, a pattern often called a *bile ductular reaction*. The neutrophils are found primarily at the edges of the portal tract, where they accompany the bile ductular proliferation (Figure 11.3). In some cases, occasional eosinophils can also be seen. Portal tract edema may be present with severe acute obstruction (Figure 11.4). Neutrophils in the dilated lumen of the bile duct proper would suggest an additional component of ascending cholangitis. The lobules may show canalicular and hepatocellular cholestasis (Figure 11.5) and sometimes will have very mild, patchy lobular, lymphocytic

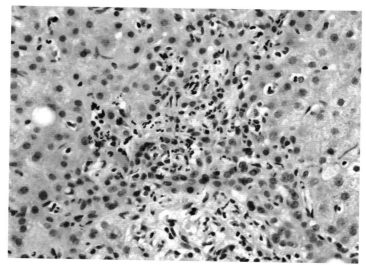

FIGURE 11.3 **Portal tract changes with obstruction, ductular reaction.** There is mild, mixed inflammation containing lymphocytes and neutrophils.

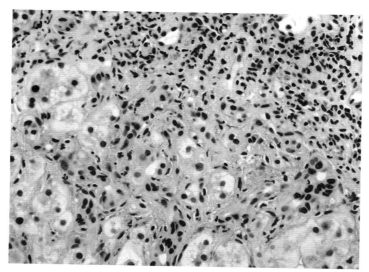

FIGURE 11.4 **Portal tract changes with obstruction, portal edema.** The light gray, myxoidlike color of the stromal is referred to as portal edema.

inflammation. Occasionally, bile infarcts may be seen (Figure 11.6); this finding is not specific for high-grade obstruction in isolation, as it can also be seen with long-standing, severe cholestasis, but outside of that setting, essentially all bile infarcts are found in the setting of high-grade obstruction.

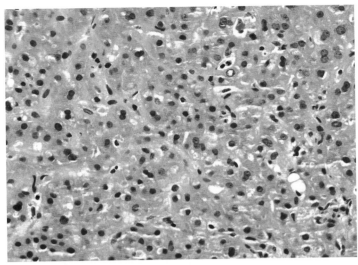

FIGURE 11.5 **Lobular cholestasis.** Moderate lobular cholestasis is present in this case of severe acute obstruction.

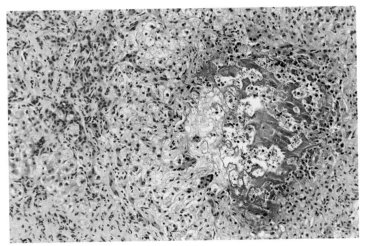

FIGURE 11.6 **Bile infarct.** A pool of extracellular, extravasated bile is seen in the periportal hepatic parenchyma.

Differential

The main histologic finding in clinically acute biliary obstruction is a bile ductular reaction, which may be accompanied by lobular cholestasis but has minimal lobular inflammatory changes. The ductular reaction, however, is not specific for acute biliary obstruction and can be seen in a few other injury patterns. Of these, the most commonly encountered in clinical practice is a bile ductular reaction associated with a marked hepatitis or a bile ductular reaction associated with vascular outflow disease. In most cases, extrahepatic biliary obstructive changes can be separated from these two possibilities by the lack of significant hepatitis or sinusoidal dilatation in the lobules, respectively. In the liver transplant population, fibrosing cholestatic hepatitis C and antibody-mediated rejection can closely mimic biliary obstruction. In these transplant situations, other histologic findings can help refine the differential, but the final clinical diagnosis requires evaluation of the extrahepatic biliary tree to exclude obstruction. In cirrhotic livers, mild bile ductular proliferation is common and nonspecific.

Special Stains

In most cases, the hematoxylin-eosin (H&E) stain findings are sufficient to generate a diagnosis and differential, but special stains can sometimes be helpful. The edematous changes in acute biliary obstruction can be highlighted with an alcian blue stain, but this is not necessary. A CK7 will highlight the proliferating bile ductules. Intermediate hepatocytes are often present, at least focally, but may not be as pronounced as seen with chronic biliary obstruction. Copper stains usually show negative results, in contrast to cases of chronic biliary obstruction or other causes of chronic cholestatic liver disease.

CHRONIC BILIARY OBSTRUCTION

Chronic Biliary Obstruction Pattern

Liver Enzymes
- Alkaline phosphatase ($\geq 2\times$ ULN) or GGT elevations ($\geq 5\times$ ULN) predominate; AST and ALT levels can be mildly elevated.
- Bilirubin levels can be elevated with end-stage disease.

Histology
- Bile ductular proliferation is the predominant pattern, but findings can be mild and patchy.
- Portal inflammation is mild with mixed lymphocytes and neutrophils.
- Long-term changes can include:
  Bile duct duplication
  Periductal fibrosis (onion-skin fibrosis)
  Fibro-obliterative duct lesions
  Ductopenia
  Cholate stasis
  Biliary cirrhosis

Clinical Findings

Chronic large bile duct obstruction is associated with elevated alkaline phosphatase levels. Serum bilirubin levels are also elevated in some cases, especially with advanced or end-stage disease. Chronic biliary tract obstruction can result from many different causes, ranging from intrahepatic stones, tumors, or parasites to mass lesions that compress the extrahepatic biliary tree, such as pancreatic tumors or enlarged hilar lymph nodes. In most cases, imaging of the liver and abdomen is pretty good at identifying extrahepatic biliary obstruction, so liver biopsies are enriched for cases with equivocal imaging findings, very early diseases where the extrahepatic changes are not well developed, or complicated clinical scenarios where tissue examination might clarify the diagnosis.

Histologic Findings

PORTAL TRACT FINDINGS. The histologic findings in chronic biliary obstruction will vary depending on the extent and duration of the obstruction. For many extrahepatic biliary tract diseases, the intrahepatic liver changes can be heterogeneous when the disease is early, so some but not all the portal tracts will show biliary obstructive changes. The portal tracts show bile ductular proliferation with mild mixed inflammation containing admixed lymphocytes and neutrophils with absent or rare plasma cells and eosinophils; there may be a few more lymphocytes than seen with acute obstruction. Of note, the bile ductular proliferation should be clearly evident on H&E stain to support the diagnosis. Bile ductular proliferations that are evident only with cytokeratin immunostains are a common and nonspecific component of the reparative response to lobular injury.

As disease progresses, portal-based fibrosis will develop (Figure 11.7). Over time, the ductular reaction often diminishes and may essentially disappear with advanced fibrosis. The bile ducts themselves also may be lost (ductopenia); it is best to confirm ductopenia with cytokeratin stains such as CK7. While not common in biopsy specimens, additional findings that can be present with long-standing, chronic biliary obstruction include bile duct duplication (Figure 11.8), onion-skin fibrosis (concentric fibrosis around bile ducts; Figure 11.9), and fibro-obliterative duct lesions (Figure 11.10). The latter two findings are seen primarily with medium-sized and larger sized portal tracts, which are only rarely sampled in liver biopsy specimens. While onion-skin fibrosis and fibro-obliterative duct lesions are best known for their association with primary sclerosing cholangitis (PSC), they indicate generic chronic large-duct obstruction and are not specific for PSC.

LOBULAR CHANGES. In chronic obstruction, the lobules show absent or minimal inflammatory, although there can be Kupffer cell hyperplasia in

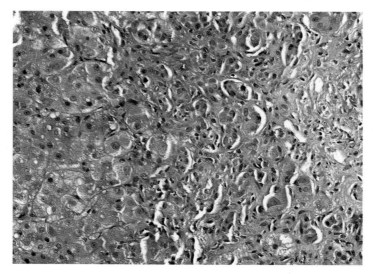

FIGURE 11.7 **Biliary fibrosis.** The portal tract shows an irregular pattern of portal fibrosis with entrapped bile ductules.

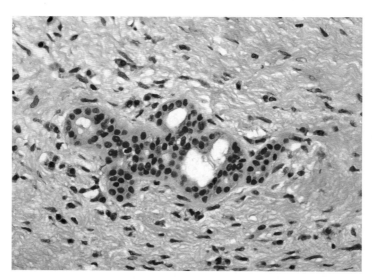

FIGURE 11.8 **Bile duct duplication.** In this case of primary sclerosing cholangitis (PSC), there are multiple profiles of the central bile duct, all clustered together.

cases with cholestasis. Lobular cholestasis can be seen in severe, long-standing disease, but it is mostly an end-stage finding. Lobular cholestasis with minimal or mild portal tract changes would be unusual for chronic biliary obstruction, and the differential would shift toward the bland lobular cholestasis pattern of injury.

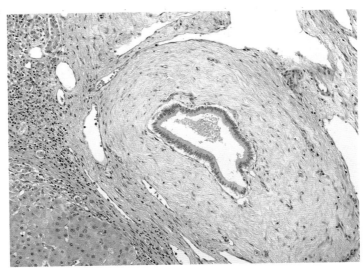

FIGURE 11.9 **Periductal or "onion-skin" fibrosis.** A medium-sized bile duct shows a concentric, lamellar pattern of fibrosis that surrounds the bile duct.

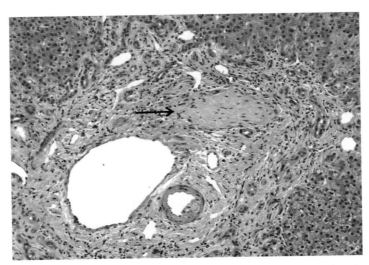

FIGURE 11.10 **Fibro-obliterative duct lesion.** From a case of primary sclerosing cholangitis, the bile duct has been replaced by a fibrous scar (arrow).

In chronic cholestatic liver disease, the zone 1 hepatocytes can show cholate stasis (Figure 11.11), characterized by mild hepatocyte swelling, occasional bits of Mallory hyaline, and patchy mild copper accumulation (Figure 11.12). A CK7 immunostain can highlight zone 1 intermediate hepatocytes in cases of subtle chronic cholestatic liver disease

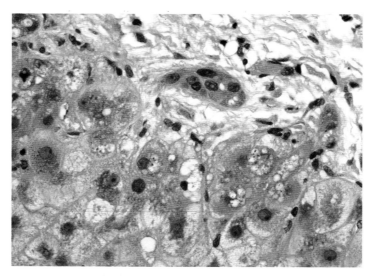

FIGURE 11.11 **Cholate stasis.** The periportal hepatocytes show swelling with granular pigment (copper) and bits of Mallory hyaline in this case of chronic cholestatic liver disease.

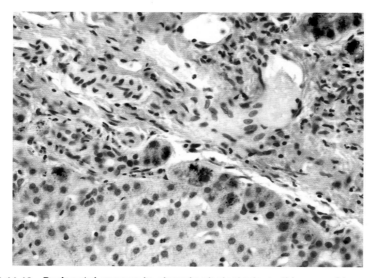

FIGURE 11.12 **Periportal copper in chronic cholestasis.** In this case of long-standing but indolent primary biliary cirrhosis/cholangitis (PBC), the periportal hepatocytes show copper accumulation on Rhodanine copper stain.

(Figure 11.13). In cirrhotic livers, the cholate stasis can often be identified at low power by paleness of the periportal hepatocytes, a finding sometimes called the *halo sign* (Figure 11.14).

Pancreatic acinar cell metaplasia can be seen in the peribiliary glands surrounding the larger portal tracts in some cases of chronic biliary tract

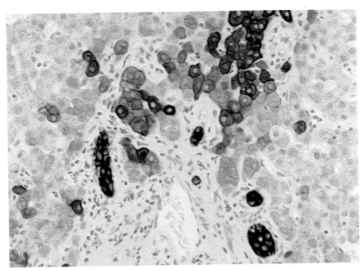

FIGURE 11.13 **CK7-positive hepatocytes in chronic cholestasis.** The periportal hepatocytes in this case of chronic cholestasis stain positive for CK7. A few ductules in the portal tract also stain strongly.

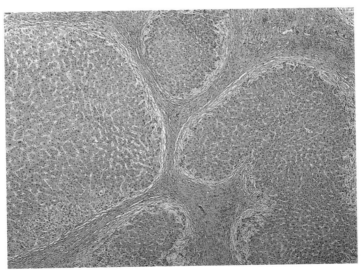

FIGURE 11.14 **Halo sign.** In this case of primary sclerosing cholangitis, the nodules are surrounded by lighter stained areas that resemble a halo and correlate with cholate stasis.

disease. Pancreatic acinar cell metaplasia is more commonly seen in surgical resection specimens than in biopsies because the larger branches of the biliary tree near the hilum are principally affected (Figure 11.15). This finding is nonspecific, however, so a diagnosis of chronic biliary tract disease should not be based primarily on this finding.[1,2]

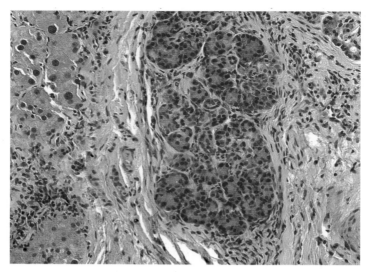

FIGURE 11.15 **Pancreatic acinar cell metaplasia.** The underlying liver disease was primary biliary cirrhosis/cholangitis (PBC), but this finding is not specific for chronic biliary tract disease.

Differential

The H&E differential depends on the pattern of injury. For specimens with a definite bile ductular reaction that is evident on H&E stain, and that have either no or mild fibrosis, the differential is influenced by the associated findings in the liver specimen. For example, when the ductular reaction is the predominant finding, this supports a diagnosis of biliary obstruction. On the other hand, a bile ductular reaction in a liver with a severely active hepatitis is most often reactive to the inflammatory changes and does not indicate obstructive biliary tract disease. As another example, a mild to focally moderate bile ductular reaction is common in cases of vascular outflow disease.[3]

In livers with advanced fibrosis or with cirrhosis, a mild bile ductular proliferation is very common and does not strongly suggest chronic biliary tract obstructive disease. CK7 staining and/or copper deposition in this setting is also nonspecific for chronic biliary obstruction. On the other hand, a liver specimen with advanced fibrosis or cirrhosis from chronic biliary tract disease is anticipated to have both copper positivity and CK7-positive intermediate hepatocytes, so the lack of these findings would argue against biliary cirrhosis.

In liver biopsies with ductopenia, the differential also depends on the degree of fibrosis. Ductopenia in livers with no fibrosis or minimal fibrosis is typically not a result of chronic obstructive biliary tract disease and has a wide differential (Chapter 2, Table 2.4). When looking at cirrhotic livers, ductopenia can sometimes be overlooked, as ductopenia preferentially affects the smallest branches of the biliary tree and large- and medium-sized bile ducts will still be present.

Lobular cholestasis in isolation should also not be overinterpreted as suggesting biliary obstruction. Lobular cholestasis can be seen in acute high-grade obstruction but is typically absent in chronic biliary obstruction, until there is either severe ductopenia or end-stage cirrhosis with clinical decompensation. Of course, cirrhosis from any cause can become cholestatic, often deeply, when there is clinical decompensation.

Immunohistochemical Stains

A CK7 immunostain can identify both intermediate hepatocytes and ductopenia. Copper stains are also helpful for identifying periportal copper deposition. Both these stains can show positive results in livers with chronic cholestatic liver disease from any cause, but they are not specific as to the cause of the chronic cholestatic liver disease. Also, as noted previously, intermediate hepatocytes and or copper deposition becomes less specific as clues to chronic cholestatic liver disease in livers with bridging fibrosis or cirrhosis.

BACTERIAL CHOLANGITIS

Ascending Cholangitis

Ascending cholangitis results from colonization and infection of the biliary tree by bacteria, most of which originate within the intestinal tract. The disease is usually triggered by some sort of anatomic defect of the biliary tree, such as biliary stones, bile duct strictures, or mass lesions, that restricts normal bile flow. Common symptoms at presentation include abdominal pain and fevers. If the ascending cholangitis is associated with acute biliary obstruction, then patients can also present with jaundice. Overall, biopsies are typically not needed for diagnosis and changes of ascending cholangitis are most encountered in surgical pathology as secondary findings in resection specimens for biliary strictures or tumors.

The medium-sized and larger sized bile ducts show collections of luminal neutrophils (Figures 11.16 and 11.17). The bile ducts are often dilated and the lining epithelium is commonly attenuated. The smaller portal tracts show the typical changes of obstruction.

Segmental Cholangiectasia

Segmental cholangiectasia is more of a surgical disease and so is rarely seen on needle biopsy specimens, but it results from recurrent or chronic bacterial infections that involve a segmental branch of the intrahepatic biliary tree.[4] Segmental cholangiectasia closely mimics cholangiocarcinoma

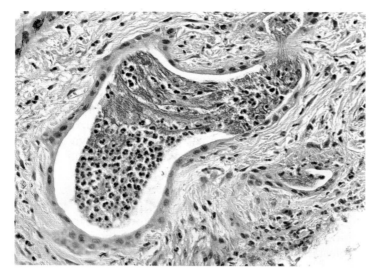

FIGURE 11.16 **Ascending cholangitis.** This large bile duct is dilated and shows attenuated epithelium. Numerous neutrophils are seen within the bile duct lumen.

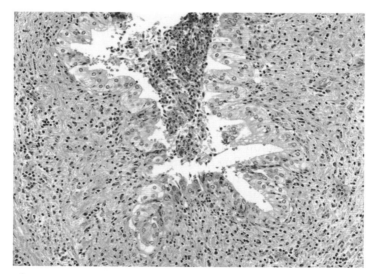

FIGURE 11.17 **Ascending cholangitis.** Another example shows neutrophils in the bile duct lumen.

or cystic biliary neoplasms on imaging studies,[4] so the clinical team is often surprised when resection specimens show negative results for neoplasm.

The disease is associated with intrahepatic biliary stones, which can sometimes be evident in the tissue specimen. The bacterial infection leads to a distinctive pattern of segmental bile duct dilatation with cystlike

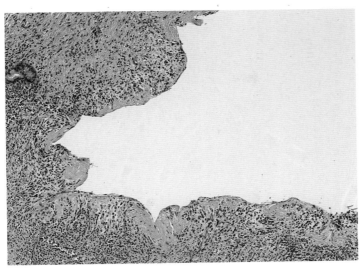

FIGURE 11.18 **Segmental cholangiectasia.** The bile duct shows saccular dilatation with chronic inflammation and fibrosis of the wall.

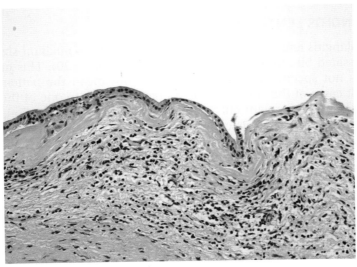

FIGURE 11.19 **Segmental cholangiectasia.** On higher magnification, the epithelium is reactive and partially denuded, with a thickened layer of subepithelial collagen.

areas of the biliary tree. These are not true cysts, but instead are irregular, saccular dilatations of the intrahepatic bile ducts, showing acute and chronic inflammation and fibrosis of the duct walls, often with a dense layer of hyalinization/fibrosis right beneath the epithelium (Figures 11.18 and 11.19).[4]

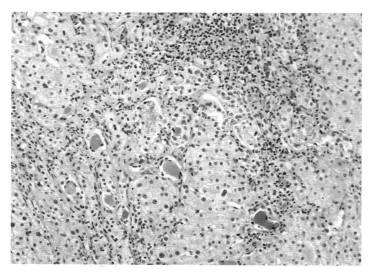

FIGURE 11.20 **Cholangitis lenta.** The bile ductules are dilated by plugs of bile. The patient had long-standing cholestasis but was not septic.

CHOLANGITIS LENTA

The cholangitis lenta pattern of injury shows small- to medium-sized plugs of inspissated bile located in bile ductules (Figure 11.20). This pattern of injury is not specific and specifically does not mean the patient is septic. Most cases of the cholangitis lenta pattern fall into one of these three categories: (1) livers with chronic high-grade biliary obstruction, such as biliary atresia; (2) liver specimens in patients with long-standing severe cholestasis from any cause, such as transplanted livers in patient with severe cholestasis resulting from liver decompensation; or (3) liver biopsy specimens from patients who have chronic, debilitating, systemic illnesses, leading to secondary liver cholestasis; such patients are at higher risk for infections in general and some in fact go on to become septic, but it is the debilitating illness that predisposes to both cholangitis and sepsis, and cholangitis lenta is not a marker of current sepsis per se.

PRIMARY SCLEROSING CHOLANGITIS

- Most common demographics: young adult men with a history of inflammatory bowel disease (IBD).
- Liver enzymes: alkaline-phosphatase-predominate pattern.
- Major clinical complications: cholangiocarcinoma, cirrhosis.

Histology

- Key pattern: biliary obstruction pattern in portal tracts. The lobules typically show no inflammation and no cholestasis.
- Useful stains: CK7 and copper stains in early disease with subtle H&E changes; CK7 in advanced disease for ductopenia.
- Variants: (1) small-duct PSC and (2) autoimmune sclerosing cholangitis.

Definition

PSC is an immune-mediated disease of the bile ducts that leads to inflammation and fibrosis of the biliary tree. The extrahepatic biliary tree is usually the primary target for inflammation and the liver parenchymal changes are at least in part secondary. In a minority of cases, however, the intrahepatic ducts are the primary target, a pattern called *small-duct PSC*. PSC should not be confused with *autoimmune sclerosing cholangitis*, which is a separate disease entity that shows overlapping features of autoimmune hepatitis and PSC.

Clinical Findings

The typical individual with PSC is a young to middle-aged-man (mean age at presentation is 37 years)[5] with idiopathic inflammatory bowel disease, usually ulcerative colitis (60%-70%) but sometimes Crohn disease (10%).[5] On the other hand, about 20% of individuals with PSC will not have a diagnosis of idiopathic inflammatory bowel disease. The diagnosis of PSC is established by imaging studies of the extrahepatic biliary tree, which show both strictures and dilatation of the bile ducts, leading to a "beaded" appearance. About 70% to 80% of individuals will also have positive serologic test results for perinuclear antineutrophil cytoplasmic antibodies (p-ANCAs), but this test is not specific and imaging studies are needed to make the diagnosis. Major distinguishing features between PSC, primary biliary cirrhosis/cholangitis (PBC), and autoimmune hepatitis are shown in Table 11.2.

PSC is a major risk factor for cholangiocarcinomas arising in the liver hilum, extrahepatic biliary tree, or the largest branches of the intrahepatic biliary tree. When the liver becomes cirrhotic, there is also an increased risk for hepatocellular carcinoma and peripheral cholangiocarcinomas. An increased risk for gallbladder adenocarcinoma is also reported. For example, one study followed 2616 patients with PSC for a median of 14.5 years; 594 patients developed cholangiocarcinomas (23%), 59 developed hepatocellular carcinomas (2%), and 58 developed gallbladder adenocarcinomas (2%).[5]

TABLE 11.2	Major Features of PBC, PSC, and AIH		
Findings	**PSC**	**PBC**	**AIH**
Gender	Male 5:1 Female	Female 8:1 Male	Female 10:1Male
Age range at presentation for typical cases (years)	20-40	40-60	20-60
Clinical associations	Inflammatory bowel disease (80%)	Autoimmune thyroiditis, Sjogren syndrome	Other autoimmune conditions (40%)
Liver enzyme elevation pattern	"biliary" with Alk phos/GGT predominate	"biliary" with Alk phos/GGT predominate	"hepatitic" with AST/ALT predominate
Autoantibody	pANCA[a]	AMA	ANA, ASMA (type 1)
% Positive	50%-80% Positive	90%-95% Positive	LKM (type 2) 80%-90% For at least one marker
Major histologic patterns of injury	Early: biliary obstruction pattern Late: onion-skin fibrosis, fibro-obliterative duct lesion, ductopenia	Early: portal-based inflammation with bile duct injury, florid duct lesions, granulomas Late: few or no florid duct lesions, ductopenia	Hepatitic pattern of injury with significant lobular hepatitis. Plasma-cell-rich portal inflammation. Minimal bile duct changes.
Plasma cells	Not prominent in peripheral needle biopsies	Prominent in about 50% of cases IgM-positive plasma cells are equal or greater than IgG in most cases	Prominent in 80% of cases IgG-positive plasma cells are greater than IgM in essentially all cases
Cirrhotic pattern	Biliary pattern of cirrhosis	Biliary pattern of cirrhosis	Often nondescript cirrhosis with minimal to mild inflammation

AIH, autoimmune hepatitis; Alk phos, alkaline phosphatase; ALT, alanine transaminase; AMA, anti-mitochondrial antibody; ANA, antinuclear antibody; ASMA, anti-smooth muscle antibody; AST, aspartate transaminase; GGT, γ-glutamyltransferase; pANCA, perinuclear antineutrophil cytoplasmic antibody; PBC, primary biliary cirrhosis/cholangitis; PSC, primary sclerosing cholangitis.
[a]pANA is not very sensitive or specific.

Histologic Findings

PSC tends to progress slowly and individuals can be diagnosed at various stages of disease; thus, the histologic findings will vary accordingly. In very early disease, the liver can show minimal nonspecific changes, despite evidence for PSC by imaging studies. As the disease progresses, the findings are essentially those of chronic biliary obstruction. The portal tracts show patchy to diffuse bile ductular proliferation with mild mixed portal inflammation, including neutrophils that are accentuated near the proliferating bile ductules (Figures 11.21 and 11.22). Minimal to sometimes mild lymphocytic inflammation can also be seen within the portal tracts (Figure 11.23), especially in later cases. The bile ducts proper might show occasional inflammatory cells and reactive changes, but a more diffuse lymphocytic cholangitis suggests other disease processes, such as a drug reaction. The lobules generally show minimal nonspecific changes (Figure 11.24) and are not cholestatic. As an exception to this typical pattern, PSC can show mild lobular hepatitis when presenting in children and may also have increased lymphocytic inflammation in the portal tracts.

As the disease progresses, the liver will begin to scar down. The fibrosis is portal-based. Early on, the fibrotic portal tracts often have a more irregular outline than that seen in chronic viral hepatitis or autoimmune hepatitis. The fibrosis can progress to bridging fibrosis and cirrhosis. Liver biopsies with advanced fibrosis often show ductopenia and sometimes have findings of onion-skin fibrosis and/or fibro-obliterative duct lesions. While none of these are specific for PSC, they do support a diagnosis of chronic biliary tract obstruction. Of note, onion-skin fibrosis

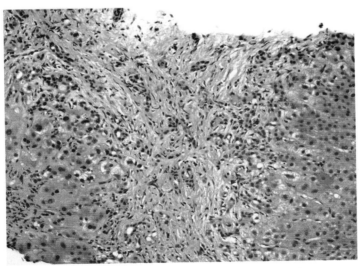

FIGURE 11.21 **Primary sclerosing cholangitis.** The portal tract shows bile ductular proliferation, mild inflammation, and fibrosis; the patient also had ulcerative colitis.

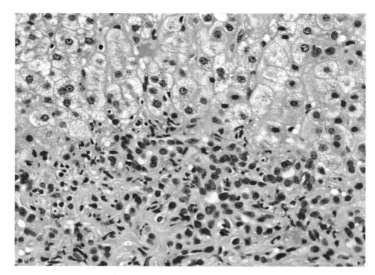

FIGURE 11.22 **Primary sclerosing cholangitis.** The proliferating bile ductules are accompanied by mild neutrophilic inflammation.

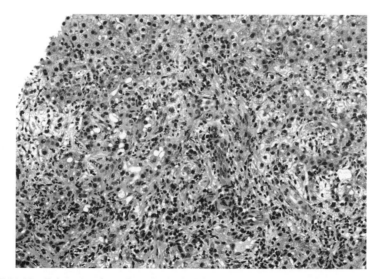

FIGURE 11.23 **Primary sclerosing cholangitis.** The portal tracts show bile ductular proliferation and mixed inflammation, including mild lymphocytic inflammation and rare plasma cells. The patient also had Crohn disease.

and/or fibro-obliterative duct lesions can be seen in other diseases, such as ischemic strictures, chronic hepatolithiasis,[6] segmental cholangiectasia,[4] sarcoidosis with a biliary obstruction pattern of injury,[7] and MDR3 deficiency.[8] As an additional caveat, onion-skin fibrosis can be easily overdiagnosed, especially when the pathologist knows the patient has ulcerative

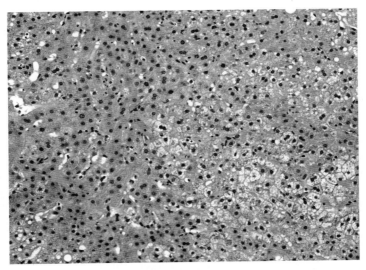

FIGURE 11.24 **Primary sclerosing cholangitis.** The lobules show minimal nonspecific reactive changes.

colitis and is specifically looking for changes of PSC. As a general rule of thumb, onion-skin fibrosis is typically seen in association with other histologic findings of obstructive biliary tract disease and should be interpreted cautiously if it is the only finding in the biopsy.

Fibrosis Staging

Currently there is no widely used fibrosis staging systems specifically designed for PSC. This is mostly because fibrosis can be adequately staged by classifying the biopsy as having no fibrosis, portal fibrosis, bridging fibrosis, or cirrhosis, with the addition of modifiers as needed, for example, "focal early bridging fibrosis" or "extensive bridging fibrosis." Formal staging systems also work well, including the Ishak, Metavir, and Batts-Ludwig.

Differential

Infections of the extrahepatic biliary tree, such as Isospora belli, are rare but can closely mimic PSC on imaging studies; the diagnosis can be clarified in many cases by biopsy of the extrahepatic biliary tree.[9] Syphilis can also rarely cause bile duct strictures, mimicking PSC on imaging,[10] with plasma cell- and neutrophil-rich inflammation around large bile ducts, as well as mild bile ductular proliferation in the smaller ducts. IgG4 sclerosing cholangitis is discussed separately later. Ischemic cholangitis can also lead to biliary tract disease that closely mimics PSC.[11] The vast majority of ischemic cholangitis cases occur in the setting of liver transplantation or after major abdominal surgery with inadvertent injury to the hepatic artery. At the histologic level, the biopsy findings are sufficiently similar between primary and secondary forms of obstructive biliary tract disease that correlation with clinical findings and imaging studies is necessary.

SMALL-DUCT PRIMARY SCLEROSING CHOLANGITIS

Definition

A diagnosis of small-duct PSC requires the following: (1) liver histologic findings typical of PSC, (2) imaging studies showing no evidence for typical large-duct PSC in the extrahepatic biliary tree, and (3) exclusion of other causes of chronic biliary tract disease, including infections, drug effect, cystic fibrosis, IgG4-related disease, and PBC. While the imaging findings of the extrahepatic biliary tree are normal or near normal, imaging studies commonly show abnormalities of the larger intrahepatic bile ducts.[12] Most, but not all, individuals will also have ulcerative colitis.[13] Patients without inflammatory bowel disease appear to have different genetic risk factors than those with inflammatory bowel disease.[14]

Clinical Findings

Small-duct PSC is seen in 13% of children with PSC and 5% of adults with PSC.[15,16] The clinical findings are generally similar to those seen with large-duct PSC. In one study, 88% of individuals with small-duct PSC had inflammatory bowel disease, of which 61% had ulcerative colitis.[17] The small-duct pattern of disease may be somewhat enriched in individuals who have sclerosing cholangitis in the setting of Crohn disease.[18] One study suggested individuals with autoimmune sclerosing cholangitis (overlap syndrome between PSC and autoimmune hepatitis) have a higher prevalence of small-duct PSC.[19]

A proportion of individuals with small-duct PSC will eventually develop typical large-duct PSC,[13,20,21] up to 55% in some studies.[22] In many cases, however, small-duct PSC does not appear to be an "early stage" of classic large-duct PSC. Instead, it appears to be a closely related but distinct entity. The overall prognosis is better than that for large-duct PSC, with fewer individuals progressing to cirrhosis or to cholangiocarcinoma.[17,20] Interestingly, many of the individuals who develop cholangiocarcinoma will have first transitioned to large-duct PSC.[17] Also of note, small-duct PSC can recur after transplantation.[17]

Histologic Findings

The histologic findings in peripheral needle biopsy specimens are essentially the same as for large-duct PSC (Figure 11.25). As is true for all liver diseases, the biopsy findings will vary depending on the length and severity of the injury as well as the fibrosis stage.

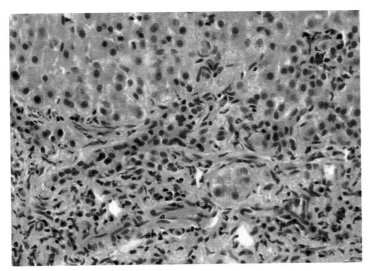

FIGURE 11.25 **Primary sclerosing cholangitis (PSC), small-duct variant.** Imaging was negative for the findings of typical PSC, while the biopsy showed patchy, moderate bile ductular proliferation and mild, predominantly neutrophilic inflammation.

IGG4 SCLEROSING CHOLANGITIS

Definition

IgG4 sclerosing cholangitis is a chronic autoimmune inflammatory disease of the biliary tree associated with increased serum IgG4 levels and increased numbers of IgG4-positive plasma cells in the liver. In essentially all cases, it is a manifestation of systemic IgG4-related disease. In contrast to PSC, the biliary strictures in IgG4 disease are steroid responsive and show improvement within 4 to 6 weeks of starting therapy.

Of note, a diagnosis is not made by histology alone but requires the following constellation of findings: (1) compatible clinical and imaging findings, (2) elevated serum IgG4 levels (>135 mg/dL), (3) compatible histology, and (4) steroid responsiveness of the liver disease.

Clinical Findings

There is a male predominance and the mean age at presentation is in the mid-60s,[23] which is about 20 years older than the average age of first presentation for PSC.[23] In contrast to PSC, IgG4 sclerosing cholangitis commonly presents with clinically evident acute biliary tract obstructive disease (in approximately 75% of cases).[23,24] Another important presentation is that of a hilar mass that closely mimics cholangiocarcinoma on imaging studies, or that of an inflammatory pseudotumor within the liver.

IgG4 sclerosing cholangitis is strongly associated with type 1 autoimmune pancreatitis (greater than 90% of cases) but is not associated with ulcerative colitis. Overall, about 60% of patients with systemic IgG4 disease will have liver involvement.[25] Serum IgG4 levels that are greater than 135 mg/dL support a diagnosis of IgG4 disease. The cholangiographic findings in IgG4 sclerosing cholangitis are not specific but show variable degrees of intrahepatic and extrahepatic biliary strictures.[23] The strictures in IgG4 sclerosing cholangitis are steroid responsive, in contrast to the strictures of PSC, so the proper diagnosis has important clinical consequences.

Histologic Findings

Histology of IgG4 Sclerosing Disease

- Four main patterns are seen in liver biopsies:
  Mild nonspecific portal inflammation
  Biliary obstruction pattern
  Inflammatory pseudotumor
  Hepatitic pattern (rare)
- Increased number of IgG4-positive plasm cells in the portal tracts.

The histologic findings depend considerably on the presentation; patients who present with clinical signs or symptoms have more striking histologic findings—typically that of biliary obstruction—than those who present primarily because of disease involvement in other organs. In the latter setting, the histologic findings are generally mild and nonspecific, with mild portal inflammation, equivocal ductular proliferation, and no lobular inflammation or cholestasis. There is often no increase in IgG4-positive plasma cells.

BILIARY OBSTRUCTION PATTERN. For patients who present with clinical disease of the pancreas or liver, the histologic findings typically show a biliary obstruction pattern of injury (Figure 11.26), which can be very similar to PSC. The most common pattern of injury is mild portal tract inflammation and a mild to moderate bile ductular reaction. There can be a wide variety of additional changes in liver biopsies, including lobular cholestasis (seen in cases with more rapid onset of biliary obstruction) and mild and patchy lymphocytic lobular hepatitis. Onion-skin fibrosis and bile duct duplication have been reported,[23,24] but ductopenia or fibro-obliterative duct lesions would be unusual for IgG4 sclerosing cholangitis. If larger portal tracts are sampled (Figure 11.27), the biopsy may show moderate, patchy periductal lymphocytic inflammation that is enriched for plasma cells and may have scattered eosinophils. In a subset of biopsies, the portal tracts will be sufficiently inflamed and edematous to form irregular fibroinflammatory nodules that can be seen grossly in resections or wedge biopsies. Histologically, these

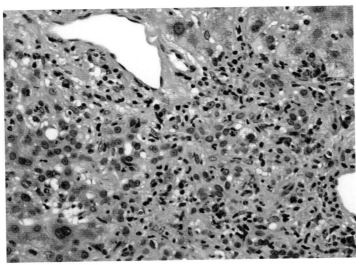

FIGURE 11.26 **IgG4 sclerosing disease.** The patient had a history of IgG4 pancreatic disease with elevated serum IgG4 levels. The liver biopsy showed patchy bile duct obstructive changes.

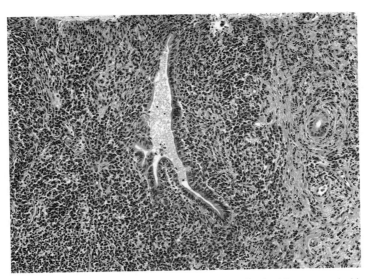

FIGURE 11.27 **IgG4 sclerosing disease.** A large-sized bile duct is surrounded by a dense lymphoplasmacytic infiltrate.

enlarged, inflamed, and edematous portal tracts can have an irregular or stellate profile. A storiform pattern of portal fibrosis can be seen in some portal tracts, but advanced fibrosis is rare in IgG4 disease.[24] Obliterative phlebitis is a rare finding in nonmass-directed biopsy specimens, but when present, it favors IgG4 sclerosing cholangitis over PSC.

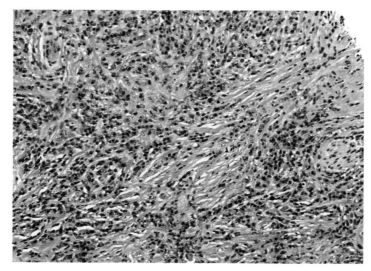

FIGURE 11.28 **IgG4 sclerosing disease.** In this case, the biopsy shows an inflammatory pseudotumor pattern.

INFLAMMATORY PSEUDOTUMOR PATTERN. Cases that present as mass lesions typically show the histology of an inflammatory pseudotumor, with dense fibrosis and chronic inflammation consisting of lymphocytes and plasma cells (Figure 11.28). The fibrosis can be admixed with atrophic cords of hepatocytes and bile ductules. Storiform fibrosis and central vein phlebitis can often be seen. A ductular proliferation is commonly present at the interface with the normal liver. Larger bile ducts, when sampled, show inflammatory and reactive changes. Immunostains will show increased numbers of IgG4-positive plasma cells, in contrast to other causes of inflammatory pseudotumors.

HEPATITIC PATTERN. Rare cases show a hepatitic pattern of injury (without features of biliary tract disease) that histologically looks like autoimmune hepatitis but has prominent IgG4-positive plasma cells in the portal tracts.[26] Patients with a hepatitic pattern of injury, who also have elevated serum IgG4 levels, are more likely to have systemic IgG4 disease, while patients who have increased tissue IgG4 levels, but normal serum levels, appear to have a variant of autoimmune hepatitis.[27] In any case, patients are usually treated for ordinary autoimmune hepatitis, with good response.[28]

Immunohistochemistry

Immunohistochemistry is used to identify increased numbers of IgG4-positive plasma cells (Figure 11.29). A commonly used cutoff for biopsy specimens is greater than 10 IgG4-positive plasma cells per high-power field (HPF), in at least one HPF.[23] This cutoff is very useful, as it has useful specificity, but it is seen in only 50% to 60% of peripheral biopsies in

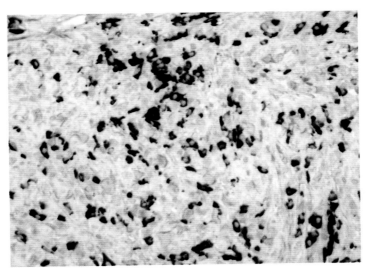

FIGURE 11.29 **IgG4 sclerosing disease, IgG4 immunostain.** There are increased numbers of IgG4-positive plasma cells.

patients with IgG4 sclerosing cholangitis, while another 20% to 30% of cases will have between 1 and 10 positive plasma cells per HPF and 10% of cases will have none. As a general rule of thumb, the number of IgG4-positive plasma cells reflects the size of the sampled portal tract and the degree of chronic lymphoplasmacytic inflammation. For example, a small peripheral portal tract with only few plasma cells will not have as many IgG4-positive plasma cells, even if the liver as a whole shows classic IgG4-related disease.

Also, of note, IgG4-positive plasma cells in liver biopsies are not specific for IgG4 sclerosing cholangitis, even at high levels. For example, the inflammation adjacent to liver abscesses can show increased IgG4-positive plasma cells (Figure 11.30). As another example, one study of liver explants in patients with PSC showed that 22% of cases were associated with elevated serum IgG4 levels and 23% of cases had inflamed, large hilar bile ducts with greater than 10 positive plasma cells per HPF on immunostaining, yet the combined clinical-histologic diagnosis was felt to be PSC and not Ig4 disease.[29] Thus, the final diagnosis is only achieved by combining the entire set of clinical, histologic, imaging, and laboratory findings.

Differential

Liver biopsy findings with IgG4 sclerosing cholangitis may show significant overlap with PSC. Clinical findings (Table 11.3) and immunostains can help refine the differential. When presenting as mass lesions, the differential is the same as that of any other inflammatory pseudotumor, including a healing abscess, syphilis, and Hodgkin disease.

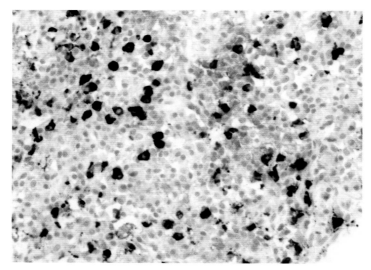

FIGURE 11.30 **Wall of an abscess, IgG4 immunostain.** There are increased numbers of IgG4-positive plasma cells, but the histologic and imaging findings were that of an abscess and not IgG4 disease.

TABLE 11.3 Comparison of Primary Sclerosing Cholangitis and IgG4 Sclerosing Cholangitis

Feature	Primary Sclerosing Cholangitis	IgG4 Sclerosing Cholangitis
Gender	Male predilection	Male predilection
Common age at presentation (years)	10-50	Often >50
Common presentation	Chronic biliary tract disease	Acute obstructive jaundice
Disease associations	Ulcerative colitis Crohn disease	Type 1 autoimmune pancreatitis Sclerosing sialadenitis Sclerosing mesenteritis, nephritis
Response to steroids	No	Yes
Serum IgG4 level elevations	20%	100%
Cholangiogram findings	Bandlike or beaded appearance	Segmental strictures, often in the distal third of common bile duct
Erosions of the ductal epithelium of large hilar ducts	Favors primary sclerosing cholangitis	

TABLE 11.3 **Comparison of Primary Sclerosing Cholangitis and IgG4 Sclerosing Cholangitis (Continued)**

Feature	Primary Sclerosing Cholangitis	IgG4 Sclerosing Cholangitis
Neutrophils in the duct lumen of large hilar duct	Favors primary sclerosing cholangitis. Superimposed ascending cholangitis should also be excluded.	
Onion-skin fibrosis	Favors primary sclerosing cholangitis	
Ductopenia	Favors primary sclerosing cholangitis	
Fibro-obliterative duct lesions	Favors primary sclerosing cholangitis	
Advanced fibrosis	Favors primary sclerosing cholangitis	
Storiform fibrosis		Favors IgG4 sclerosing cholangitis
Obliterative venopathy		Favors IgG4 sclerosing cholangitis
Fibroinflammatory portal nodules		Favors IgG4 sclerosing cholangitis
IgG4 immunostaining		>10 per HPF favors IgG4 sclerosing cholangitis

HPF, high-power field.

SCLEROSING CHOLANGITIS WITH GRANULOCYTIC EPITHELIAL LESION

Definition

Granulocytic epithelial lesions show neutrophilic inflammation and injury of intrahepatic bile ducts.

Clinical Findings

Our understanding of this histologic finding is limited by the few numbers of reported cases, but this pattern may be linked to type 2 autoimmune pancreatitis, at least in some cases, and is steroid responsive.[30] To date, most cases have been reported in children with inflammatory bowel disease and radiographic strictures of the intrahepatic bile ducts, with or without stricturing of the extrahepatic bile ducts.[30] Many cases show significant clinical, radiologic, and histologic overlap with autoimmune sclerosing cholangitis. In this regard, serum antinuclear antibody (ANA) titers can also be positive, sometimes strongly. Serum IgG4 levels are normal, but total IgG levels can be elevated.

Histologic Findings

A granulocytic epithelial lesion consists of a bile duct with neutrophilic infiltration of the duct epithelium (Figure 11.31, eFig. 11.1), with epithelial injury and/or epithelial disruption. The involved duct should be the bile duct proper and not the proliferating bile ductules at the edges of the portal tract. Also, numerous neutrophils in the lumen of a dilated duct would suggest ascending cholangitis, not a granulocytic epithelial lesion.

Only a few cases have been reported,[30,31] so the full range of histologic findings is not clear, but the reports indicate that granulocytic epithelial lesions have a patchy distribution, affecting, on average, only 1 in 10 portal tracts. The changes in the remaining portal tracts are less specific and show mild to moderate portal chronic inflammation with patchy interface activity and generally mild and focal bile ductular reactions. Scattered eosinophils in the portal infiltrates are common and plasma cells are prominent in most cases. Immunostains for IgG4 disease typically show two or less positive cells per HPF. Bile duct loss is uncommon, but onion-skin fibrosis can be seen in a subset of cases.

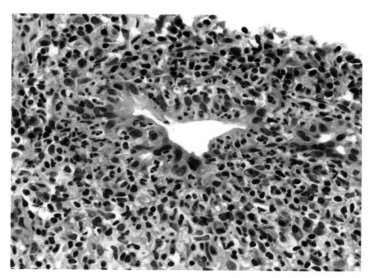

FIGURE 11.31 Granulocytic epithelial lesion (GEL). Neutrophilic inflammation is seen in this medium-sized portal tract.

Differential Diagnosis

The differential is primarily between liver changes in the setting of type 2 autoimmune pancreatitis and autoimmune sclerosing cholangitis. Based on the scant literature and personal anecdotal experience, most cases seem to best fit for autoimmune sclerosing cholangitis. Laboratory testing and imaging of the pancreas can be helpful to rule out pancreatic disease. Focal granulocytic epithelial lesions can also rarely be seen in PBC as well as infections of the biliary tree, such as syphilis. Thus, this lesion is best interpreted in the context of the findings in the remainder of the liver biopsy specimen.

PRIMARY BILIARY CIRRHOSIS/CHOLANGITIS

- Most common demographics: middle-aged women
- Not associated with IBD
- Serology: AMA M2 positive in 90%-95%
- Major clinical complications: cirrhosis

Histology
- Key patterns: patchy but usually moderate portal inflammation with bile duct lymphocytosis and injury, florid duct lesions (50%), and epithelioid granulomas may be seen in the lobules (20%) or portal tracts (40%).
- Useful stains: CK7 and copper stains in early disease with subtle H&E changes; CK7 in advanced disease for ductopenia.
- Variants: (1) AMA-negative PBC, (2) early ductopenic variant, and (3) PBC-autoimmune hepatitis overlap.

Definition

An autoimmune form of chronic cholangitis with inflammatory destruction of medium-sized intrahepatic bile ducts.

Nomenclature

Recently, medical terminology activists found offense with the name *primary biliary cirrhosis*, formed a committee, and had the disease renamed in order to alleviate the offense. This committee chose the name *primary biliary cholangitis*, a name inspired perhaps by the committee's love of tautologies but mostly because they found the medical term *cholangitis* less offensive than *cirrhosis*. Their dismay at the original term was directed at the confusion they thought it engendered. They were concerned that there was trouble understanding that patients with PBC have a range of outcomes, not all of whom develop cirrhosis. To sort this out for us, they shared their time and wisdom and renamed the disease. In that same magnanimous spirit, I have also decided to rename a few liver terms that are not perfect (Table 11.4). I did not have a large, federally funded committee to help me with the renaming process–although I am certainly open to such funding in the future–but I have done my best. Until these new names catch on, I have decided to stick with the older names throughout

TABLE 11.4 Efforts to Improve Medical Liver Terminology (EIMLT)[a]		
Original Term	Flaw in the Term	Proposed New Name
Zones 1, 2, and 3	These numbers imply primacy–who does not prefer to come in 1st rather than 3rd? This does not seem fair, as all hepatocytes contribute to health. Also, terminology that traces blood flow is unfair to bile flow, which moves in the opposite direction through no fault of its own.	Renamed after the primary colors, red, yellow, and blue–making it then the "red zone, yellow zone, and blue zone," respectively.
Bile ductules	They are not really "bile ducts that are small," but instead are part of the reparative response to injury, involving activation and proliferation of stem cells.	Portal tract stem cell proliferation in response to injury (PTSCPRI)
Biliary adenofibroma	It is not really a fibroma that has glands, but an adenoma that has fibrosis.	Biliary fibroadenoma that was previously known as biliary adenofibroma (BFAAKABAF)
Primary biliary cholangitis	It is a tautology, and the whole notion of primary vs secondary is archaic because by "primary" we mean simply that we do not know the cause.	Immune-mediated destruction of medium-sized intrahepatic bile ducts (IMDMSIBD)

[a]For well-established medical terminology, such as "primary biliary cirrhosis," the decision to have them undergo cosmetic surgery and give them a new name is a difficult balancing act; while I personally do not see any forward medical progress in these activities, apparently several powerful committees did, including several major clinical gastrointestinal and clinical liver societies, all of which rather quickly jumped aboard to approve the name change for primary biliary cirrhosis. Pathologists were notably left out of the process, perhaps because we actually see the tissue and know that *primary biliary cholangitis* does not really capture the essence of the histologic disease, but then again, the name change was not prompted by scientific concerns. But if you cannot beat them join them, as the saying goes. So let us get started and change them names!

the book. Likewise, to be inclusive to both sides, I have used the back-slash technique whenever having to spell out the full name for PBC as follows: primary biliary cirrhosis/cholangitis.

On a more serious note, it seems most reasonable to change well-established medical terminology very sparingly and only in response to advancements in the *classification* of a disease to such a degree that older terminology is no longer tenable. As one example, cirrhosis used to be classified by the size of the cirrhotic nodules because etiologies were unknown in so many cases, but it is now classified by etiology; the older terminology is no longer useful because the way we classify the disease has changed. In other words, changes to the name of a well-established disease seem most justifiable when the name change has the specific function of improving disease classification, not because an expert(s) believes their understanding of the disease is better than those who first discovered and named it. In fact, it is fully understood that improvements in scientific understandings of a disease have been rapid over the past few decades, and this hopefully will continue in a robust fashion; however, pushes to change names solely because the disease is better understood today than it was yesterday are excessive when they are functionally meaningless and solely cosmetic. At least that is what this author thinks.

Clinical Findings

The typical individual with PBC is a middle-aged woman of northern European ancestry who presents with cholestatic itching, or is identified by abnormal liver enzyme levels, often as an incidental finding. The male-to-female ratio is approximately 10:1. PBC is essentially unheard of in children. Other common coexisting autoimmune diseases include autoimmune thyroiditis (11%), Sjögren syndrome (8%), scleroderma (3%), rheumatoid arthritis (3%), and systemic lupus erythematosus (2%).[32] Sjögren syndrome is also strongly associated with autoimmune gastritis,[33] and a link between PBC and autoimmune gastritis has been postulated but is more controversial.[34,35]

Laboratory testing shows predominately alkaline phosphatase elevations, although AST and ALT levels are often mildly elevated as well. Serum cholesterol levels can be elevated, and individuals are at increased risk for osteopenia. Most patients have serum hypergammaglobulinemia with an increase in the IgM fraction. About 10% of individuals also have elevated serum IgG levels. Of most diagnostic use, the serum is typically positive for antimitochondrial antibody (AMA). Antibodies to the M2 fraction are most specific, and approximately 90% to 95% of individuals with PBC are positive to those antibodies. The antibody is directed against a mitochondrial protein, the E2 subunit of pyruvate dehydrogenase. Serum ANA is also positive in about one-third of individuals, with titers typically in the low range to midrange.

Treatment with ursodeoxycholic acid (UDCA) can significantly delay fibrosis progression and is the mainstay of treatment. Liver transplant is available for decompensated cirrhosis.

Histologic Findings

At low power, the biopsy findings are predominately portal based (Figure 11.32). Epithelioid, noncaseating granulomas are found in the portal tracts in approximately 40% of cases (Figure 11.33) and/or the lobules in approximately 20% of cases (Figure 11.34).

EARLY NONSPECIFIC CHANGES. The biopsy findings can be very mild in early disease, with mild nonspecific portal lymphocytic inflammation, no apparent bile duct injury, and mild nonspecific lobular changes. CK7 and copper stains are used to detect early changes of chronic cholestasis, looking for CK7-positive intermediate hepatocytes and periportal copper deposition, respectively. In cases with nonspecific H&E changes, deeper levels are also useful, as the histologic features of early PBC can be sufficiently patchy that a biopsy shows only mild and nonspecific changes on initial levels, but shows typical features of PBC on deeper levels. A good approach to cases with convincingly positive AMA test result and minimal biopsy findings is to indicate that the biopsy findings are nonspecific and mild, but still consistent with PBC in the right clinical setting. Studies that follow patients with AMA positivity and no clinical or biochemical evidence for liver disease have found that about 10% will develop PBC over time.[36]

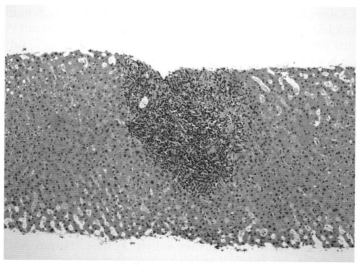

FIGURE 11.32 **Primary biliary cirrhosis/cholangitis (PBC).** At low power, the portal-based nature of the disease is evident.

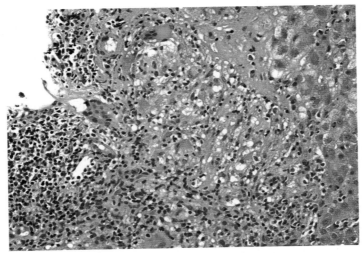

FIGURE 11.33 **Primary biliary cirrhosis/cholangitis (PBC), portal tract granuloma.** A large granuloma is seen in the portal tracts.

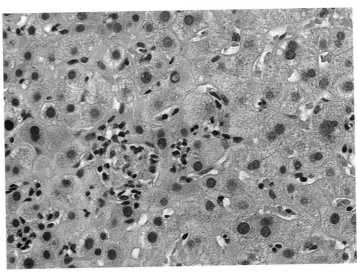

FIGURE 11.34 **Primary biliary cirrhosis/cholangitis (PBC), lobular granuloma.** A small lobular granuloma and mild lymphocytic lobular inflammation is seen.

PORTAL TRACT CHANGES. The portal tract findings can vary considerably within any given biopsy, especially with early disease. In general, the smaller branches of the portal tracts show only mild nonspecific lymphocytic inflammation. In the medium-sized portal tracts, the inflammation can be moderate to marked, and there can be mildly to moderately prominent plasma cells. Eosinophils can be mildly prominent in occasional cases.

There is frequently some degree of interface activity in the larger, inflamed portal tracts. Note that the presence of mild interface activity is completely typical of PBC in those portal tracts that have moderate or greater inflammation and does not suggest an additional component of autoimmune hepatitis.

The bile ducts in the inflamed, medium-sized portal tracts can show active injury, with bile duct lymphocytosis and reactive epithelial changes (Figure 11.35, eFig. 11.2). The reactive changes can range from a mild disorganization of the usually tidy and aligned biliary epithelial cells, to apoptosis, to a distinctive but mild epithelial oncocytosis. When the bile duct injury is associated with a cuff of histiocyte-rich or granulomatous inflammation, then the lesion is referred to as a *florid duct lesion* (Figures 11.36 and 11.37). Well-formed granulomas can be seen with florid duct lesions but are not required. Likewise, there can be granulomas in portal tracts that have no features of a florid duct lesion.

Cases of PBC with significant portal inflammation can also show patchy but mild bile ductular proliferation. In time, the livers can become increasingly ductopenic and increasingly fibrotic.

LOBULAR CHANGES. The hepatic lobules often show minimal to mild, patchy lobular lymphocytic inflammation with occasional apoptotic bodies. Inflammation that reaches the diffusely mild or greater level is unusual in PBC and suggests an additional disease process. The lobules in some cases can also show nodular regenerative hyperplasia (NRH). In livers with cholestasis, especially those with ductopenia and/or advanced fibrosis, the

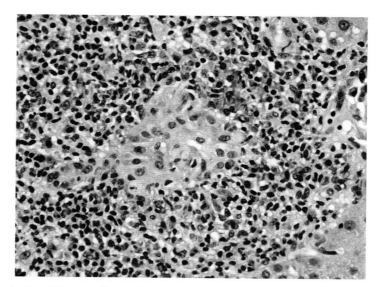

FIGURE 11.35 **Primary biliary cirrhosis/cholangitis (PBC), bile duct injury.** The bile duct shows mild lymphocytosis and reactive changes, surrounded by a dense cuff of inflammation.

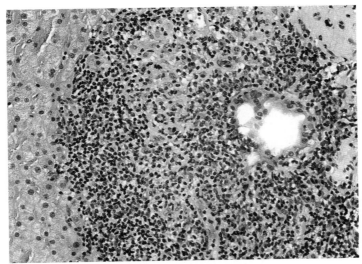

FIGURE 11.36 **Primary biliary cirrhosis/cholangitis (PBC), florid duct lesion.** An injured bile duct is surrounded by a dense lymphoplasmacytic infiltrate with numerous plasma cells, and a focus of numerous histiocytes, giving a focal "granulomatous" appearance.

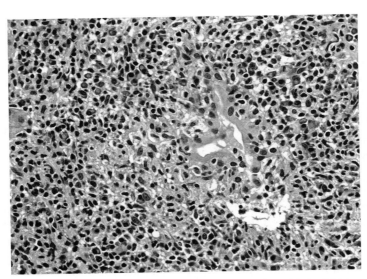

FIGURE 11.37 **Primary biliary cirrhosis/cholangitis (PBC), florid duct lesion.** Another example.

zone 1 hepatocytes can show cholate stasis on H&E staining, with swelling, occasional Mallory bodies, and mild periportal copper accumulation. Finally, the hepatocytes can rarely show a giant cell transformation of the zone 3 hepatocytes (Figure 11.38).[37] This giant cell change is typically not associated with significant lobular inflammation. There is no clinical

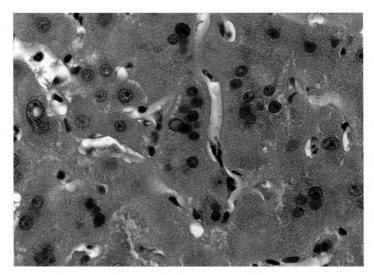

FIGURE 11.38 **Primary biliary cirrhosis/cholangitis (PBC), giant cell change.** The hepatocytes show focal giant cell transformation.

significance to this finding, and it should not be equated with adult giant cell hepatitis.

PBC STAGING. Early PBC staging systems combined inflammatory grading and fibrosis staging into one system, an approach that is now recognized as suboptimal. Additional staging systems have been proposed[38] and work well, but none have become widely used, mostly because fibrosis staging with the standard systems of Ishak, Metavir, or Batts-Ludwig also works great. When using these standard staging systems, the biopsy report should also comment on the degree of inflammation (grade) and whether or not there is ductopenia.

Prematurely Ductopenic Variant of PBC

In a small proportion of PBC cases (eFig. 11.3), the liver can show extensive ductopenia early in the course of the disease.[39] The livers can become deeply cholestatic despite the lack of cirrhosis and individuals can require transplant for pruritus. This variant has been reported in essentially a single small study, so information remains sparse, but other causes of ductopenia should be carefully excluded before making this diagnosis.

AMA-Negative PBC

After a complete clinical, laboratory, and histologic evaluation, about 5% to 10% of individuals will be given a final diagnosis of PBC despite being AMA negative. AMA-negative PBC is sometimes referred to as *autoimmune cholangiopathy*, but the term can be confusing and its use has been steadily dropping over the recent years. In some of these patients, AMA testing will show positive result over time. To date, no differences have been identified in the overall histologic findings or the clinical course in AMA-negative PBC versus AMA-positive PBC.[40,41]

PBC and Autoimmune Hepatitis Overlap Syndrome

This entity is considered in more detail in Chapter 10, but by brief review, a small proportion of individuals with PBC will have histologic findings that suggest an additional component of autoimmune hepatitis; this disease pattern is called PBC–autoimmune hepatitis overlap syndrome. The frequency in the literature depends on how the two components are defined, varying from less than 1% to nearly 10%. At a practical diagnostic level, positivity for ANA and/or anti-smooth muscle antibody (ASMA), as well as elevated serum gammaglobulin levels, are present in nearly all cases of overlap syndrome, but they are also present in many cases of PBC that do not have the overlap syndrome. Thus, serologic autoimmune markers are sensitive but lack specificity. Serum ALT levels in cases of the overlap syndrome are typically elevated 5× greater than the ULN and serum gammaglobulin levels are elevated 2× the ULN.

The main histologic finding that suggests PBC–autoimmune hepatitis overlap, versus PBC alone, is the presence of more lobular hepatitis than that is typical for PBC. In PBC, the lobular inflammation tends to range from minimal to mild and patchy, but is not diffuse-mild or greater. Another potential clue can be the amount of portal inflammation, which can be moderate and diffuse in untreated autoimmune hepatitis, versus PBC that can have patchier portal inflammation. Interface activity is common in PBC and its presence does not strongly suggest overlap syndrome per se. On the other hand, finding diffuse portal inflammation that is accompanied by diffuse interface activity would suggest an autoimmune hepatitis component. In PBC, the portal inflammation and interface activity is most striking in the medium-sized (septal) portal tracts.

Supplementary Stains

Immunostains can be helpful to look for bile duct loss, such as CK19, or CK7. CK7 is also helpful in supporting a diagnosis of chronic cholestatic liver disease when it identifies zone 1 intermediate hepatocytes. Rhodanine can identify copper deposition in periportal hepatocytes. Acid-fast bacteria (AFB) and Grocott-Gomori methenamine silver (GMS) stains can help exclude infection when there are granulomas. AFB and GMS stains are not necessary in patients with known PBC unless there are unusual findings, such as caseation, unusually large granulomas, or larger numbers of granulomas.

In cases with moderate to marked plasma-cell–rich portal inflammation, the differential is often between autoimmune hepatitis and PBC. In these cases, immunophenotyping the portal plasma cells can be helpful, using immunostains for IgG and IgM.[42-44] IgG-positive plasma cells are plentiful in both, but IgM-positive plasma cells are equal or greater in number in most cases of PBC, while IgG plasma cells greatly outnumber IgM plasma cells in most cases of PBC (Figures 11.39 and 11.40). When using these stains, it is helpful to identify several portal tracts that have the greatest degree of chronic inflammation and compare the numbers of IgG- and IgM-positive

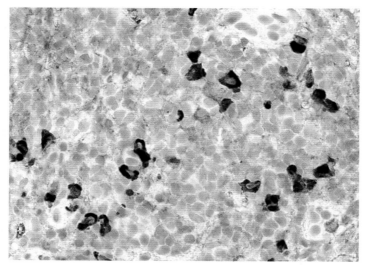

FIGURE 11.39 **Primary biliary cirrhosis/cholangitis (PBC), immunostain for IgG in PBC.** Numerous IgG-positive plasma cells are seen, but an image from the same field shows more IgM-positive plasma cells (see Figure 11.40).

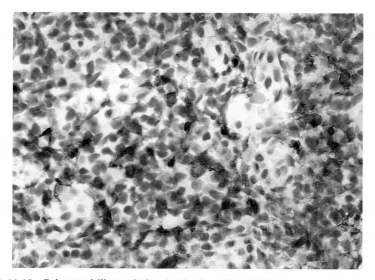

FIGURE 11.40 **Primary biliary cirrhosis/cholangitis (PBC), immunostain for IgM in PBC.** Numerous IgM-positive plasma cells are seen, and they are more numerous than IgG-positive plasma cells (see Figure 11.39).

plasma cells in the exact same portal tracts. The IgG and IgM antibodies often have high background in liver sections, so it can be helpful to have the laboratory lower the antibody titer. Alternatively, with experience, interpretation can focus on the bright and strong staining and ignore the background. As caveats, these stains should always be interpreted in the context of the H&E staining and clinical findings; also, they have not been shown to be useful in identifying PBC–autoimmune hepatitis overlap syndromes.

Differential

The differential for PBC will vary considerably depending on the histologic findings and can be broadly classified into several patterns.

- *Almost normal liver.* Some biopsies in patients with positive AMA serologies are almost normal or have minimal nonspecific changes. In these cases, CK7 and copper stains are important ancillary tests to look for evidence of chronic cholestatic liver disease. If these stains are negative, and if there are no other findings of PBC, then the best approach is to include in the surgical pathology note or comment section that careful follow-up is warranted, as about 10% of these patients will go on to develop typical features of PBC.
- *Florid duct lesion.* If the biopsy shows a classic florid duct lesion, then the differential is largely that of PBC versus a DILI, as some drug reactions, including herbal remedies,[45] can closely mimic PBC based on histology.
- *Granulomas and no other specific findings.* If the biopsy mainly shows granulomas without a florid duct lesion, then the differential is focused on granulomas of the liver (see Chapter 7).
- *Nonspecific chronic hepatitis pattern.* Many biopsies show mild to focally moderate portal chronic inflammation without granulomas and no bile duct lymphocytosis or injury. In these cases, the diagnosis is reached by the positive result for AMA, compatible clinical findings, and biopsy findings that do not strongly suggest any other disease process. The differential is primarily DILI and chronic viral hepatitis.

Additional histologic findings that further support the possibility of chronic cholestatic liver disease include periportal copper accumulation, intermediate hepatocytes, and ductopenia. Well-developed onion-skin fibrosis or a fibro-obliterative duct lesion would suggest chronic obstructive biliary tract disease, such as PSC, and not PBC. However, occasional cases of PBC can have focal equivocal onion-skin fibrosis (Figure 11.41). An elevated serum IgM level or increased IgM-positive plasma cells in the portal infiltrates can also help support the diagnosis of PBC.

- *AMA positive serologies in the setting of fatty liver disease.* Overall, about 2% of patients with fatty liver disease will have a positive result for serum AMA, and most of these patients lack histologic findings of PBC.[46,47]

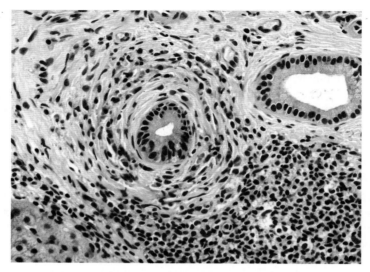

FIGURE 11.41 **Primary biliary cirrhosis/cholangitis (PBC).** This case shows focal equivocal periductal fibrosis.

OTHER CAUSES OF CHRONIC BILIARY TRACT DISEASE

A number of additional conditions can lead to varying degrees of chronic injury to the biliary tree, some of which can present with an obstructive histologic pattern of injury. These conditions are much less common than the entities discussed earlier and, in nearly all cases, require clinical findings to establish the diagnosis. Nonetheless, the biopsy findings can help guide the clinical workup in cases of liver disease of unknown cause. In the end, a small subset of cases of chronic biliary tract disease defy classification on both the biopsy and clinical workup and the cause only becomes apparent, if it does at all, with the subsequent development of more typical clinical or histologic findings. When facing one of these difficult cases remember to include parasitic and other infections of the biliary tree in your differential.

Cystic Fibrosis

Cystic fibrosis is considered in more detail in Chapter 17, but one of its histologic manifestations is patchy biliary obstructive type changes, with bile ductular proliferation and mixed portal inflammation. Inspissated secretions are only rare seen on biopsy (Figure 11.42) but can be seen in the larger ducts of the liver and explain the focal obstructive changes seen on biopsy. In most cases, the clinical diagnosis of cystic fibrosis is known at the time of biopsy.

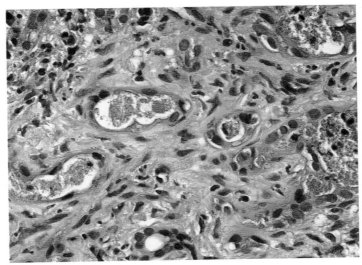

FIGURE 11.42 **Cystic fibrosis.** A portal tract shows a bile ductular reaction consistent with obstructive changes. Inspissated material can also be seen within some of ductules.

Vasculitis-Induced Chronic Biliary Tract Disease

Various causes of systemic vasculitis can involve the liver. When the vasculitis injures the hepatic artery, this can in turn lead to ischemic injury to the bile ducts and a chronic cholestatic pattern of liver injury, one that can mimic PSC or can have a ductopenia pattern.

Vasculitis-induced chronic biliary tract disease can be illustrated by the example of the Kawasaki syndrome. Kawasaki syndrome is a systemic inflammatory condition of unclear cause, but it appears to have an autoimmune and possibly an infectious basis. Medium-sized arteries and veins become inflamed and injured; if hepatic arteries are involved, this can lead to ischemic injury to the biliary tree. Overall, involvement of the liver is not a prominent part of the clinical disease. The liver is frequently involved, however, at some point during the course of the disease, and liver disease can rarely be the dominant clinical feature. Biopsies show nonsuppurative, inflammatory/fibrotic destruction of the biliary tree secondary in part to ischemia. These areas are not always sampled on biopsy, but biopsies commonly show patchy changes of bile duct obstruction (Figure 11.43).[48-50]

HIV-Associated Cholangiopathy

HIV/AIDS cholangiopathy is a somewhat loosely used term to describe various degrees of unexplained chronic biliary tract disease in individuals with HIV infection. The histologic changes vary from mild bile duct lymphocytosis and injury to findings that closely resemble PSC (Figure 11.44),

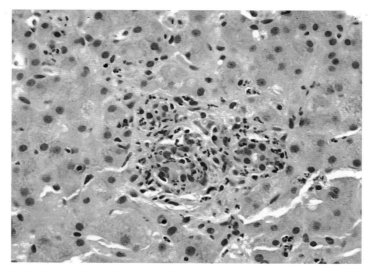

FIGURE 11.43 **Kawasaki syndrome.** The liver biopsy shows patchy bile ductular proliferation and mild neutrophil-predominant portal inflammation.

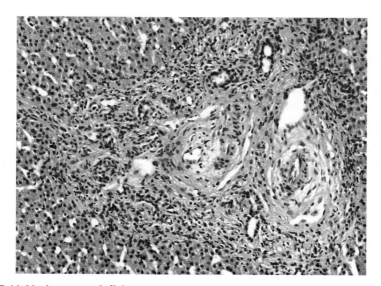

FIGURE 11.44 **Immune-deficiency-associated sclerosing cholangitis.** The patient did not have HIV but had an inherited severe immune deficiency and developed sclerosing cholangitis that was clinically thought to be infection related. The liver biopsy showed mild bile ductular proliferation with mild portal fibrosis.

with ductular proliferation and mixed portal inflammation. Fibrosis is usually mild or absent unless there is an additional underlying chronic liver disease, such as chronic hepatitis C or fatty liver disease.

The cause is thought to be infectious in most cases, although a specific agent is only rarely identified by routine clinical methods. One study used molecular methods and found a high proportion of cases were associated with various protozoa.[51] Some authors also include ductopenic injury as part of the HIV/AIDS cholangiopathy spectrum, but drug effects have to be carefully excluded in this setting. Rare reports suggest some cases of ductopenia in the setting of AIDS are related to cytomegalovirus (CMV) infection.[52]

Chemotherapy and Immunotherapy

Infusion of chemotherapy through the hepatic artery can lead to arterial injury and secondary ischemic injury to the bile ducts, with bile duct strictures that resemble PSC.[53] There also have been multiple reports of patients developing typical histologic and imaging features of PSC following checkpoint inhibitor therapy for lung adenocarcinoma.[54,55] Rare cases of DILI from checkpoint inhibitors can also resemble PBC.[56]

Severely Ill Patients

Severely ill patients, such as those with septic shock or trauma-related shock, can develop a secondary sclerosing cholangitis caused by biliary ischemia.[57,58] The cholangiopathy can continue, and even worsen, after patients recover from their primary illnesses. Imaging studies show strictures that mimic PSC. Endoscopic retrograde cholangiopancreatography (ERCP) can also demonstrate black-pigmented casts within the bile ducts.[59]

Only limited descriptions of the pathologic findings are available, but the biopsies generally mimic PSC, with mixed neutrophilic and lymphocytic portal inflammation, bile ductular proliferation, and portal fibrosis. The lobules are variably cholestatic but generally have little or no inflammation. The prognosis is unfavorable, with many individuals showing rapid fibrosis progression and liver decompensation.[57,59]

CONGENITAL HEPATIC FIBROSIS AND CAROLI DISEASE

Definition

Congenital hepatic fibrosis is generally considered to be a part of the spectrum of disease seen with autosomal recessive polycystic kidney disease, although in rare cases the findings are limited to the liver. The bile ducts show structural abnormalities secondary to defective remodeling of the ductal plate during organogenesis. Congenital hepatic fibrosis is associated with mutations in *PKHD1*, the gene that codes for fibrocystin. Fibrocystin is a receptor-like protein involved in the embryogenesis of tubules in the liver and kidney. Patients present as children and young adults.

CAROLI DISEASE was originally defined as an autosomal recessive disease with macroscopically visible, fusiform dilations of the biliary tree, sometimes called "cysts," in a liver that was without other imaging or histologic changes of congenital hepatic fibrosis. On the other hand, if the background liver showed changes of congenital hepatic fibrosis, then the term *Caroli syndrome* was used. These distinctions were made historically because Caroli syndrome was clearly part of the autosomal recessive polycystic kidney disease spectrum, while Caroli disease did not seem to be, and was instead thought to result from other mutation patterns. Currently, however, it appears that both are part of the spectrum of changes seen with autosomal recessive polycystic kidney disease.[60]

Clinical Findings

Congenital hepatic fibrosis is inherited in an autosomal recessive pattern most often, but there have been rare reports of autosomal dominant and X-linked recessive inheritance patterns. The microscopic features of congenital hepatic fibrosis are present at birth, but fibrosis is generally lacking. Over time, however, fibrosis can develop and there can be progression to advanced fibrosis, associated with portal hypertension and liver decompensation. The rate of progression varies significantly, even within families, and is difficult to predict. Even with advanced fibrosis, the liver often does not develop the typical well-defined nodularity of cirrhosis, even though the changes are functionally equivalent.

Histologic Findings

The primary histologic findings are in the portal tracts. The bile ducts are abnormally organized, with ductlike structures located circumferentially around the portal tract. These ducts often show abnormal branching (Figure 11.45). The portal veins are typically hypoplastic and can sometimes be absent (Figure 11.46).

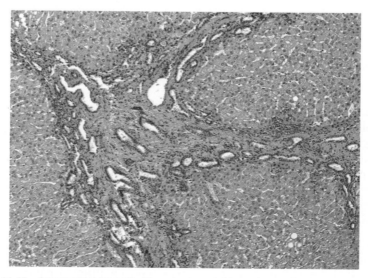

FIGURE 11.45 **Congenital hepatic fibrosis.** A portal tract shows abnormal bile ducts with open lumens and interanastomosing channels, located at the edges of the portal tracts.

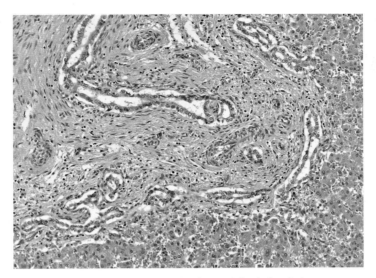

FIGURE 11.46   **Congenital hepatic fibrosis.** The portal vein is missing.

The portal tracts over time can become large and bulbous due to fibrosis. Bridging fibrosis and cirrhosis can develop. In some cases with severe fibrosis, well-developed cirrhotic nodules may not be apparent.

In a subset of cases, as noted earlier, congenital hepatic fibrosis can be associated with macroscopic intrahepatic cystlike structures that actually represent fusiform dilatations of the biliary tree. These areas often have superimposed cholangitic features with ulceration and acute inflammation.

POLYCYSTIC LIVER DISEASE

Polycystic liver disease will not be discussed in detail here, as it is usually not biopsied. In general, macroscopic cystic liver disease is associated with autosomal dominant polycystic kidney disease, but not with autosomal recessive polycystic kidney disease. The liver shows numerous unilocular cysts lined by biliary type epithelium (Figure 11.47). The cysts do not connect to the bile duct proper. von Meyenburg complexes are present in the background liver in the autosomal dominant form of polycystic liver disease (Figure 11.48). On the other hand, most von Meyenburg complexes encountered in surgical pathology are sporadic and not associated with polycystic liver disease. Autosomal recessive polycystic liver disease shows congenital hepatic fibrosis with diffuse ductal plate malformations.

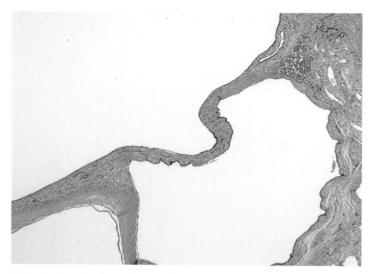

FIGURE 11.47 **Polycystic liver disease in a case of autosomal dominant polycystic kidney disease.** Large unilocular cysts are seen.

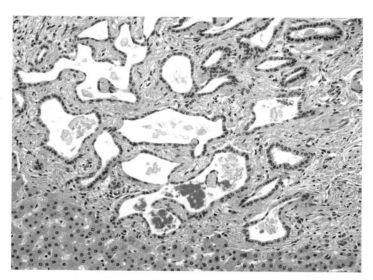

FIGURE 11.48 **von Meyenburg complex (VMC).** This case of polycystic liver disease showed numerous VMC in the background liver.

GIANT CELL TRANSFORMATION OF BILE DUCTS

This rare finding is of unknown significance (Figure 11.49) but can be seen in occasional liver explants and rarely on biopsies. In most cases, the livers are cirrhotic with active bile ductular proliferations, and, in some cases,

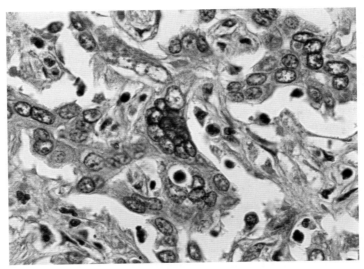

FIGURE 11.49 **Giant cell transformation of bile ducts/ductules.** The liver had patchy but striking giant cell transformation of the bile ducts.

this appears to result from hepatocytes undergoing ductular metaplasia. Giant cell change in bile duct epithelium has also been reported in the liver after heart transplant, perhaps related to human herpesvirus 6 (HHV-6) infection.[61]

REFERENCES

1. Kuo FY, Swanson PE, Yeh MM. Pancreatic acinar tissue in liver explants: a morphologic and immunohistochemical study. *Am J Surg Pathol.* 2009;33:66-71.

2. Pedica F, Heaton N, Quaglia A. Peribiliary glands pathology in a large series of end-stage alcohol-related liver disease. *Virchows Arch.* 2020;477:817-823.

3. Kakar S, Batts KP, Poterucha JJ, et al. Histologic changes mimicking biliary disease in liver biopsies with venous outflow impairment. *Mod Pathol.* 2004;17:874-878.

4. Zhao L, Hosseini M, Wilcox R, et al. Segmental cholangiectasia clinically worrisome for cholangiocarcinoma: comparison with recurrent pyogenic cholangitis. *Hum Pathol.* 2015;46:426-433.

5. Weismuller TJ, Trivedi PJ, Bergquist A, et al. Patient age, sex, and inflammatory bowel disease phenotype associate with course of primary sclerosing cholangitis. *Gastroenterology.* 2017;152:1975-1984 e8.

6. Nakanuma Y, Yamaguchi K, Ohta G, et al. Pathologic features of hepatolithiasis in Japan. *Hum Pathol.* 1988;19:1181-1186.

7. Nakanuma Y, Kouda W, Harada K, et al. Hepatic sarcoidosis with vanishing bile duct syndrome, cirrhosis, and portal phlebosclerosis. Report of an autopsy case. *J Clin Gastroenterol.* 2001;32:181-184.

8. Wendum D, Barbu V, Rosmorduc O, et al. Aspects of liver pathology in adult patients with MDR3/ABCB4 gene mutations. *Virchows Arch.* 2012;460:291-298.

9. Walther Z, Topazian MD. Isospora cholangiopathy: case study with histologic characterization and molecular confirmation. *Hum Pathol.* 2009;40:1342-1346.

10. Ilkova F, Attila T. Cholangiopathy associated with syphilis. *Am J Gastroenterol.* 2019;114:1570.

11. Deltenre P, Valla DC. Ischemic cholangiopathy. *Semin Liver Dis.* 2008;28:235-246.

12. Boberg KM, Schrumpf E, Fausa O, et al. Hepatobiliary disease in ulcerative colitis. An analysis of 18 patients with hepatobiliary lesions classified as small-duct primary sclerosing cholangitis. *Scand J Gastroenterol.* 1994;29:744-752.

13. Broome U, Glaumann H, Lindstom E, et al. Natural history and outcome in 32 Swedish patients with small duct primary sclerosing cholangitis (PSC). *J Hepatol.* 2002;36:586-589.

14. Naess S, Bjornsson E, Anmarkrud JA, et al. Small duct primary sclerosing cholangitis without inflammatory bowel disease is genetically different from large duct disease. *Liver Int.* 2014;34:1488-1495.

15. Deneau MR, El-Matary W, Valentino PL, et al. The natural history of primary sclerosing cholangitis in 781 children: a multicenter, international collaboration. *Hepatology.* 2017;66:518-527.

16. Eaton JE, McCauley BM, Atkinson EJ, et al. Variations in primary sclerosing cholangitis across the age spectrum. *J Gastroenterol Hepatol.* 2017;32:1763-1768.

17. Bjornsson E, Boberg KM, Cullen S, et al. Patients with small duct primary sclerosing cholangitis have a favourable long term prognosis. *Gut.* 2002;51:731-735.

18. Halliday JS, Djordjevic J, Lust M, et al. A unique clinical phenotype of primary sclerosing cholangitis associated with Crohn's disease. *J Crohns Colitis.* 2012;6:174-181.

19. Olsson R, Glaumann H, Almer S, et al. High prevalence of small duct primary sclerosing cholangitis among patients with overlapping autoimmune hepatitis and primary sclerosing cholangitis. *Eur J Intern Med.* 2009;20:190-196.

20. Angulo P, Maor-Kendler Y, Lindor KD. Small-duct primary sclerosing cholangitis: a long-term follow-up study. *Hepatology.* 2002;35:1494-1500.

21. Wee A, Ludwig J. Pericholangitis in chronic ulcerative colitis: primary sclerosing cholangitis of the small bile ducts? *Ann Intern Med.* 1985;102:581-587.

22. Ringe KI, Bergquist A, Lenzen H, et al. Clinical features and MRI progression of small duct primary sclerosing cholangitis (PSC). *Eur J Radiol.* 2020;129:109101.

23. Deshpande V, Sainani NI, Chung RT, et al. IgG4-associated cholangitis: a comparative histological and immunophenotypic study with primary sclerosing cholangitis on liver biopsy material. *Mod Pathol.* 2009;22:1287-1295.

24. Nishino T, Oyama H, Hashimoto E, et al. Clinicopathological differentiation between sclerosing cholangitis with autoimmune pancreatitis and primary sclerosing cholangitis. *J Gastroenterol.* 2007;42:550-559.

25. Zen Y, Kawakami H, Kim JH. IgG4-related sclerosing cholangitis: all we need to know. *J Gastroenterol.* 2016;51:295-312.

26. Lee HE, Zhang L. Immunoglobulin G4-related hepatobiliary disease. *Semin Diagn Pathol.* 2019;36:423-433.

27. Minaga K, Watanabe T, Chung H, et al. Autoimmune hepatitis and IgG4-related disease. *World J Gastroenterol.* 2019;25:2308-2314.

28. Canivet CM, Anty R, Patouraux S, et al. Immunoglobulin G4-associated autoimmune hepatitis may be found in Western countries. *Dig Liver Dis.* 2016;48:302-308.

29. Zhang L, Lewis JT, Abraham SC, et al. IgG4+ plasma cell infiltrates in liver explants with primary sclerosing cholangitis. *Am J Surg Pathol.* 2010;34:88-94.

30. Zen Y, Grammatikopoulos T, Heneghan MA, et al. Sclerosing cholangitis with granulocytic epithelial lesion: a benign form of sclerosing cholangiopathy. *Am J Surg Pathol.* 2012;36:1555-1561.

31. Grammatikopoulos T, Zen Y, Portmann B, et al. Steroid-responsive autoimmune sclerosing cholangitis with liver granulocytic epithelial lesions. *J Pediatr Gastroenterol Nutr.* 2013;56:e3-e4.

32. Efe C, Torgutalp M, Henriksson I, et al. Extrahepatic autoimmune diseases in primary biliary cholangitis: prevalence and significance for clinical presentation and disease outcome. *J Gastroenterol Hepatol*. 2021;36:936-942.

33. Melchor S, Sanchez-Piedra C, Fernandez Castro M, et al. Digestive involvement in primary Sjogren's syndrome: analysis from the Sjogrenser registry. *Clin Exp Rheumatol*. 2020;38(suppl 126):110-115.

34. Dohmen K, Shigematsu H, Miyamoto Y, et al. Atrophic corpus gastritis and *Helicobacter pylori* infection in primary biliary cirrhosis. *Dig Dis Sci*. 2002;47:162-169.

35. Floreani A, Biagini MR, Zappala F, et al. Chronic atrophic gastritis and Helicobacter pylori infection in primary biliary cirrhosis: a cross-sectional study with matching. *Ital J Gastroenterol Hepatol*. 1997;29:13-17.

36. Zandanell S, Strasser M, Feldman A, et al. Low rate of new-onset primary biliary cholangitis in a cohort of anti-mitochondrial antibody-positive subjects over six years of follow-up. *J Intern Med*. 2020;287:395-404.

37. Watanabe N, Takashimizu S, Shiraishi K, et al. Primary biliary cirrhosis with multinucleated hepatocellular giant cells: implications for pathogenesis of primary biliary cirrhosis. *Eur J Gastroenterol Hepatol*. 2006;18:1023-1027.

38. Hiramatsu K, Aoyama H, Zen Y, et al. Proposal of a new staging and grading system of the liver for primary biliary cirrhosis. *Histopathology*. 2006;49:466-478.

39. Vleggaar FP, van Buuren HR, Zondervan PE, et al. Jaundice in non-cirrhotic primary biliary cirrhosis: the premature ductopenic variant. *Gut*. 2001;49:276-281.

40. Liu B, Shi XH, Zhang FC, et al. Antimitochondrial antibody-negative primary biliary cirrhosis: a subset of primary biliary cirrhosis. *Liver Int*. 2008;28:233-239.

41. Invernizzi P, Crosignani A, Battezzati PM, et al. Comparison of the clinical features and clinical course of antimitochondrial antibody-positive and -negative primary biliary cirrhosis. *Hepatology*. 1997;25:1090-1095.

42. Daniels JA, Torbenson M, Anders RA, et al. Immunostaining of plasma cells in primary biliary cirrhosis. *Am J Clin Pathol*. 2009;131:243-249.

43. Moreira RK, Revetta F, Koehler E, et al. Diagnostic utility of IgG and IgM immunohistochemistry in autoimmune liver disease. *World J Gastroenterol*. 2010;16:453-457.

44. Cabibi D, Tarantino G, Barbaria F, et al. Intrahepatic IgG/IgM plasma cells ratio helps in classifying autoimmune liver diseases. *Dig Liver Dis*. 2010;42:585-592.

45. Elbl C, Terracciano L, Stallmach TK, et al. Herbal drugs mimicking primary biliary cirrhosis. *Praxis*. 2012;101:195-198.

46. Loria P, Lonardo A, Leonardi F, et al. Non-organ-specific autoantibodies in nonalcoholic fatty liver disease: prevalence and correlates. *Dig Dis Sci*. 2003;48:2173-2181.

47. Ravi S, Shoreibah M, Raff E, et al. Autoimmune markers do not impact clinical presentation or natural history of steatohepatitis-related liver disease. *Dig Dis Sci*. 2015;60:3788-3793.

48. Amano S, Hazama F, Kubagawa H, et al. General pathology of Kawasaki disease. On the morphological alterations corresponding to the clinical manifestations. *Acta Pathol Jpn*. 1980;30:681-694.

49. Bader-Meunier B, Hadchouel M, Fabre M, et al. Intrahepatic bile duct damage in children with Kawasaki disease. *J Pediatr*. 1992;120:750-752.

50. Gear JH, Meyers KE, Steele M. Kawasaki disease manifesting with acute cholangitis. A case report. *S Afr Med J*. 1992;81:31-33.

51. Netor Velasquez J, Marta E, Alicia di Risio C, et al. Molecular identification of protozoa causing AIDS-associated cholangiopathy in Buenos Aires, Argentina. *Acta Gastroenterol Latinoam*. 2012;42:301-308.

52. Tyagi I, Puri AS, Sakhuja P, et al. Co-occurrence of cytomegalovirus-induced vanishing bile duct syndrome with papillary stenosis in HIV infection. *Hepatol Res*. 2013;43:311-314.

53. Phongkitkarun S, Kobayashi S, Varavithya V, et al. Bile duct complications of hepatic arterial infusion chemotherapy evaluated by helical CT. *Clin Radiol.* 2005;60:700-709.

54. Nabeshima S, Yamasaki M, Matsumoto N, et al. Atezolizumab-induced sclerosing cholangitis in a patient with lung cancer: a case report. *Cancer Treat Res Commun.* 2020;26:100270.

55. Yoshikawa Y, Imamura M, Yamaoka K, et al. A case with life-threatening secondary sclerosing cholangitis caused by nivolumab. *Clin J Gastroenterol.* 2021;14:283-287.

56. Zen Y, Chen YY, Jeng YM, et al. Immune-related adverse reactions in the hepatobiliary system: second-generation check-point inhibitors highlight diverse histological changes. *Histopathology.* 2020;76:470-480.

57. Engler S, Elsing C, Flechtenmacher C, et al. Progressive sclerosing cholangitis after septic shock: a new variant of vanishing bile duct disorders. *Gut.* 2003;52:688-693.

58. Zilkens C, Friese J, Koller M, et al. Hepatic failure after injury—a common pathogenesis with sclerosing cholangitis? *Eur J Med Res.* 2008;13:309-313.

59. Kulaksiz H, Heuberger D, Engler S, et al. Poor outcome in progressive sclerosing cholangitis after septic shock. *Endoscopy.* 2008;40:214-218.

60. Gunay-Aygun M. Liver and kidney disease in ciliopathies. *Am J Med Genet C Semin Med Genet.* 2009;151C:296-306.

61. Randhawa PS, Jenkins FJ, Nalesnik MA, et al. Herpesvirus 6 variant A infection after heart transplantation with giant cell transformation in bile ductular and gastroduodenal epithelium. *Am J Surg Pathol.* 1997;21:847-853.

12

PEDIATRIC CHOLESTATIC LIVER DISEASE

BILIARY ATRESIA

Definition

Biliary atresia results from inflammatory or toxin-mediated destruction of the extrahepatic biliary tree, leading to bile duct atresia in the first weeks to months of life. The location of injury is used to subdivide biliary atresia into three types (although several other classifications are also in use).[1] Type 1 (about 5% of cases) has patent right and left hepatic ducts and a patent common hepatic duct, but the common bile duct is atretic, often below the cystic duct confluence (Figure 12.1). The right and left and common hepatic ducts can be dilated, and the gall bladder often has bile. Type 2 biliary atresia (about 2% of cases) has the atresia located at the common hepatic duct. In type 2 biliary atresia, the right and left ducts above the atretic area can be dilated, but the gall bladder is empty because it is located below the atretic area. The most common pattern of biliary atresia is type 3 (>90%), where the right and left hepatic ducts are atretic as they exit the liver at the porta hepatis. Some residual small bile ducts in the porta hepatis may remain, but the main bile ducts are fibrotic/atretic. The histology of the liver is similar in all of these types of biliary atresia on needle biopsy, but it is useful to know these patterns when correlating the imaging findings with the histological findings.

Clinical Findings

Most infants with biliary atresia are term infants with normal birth weights. Infants present within the first 1 to 6 weeks of life with jaundice, pale stools, and dark urine. Other findings include pruritus and failure to thrive. Failure to thrive can manifest as poor weight gain or excessive feeding.[2] Serum abnormalities included conjugated hyperbilirubinemia, high gamma-glutamyltransferase (GGT) levels, high alkaline phosphatase levels, and elevated cholesterol but normal triglyceride levels.

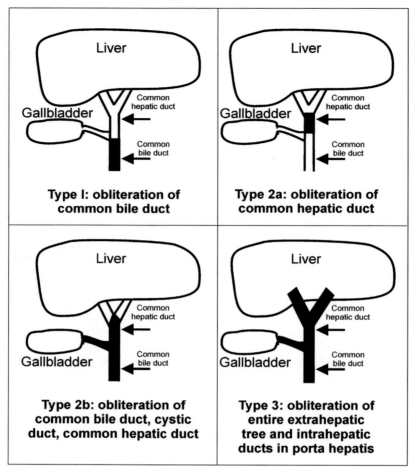

FIGURE 12.1　Anatomic subtypes of biliary atresia.

Associated anomalies are present in about 20% cases. The most common (10% of total cases) is called the *biliary atresia–splenic malformation syndrome*, which is associated with polysplenia, asplenia, or a double spleen.[2] Other associated malformations with this syndrome include situs in versus, a preduodenal portal vein, intestinal malrotation, absent vena cava, cardiac anomalies, and pancreas anomalies.

Etiology

The etiology is unknown, although many possibilities have been proposed, including viral infections that break tolerance, leading to immune destruction of the biliary tree, and toxin exposure in utero. An outbreak of biliary atresia in lambs was associated with toxin exposure,[3] but currently no specific toxin has been associated with human cases.

Treatment

Treatment currently is focused on surgical intervention called a *Kasai procedure*, or *hepatoportoenterostomy*, where the remnants of the extrahepatic tree are removed and a loop of the duodenum is attached to the hilum of the liver. The Kasai procedure is not curative in most cases but can prolong life and is an important bridge to liver transplantation. The best outcomes for the Kasai procedure are observed in younger individuals, usually defined as those less than 60 days of age.

Imaging Findings

Ultrasound typically shows an enlarged liver with no dilatation of the common bile duct. The gall bladder is commonly absent or contracted but can be present and appear relatively normal in the subset with type 1 atresia. A hepatobiliary iminodiacetic acid (HIDA) scan typically shows good hepatic uptake but reduced or absent intestinal excretion within 24 hours. Of note, reduced or absent intestinal excretion on HIDA scans is not specific for biliary atresia and can be seen in other pediatric cholestatic liver diseases. Endoscopic retrograde cholangiopancreatography or magnetic resonance retrograde cholangiopancreatography can be helpful in some cases.[4,5] In the end, the diagnosis usually requires a multidisciplinary approach, often including a liver biopsy.

Histological Findings

The histological findings in biliary atresia depend on when the biopsy is performed in the course of the disease. The earliest biopsies (days after birth) show the least specific findings, with variable cholestasis, extramedullary hematopoiesis, and little if any bile ductular proliferation. Fortunately, most biopsies are not obtained in this earliest phase of the disease.

PORTAL TRACTS. Liver biopsies obtained early in the disease course can have very mild changes, but bile ductular proliferation is the major finding in most cases performed outside the very earliest time frame (Figure 12.2). The portal tracts often have a prominent hepatic artery (Figure 12.3) and some degree of portal fibrosis (Figure 12.4). The hepatic artery appears prominent because of thickening of the muscular wall. This finding is not specific for biliary atresia, however, and can be seen in a number of different cholestatic liver diseases. The bile ductular proliferation varies in intensity depending on the time of the biopsy from disease onset, but in most cases it is the dominant histological finding. In some cases, bile plugs can be seen in the proliferating bile ductules or in the bile ducts.

In a subset of approximately 30% of cases,[6-8] the ductular reaction has a pattern that suggests a ductular plate malformation (Figure 12.5), with proliferating bile ductules forming a circular structure that resembles the early bile ducts in liver organogenesis. The significance of this finding

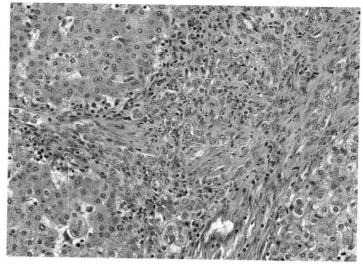

FIGURE 12.2 **Biliary atresia.** The portal tracts show marked bile ductular proliferation.

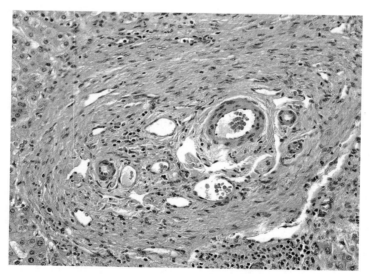

FIGURE 12.3 **Biliary atresia.** The hepatic artery appears prominent. The bile duct proper is absent, but there is a ductular proliferation at the periphery of this portal tract (outside the field of this image).

is unclear. These biliary changes that resemble ductal plate malformation are not associated with the biliary atresia-splenic malformation syndrome.[9] Some authors have suggested it represents an intrauterine start to the biliary atresia,[10] whereas others have suggested a worse prognosis.[7,11] The prognostic, significance of this finding, however, has not been validated by others.[8,12]

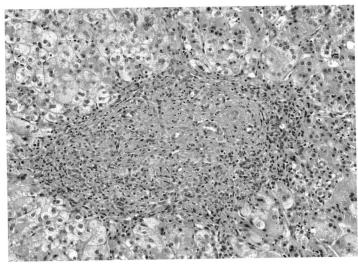

FIGURE 12.4 **Portal fibrosis.** Portal fibrosis is easily seen, even without a trichrome stain.

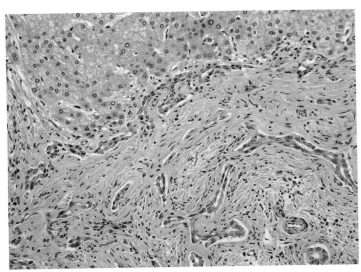

FIGURE 12.5 **Biliary atresia.** In this case of biliary atresia, focal portal tracts showed changes similar to a ductal plate malformation.

The hepatic lobules show cholestasis with relatively little to no inflammatory changes. Extramedullary hematopoiesis is common and can mimic a lobular and/or portal hepatitis. The hepatocytes can also show giant cell transformation. The amount of fibrosis varies depending on the time of the biopsy. Earliest biopsies may show little or no fibrosis, but, in most cases, there is at least mild portal fibrosis. Bridging fibrosis and cirrhosis have a worse prognosis.

CYSTIC BILIARY ATRESIA. About 4% of patients with biliary atresia also have hilar cysts that can resemble ordinary choledochal cysts.[13] Biopsies of the background liver in cases of cystic biliary atresia are very helpful, as they show the typical changes of large duct obstruction. The cystic areas in biliary atresia tend to have denuded/absent epithelium with a dense subepithelial layer of fibrosis and foci of myofibroblastic proliferation. In contrast, conventional choledochal cysts tend to be lined by intact biliary epithelium, have walls composed of bland stromal tissue that lacks dense fibrosis, and some will have irregular bundles of smooth muscle.[13] The cyst content contains frank bile in about 20% of cases of cystic biliary atresia.[14] About 75% of cases of cystic biliary atresia are associated with type 3 biliary atresia, but types 1 and 2 can also show cystic change.[14]

HILAR PLATE. A small portion of liver hilum is removed during the Kasia procedure. Histological evaluation typically shows several small bile ducts, occasional peribiliary glands, and lymphocytic inflammation, embedded in a background of fibrous and connective tissue. There often are foci of myofibroblastic proliferation.

IMMUNOSTAINS. The proliferating bile ductules seen on the liver biopsies in most cases of biliary atresia are CD56 positive (Figure 12.6), whereas CD56-positive bile ducts are only rarely observed in other causes of pediatric cholestatic liver disease.[15-18] Immunostains for CD56 can be helpful diagnostically[19] but should be used in conjunction with the hematoxylin-eosin (H&E) findings. CK7 stains highlight the bile ductular proliferation as well as intermediate hepatocytes. To date, no other immunostains have been consistently found to be useful.

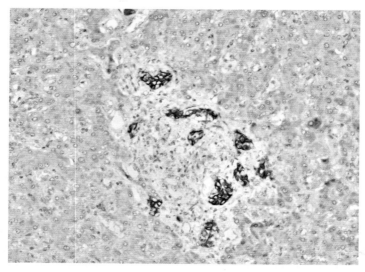

FIGURE 12.6 **Biliary atresia, CD56.** The bile ductules are strongly positive for CD56.

PROGNOSTIC INFORMATION. The histological findings in the liver biopsy and evaluation of the hilar plate removed during the Kasai procedure have both been reported to have prognostic information. Fundamentally, they all reflect to varying degrees the severity of the disease. Liver biopsies with more ductular proliferation and more fibrosis tend to have a worse prognosis. Hilar plate sections with large bile ducts (less atretic) tend to have a better prognosis.

Differential

Choledochal cysts and cystic biliary atresia can appear similar on imaging studies, and liver biopsies can be helpful in making a definitive diagnosis. Although the background liver in cases of choledochal cysts can show bile ductular proliferation, the bile ductular proliferation is typically mild and focal and fibrosis is absent or mild. Bridging or worse fibrosis favors biliary atresia.[20] In biliary atresia, the bile ducts and ductules are also typically CD56 positive.[16]

The histological differential for biliary atresia often includes neonatal hepatitis (Table 12.1). In both diseases, giant cell transformation can be present and there often is lobular cholestasis. Moderate or marked bile ductular proliferation, as well as portal fibrosis, favors biliary atresia over neonatal hepatitis. Of note, about 25% of cases of neonatal hepatitis have a patchy, mild bile ductular proliferation[21] and in some cases the histological findings may show substantial overlap with the early changes of biliary atresia. In fact, up to 10% of biopsies initially diagnosed as neonatal hepatitis are eventually diagnosed as biliary atresia[21]; these biopsies typically were taken in the course of the disease. Nonetheless, a biopsy diagnosis of biliary atresia is possible in most cases, with moderate or severe bile ductular proliferation, bile plugs in the bile ducts or proliferating ductules, and portal fibrosis all favoring biliary atresia.[6,22]

NEONATAL HEPATITIS

Definition

Neonatal hepatitis is an important cause of cholestasis in infants. Neonatal hepatitis is a histological pattern of injury that can be diagnosed only on biopsy. The biopsy shows lobular cholestasis as the predominant finding, often with giant cell transformation of the hepatocytes, but without evidence for biliary atresia or paucity of intrahepatic bile ducts. Most cases with this pattern were formerly classified as *neonatal giant cell hepatitis*, but the term has been broadened since cases without giant cell transformation have essentially the same differential diagnosis.

Clinical Findings

Clinically, infants with neonatal hepatitis demonstrate elevated levels of conjugated bilirubin and have normal biliary trees by imaging studies. The clinical picture can often be confusing, and liver biopsies are an important part of the diagnostic algorithm.

TABLE 12.1 Major Patterns in Biliary Atresia, Neonatal Hepatitis, and Paucity of Intrahepatic Bile Ducts

Histology	Biliary Atresia	Neonatal Hepatitis	Paucity of Intrahepatic Bile Ducts
Major injury pattern	Extrahepatic biliary obstruction	Lobular cholestasis with giant cell transformation of hepatocytes	Paucity of bile ducts
Bile ductular proliferation	Prominent Typically CD56 positive	Patchy, mild; present in 25% of cases Typically CD56 negative	Minimal or absent
Giant cell changes of hepatocytes	20%, patchy, mild	Most cases (about 90%); range from mild to marked	10%, patchy, minimal
Paucity of bile ducts (should be confirmed with immunostain, eg, CK7)	Absent in most cases, present only with advanced fibrosis	Absent; some ducts can be hypoplastic but no duct loss	Present
Lobular cholestasis	Common	Common	Absent or mild at presentation
Bile duct or bile ductular cholestasis	50%-75%	10%	Absent
Fibrosis	Portal fibrosis is common; there can be bridging fibrosis or cirrhosis especially in older children	No fibrosis in most cases; if there is fibrosis, genetic diseases should be carefully excluded	None at presentation; fibrosis can develop slowly over time

Etiology

Neonatal hepatitis is a pattern of injury that can be associated with a wide variety of injuries, including infections and genetic diseases (Table 12.2). A cause can be found in approximately half of cases, but the remainder is idiopathic despite full clinical and histological evaluation. Of the known etiological associations, one of the most common is pituitary abnormalities that lead to a lack of normal hormone production.[21]

TABLE 12.2 Etiologies in Neonatal Hepatitis	
Etiology	Approximate %
Idiopathic	50%
Hypopituitarism	16%
Biliary atresia	8%
Alagille syndrome	6%
Genetic with known gene defects	
Bile salt deficiencies (especially BSEP)	6%
Neonatal hemochromatosis[21,23]	5%
Cystic fibrosis	2%
Alpha-1-antitrypsin deficiency, PiZZ[21,24]	2%
Type 2 Gaucher disease[25]	<1%
Mutations with 5beta-reductase deficiency[26]	<1%
Mutations leading to cholesterol 27-hydroxylase deficiency[27]	<1%
2-Methylacyl-CoA racemase deficiency[28]	<1%
Mitochondrial DNA depletion[29]	<1%
Familial hemophagocytic lymphohistiocytosis[30]	<1%
Infection	
CMV	2%
Echovirus	2%
Paramyxoviral-like inclusions[31]	
HHV6[32]	
Rubella[33]	
Immune system dysregulation	
Autoimmune hepatitis	2%
SCID	2%
Neonatal lupus erythematosus[34]	<1%
Juvenile xanthogranulomas[35]	<1%

References are from Torbenson et al.,[21] unless otherwise noted.
CMV, cytomegalovirus; HHV, human herpesvirus; SCID, severe combined immunodeficiency.

Histological Findings

As an overview, neonatal hepatitis shows mild to moderate lobular cholestasis, typically with syncytial giant cell transformation of the hepatocytes, and variable but generally mild inflammation.[36] In addition to these positive findings, the biopsies lack the marked biliary obstructive changes of biliary atresia or the reduction in bile duct numbers that defines the various syndromes leading to paucity of intrahepatic bile ducts.

LOBULAR FINDINGS. The lobules show mild to moderate and only rarely marked cholestasis. The cholestasis can be canalicular or hepatocellular or a combination (Figure 12.7). Giant cell change is commonly a striking finding at low power and often dominates the histology (Figure 12.8); on average, about 40% of the hepatocytes are affected, although the percentage can range from as low as 1% to as high as 90%. In most

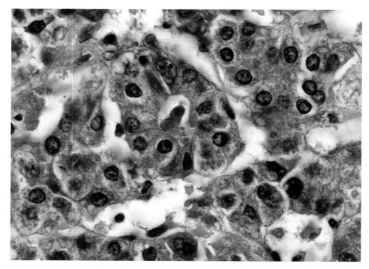

FIGURE 12.7 **Neonatal hepatitis.** The lobules show moderate cholestasis.

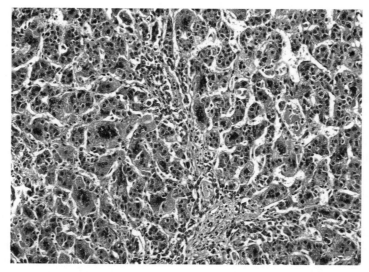

FIGURE 12.8 **Neonatal hepatitis, giant cells.** The hepatocytes show striking giant cell transformation on low power.

cases, the hepatocytes with giant cell transformation have either a predominately zone 3 distribution (one-third of cases) or an azonal pattern, with no discernible zonation (two-thirds of cases). A zone 1 predominate pattern is only rarely observed. Hepatocytes with giant cell change have between 4 and 10 nuclei (Figure 12.9), although examples with up to 20 nuclei can occasionally be found. Giant hepatocytes often have abundant amphophilic cytoplasm that resembles endoplasmic reticulum proliferation, with a peripheral localization of nuclei (Figure 12.10). Other giant hepatocytes have a homogenous, eosinophilic cytoplasm with centrally located nuclei (Figure 12.11). Both forms can be found in a single biopsy, although there often is a relative prominence of one of the morphologies.

Extramedullary hematopoiesis is present in the lobules in approximately three-fourths of cases and includes both myelopoiesis and erythropoiesis (Figure 12.12). Lobular lymphocytic inflammation is mild or absent in nearly all cases. A small subset of cases also show fatty change.[21,37]

PORTAL TRACT CHANGES. Portal lymphocytic inflammation is absent or mild in the vast majority of cases, but the portal tracts often show mild to moderate cellularity composed of myelopoiesis, including numerous eosinophils and metamyelocytes.

Bile ductular proliferation is evident on H&E stains in about 25% of cases but is focal and mild, in contrast to biliary atresia. Septal-sized bile ducts are only rarely sampled but can demonstrate mild epithelial

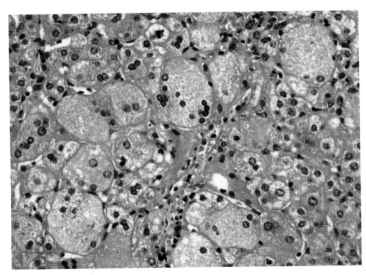

FIGURE 12.9 **Neonatal hepatitis, giant cells.** The lobules show giant cells and cholestasis. The giant cells in this case clustered in zone 3. An etiology was identified in this case: neonatal hepatitis B infection.

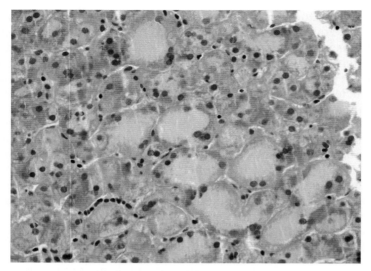

FIGURE 12.10 **Neonatal hepatitis, giant cells.** These giant cells have distinctive gray color to their cytoplasm.

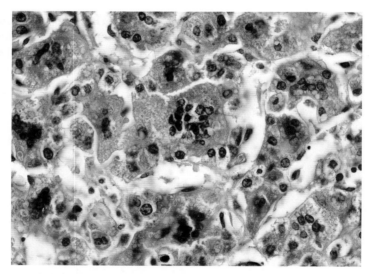

FIGURE 12.11 **Neonatal hepatitis.** These giant cells have eosinophilic cytoplasm.

lymphocytosis and equivocal epithelial injury. Small bile ducts can appear hypoplastic and be difficult to identify on H&E stain,[21,38] and cytokeratin immunostains are useful to rule out true ductopenia.

FIBROSIS AND IRON ACCUMULATION. Fibrosis is present in about one-third of biopsy specimens. Fibrosis is usually mild, but a subset of cases can show bridging fibrosis. Livers with bridging fibrosis often show marked

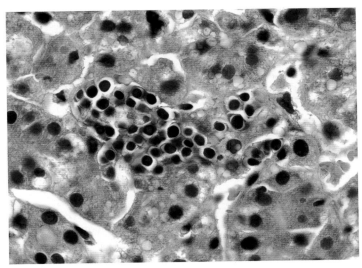

FIGURE 12.12 **Neonatal hepatitis, extramedullary hematopoiesis.** A discrete cluster of cells with round hyperchromatic nuclei and scant cytoplasm is seen.

pericellular fibrosis. Isolated mild pericellular fibrosis can also be seen. A small series of cases has been published where reversed blood flow in the portal vein was associated with rapid fibrosis progression.[39]

Iron stains are negative in one-third of cases, and most of the remaining show minimal iron in hepatocytes, Kupffer cells, or both. In a subset of about 5% of cases, there can be more substantial hepatocellular iron accumulation; these latter cases may also have bile ductular iron deposition if there were prior episodes of massive liver necrosis and subsequent regeneration. Neonatal hemochromatosis should be carefully excluded by correlation with clinical findings and looking for evidence of iron deposition in other organs, either by biopsy or by imaging.

PAUCITY OF INTRAHEPATIC BILE DUCTS

Definition

Paucity of intrahepatic bile ducts is a pathology diagnosis but not a distinctive entity. Similar to neonatal hepatitis, paucity of intrahepatic bile ducts represents a pattern of injury that can be associated with many different causes, including many that are nonsyndromic (Table 12.3).

Clinical Findings

Neonates typically present with jaundice and elevated conjugated bilirubin levels in the first weeks to month of life. Patients may have acholic stools and HIDA scans often fail to excrete tracer into the duodenum, mimicking biliary atresia.[40]

TABLE 12.3 Nonsyndromic Causes of Paucity of Intrahepatic Bile Ducts in Neonates	
Cause	Comment and/or Reference
Infection	
CMV	
Hepatitis B	
Rubella	
Syphilis	
Metabolic	
Alpha-1-antitrypsin deficiency	
Bile salt deficiency	Most commonly ABCB11(BSEP) deficiency in the setting of a neonatal giant cell hepatitis pattern
Cystic fibrosis	Usually has some mild ductular proliferation
Hypopituitary disease	Often in the setting of a neonatal giant cell hepatitis pattern
Genetic	
Trisomy 11	
Trisomy 18	
Trisomy 21	
Monosomy X	

The list continues to grow and this table is not exhaustive.

Alagille syndrome makes up a distinct subset of cases of paucity of intrahepatic bile ducts. Alagille syndrome is associated with *JAG1* mutations, and patients have other congenital abnormalities, including butterfly vertebrae, cardiovascular anatomic abnormalities, hypothyroidism, and pancreas insufficiency.[41] In some cases where Alagille syndrome is diagnosed on clinical grounds, bile duct loss may not be evident on biopsy. One large study, for example, found that about 25% of liver biopsies did not have ductopenia, despite a firm clinical diagnosis of Alagille syndrome.[40]

Histological Findings

PORTAL TRACTS. The portal tracts show hypoplastic bile ducts and/or bile duct loss (Figures 12.13 and 12.14). The portal tracts commonly show nonspecific lymphocytic inflammation that may include rare eosinophils or plasma cells. The inflammation can range from mild to focally moderate and can sometimes obscure residual bile ducts. An immunostain for cytokeratin can help identify the bile duct loss. The portal tracts also may have focal, mild bile ductular proliferation (Figure 12.15). In some cases, the ductular proliferation can have a metaplastic phenotype, with the ductules

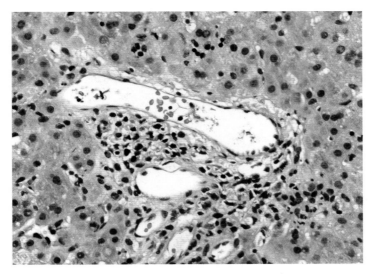

FIGURE 12.13 **Paucity of intrahepatic bile duct.** No bile duct is seen in the portal tract in this case of Alagille syndrome. There is mild nonspecific portal inflammation.

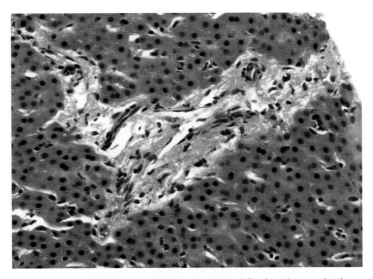

FIGURE 12.14 **Paucity of intrahepatic bile duct.** No bile duct is seen in the portal tract in this case of Alagille syndrome.

also staining for hepatocyte markers (Figures 12.16 and 12.17). The bile duct loss initially affects the smaller branches of the biliary tree and can be patchy. Larger portal tracts, although uncommonly sampled, have intact bile ducts (Figure 12.18). Bile duct loss may not develop in some cases until after the first year or second year of life.

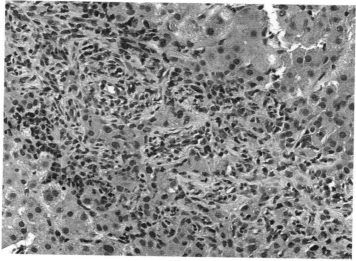

FIGURE 12.15 **Paucity of intrahepatic bile duct**. Bile ducts were absent in this biopsy, but a patchy bile ductular proliferation was present. The ductules appear "metaplastic" with a combined hepatic and ductular appearance.

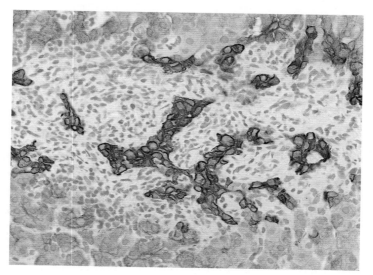

FIGURE 12.16 **Paucity of intrahepatic bile duct**. The metaplastic ductular reaction (see prior image) was positive for both cytokeratin AE1/3 and Hepar1 (see Figure 12.17).

Liver fibrosis is unusual in neonates with paucity of intrahepatic bile ducts, and the presence of clear fibrosis would favor biliary atresia. Progressive fibrosis, however, can develop later in some cases of paucity of intrahepatic bile ducts, more commonly with the Alagille syndrome.

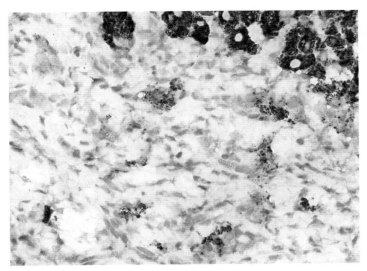

FIGURE 12.17 **Paucity of intrahepatic bile duct.** The metaplastic ductular reaction is Hepar1 positive (see Figures 12.15 and 12.16).

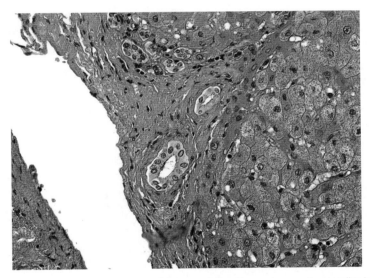

FIGURE 12.18 **Alagille syndrome.** In this case of Alagille syndrome, the smaller bile ducts were absent, but larger septal-sized bile ducts are still present.

LOBULAR FINDINGS. The lobules show canalicular and hepatocellular cholestasis with sparse inflammation and often mild giant cell transformation of the hepatocytes (Figure 12.19). Extramedullary hematopoiesis in the lobules is common and occasionally can be striking.

The bile canaliculi in children begin to show CD10 expression at around 2 years of age, but there can be persistent absence of CD10 staining in children with Alagille syndrome who are older than 2 years (Figure 12.20).[42]

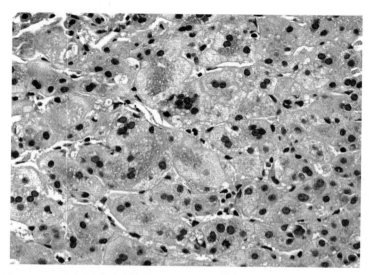

FIGURE 12.19 **Alagille syndrome.** There is patchy mild giant cell transformation and mild cholestasis.

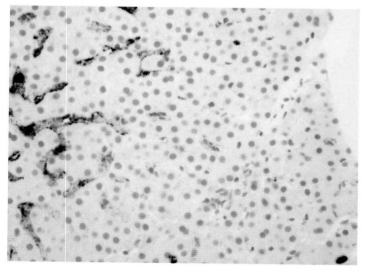

FIGURE 12.20 **Alagille syndrome, CD10.** The normal CD10 canalicular staining pattern is patchy and disrupted.

Key Distinguishing Features of the Major Neonatal Cholestatic Liver Diseases

Biopsies play an important role in evaluating infants with elevated conjugated bilirubin levels. Although there is histological overlap between all of the major patterns of cholestatic injury in pediatric livers, careful attention to the biopsy findings and correlation with the clinical and imaging findings can lead to the proper diagnosis in most cases (Table 12.1). Biliary atresia should have large-duct obstructive-type changes as the predominant finding, with no loss of the actual bile ducts (bile duct loss can develop in cases with advanced fibrosis but is typically not present at first presentation), a ductular proliferation, and often at least mild portal fibrosis. The lobules can have giant cell transformation in any pediatric cholestatic liver disease, but this is often the dominant pattern in cases of neonatal hepatitis. In neonatal hepatitis, there should be no strong evidence for biliary obstructive changes. The lobules are relatively uninflamed in neonatal hepatitis, although extramedullary hematopoiesis can be prominent. Mild bile duct hypoplasia can be seen, but there should be no established bile duct loss. Fibrosis can be present but is usually focal and mild; the fibrosis may include both portal and pericellular patterns. In paucity of intrahepatic bile ducts, loss of bile ducts is the major histological finding. The portal tracts can show mild inflammation and can also have a mild and patchy bile ductular proliferation, but the bile ductular proliferation does not reach the levels of biliary atresia.

FAMILIAL CHOLESTASIS OVERVIEW

Terminology for Progressive Familial Intrahepatic Cholestasis

- **Familial intrahepatic cholestasis (FIC) deficiency**
  - Results from *ATP8B1* mutations
  - Formerly called BRIC1 or progressive familial intrahepatic cholestasis 1 (PFIC1) based on the clinical course
  - Historical terms: Byler disease and Greenland familial cholestasis
- **Bile salt export pump (BSEP) deficiency**
  - Results from *ABCB11* mutations
  - Formerly called BRIC2 or PFIC2 based on clinical course
  - Historical term is Byler syndrome
- **Multiple drug resistance 3 (MDR3) deficiency**
  - Results from *ABCB4* mutations
  - Formerly called BRIC3 or PFIC3 based on clinical course
- **Other very rare causes**
  - Mutations in *TJP2*, *NR1H4* (encodes FXR), and *MYO5B*

Abbreviations: BRIC, benign recurrent intrahepatic cholestasis; PFIC, progressive familial intrahepatic cholestasis.

Overview

Familial causes of pediatric intrahepatic cholestatic liver disease are inherited in an autosomal recessive manner. Historically, this group of liver diseases was classified by the clinical course into *benign recurrent intrahepatic cholestasis* or *progressive familial intrahepatic cholestasis*. This differentiation was based on whether the elevated bilirubin levels were episodic or persistent, with the persistent form more strongly associated with fibrosis progression. However, the advent of improved genetics-based understanding has led to reclassification of these diseases based on the underlying genetics. Because of this improved understanding, these diseases are now commonly referred to by their specific molecular changes, for example, *FIC1 deficiency*, instead *of progressive intrahepatic cholestasis 1*.

In addition to the three most common mutations (*ATPB81, ABCB11, ABCB4*), other very rare mutations have been identified, including mutations in *TJP2*,[43] *NR1H4*,[44] and *MYO5B*.[45] Of interest, *NR1H4* encodes a protein (FXR) that is a negative regulator of BSEP, whereas *MYO5B* mutations lead to incorrect localization of BSEP protein.[46] Finally, a small proportion of cases with progressive familial intrahepatic cholestasis still do not have mutations in known genes, suggesting that other genes remain to be identified. Also of note, all of the three major genes with mutations are also associated with intrahepatic cholestasis of pregnancy in heterozygotes.

Serum Findings

Serum conjugated bilirubin levels are elevated in all of the different types of familial intrahepatic cholestasis. Elevated serum GGT levels favor ABCB4 mutations, whereas elevated serum alpha-fetoprotein (AFP) levels favor *ABCB11* or *FXR* mutations. The aspartate aminotransferase and alanine aminotransferase (ALT) levels are also typically elevated, usually in the mild range. Somewhat higher levels of ALT elevations are seen more commonly with *ABCB11* mutations ($5\times$ or more of normal).

Histological Findings

The histological findings show significant overlap, but there are some broad patterns that can be informative. FIC1 deficiency tends to show bland lobular cholestasis as the predominant histological pattern, BSEP deficiency tends to show a neonatal hepatitis pattern with prominent hepatocyte giant cell transformation, whereas MDR3 deficiency tends to resemble large-duct-type biliary obstruction. These patterns can be very helpful but are not highly specific. When combined with immunostains and/or with electron microscopy, however, the entire set of findings can be highly suggestive and, in some cases, diagnostic. Adding in the clinical and laboratory findings further clarifies the diagnosis in most cases. Table 12.4 summarizes many of the key features of the most common causes of familial intrahepatic cholestasis.

TABLE 12.4 Summary of Key Clinical, Laboratory, and Pathology Findings in Diseases of Bile Salt Deficiency

Finding	ATPB81 Deficiency	ABCB11 (BSEP) Deficiency	ABCB4 (MDR3) Deficiency	TJP2 Mutations	NR1H4 Mutations	MYO5B Mutations
Clinical progression	Moderate	Moderate to rapid	Variable	Rapid	Rapid	Slow
Extrahepatic findings	Diarrhea, pancreatic disease, hearing loss	None	None	Respiratory and neurological disease	Early onset coagulopathy	Some may have intestinal disease from microvillous inclusions disease
Risk of hepatocellular and cholangiocarcinoma	Not reported to date	Yes	Not reported to date	Yes, can be present at birth	Not reported to date	Not reported to date
Serum	• Elevated conjugated bilirubin • Normal or low GGT • Normal AFP • ALT elevations mild	• Elevated conjugated bilirubin • Normal or low GGT • Elevated AFP • ALT elevations mild to moderate	• Elevated conjugated bilirubin • Elevated GGT • Normal AFP • ALT elevations mild	• Elevated conjugated bilirubin • Low GGT	• Elevated conjugated bilirubin • Normal GGT • High AFP • ALT elevations mild	• Elevated conjugated bilirubin • Normal to low GGT • Normal AFP • ALT elevations mild

(Continued)

TABLE 12.4 Summary of Key Clinical, Laboratory, and Pathology Findings in Diseases of Bile Salt Deficiency (Continued)

Finding	ATPB81 Deficiency	ABCB11 (BSEP) Deficiency	ABCB4 (MDR3) Deficiency	TJP2 Mutations	NR1H4 Mutations	MYO5B Mutations
Main histological findings	Bland lobular cholestasis	• Giant cell transformation • Lobular cholestasis • Subset with paucity of intrahepatic ducts	• Lobular cholestasis • Bile ductular proliferation	• Lobular cholestasis	• Lobular cholestasis • Bile ductular proliferation • Giant cell transformation	• Lobular cholestasis • Giant cell transformation
Electron microscopy	Coarse granular bile	Amorphous to filamentous bile	No distinctive findings	Unknown	Unknown	Unknown
Immunohistochemistry		Reduction or loss of BSEP	Reduction or loss of MDR3	Absence of TJP		BSEP and MDR3 present but abnormal staining

ATP8B1 Mutations/FIC Deficiency

DEFINITION

FIC deficiency is caused by *ATP8B1* mutations and was previously called Byler disease and Greenland familial cholestasis. FIC deficiency can be associated with benign recurrent patterns of cholestasis, as well as cholestatic injury associated with progressive fibrosis, depending in part on the type and location of the mutation. Over 50 different mutations have been reported. Missense mutations tend to correlate with the benign recurrent pattern of cholestasis, whereas nonsense and frameshift mutations tend to correlate with the fibrosis-progressing pattern of cholestasis. This suggests residual activity in the missense mutated proteins, but the genotype-phenotype correlation is imperfect, even for individuals with the same mutation, indicating an important role for other factors in gene penetrance, including environment and other genetic changes. *ATP8B1* encodes for an aminophospholipid-transporting ATPase, and cholestatic liver disease is thought to result from impaired translocation of aminophosholipids across cellular membranes into the bile.

CLINICAL FINDINGS

Infants present with conjugated bilirubinemia and pruritus. Serum GGT levels are normal or low despite the elevated bilirubin. The elevated bilirubin levels can be episodic or persistent. Extrahepatic disease may be present, including diarrhea, pancreatic disease, and loss of hearing. Fat malabsorption can lead to malnutrition and vitamin deficiencies. If patients undergo liver transplantation, the liver allograft can develop de novo macrovesicular steatosis or steatohepatitits.[47,48]

HISTOLOGICAL FINDINGS

The histological findings are not specific but typically show a canalicular pattern of cholestasis, often with bile that appears pale, with little or no hepatocellular cholestasis (Figure 12.21). Bile duct obstructive changes are not seen and neither is ductopenia. Mild cholate stasis and occasional balloon cells may be present, but giant cell transformation is relatively rare. Inflammation is mild or absent. Fibrosis is generally rare in biopsies of infants, even in those who eventually progress to substantial fibrosis.

ELECTRON MICROSCOPIC FINDINGS

On electron microscopy, the bile is coarse and granular, a finding at one time referred to as "Byler bile."

ABCB11 Mutations/BSEP Deficiency

DEFINITION

ABCB11 mutations can cause both a benign recurrent pattern of cholestasis and a cholestatic injury pattern associated with progressive fibrosis. *ABCB11* codes for the BSEP protein, and mutations lead to impaired canalicular transport of bile salts. Over 100 mutations have been reported.

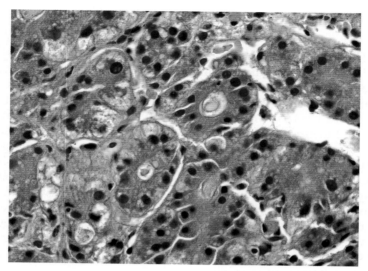

FIGURE 12.21 **FIC deficiency.** The lobules show cholestatic rosettes and pale bile.

CLINICAL FINDING

Infants present with conjugated bilirubinemia. The elevated bilirubin levels can be episodic or persistent. The serum GGT levels are normal or low despite the elevated bilirubin. Serum AFP levels are commonly elevated in infants with BSEP deficiency,[49] in contrast to FIC1 deficiency where levels are typically normal. Individuals with BSEP deficiency have a high life-time frequency of cholelithiasis. Patients with fibrosis progression are at risk for cholangiocarcinoma and hepatocellular carcinoma.

HISTOLOGICAL FINDINGS

The histological findings vary, but the majority of cases show lobular cholestasis and most show a neonatal hepatitis pattern, at least in biopsies of infants and young children. Inflammation is mild in most cases but occasionally can be moderate (Figure 12.22). There tends to be more inflammation and less giant cell transformation in BSEP deficiency than is seen in cases of idiopathic neonatal hepatitis, although there is histological overlap. Obstructive changes are not seen and neither is ductopenia.

IMMUNOSTAINS

Immunostains for BSEP proteins can be useful but are not widely available. Reduced or absent BSEP staining strongly supports a diagnosis of ABCB11 deficiency, but a normal BSEP staining pattern does not completely exclude ABCB11 deficiency, as some mutations affect the protein function and not its overall expression.

ELECTRON MICROSCOPIC FINDINGS

On electron microscopy, the bile is finely granular and somewhat amorphous or can appear filamentous. The coarse, granular bile typical of ATP8B1 deficiency is not seen.

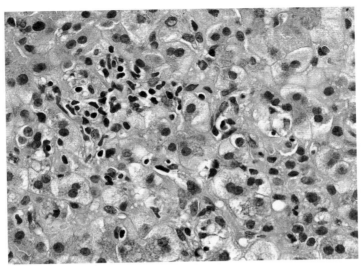

FIGURE 12.22 **BSEP (*ABCB11*) deficiency.** The biopsied moderate lobular cholestasis and patchy moderate lobular hepatitis pattern.

ABCB4 Mutations/MDR3 Deficiency

DEFINITION
ABCB4 codes for the MDR3 protein, and mutations lead to impaired canalicular translocation of phosphatidylcholine. MDR3 deficiency is most commonly associated with a cholestatic injury pattern associated with progressive fibrosis, but there is wide phenotypic variation.

CLINICAL FINDINGS
The average age at presentation for MDR3 deficiency is somewhat older than for FIC or BSEP deficiency, with a mean age of about 3 years and some cases presenting as adults, although presentation in infancy also occurs. Individuals present with conjugated bilirubinemia. The serum GGT levels are elevated (in contrast to *ATP8B1* and *ABCB11* deficiency). Individuals are at increased life time risk for cholelithiasis because of low phospholipid concentrations in the bile. Some patients present in late teenage years with cryptogenic cirrhosis.[50]

Also of note, heterozygosity for *ABCB4* mutations has been linked to cryptogenic cirrhosis in adults (often with a biliary pattern of cirrhosis), drug-induced cholestasis in adults, and recurrent gallstones.[51] Cholesterol crystals in the bile ducts, often associated with a macrophage infiltrate, is an uncommon but useful clue to the possibility of *ABCB4* mutations in adults with unexplained chronic cholestatic liver disease.[52]

HISTOLOGICAL FINDINGS
The histological findings vary, but all show lobular cholestasis. In contrast to cases with *ATP8B1* or *ABCB11* mutations, biopsies in the setting of *ABCB4* mutations often show a bile ductular proliferation that can dominate the

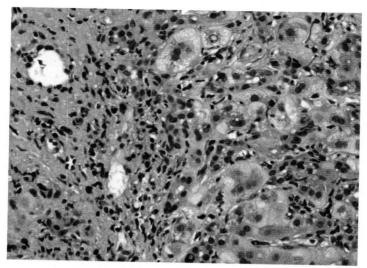

FIGURE 12.23 **PFIC3 (*ABCB4* deficiency).** The portal tracts showed bile ductular proliferation that extended into the lobules.

histological findings (Figure 12.23). Imaging of the extrahepatic biliary tree is important to rule out downstream biliary obstruction. Portal and lobular inflammation is mild or absent. Fibrosis progression is variable, but some cases can show rapid progression, with cirrhosis by age 20 years.

IMMUNOSTAINS

Immunostains for MDR3 proteins are not widely available but can be useful. The overall interpretation is similar to that of BSEP staining. Reduced or absent MDR3 staining strongly supports a diagnosis of MDR3 deficiency, but a normal MDR3 staining pattern does not completely exclude deficiency, as some mutations affect the protein's function and not the overall expression.

INHERITED DEFECTS IN BILIRUBIN METABOLISM

There are five main genetic diseases of bilirubin metabolism: Rotor syndrome, Dubin-Johnson syndrome, Gilbert syndrome, and Crigler-Najjar syndrome types I and II (Table 12.5). These diseases as a group are not specifically pediatric but are included in this section because of Crigler-Najjar syndrome type 1.

In the Crigler-Najjar syndrome type 1, jaundice develops in the first few days of life and persists. If untreated, infants can develop neurological complications from the chronically elevated bilirubin levels. Published biopsy data are limited, but biopsies typically show lobular cholestasis with relatively little inflammation (Figure 12.24). Bile ductular proliferation tends to be absent to minimal.

TABLE 12.5 The Five Major Inherited Defects in Bilirubin Metabolism

Disease	Disease Course	Inheritance	Gene	Bilirubin Elevations	Histological Findings
Rotor syndrome	Minimal to mild	Autosomal recessive	SLCO1B1 SLCO1B3	Conjugated	May be cholestatic if biopsied during an episode of jaundice Lipofuscin, often light but heavy in about one-fourth of patients
Dubin-Johnson syndrome	Minimal to mild	Autosomal recessive	ABCC2	Conjugated	May be cholestatic if biopsied during an episode of jaundice Hepatocytes also show dense brown and granular lipofuscin related pigment
Gilbert syndrome	Minimal to mild	Autosomal recessive	UGT1A1	Unconjugated	May be cholestatic if biopsied during an episode of jaundice Lipofuscin, often light
Crigler-Najjar syndrome type II	Mild to moderate	Autosomal recessive	UGT1A1	Unconjugated	May be cholestatic if biopsied during an episode of jaundice No distinctive pigment accumulation
Crigler-Najjar syndrome type I	Severe	Autosomal recessive	UGT1A1	Unconjugated	May be cholestatic if biopsied during an episode of jaundice No distinctive pigment accumulation

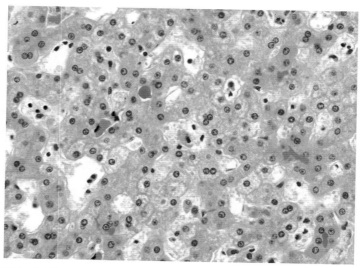

FIGURE 12.24   **Crigler-Najjar syndrome, type 1.** Moderate lobular cholestasis is seen.

In type II Crigler-Najjar syndrome, the bilirubin levels are lower and may escape diagnosis until later in life. Bilirubin levels can usually be managed with phenobarbital therapy. Both types of Crigler-Najjar syndrome, as well as Gilbert syndrome, result from genetic mutations in *UGT1A1*. The different clinical manifestations are a reflection of the amount of residual gene activity for a given mutation. In type II Crigler-Najjar syndrome, the biopsy findings can be normal but can also show lobular cholestasis with minimal or absent inflammatory changes. Although the mechanism is unclear, biopsies also commonly show mild to moderate hepatocellular iron deposition. In one study, 10 of 15 (67%) of biopsies with type II Crigler-Najjar syndrome showed iron deposition, with a zone 1 predominance.[53] Rare cases of type II Crigler-Najjar syndrome can also progress to bridging fibrosis[54] or cirrhosis.[55] In some cases, the cirrhosis can be clinically cryptogenic; the best clue is a history of unconjugated hyperbilirubinemia and a biliary pattern of cirrhosis in a teenaged or young adult.

In Rotor syndrome, Dubin-Johnson syndrome, and Gilbert syndrome, individuals are generally asymptomatic but can have episodes of jaundice when placed under stress from various illnesses such as infections, hemolysis, or medications. Rotor syndrome and Dubin-Johnson syndrome primarily have elevations in conjugated bilirubin levels, whereas Gilbert syndrome primarily has elevations in unconjugated bilirubin levels. They generally do not require treatment. Histologically, the liver may show cholestatic changes when biopsied, but distinctive pigment is seen only with Dubin-Johnson syndrome, where the pigment is a coarse brown lipofuscin-type of

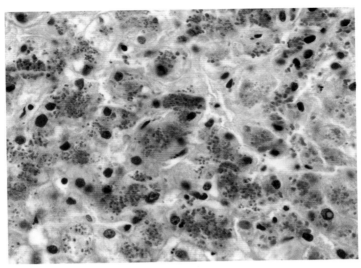

FIGURE 12.25 **Dubin-Johnson syndrome.** The hepatocytes show abundant coarse brown pigment.

pigment (Figure 12.25). There can be significant histological overlap with the more mundane lipofuscin seen in routine biopsies, so a diagnosis is best made by combining clinical and histological findings.

Lipofuscin is also common in Gilbert syndrome. In one study, 20% of liver biopsies in the setting of Gilbert syndrome showed lipofuscin in hepatocytes (Figure 12.26).[56] Also of note, biopsies with Gilbert syndrome often have mild nonspecific inflammatory changes with mild portal lymphocytic inflammation and minimal lobular inflammation.[57]

OTHER CAUSES OF NEONATAL CHOLESTASIS

Even after excluding the pediatric diseases discussed in prior sections (biliary atresia, paucity of intrahepatic bile ducts, neonatal hepatitis, familial intrahepatic cholestasis, etc), a wide variety of additional diseases can present with a predominantly cholestatic pattern in infants and children. These latter cases show predominantly lobular cholestasis, which can be severe, with no changes to suggest obstruction, mild or absent inflammatory changes, and minimal or absent giant cell change.

Genetic Causes of Neonatal Cholestasis

One important cause is alpha-1-antitrypsin deficiency, which only rarely presents in infancy, but, when it does, the majority of infants have liver disease. The histological findings vary and can include a neonatal hepatitis pattern or a paucity of intrahepatic bile ducts pattern. Intrahepatic globules of alpha-1-antitrypsin protein are often absent until about 3 to 4 months

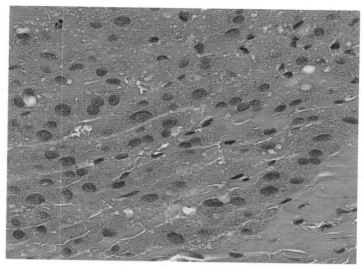

FIGURE 12.26 **Gilbert syndrome.** Marked lipofuscin accumulation is seen within the hepatocytes.

of life, at which time they are generally present at least focally. The diagnosis is made by measuring the total serum levels of alpha-1-antitrypsin and by electrophoresis to characterize the Pi type. The ZZ pattern is the most common phenotype of alpha-1-antitrypsin deficiency presenting in infancy.

Niemann-Pick disease type C can also present clinically with a conjugated hyperbilirubinemia. Ascites may be found at presentation. In some cases, the biopsies can have features that suggest obstruction. Pericellular fibrosis is often present. The abnormal Kupffer cells typical of Niemann-Pick disease type C are often not present in infants.

There are many other rare genetic/metabolic causes of neonatal cholestasis, including Aageneas syndrome, North American Indian familial cholestasis (also called North American Indian childhood cirrhosis), and the Zellweger syndrome. A number of primary disorders of bile acid synthesis have also been reported, all of which are very rare. Glucose 6-phosphatase dehydrogenase deficiency can occasionally present as neonatal cholestasis.[58] Finally, a number of primary disorders of the pituitary, all leading to hypopituitarism, can lead to a bland lobular cholestasis.

Other Causes

Other causes of bland lobular cholestasis include medication effects as well as total parenteral nutrition. Sepsis can also lead to a bland lobular cholestatic pattern. In fact, even localized infections outside the liver can sometimes lead to cholestatic changes in the liver.

REFERENCES

1. Superina R, Magee JC, Brandt ML, et al. The anatomic pattern of biliary atresia identified at time of Kasai hepatoportoenterostomy and early postoperative clearance of jaundice are significant predictors of transplant-free survival. *Ann Surg.* 2011;254:577-585.
2. Hartley JL, Davenport M, Kelly DA. Biliary atresia. *Lancet.* 2009;374:1704-1713.
3. Harper P, Plant JW, Unger DB. Congenital biliary atresia and jaundice in lambs and calves. *Aust Vet J.* 1990;67:18-22.
4. Negm AA, Petersen C, Markowski A, et al. The role of endoscopic retrograde cholangiopancreatography in the diagnosis of biliary atresia: 14 years' experience. *Eur J Pediatr Surg.* 2018;28:261-267.
5. Wang L, Yang Y, Chen Y, et al. Early differential diagnosis methods of biliary atresia: a meta-analysis. *Pediatr Surg Int.* 2018;34:363-380.
6. Rastogi A, Krishnani N, Yachha SK, et al. Histopathological features and accuracy for diagnosing biliary atresia by prelaparotomy liver biopsy in developing countries. *J Gastroenterol Hepatol.* 2009;24:97-102.
7. Shimadera S, Iwai N, Deguchi E, et al. Significance of ductal plate malformation in the postoperative clinical course of biliary atresia. *J Pediatr Surg.* 2008;43:304-307.
8. Arii R, Koga H, Arakawa A, et al. How valuable is ductal plate malformation as a predictor of clinical course in postoperative biliary atresia patients? *Pediatr Surg Int.* 2011;27:275-277.
9. Pacheco MC, Campbell KM, Bove KE. Ductal plate malformation-like arrays in early explants after a Kasai procedure are independent of splenic malformation complex (heterotaxy). *Pediatr Dev Pathol.* 2009;12:355-360.
10. Tan CE, Driver M, Howard ER, et al. Extrahepatic biliary atresia: a first-trimester event? Clues from light microscopy and immunohistochemistry. *J Pediatr Surg.* 1994;29:808-814.
11. Low Y, Vijayan V, Tan CE. The prognostic value of ductal plate malformation and other histologic parameters in biliary atresia: an immunohistochemical study. *J Pediatr.* 2001;139:320-322.
12. Vukovic J, Grizelj R, Bojanic K, et al. Ductal plate malformation in patients with biliary atresia. *Eur J Pediatr.* 2012;171:1799-1804.
13. Lobeck IN, Sheridan R, Lovell M, et al. Cystic biliary atresia and choledochal cysts are distinct histopathologic entities. *Am J Surg Pathol.* 2017;41:354-364.
14. Caponcelli E, Knisely AS, Davenport M. Cystic biliary atresia: an etiologic and prognostic subgroup. *J Pediatr Surg.* 2008;43:1619-1624.
15. Sira MM, El-Guindi MA, Saber MA, et al. Differential hepatic expression of CD56 can discriminate biliary atresia from other neonatal cholestatic disorders. *Eur J Gastroenterol Hepatol.* 2012;24:1227-1233.
16. Okada T, Itoh T, Sasaki F, et al. CD56-immunostaining of the extrahepatic biliary tree as an indicator of clinical outcome in biliary atresia: a preliminary report. *Turk J Pediatr.* 2008;50:542-548.
17. Torbenson M, Wang J, Abraham S, et al. Bile ducts and ductules are positive for CD56 (N-CAM) in most cases of extrahepatic biliary atresia. *Am J Surg Pathol.* 2003;27:1454-1457.
18. Okada T, Itoh T, Sasaki F, et al. Comparison between prenatally diagnosed choledochal cyst and type-1 cystic biliary atresia by CD56-immunostaining using liver biopsy specimens. *Eur J Pediatr Surg.* 2007;17:6-11.
19. Krishna OH, Sultana N, Malleboyina R, et al. Efficacy of the seven feature, fifteen point histological scoring system and CD56 in interpretation of liver biopsies in persistent neonatal cholestasis: a five-year study. *Indian J Pathol Microbiol.* 2014;57:196-200.
20. Okada T, Sasaki F, Cho K, et al. Histological differentiation between prenatally diagnosed choledochal cyst and type I cystic biliary atresia using liver biopsy specimens. *Eur J Pediatr Surg.* 2006;16:28-33.

21. Torbenson M, Hart J, Westerhoff M, et al. Neonatal giant cell hepatitis: histological and etiological findings. *Am J Surg Pathol.* 2010;34:1498-1503.

22. Russo P, Magee JC, Anders RA, et al. Key histopathologic features of liver biopsies that distinguish biliary atresia from other causes of infantile cholestasis and their correlation with outcome: a multicenter study. *Am J Surg Pathol.* 2016;40:1601-1615.

23. Hoogstraten J, de Sa DJ, Knisely AS. Fetal liver disease may precede extrahepatic siderosis in neonatal hemochromatosis. *Gastroenterology.* 1990;98:1699-1701.

24. Ghishan FK, Greene HL. Liver disease in children with PiZZ alpha 1-antitrypsin deficiency. *Hepatology.* 1988;8:307-310.

25. Elias AF, Johnson MR, Boitnott JK, et al. Neonatal cholestasis as initial manifestation of type 2 Gaucher disease: a continuum in the spectrum of early onset Gaucher disease. *JIMD Rep.* 2012;5:95-98.

26. Lemonde HA, Custard EJ, Bouquet J, et al. Mutations in SRD5B1 (AKR1D1), the gene encoding delta(4)-3-oxosteroid 5beta-reductase, in hepatitis and liver failure in infancy. *Gut.* 2003;52:1494-1499.

27. Clayton PT, Verrips A, Sistermans E, et al. Mutations in the sterol 27-hydroxylase gene (CYP27A) cause hepatitis of infancy as well as cerebrotendinous xanthomatosis. *J Inherit Metab Dis.* 2002;25:501-513.

28. Setchell KD, Heubi JE, Bove KE, et al. Liver disease caused by failure to racemize trihydroxycholestanoic acid: gene mutation and effect of bile acid therapy. *Gastroenterology.* 2003;124:217-232.

29. Muller-Hocker J, Muntau A, Schafer S, et al. Depletion of mitochondrial DNA in the liver of an infant with neonatal giant cell hepatitis. *Hum Pathol.* 2002;33:247-253.

30. Chen JH, Fleming MD, Pinkus GS, et al. Pathology of the liver in familial hemophagocytic lymphohistiocytosis. *Am J Surg Pathol.* 2010;34:852-867.

31. Hicks J, Barrish J, Zhu SH. Neonatal syncytial giant cell hepatitis with paramyxoviral-like inclusions. *Ultrastruct Pathol.* 2001;25:65-71.

32. Domiati-Saad R, Dawson DB, Margraf LR, et al. Cytomegalovirus and human herpesvirus 6, but not human papillomavirus, are present in neonatal giant cell hepatitis and extrahepatic biliary atresia. *Pediatr Dev Pathol.* 2000;3:367-373.

33. Stern H, Williams BM. Isolation of rubella virus in a case of neonatal giant-cell hepatitis. *Lancet.* 1966;1:293-295.

34. Silverman E, Jaeggi E. Non-cardiac manifestations of neonatal lupus erythematosus. *Scand J Immunol.* 2010;72:223-225.

35. Dehner LP. Juvenile xanthogranulomas in the first two decades of life: a clinicopathologic study of 174 cases with cutaneous and extracutaneous manifestations. *Am J Surg Pathol.* 2003;27:579-593.

36. Cho SJ, Perito ER, Shafizadeh N, et al. Dialogs in the assessment of neonatal cholestatic liver disease. *Hum Pathol.* 2021;112:102-115.

37. Tazawa Y, Abukawa D, Maisawa S, et al. Idiopathic neonatal hepatitis presenting as neonatal hepatic siderosis and steatosis. *Dig Dis Sci.* 1998;43:392-396.

38. Reiterer EE, Zenz W, Deutsch J, et al. Congenital hypopituitarism and giant cell hepatitis in a three month old girl. Article in German. *Klin Pädiatr.* 2002;214:136-139.

39. Yokoyama S, Kasahara M, Fukuda A, et al. Neonatal hepatitis with hepatofugal portal flow and collateral veins: report of three cases. *Transplant Proc.* 2008;40:1461-1465.

40. Subramaniam P, Knisely A, Portmann B, et al. Diagnosis of Alagille syndrome-25 years of experience at king's college hospital. *J Pediatr Gastroenterol Nutr.* 2011;52:84-89.

41. Vajro P, Ferrante L, Paolella G. Alagille syndrome: an overview. *Clin Res Hepatol Gastroenterol.* 2012;36:275-277.

42. Byrne JA, Meara NJ, Rayner AC, et al. Lack of hepatocellular CD10 along bile canaliculi is physiologic in early childhood and persistent in Alagille syndrome. *Lab Invest.* 2007;87:1138-1148.

43. Sambrotta M, Strautnieks S, Papouli E, et al. Mutations in TJP2 cause progressive cholestatic liver disease. *Nat Genet.* 2014;46:326-328.

44. Gomez-Ospina N, Potter CJ, Xiao R, et al. Mutations in the nuclear bile acid receptor FXR cause progressive familial intrahepatic cholestasis. *Nat Commun.* 2016;7:10713.

45. Gonzales E, Taylor SA, Davit-Spraul A, et al. MYO5B mutations cause cholestasis with normal serum gamma-glutamyl transferase activity in children without microvillous inclusion disease. *Hepatology.* 2017;65:164-173.

46. Henkel SA, Squires JH, Ayers M, et al. Expanding etiology of progressive familial intrahepatic cholestasis. *World J Hepatol.* 2019;11:450-463.

47. Lykavieris P, van Mil S, Cresteil D, et al. Progressive familial intrahepatic cholestasis type 1 and extrahepatic features: no catch-up of stature growth, exacerbation of diarrhea, and appearance of liver steatosis after liver transplantation. *J Hepatol.* 2003;39:447-452.

48. Miyagawa-Hayashino A, Egawa H, Yorifuji T, et al. Allograft steatohepatitis in progressive familial intrahepatic cholestasis type 1 after living donor liver transplantation. *Liver Transpl.* 2009;15:610-618.

49. Davit-Spraul A, Fabre M, Branchereau S, et al. ATP8B1 and ABCB11 analysis in 62 children with normal gamma-glutamyl transferase progressive familial intrahepatic cholestasis (PFIC): phenotypic differences between PFIC1 and PFIC2 and natural history. *Hepatology.* 2010;51:1645-1655.

50. Goubran M, Aderibigbe A, Jacquemin E, et al. Case report: progressive familial intrahepatic cholestasis type 3 with compound heterozygous ABCB4 variants diagnosed 15 years after liver transplantation. *BMC Med Genet.* 2020;21:238.

51. Avena A, Puggelli S, Morris M, et al. ABCB4 variants in adult patients with cholestatic disease are frequent and underdiagnosed. *Dig Liver Dis.* 2021;53:329-344.

52. Wendum D, Barbu V, Rosmorduc O, et al. Aspects of liver pathology in adult patients with MDR3/ABCB4 gene mutations. *Virchows Arch.* 2012;460:291-298.

53. Sun L, Li M, Zhang L, et al. Differences in UGT1A1 gene mutations and pathological liver changes between Chinese patients with Gilbert syndrome and Crigler-Najjar syndrome type II. *Medicine (Baltimore).* 2017;96:e8620.

54. Fata CR, Gillis LA, Pacheco MC. Liver fibrosis associated with Crigler-Najjar syndrome in a compound heterozygote: a case report. *Pediatr Dev Pathol.* 2017;20:522-525.

55. Baris Z, Ozcay F, Usta Y, et al. Liver cirrhosis in a patient with Crigler Najjar syndrome. *Fetal Pediatr Pathol.* 2018;37:301-306.

56. Dawson J, Carr-Locke DL, Talbot IC, et al. Gilbert's syndrome: evidence of morphological heterogeneity. *Gut.* 1979;20:848-853.

57. Kay EW, O'Dowd J, Thomas R, et al. Mild abnormalities in liver histology associated with chronic hepatitis: distinction from normal liver histology. *J Clin Pathol.* 1997;50:929-931.

58. Mizukawa B, George A, Pushkaran S, et al. Cooperating G6PD mutations associated with severe neonatal hyperbilirubinemia and cholestasis. *Pediatr Blood Cancer.* 2011;56:840-842.

13

VASCULAR DISEASE

CONGENITAL/GENETIC ABNORMALITIES

There are many rare congenital or genetic abnormalities that cause abnormal vascular changes in the liver that are not discussed in this book because of space limitations. Instead, we focus on entities that, although still rare, are somewhat more common, and thus more likely to be seen in surgical pathology practice, or illustrate a general injury pattern.

Most genetic conditions that affect the portal vein share a constellation of findings. The individual components will vary in their severity, but all tend to show the following elements: absent or atrophic portal veins, nodular regenerative hyperplasia, abnormal arterialization of the portal tracts and lobules, focal bile ductular proliferations that may resemble downstream biliary tract disease, and a propensity to develop focal nodular hyperplasia.

Abernethy Syndrome

Abernethy syndrome is characterized by a congenitally absent portal vein with shunting of the normal intestinal and splenic blood around the liver into the inferior vena cava. There are three common anatomic subtypes:

- Type 1a malformations are more common in female patients, and the superior mesenteric vein and splenic vein drain directly and separately into the vena cava.
- Type 1b malformations have a male predominance, and the mesenteric vein and splenic vein form a common trunk vessel, which then drains into the inferior vena cava.
- The type II pattern has an intact but often hypoplastic portal vein with a shunt going from the extrahepatic portal vein to inferior vena cava, in which much portal blood flow circumvents the liver.

Of note, the type 1a/1b/II nomenclature is not universal, but these are the three basic patterns for the malformations and, overall, the most common terminology.

Histologically, portal veins are absent in the smaller and medium-sized portal tracts, with occasional hypoplastic portal veins in the larger-sized portal tracts. Nodular regenerative hyperplasia is common. The hepatic arteries often appear hypertrophied and can have prominent muscular coats. Isolated small arterioles can also be found in the hepatic lobules. Focal biliary obstruction–type changes can be present, including focal bile ductular proliferations and mild periportal hepatocyte copper deposition.[1] Fibrosis is absent or mild and limited to the portal tracts. Mass lesions can develop, including focal nodular hyperplasia[1,2] and hepatocellular carcinoma in noncirrhotic livers.[1]

VATER Syndrome

The VATER syndrome (or VACTERL syndrome) is a nonrandom association of birth defects, with most of the defects structural in nature, resulting from undefined defects in the development of the embryonic mesoderm. The etiology is unknown and probably multifactorial. Defects are found in the vertebrae, radius, heart, trachea, esophagus, anus and rectum, and kidneys. Infants can have any combination of features, and there is a wide range of severity.

The liver can be involved, and biopsies can show absent or atrophic portal veins, associated with increased numbers and prominence of arteriole profiles in the portal tracts (Figure 13.1). Overall, the liver findings are similar to that of the Abernethy syndrome, but the associated clinical findings clarify which syndrome is involved. Liver biopsies are typically performed because of unexplained enzyme elevations or portal hypertension. Just as with the Abernethy syndrome, the livers can also develop focal nodular hyperplasias.[3] Lymphatic cysts have also been described.[4] Mitochondrial respiratory chain defects have been reported in rare cases and were associated with elevated liver enzymes.[5]

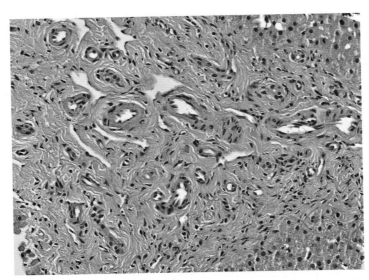

FIGURE 13.1 **VATER syndrome.** The portal tract shows small atrophic portal veins, with only small slit-like veins present. There also are increased numbers of arterial profiles.

Hereditary Hemorrhagic Telangiectasia

Hereditary hemorrhagic telangiectasia (HHT) is also known as the Osler-Weber-Rendu syndrome. HHT is an autosomal dominant genetic disorder leading to abnormal formation of blood vessels in various organs. Mutations disrupt the TGF-beta signaling pathway, and there are several subtypes based on the specific mutation. One of the subtypes is associated with *SMAD4* mutations and juvenile-type polyps of the intestinal tract. The subtype associated with *ALK1* mutations is most likely to have liver disease, but about 40% of patients with *SMAD4* mutations also develop liver arteriovenous malformations (AVMs)[6] and about 50% to 75% of all patients with HHT have at least one vascular abnormality on imaging (telangiectasias, large confluent vascular masses, perfusion abnormalities, or hepatic shunts).[7] Interestingly, HHT can recur after liver transplantation (mean of 10 years), likely as a result of intrahepatic endothelial cell microchimerism, where recipient cells colonize the donor liver and then, in time, recreate telangiectasias.[8]

Vascular telangiectasias can affect the face, oral mucosa including the tongue, and the mucosal lining of the nasal passages. Epistaxes (nose bleeds) are frequent and can be severe. The gastrointestinal (GI) tract is involved in about 20% of cases. Liver disease in the form of AVMs can be seen in 50% to 75% of individuals[9,10] and telangiectasias in 50%.[9] Large AVMs can rarely present as high-output cardiac failure secondary to shunting of blood. Histologically, AVMs show clusters of larger-caliber but thinwalled venous-like vessels that irregularly dissect the liver parenchyma (Figures 13.2 and 13.3). If the section is well orientated, direct shunting

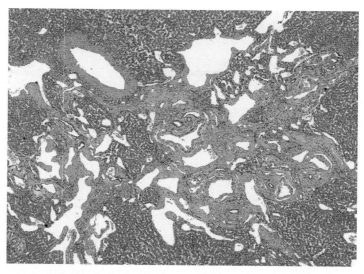

FIGURE 13.2 **Hereditary hemorrhagic telangiectasia.** At low power, the vascular shunt forms a localized lesion. Most larger shunts affect medium-sized portal tracts, as seen in this case.

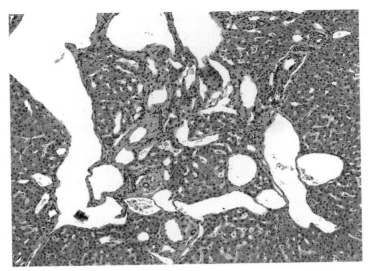

FIGURE 13.3 **Hereditary hemorrhagic telangiectasia.** Another example of the portal-based telangiectasia.

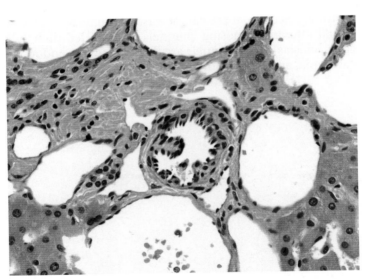

FIGURE 13.4 **Hereditary hemorrhagic telangiectasia.** The telangiectasias lead to shunting of arterial blood to venous-like structures. The precise point of the arterial-to-venous connection can be seen with perfectly oriented cuts or by serial sections; the vessel right at the shunt point is lined by reactive and somewhat epithelioid endothelial cells.

from portal arteries to venous-like structures can be seen; the vessel at the point of the shunt typically is lined by somewhat epithelioid cells (Figure 13.4). Of note, as the vascular ectasias dissect the liver parenchyma, the hepatocytes trapped within can undergo a regenerative response/reactive change that leads to patchy areas of loss of the normal reticulin framework, a finding that can lead to a misdiagnosis of hepatocellular carcinoma.

Larger AVMs can be associated with thicker-walled shunt vessels and localized areas of hemorrhage, fibrosis, and hemosiderin-laden macrophages. Imaging studies commonly demonstrate dilatation of the large hilar hepatic arteries and intrahepatic shunts. The vascular shunting can also lead to a localized hyperplastic response by the parenchyma, causing a focal nodular hyperplasia; focal nodular hyperplasias are seen in about 5% of individuals.[9]

Multiple liver lesions are present in most cases and include AVMs, focal nodular hyperplasias, mass-forming telangiectasias (focal collections of dilated interanastomosing vessels), and other vascular shunts. Livers are generally not biopsied if the diagnosis is known clinically because of an increased risk for bleeding. Some cases, however, are not diagnosed prior to the biopsy, or a biopsy is performed to exclude a malignancy. In addition, some cases of HHT have only a single liver lesion on imaging[9] and the diagnosis is not evident based on clinical findings and imaging studies.

Histologically, mass lesions in patients with HHT show several different patterns, in addition to AVMs described above. First, there can be focal nodular hyperplasias that are histologically similar to those in the sporadic setting.[11] Second, there can be vascular mass lesions with distinctive abnormal interanastomosing channels that are fed directly by portal veins (telangiectasias). The channels are thin walled, the endothelium lacks cytological atypia, and Ki-67 shows an absent or very low proliferative rate (Figures 13.5-13.7). The channels dissect the hepatic parenchyma, leaving

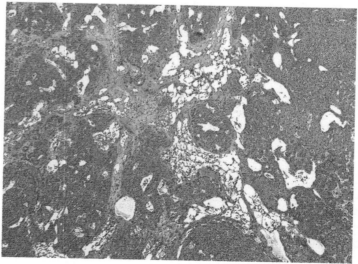

FIGURE 13.5 **Hereditary hemorrhagic telangiectasia.** An interanastomosing growth pattern is seen at low power.

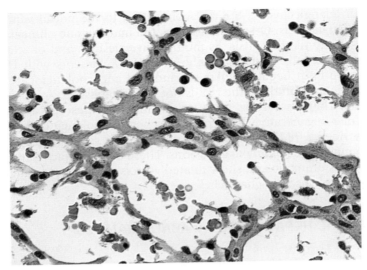

FIGURE 13.6 **Hereditary hemorrhagic telangiectasia.** At higher power, some of the shunt vessels have a hemangioma-like appearance.

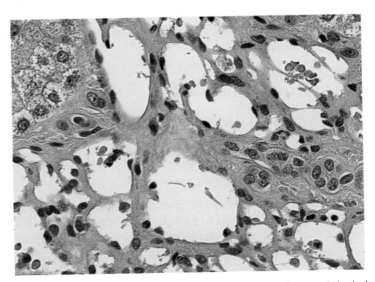

FIGURE 13.7 **Hereditary hemorrhagic telangiectasia.** There is no cytological atypia in the hemangioma-like areas.

residual portal tracts. The hepatic lobules may show mild hyperplasia but are without well-defined regenerative nodules. The histology of mass-forming telangiectasias is very distinctive, but the differential can include an anastomosing hemangioma. Anastomosing hemangiomas tend to be better circumscribed and the vascular channels are less interanastomosing than with telangiectasias. A direct connection to the portal vein may be seen in telangiectasis. On small biopsies, the imaging and clinical findings can also clarify the diagnosis, as multiple liver lesions and or telangiectasias of other organs would strongly favor HHT. Patients with HHT can also develop both hepatocellular carcinoma[12] and cholangiocarcinoma,[13] although the magnitude of the risk is not well established.

Other changes besides mass lesions include sinusoidal dilatation[11,14] and nodular regenerative hyperplasia. Ischemic cholangiopathy has also been described.[11,12] Microscopic telangiectasias are routinely present in the parenchyma outside of any mass lesions. These microscopic telangiectasias are often less dramatic and show dilated vessels with less prominent interanastomosis of vascular channels.

NONGENETIC HEPATIC INFLOW ABNORMALITIES
Portal Vein Thrombosis

Portal Vein Thrombosis, Acute
- Most common pattern of injury: macrovesicular steatosis
- Less common pattern of injury: zone 3 ischemic necrosis if there also is severe hypotension

Portal Vein Disease, Chronic
- Hepatoportal sclerosis pattern of injury
  - Portal vein atrophy/fibrosis
  - Portal vein herniation/dilatation
  - Fibrotic portal vein thrombosis
- Nodular regenerative hyperplasia

Thrombosis of the extrahepatic portal vein leads to liver injury, but the thrombi itself are not present in peripheral biopsy specimens. There are many possible causes of portal vein thrombosis, but approximately 15% of cases remain idiopathic.[15] Cirrhosis is a major risk factor (present in about 30% of cases). In noncirrhotic patients, risk factors are often grouped into these categories: (1) estrogen related (OCP use, pregnancy, etc), (2) underlying genetic thrombotic disorders, (3) intraabdominal malignancies, (4) structural abnormalities from prior surgery or procedures, including remote perinatal injury of the umbilical vein, for example, from sepsis or canalization, and (5) transient inflammatory conditions, such as pancreatitis, appendicitis, and diverticulitis. Recently, COVID-19 has been noted to cause portal vein thrombosis.[16] Extrahepatic portal vein thrombosis can often be clinically occult and manifest with portal hypertension and ascites, leading to a clinical working diagnosis of probable cirrhosis.

Histologically, acute extrahepatic portal vein thrombosis is often associated with macrovesicular steatosis (but generally not steatohepatitis).[16] Ischemic necrosis in zone 3 hepatocytes is rare unless the patient also has severe hypotension.

Chronic extrahepatic portal vein thrombosis is often associated with the hepatoportal sclerosis pattern of injury (see below). In addition, extrahepatic portal vein thrombi can rarely lead to strictures and irregularities of the extrahepatic bile ducts, a finding called *portal biliopathy*. The changes can radiographically mimic cholangiocarcinoma. Portal biliopathy is more common in noncirrhotic than cirrhotic livers and is associated with extension of the thrombosis into the mesenteric veins. Portal biliopathy is thought to develop as collaterals around the thrombosed portal vein compress the extrahepatic bile ducts. The diagnosis is usually made radiographically, and biopsies are rare. When biopsied, the portal tracts show ductular proliferation in keeping with extrahepatic bile duct obstruction.

Smaller intrahepatic branches of the portal veins, such as those at the periphery of the liver, only rarely show thrombosis but when they occur they may be seen on liver biopsy specimens, often in association with other portal tract changes and nodular regenerative hyperplasia. These small intrahepatic thrombi generally have a different differential than thrombosis of the extrahepatic portal veins. If seen as a generalized process, involving multiple portal veins, then the differential is primarily that of prothrombotic clotting disorders. Localized portal vein thrombosis involving a segmental or subsegmental portal vein can be associated with a variety of mass-forming pseudotumors such as nodular elastosis or regenerative hepatic pseudotumor. In these cases, the cause of the localized portal vein thrombosis is usually idiopathic, but search for prothrombotic risk factors can still be useful.

Idiopathic Portal Hypertension and Hepatoportal Sclerosis

Idiopathic portal hypertension or idiopathic noncirrhotic portal hypertension are the clinical terms for cases where the liver is noncirrhotic and no extrahepatic portal vein thrombosis is seen. Some cases of idiopathic portal hypertension are related to prior, remote extrahepatic portal vein thromboses that have recannulated, or are still there but radiographically occult.

The constellation of histological findings seen in idiopathic noncirrhotic portal hypertension is referred to as *hepatoportal sclerosis*. This term is not perfect, and so there have been a bunch of attempts to replace this term with ones that tend to be even more cumbersome and often less accurate, so for now we will stick with *hepatoportal sclerosis*, the standard term used by most liver pathologists.

The histological findings in hepatoportal sclerosis are often subtle. The portal veins can appear atrophic (Figure 13.8) or be completely absent. In other cases, there may be increased numbers of small-caliber portal

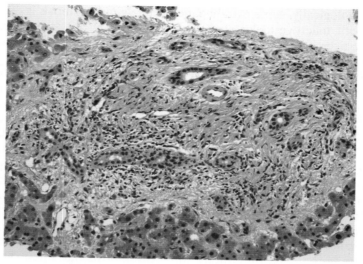

FIGURE 13.8 **Portal vein atrophy.** The portal vein is smaller than the hepatic artery.

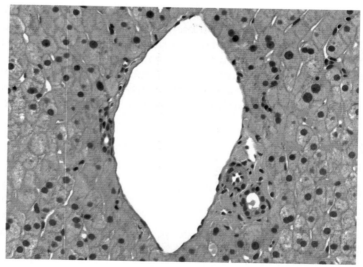

FIGURE 13.9 **Portal vein dilatation.** The portal vein is huge.

veins, portal vein dilatation (Figure 13.9), or portal vein branches that extend into the surrounding zone 1 hepatocytes (Figure 13.10), a finding called *portal vein herniation*. In rare cases, the intrahepatic portal veins can show recent thrombosis. The thrombi can also be remote and recannulated, with the vein wall showing striking muscularization (Figure 13.11). In other cases, there can be dense fibrous scars completely replacing the portal veins (Figure 13.12).

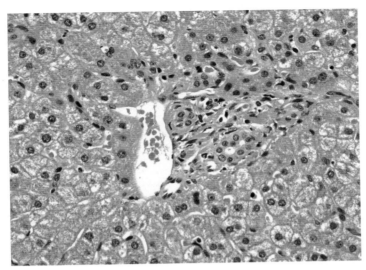

FIGURE 13.10 **Portal vein herniation.** The portal vein extends or "herniates" out of the portal tract connective tissue, into the surrounding zone 1 parenchyma.

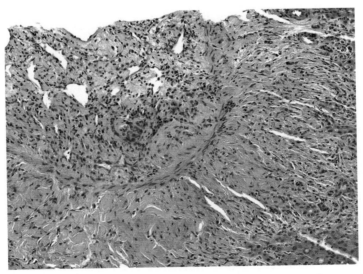

FIGURE 13.11 **Portal vein with muscular hypertrophy.** This biopsy from an individual with unexplained portal hypertension showed portal tracts with thrombosis and recanalization of the portal vein. There is striking muscular hypertrophy of the vein wall, and it resembles a large central vein.

The liver parenchyma often shows changes of nodular regenerative hyperplasia (NRH) (Figure 13.13). In fact, if the portal vein changes are subtle or equivocal, the diagnosis is strengthened by the presence of NRH; likewise, if there is no NRH in cases with subtle portal vein changes, the changes

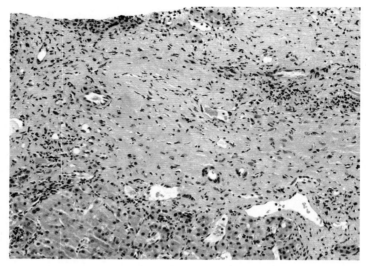

FIGURE 13.12 **Portal vein fibrosis.** The portal vein is completely replaced by a fibrous scar.

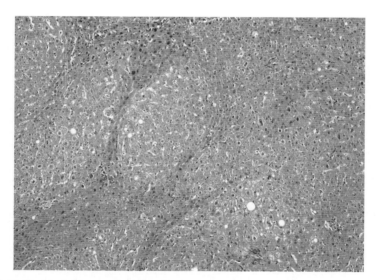

FIGURE 13.13 **Nodular regenerative hyperplasia.** Distinct nodularity without fibrosis is seen.

should be approached more circumspectly, especially if other parenchymal liver diseases are present, such as chronic hepatitis, chronic biliary tract disease, or steatohepatitis, as the portal veins in these settings can show nonspecific reactive changes. Another subtle finding can be small isolated bile ducts in the lobules (Figure 13.14), a finding called *naked ducts*. Although this finding is not specific, it is seen in about 40% of hepatoportal sclerosis cases,[17] whereas naked bile ducts are relatively rare in other conditions.

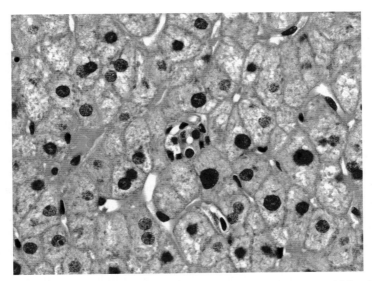

FIGURE 13.14 **Naked bile duct.** A small isolated bile duct is seen in the middle of the lobule. This finding is also called a *portal tract remnant.*

Hepatic Artery Disease

Hepatic Artery Disease, Acute
- Mild or intermittent disease: increased hepatic apoptosis and mitosis
- Severe arterial disease:
  - widespread necrosis can occur, especially if there also is reduced portal vein blood flow
  - focal subcapsular infarcts can occur with intrahepatic arterial thrombosis affecting the smaller branches of the hepatic artery

Hepatic Artery Disease, Chronic
- Bile ductular proliferation as a result of ischemic biliary strictures
- Ductopenia due to chronic biliary ischemia

Hepatic artery disease is rare, but the most common causes are thrombosis or vasculitis. Hepatic artery strictures/stenosis are seen mostly in the setting of liver transplantation. In the nontransplanted liver, hepatic arterial injury is very rare but may occur after severe pancreatitis with suppurative acute cholangitis, following intraarterial chemotherapy, or after surgery (such as resections of hilar tumors) or other abdominal interventions (such as radiofrequency ablation for hepatocellular carcinoma). Rare idiopathic cases have also been reported.[18] In the nontransplanted liver, the extrahepatic portal vein usually carries sufficient blood flow to compensate for the loss of the extrahepatic arterial blood supply (through retrograde blood flow from the portal circulation), but there can be ischemic injury if there are other comorbid conditions such as hypotension. In addition, injury to the smaller intrahepatic branches of the liver often leads to focal areas of subcapsular infarction.

The pathological findings will vary depending on the location of the vascular injury and the clinical setting. With liver transplantation, where the changes have been best described, early histological findings following hepatic artery thrombosis include increased lobular spotty necrosis and increased numbers of mitotic figures with little or no inflammation.[19,20] Severe arterial compromise can lead to intrahepatic infarcts in both liver allografts and in some nontransplant settings, such as malignant hypertension (Figure 13.15). Long-term hepatic artery compromise can lead to chronic biliary tract disease, including bile duct strictures and bile duct loss. The bile duct disease results from the loss of arterial blood flow, as bile ducts obtain most of their blood supply from the hepatic arteries.

A true arteritis is very rare but is mostly likely to occur as part of a systemic vasculitis, such as polyarteritis nodosa. The arteries show fibrinoid necrosis, sometimes leading to a vaguely granulomatous appearance, with artery-centered inflammation composed of mixed lymphocytes, plasma cells, and neutrophils (Figure 13.16). The differential can include arterial hyalinosis, but this pattern results from hypertension and diabetes mellitus and is not associated with inflammatory destruction of the hepatic artery.

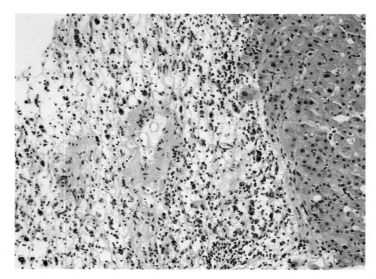

FIGURE 13.15 **Hepatic artery disease.** This patient with malignant hypertension had hypodense lesions throughout the liver. A biopsy showed subacute zone 3 necrosis affecting most zone 3 regions.

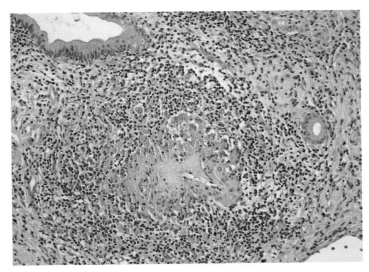

FIGURE 13.16 **Hepatic artery disease.** This case of polyarteritis nodosa shows inflammatory destruction of the hepatic artery.

SINUSOIDAL DISEASE

Sinusoidal disease can impair normal blood flow through the liver by physically blocking the sinusoids.

Histological Findings in Sinusoidal Obstructive Disease

- Sinusoidal congestion, dilatation
- Occlusion of terminal central veins (not always present)
- Perivenular/pericellular fibrosis, with long-standing disease

---

Sinusoidal Obstructive Syndrome

Some years ago, the term *sinusoidal obstruction syndrome* was chosen by a small group to replace the venerable term *veno-occlusive disease* because the veins are not always histologically occluded in a biopsy specimen. Although this fact was reasonably well understood by pathologists, who successfully used the term veno-occlusive disease for a very long time, the term caused unhappiness to some, who pushed to change the terminology and prevent future confusion. Whether or not much confusion was there to begin with is a matter of debate (not really, nobody was confused), but sinusoidal obstruction syndrome is a fine enough term and should serve just as usefully as veno-occlusive disease, at least until yet another group in the future decides to change the name to something else, probably longer and vaguer.

Sinusoidal obstruction syndrome/veno-occlusive disease (SOS/ VOD) is caused by toxic or inflammatory injury to the endothelium of the sinusoids and/or central veins. Obliteration of the central veins is present in about 50% of liver biopsies of SOS/VOD, and, despite the new moniker of SOS, can be a key histological finding. Potential etiologies include herbal teas or remedies, bone marrow transplantation, and drugs used for chemotherapy. Total body or hepatic radiation therapy is also a risk factor. Many recent cases in the literature have been associated with oxaliplatin therapy for colon carcinoma, but the frequency of chemotherapy-related SOS/VOD varies substantially in the literature. This reflects differences in both clinical protocols for chemotherapy as well as diagnostic practices by pathologists, as some pathologists appear to have relatively low thresholds. For example, mild and patchy sinusoidal dilatation in resection specimens is very common, even in cases without histories of chemotherapy, and can sometimes be overinterpreted as SOS/VOD. On the other hand, this disease pattern can occasionally be underrecognized.

Histologically, the SOS/VOD pattern of injury from chemotherapy manifests as sinusoidal dilatation and congestion (Figure 13.17; eFig. 13.1). These changes typically have a zone 3 distribution, often with "bridging congestion" on resection specimens or large biopsy specimens (Figure 13.18). The zone 3 hepatocytes often show atrophy and occasionally small foci of acidophil bodies. Increased Kupffer cell iron accumulation can be present in long-standing disease. In addition, the central veins may show fibrous obliteration by loose and finely reticulated collagen, a finding that is often best seen on trichrome stain (Figure 13.19). The lobules show little or no

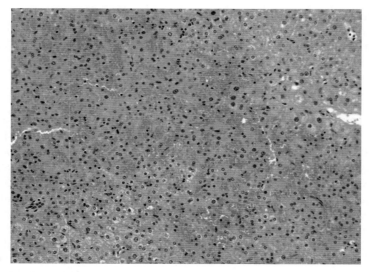

FIGURE 13.17 **Sinusoidal obstructive syndrome.** The zone 3 region shows marked sinusoidal dilation and congestion.

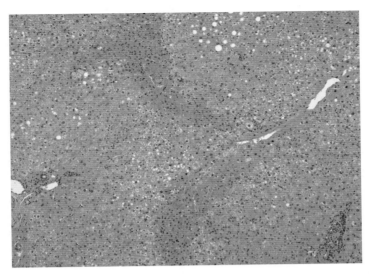

FIGURE 13.18 **Sinusoidal obstructive syndrome.** At low power, the liver shows "bridging congestion."

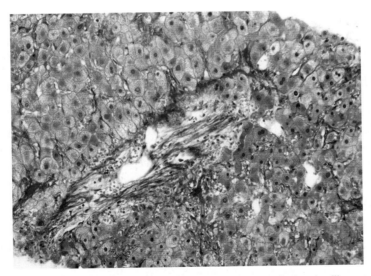

FIGURE 13.19 **Sinusoidal obstructive syndrome with central vein fibrous obliteration.** A trichrome stain shows partial obliteration of the central vein by fine reticulated collagen.

inflammation. Nodular regenerative hyperplasia and peliosis hepatis also may be present. Later, the liver can show marked central vein scarring in severe and long standing disease, with less prominent sinusoidal dilatation.

Histological changes in SOS/VOD from non–chemotherapy-related drugs, for example, from herbal remedies, can have also mild lymphocytic

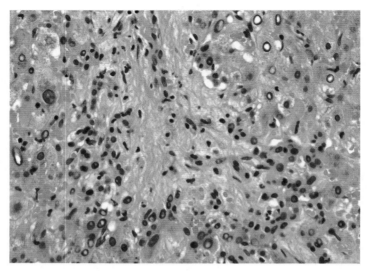

FIGURE 13.20 **Sinusoidal obstructive syndrome.** This biopsy showed veno-occlusion of the small central veins, with mild inflammatory changes, and was associated with herbal tea use.

inflammation in the scarred central veins (Figure 13.20). The portal tracts also commonly show mild, predominately lymphocytic inflammation. Sinusoids are commonly dilated and congested, but this component is often less dramatic than that of chemotherapy-related SOS/VOD.

The differential for SOS/VOD can include cautery effect in resection specimens or wedge biopsies. In these cases, the sinusoids can show artifactual dilation, often dramatic, due to the cautery (eFig. 13.2). The sinusoidal dilation can sometimes even retain a zone 3 pattern, although usually the changes show no zonal associations. The sinusoids typically do not contain blood but instead are empty or have a gray amphophilic material (eFig. 13.2).

Radiation Changes

Radiation to the liver is performed in some medical centers prior to resection of primary liver carcinoma, usually cholangiocarcinoma, or for metastatic carcinoma to the liver. Within the radiation field, the liver may show a distinctive pattern of injury, with the sinusoids and central veins distended and blocked by fine, edematous collagen (Figure 13.21). The hepatocytes often show atrophy. Larger hepatic arteries can show foam cell arteriopathy (Figure 13.22).

Sickle Cell Disease

Patients with sickle cell anemia are generally not biopsied during sickle cell crisis, and the clinical diagnosis is usually known before the biopsy. Instead, most biopsies tend to be performed to assess for iron overload

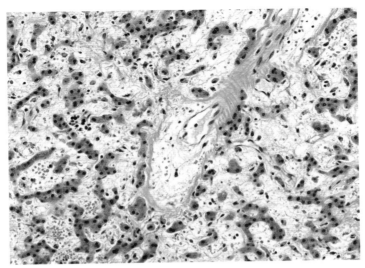

FIGURE 13.21 **Radiation changes**. The sinusoids are obstructed by a fine, edematous matrix.

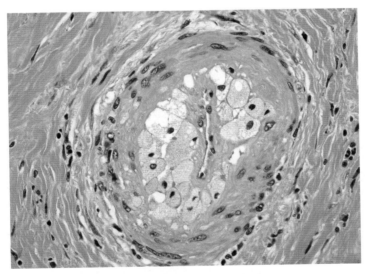

FIGURE 13.22 **Radiation changes**. Foam cell arteriopathy is seen.

secondary to transfusions or sometimes to stage the liver fibrosis. In some cases, patients with clinically unknown sickle cell trait are first diagnosed on liver biopsy, but this is rare, even in populations with a high frequency of sickle cell disease.

The predominant histological finding is typically iron overload, with moderate to marked hepatocellular and Kupffer cell iron accumulation. The sinusoids often show congestion (Figure 13.23), and erythrophagocytosis is

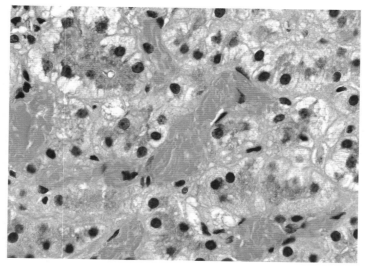

FIGURE 13.23 **Sickle cell anemia, congestion.** The sinusoids show diffuse congestion at low power.

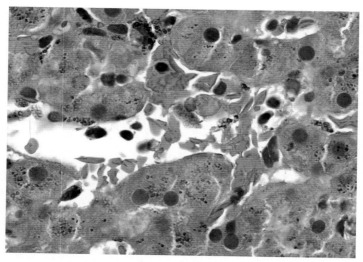

FIGURE 13.24 **Sickle cell anemia, sickled red blood cells.** At higher magnification, sickled red blood cells can be seen in the sinusoids.

found in most cases with sufficient searching (Figure 13.24). Some cases may also show mild biliary tract obstructive-type changes, as passage of small biliary stones is common. With improved medical management and improvements in life-spans, liver cirrhosis secondary to the iron overload is of increasing clinical concern (eFig. 13.3). The fibrosis progresses from portal fibrosis to bridging fibrosis to cirrhosis. Approximately 10% to 20% of individuals will develop liver cirrhosis.[21,22]

Other findings may be seen in autopsy studies but are rare in biopsy specimens, because biopsies are typically not performed in the clinical setting of acute hepatic sickle cell crisis. These findings can range from varying degrees of cholestasis and sinusoidal congestion to frank ischemic-type necrosis. In the rare event of acute hepatic sequestration, there is marked sinusoidal congestion with numerous sickled red blood cells and marked lobular cholestasis. Acute hepatic sequestration differs from acute hepatic sickle cell crisis because the former is also accompanied by a marked drop in the hematocrit, secondary to blockage of the sinusoids by sickled red blood cells, and this leads to massive sequestration of blood within the liver.

Other Causes of Sinusoidal Obstruction

Other rare diseases that can lead to the blockage of sinusoidal blood flow include widespread tumor involvement of the liver, most commonly breast carcinoma, pancreatic ductal carcinoma, or melanoma. Amyloidosis can also impair blood flow when the deposits are massive.

VASCULAR OUTFLOW DISEASE

Vascular Outflow Disease

- Main findings: sinusoidal congestion, dilatation
- Additional findings
  - Hepatocyte atrophy in zone 3
  - Reactive bile ductular proliferation in portal tracts, usually mild
  - Occlusion/thrombosis of larger central veins (rarely present in biopsy material)
  - Kupffer cell predominant secondary iron deposition (in long-standing cases)
- Perivenular/pericellular fibrosis with long-standing disease

The core histological pattern of vascular outflow disease consists of varying degrees of sinusoidal dilation, sinusoidal congestion, hepatocyte atrophy and/or dropout in zone 3, and zone 3 fibrosis in long-standing cases. There often is patchy, mild bile ductular proliferation in the portal tracts, which may be accompanied by mild mixed inflammation.[23] Nonetheless, the overall inflammatory changes tend to be minimal to absent. There can be histological overlap with the SOS/VOD, but the combined clinical history (eg, history of heart failure), imaging findings, and histology lead to the correct diagnosis.

Very mild and patchy sinusoidal dilatation is often a nonspecific finding that may simply reflect mild volume overload at the time of liver biopsy

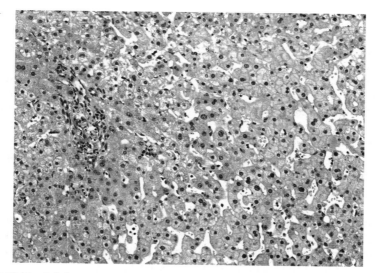

FIGURE 13.25 **Subtle zone 3 vascular out flow disease.** The sinusoidal dilatation is mild and of uncertain significance.

or can be a processing artifact. Histological changes that increase one's confidence in a diagnosis of vascular outflow obstruction include diffuse sinusoidal dilatation throughout the biopsy, sinusoidal dilatation that at least focally reaches the moderate level somewhere in the biopsy, zone 3 hepatocyte atrophy or dropout, zone 3 fibrosis, or zone 3 intermediate hepatocytes on CK7. Finding CK7-positive zone 3 intermediate hepatocytes can be particularly helpful when other H&E findings are subtle and you are on the fence (Figures 13.25 and 13.26).

Budd-Chiari Syndrome

Budd-Chiari syndrome is caused by occlusion of the hepatic veins. The current definition includes all causes of occlusion and the location can range from the medium and larger-sized intrahepatic veins to the inferior vena cava. The histological findings in peripheral biopsies are generally not specific, so heart disease and SOS/VOD need to be excluded.

The classic symptoms are not always present but, with acute cases, include abdominal pain, hepatomegaly, and recent-onset ascites. Many cases develop slowly and the patient can present with ascites suggestive of cirrhosis. The majority of cases of primary Budd-Chiari syndrome are caused by thrombosis of the hepatic veins secondary to myeloproliferative disorders or clotting disorders (Table 13.1), but compression of the hepatic veins by nearby mass lesions also can lead to secondary Budd-Chiari syndrome. In 40% to 50% of cases, more than one predisposing factor is present. Also, of note, about 25% of cases have a coexisting portal vein thrombus.

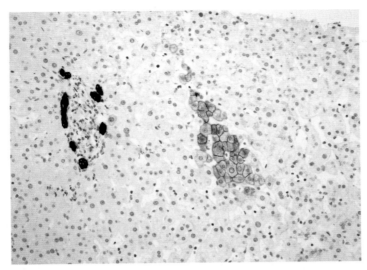

FIGURE 13.26 Subtle zone 3 vascular outflow disease, CK7. Focal zone 3 staining of hepatocytes is seen; bile ductules are also positive in the adjacent portal tract. Further workup identified right-sided heart failure. Same case and same field as the preceding image.

TABLE 13.1 **Risk Factors for Budd-Chiari Syndrome**	
Risk	**Approximate Percent of All Cases**
Anti-phospholipid antibodies	25
Hyperhomocysteinemia	25
Paroxysmal nocturnal hemoglobinuria	20
Factor V Leiden mutation	10
Protein C deficiency	3
Protein S deficiency	3
Prothrombin mutation	3
Antithrombin deficiency	3
Polycythemia vera	30
Essential thrombocythemia	10
Other	10
Oral contraceptives	25
Recent pregnancy (prior 3 months)	5
Systemic inflammatory diseases (eg, connective tissue disease, inflammatory bowel disease, sarcoidosis, vasculitis)	25

The percentages do not add up to 100 because a large proportion of cases have more than one risk factor.

Histologically, thrombi are typically not seen on peripheral liver biopsies. Instead, the main finding is that of sinusoidal dilatation and congestion. Rarely, the thrombus can originate in the medium or larger-sized intrahepatic veins (or propagate in from outside the liver) and be sampled on liver biopsy (Figure 13.27). The zone 3 hepatocytes are often atrophic, and there can be hepatocyte dropout (Figure 13.28). Acute obstruction can cause extravasation of red blood cells into the space of Disse; this finding can occasionally be prominent and confidently

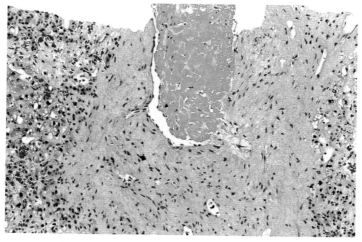

FIGURE 13.27 **Budd-Chiari, thrombi.** A thrombus is seen in the central vein in this case of acute Budd-Chiari syndrome.

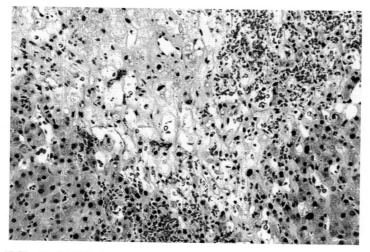

FIGURE 13.28 **Budd-Chiari, zone 3 dropout.** In this case, there is zone 3 hepatocyte dropout and a small atrophic central vein.

identified, but in most cases red blood cell extravasation is focal and equivocal and the diagnosis of vascular outflow disease is best made by looking for other findings, such as marked zone 3 congestion (eFig. 13.4). Zone 3 ischemic necrosis is a rare finding, but it can be seen in cases of severe, acute Budd-Chiari syndrome. Central vein/zone 3 pericellular fibrosis is common in long-standing disease. The portal tracts may show mild and patchy bile ductular proliferation. Mild nonspecific inflammation can be seen in both the lobules and portal tracts but is not a prominent finding.

Heart Failure

Congestive heart failure or chronic lung disease with right-sided heart failure can lead to congestive hepatopathy of the liver. The sinusoids are dilated and often congested, lined by atrophic zone 3 hepatocytes (Figure 13.29; eFig. 13.5). With sufficient time, there can be zone 3 hepatocyte drop-out and fibrosis. Kupffer cell hyperplasia and iron deposits are common (eFig. 13.6). The sinusoidal dilation often becomes less pronounced as fibrosis progresses to advanced fibrosis and cirrhosis. In a subset of cases, long-standing chronic outflow disease can also be associated with the development of pseudo–ground glass inclusions in the hepatocytes (Figure 13.30). The mechanism for the development of these inclusions is unclear, but they are a nonspecific reactive change and do not influence clinical outcomes. A specific staging system can be useful for congestive hepatopathy,[24] although more general staging systems also work well, including Ishak, Batts-Ludwig, and Metavir. Fibrosis can be patchy with congestive heart disease, so small biopsies should be interpreted cautiously.

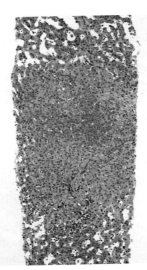

FIGURE 13.29 **Congestive heart failure.** At low power, the zone 3 dilatation (top and bottom of image) stands out on this biopsy of an individual with chronic congestive heart failure. In contrast, the zone 1 region (center of image) has normal sinusoidal spacing.

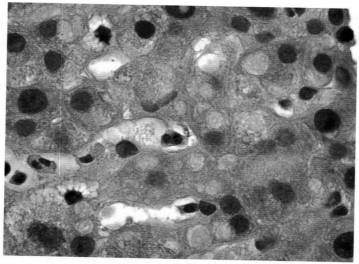

FIGURE 13.30 **Congestive heart failure.** A subset of individuals with chronic vascular out-flow disease can develop pseudo-ground glass inclusions.

Other Causes of Sinusoidal Dilatation

Sinusoidal dilatation and congestion, even when prominent, are not specific for vascular outflow disease and can result from a wide variety of causes (Table 13.2). In most of these cases, the etiology is not evident by histology and requires clinical correlation.

NODULAR REGENERATIVE HYPERPLASIA

Nodular regenerative hyperplasia develops in livers with altered patterns of blood flow that disrupt the normal balance between hepatic vein and hepatic arterial inflow to the liver. Nodular regenerative hyperplasia is commonly associated with significantly elevated alkaline phosphatase levels but normal or mildly elevated aspartate aminotransferase and alanine aminotransferase levels. There are a wide variety of clinical and pathological associations (Table 13.3). Nodular regenerative hyperplasia is a diffuse parenchymal finding. When the nodularity is heavily accentuated in the hilar region, the term *nodular transformation* is used.

The gross and imaging findings in cases of nodular regenerative hyperplasia can mimic cirrhosis. However, histologically there is no evidence for cirrhosis and typically no fibrosis at all. The hepatic parenchyma instead shows a diffuse nodularity that results from small atrophic hepatocytes, usually located in zone 3, that contrast with the normal-sized to slightly enlarged hepatocytes in zones 1 and 2. These changes are highlighted nicely by a reticulin stain (Figure 13.31), which shows the compressed and smaller zone 3 hepatic plates juxtaposed with the normal-to-wider hepatic plates in zones 1 and 2.

TABLE 13.2   Diseases Associated With Sinusoidal Dilation and Congestion

Diagnoses	Representative Reference or Comment
Vascular outflow disease	
Budd-Chiari	
Heart disease	
Drug effect	
Estrogen	[25]
Azathioprine	[26]
Chemotherapy such as oxaliplatin	
Autoimmune disease	
Rheumatoid arthritis	[27]
Antiphospholipid syndrome	[28]
Takayasu arteritis	[29]
Castleman disease	[30]
Crohn disease	[31]
Still disease	[32]
Sarcoidosis	[32]
Paraneoplastic syndrome	
Hodgkin lymphoma	[33]
Renal cell carcinoma	[34]
Systemic infections	
HIV	[35]
Brucellosis	[31]
Tuberculosis	[31]
Other	
Heroin use	[36]
Sickle cell anemia	
Hemophagocytosis syndrome	[37]

Nodular regenerative hyperplasia can be seen with or without portal tract vascular changes, including hepatoportal sclerosis or other vascular abnormalities such as portal vein wall hypertrophy (eFig. 13.7). Nodular regenerative hyperplasia is easy to overdiagnose, since many times the reticulin stain is not completely "normal" and the patient may be known to have risk factors for nodular regenerative hyperplasia. A good way to confirm the diagnosis is to make sure the alkaline phosphatase shows disproportionate elevations; also, in essentially all cases, the parenchymal nodularity is evident on H&E, at least in retrospect after the reticulin stain

TABLE 13.3 **Diseases Associated With Nodular Regenerative Hyperplasia**

Diagnoses	Representative Reference or Comment
Familial	This is very rare[38]
Medications	
Azathioprine	Commonly seen with high-dose therapy for inflammatory bowel disease[39]
Didanosine	[40]
Stavudine	[40]
Oxaliplatin	[41]
Immune dysfunction	
Hypogammaglobulinemia	[42]
Common variable immunodeficiency	[43]
HIV infection	
Myasthenia gravis	[44]
Rheumatoid arthritis	[45]
Systemic lupus erythematosus	[46]
Chronic granulomatous disease	[47]
Castleman disease	
Celiac disease	[48]
Tumors	
Hepatocellular carcinoma	In the literature, it is often not clear if there is another underlying liver disease causing both NRH and HCC
Carcinoid tumor	[49]
Hodgkin lymphoma	
Non-Hodgkin lymphoma	
Chronic lymphocytic leukemia	
Chronic myelogenous leukemia	
Multiple myeloma	
Aplastic anemia	
Prothrombotic disorders	Commonly associated with portal vein thrombosis
Others	
Chronic heart disease	Mostly congestive heart failure
Genetic syndromes with associated abnormalities in liver blood flow	Abernathy syndrome, Turner syndrome
Liver allograft	

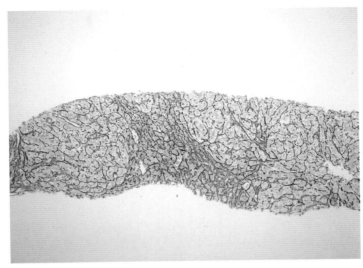

FIGURE 13.31 **Nodular regenerative hyperplasia, reticulin stain.** There is distinct parenchymal nodularity.

is examined. In fact, if either of these two features are not present, then the diagnosis should be carefully considered. Sharing the case with a colleague can also be helpful, at least if you have a good one.

Nodular regenerative hyperplasia can also develop de novo after liver transplantation.[50-52] The full significance of this finding has not been well established, but the development of nodular regenerative hyperplasia in the first few years after transplantation may increase the risk for subsequent development of portal hypertension.[51] In many cases, the etiology is idiopathic, but azathioprine is a potential cause.[52]

PELIOSIS HEPATIS

Peliosis hepatis is defined by localized areas of sinusoidal dilation that form varied-sized cavities, leading to distinct, blood-filled pools or lakes (Figure 13.32). There is a wide range of etiologies, but the most common are chronic debilitating diseases (eg, untreated mycobacterium tuberculosis, cancer), medication effects, or bacillary peliosis associated with *Bartonella henselae* infection, especially in immunosuppressed persons. The most common medications associated with peliosis hepatis are oral contraceptives, androgens, and azathioprine.

The liver is the most common organ affected by peliosis, but there can be peliosis in the spleen, bone marrow, lymph nodes, and very rarely other organs such as the GI tract, adrenals, and kidney.[53] Liver involvement can be focal or diffuse, with hepatomegaly present in most cases with diffuse disease.

The vascular lakes connect directly to the sinusoids and/or the central veins. The vascular lakes usually have liquid blood, but there can be

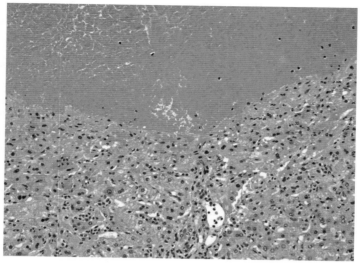

FIGURE 13.32 **Peliosis hepatis.** This large pool of blood was visible grossly to surgeon (hundreds of small lesions) when a wedge biopsy was performed. The individual had a chronic debilitating illness.

early thrombosis and organization at the edges. The vascular lakes typically lack an endothelial lining, although larger vascular lakes can develop a discontinuous layer of endothelial cells over time. The background liver is typically noncirrhotic and is without significant inflammation or findings to suggest SOS/VOD or vascular outflow disease.

HEREDITARY LYMPHEDEMA

Hereditary lymphedema is a rare, heterogenous set of diseases that have a number of syndromic names such as *lymphedema cholestasis syndrome, Emberger syndrome, Milroy syndrome,* and *Hennekam syndrome.* Disease patterns can also be organized by age at presentation. The infant forms (type I) include Milroy disease and Norwegian lymphedema cholestasis syndrome. Some of these patients will present clinically with neonatal cholestasis that over time becomes more episodic and then resolves over the next few years,[54] although cholestasis can reemerge after surgery or other significant medical stressors, during pregnancies, and sometimes without any clear trigger.[55] Type II disease presents at puberty and includes *Meige disease.* Adult presentation is called *lymphedema tarda,* and many patients present in their 30s or later.

The inheritance patterns include autosomal recessive, autosomal dominant, and X linked. In addition, disease penetrance ranges from low to high, with some evidence that disease penetrance may be higher in women. There are dozens of different mutations, but most cluster into the FGFR3 or RAS signaling pathways.

The lymphatic abnormalities can be broadly classified as (1) functional impairment with intact lymphatics, but lymph is poorly absorbed at the "blind end loop" start point of the lymphatics or (2) structurally disorganized lymphatics including valves that do not function.

Clinically, the degree of lymphedema varies considerably. There can be peripheral subcutaneous lymphedema, ascites, and, less commonly, pleural and pericardial effusions. Treatment is focused on alleviating syndromes and includes compression therapies and lymphatic drainage.

Histological findings are only sparsely reported in the literature, but the changes appear to depend on whether the mutation leads to functional impairment or disorganized lymphatics. Functional impairment often presents in early childhood and can show a bland cholestatic injury pattern in infants without features of biliary obstruction.[56] Some patients can progress to cirrhosis in early childhood.[55,56] Children with Milroy disease can also show a congestive hepatopathy pattern of injury. In adults, patients often present with recurrent lower extremity edema and/or unexplained ascites, and the liver may be biopsied to rule out parenchymal disease or cirrhosis. On biopsy, the histological findings can be very subtle, but all revolve around disorganization of the lymphatics and vasculature, often including the smaller branches of the hepatic arteries.[57] Changes are seen in the smallest branches of the hepatic arteries and include arterial dilatation, material that appears to be lymph in arteries, arterial endothelium that is very reactive and almost epithelioid in appearance, and glomeruloid structures in small vessels (Figure 13.33). Other rare presentations include secondary sclerosing cholangitis, resulting from dilated lymphatics obstructing the bile duct.[58]

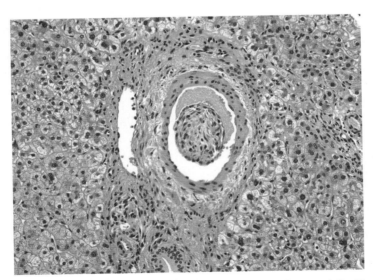

FIGURE 13.33 **Hereditary lymphedema.** The patient presented as an adult with a history of recurrent ascites and lower leg edema. The biopsy showed subtle changes in the vasculature, including focal glomeruloid-type changes in the hepatic arteries.

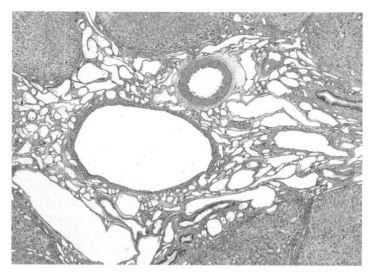

FIGURE 13.34 **Cirrhotic liver with marked but nonspecific dilatation of lymphatics.**

In terms of diagnostic pitfalls, in some cirrhotic livers, there can be marked dilatation of the lymphatics in patients without genetic lymphatic abnormalities (Figure 13.34).

PARTIAL NODULAR TRANSFORMATION

Partial nodular transformation is a very rare condition that essentially looks like nodular regenerative hyperplasia, but in contrast to diffuse changes in nodular regenerative hyperplasia, the nodules are localized primarily to the liver hilum and the nodules tend to be larger than seen in typical nodular regenerative hyperplasia. This pattern is found most commonly at autopsy, where it has been associated with portal vein thrombosis[59,60] or hypoplastic portal veins.[61] Patients often have portal hypertension, which can be severe. Some cases of primary sclerosing cholangitis can also show this pattern.

PSEUDOTUMORS AND TUMORS ASSOCIATED WITH VASCULAR FLOW ABNORMALITIES

Ischemic Infarcts

Localized ischemic infarcts in cirrhotic livers can lead to mass-forming lesions visible on imaging, which can mimic malignancy. These lesions were at one time called *hypoxic pseudolobular necrosis*,[62] but the term never really caught on; instead, the findings are reported out using descriptive terminology. Most cases are seen at autopsy, but it can occasionally be the target of a biopsy. The lesions tend to be either an infarcted macroregenerative nodule or a circumscribed aggregate of cirrhotic nodules that have underwent necrosis. In some cases, a rim of viable hepatocytes remains at the edge of the mostly necrotic macroregenerative nodule/cirrhotic nodule. Most cases occur in patients with shock, severe GI bleeding, or other causes of liver hypoperfusion. Presumably, the hypoperfusion is sufficient to cause local necrosis of vulnerable hepatocytes but not enough to cause massive necrosis.

Macroregenerative Nodules

Macroregenerative nodules can be seen in cases of chronic vascular outflow disease such as Budd-Chiari syndrome.[63,64] Large regenerative nodules can also develop in noncirrhotic livers that have underwent massive liver necrosis.

Focal Nodular Hyperplasia

Focal nodular hyperplasia (FNH) can be seen with a wide variety of vascular flow abnormalities of different etiologies, both genetic and acquired, all that lead to localized vascular shunting. Etiologies include generalized vascular inflow diseases, such as Abernathy syndrome,[1,2] as well as intraparenchymal diseases with focal vascular shunts, as well as chronic outflow diseases, such as Budd-Chiari syndrome or chronic congestive liver disease.[63-65] In all of these settings, the FNH have similar morphologies and immunohistochemical staining patterns to sporadic FNH. The diagnosis is made in the usual way.

Segmental Atrophy and Nodular Elastosis

This pseudotumor is considered in detail in Chapter 20 and is most commonly seen as a mass lesion in the periphery of the liver. The lesion is associated with intrahepatic vascular thrombi that leads to segmental parenchymal collapse and parenchymal extinction.[66] The affected segment forms a mass-like lesion that varies in size from 1 to 10 cm and typically is subcapsular in location. The lesion evolves through a series of stages, starting with parenchymal collapse, bile ductular proliferation, and mixed inflammation. The next stage shows decreased inflammation and ductular proliferation with the frequent formation of secondary biliary retention cysts and increased parenchymal elastosis. The next stage shows increasing elastosis, until this dominates the histological findings, whereas the final stage shows replacement by collagen, leaving a nodular scar.

Regenerative Hepatic Pseudotumor

The regenerative hepatic pseudotumor is discussed and illustrated in Chapter 20. It is caused by focal intrahepatic vascular thrombi that lead to areas of hypoperfusion with vague parenchymal nodularity, resulting in mass-like lesions visible on imaging, although they are often hard to see on gross examination. Histologically, lesions do not have well-defined borders but instead blend into the background liver parenchyma. The lesion is composed of benign hepatocytes and at low power shows mild sinusoidal dilatation and vague nodularity without fibrosis. Portal tracts are present throughout the pseudotumor but often have abnormal spacing. They may also show mild bile ductular proliferation and variable vascular changes, such as increased arterial profiles or portal vein abnormalities.[67] The lesions can have abnormal thick-walled vessels but lack other findings of focal nodular hyperplasia. Depending on sampling, thrombi can be seen in the intrahepatic portal vein or central veins, and prothrombotic disorders should be excluded. In some cases, aberrant arterioles can be found in the lobules.

Hepatic Adenomas

Hepatic adenomas can also arise in the setting of chronic vascular disease, such as Budd-Chiari syndrome. The diagnosis is made in the usual way, and the adenomas can be any of the different known subtypes.[68]

Hepatocellular Carcinoma

Hepatocellular carcinoma has been reported in a wide variety of chronic vascular diseases of the liver. Cirrhosis, or even advanced fibrosis, is not always present. The diagnosis is made in the usual way.

REFERENCES

1. Lisovsky M, Konstas AA, Misdraji J. Congenital extrahepatic portosystemic shunts (Abernethy malformation): a histopathologic evaluation. *Am J Surg Pathol.* 2011;35:1381-1390.
2. Osorio MJ, Bonow A, Bond GJ, et al. Abernethy malformation complicated by hepatopulmonary syndrome and a liver mass successfully treated by liver transplantation. *Pediatr Transpl.* 2011;15:E149-E151.
3. Chawla A, Kahn E, Becker J, et al. Focal nodular hyperplasia of the liver and hypercholesterolemia in a child with VACTERL syndrome. *J Pediatr Gastroenterol Nutr.* 1993;17:434-437.
4. Distefano G, Rodono A, Smilari P, et al. The VACTERL association: a report of a clinical case with hepatic cystic lymphangiectasis. Article in Italian. *Pediatr Med Chir.* 1998;20:223-226.
5. Thauvin-Robinet C, Faivre L, Huet F, et al. Another observation with VATER association and a complex IV respiratory chain deficiency. *Eur J Med Genet.* 2006;49:71-77.
6. Wain KE, Ellingson MS, McDonald J, et al. Appreciating the broad clinical features of SMAD4 mutation carriers: a multicenter chart review. *Genet Med.* 2014;16:588-593.
7. Welle CL, Welch BT, Brinjikji W, et al. Abdominal manifestations of hereditary hemorrhagic telangiectasia: a series of 333 patients over 15 years. *Abdom Radiol (NY).* 2019;44:2384-2391.
8. Dumortier J, Dupuis-Girod S, Valette PJ, et al. Recurrence of hereditary hemorrhagic telangiectasia after liver transplantation: clinical implications and physiopathological insights. *Hepatology.* 2019;69:2232-2240.
9. Scardapane A, Ficco M, Sabba C, et al. Hepatic nodular regenerative lesions in patients with hereditary haemorrhagic telangiectasia: computed tomography and magnetic resonance findings. *Radiol Med.* 2013;118:1-13.

10. Giordano P, Lenato GM, Suppressa P, et al. Hereditary hemorrhagic telangiectasia: arteriovenous malformations in children. *J Pediatr*. 2013;163:179-186.e1-e3.

11. Brenard R, Chapaux X, Deltenre P, et al. Large spectrum of liver vascular lesions including high prevalence of focal nodular hyperplasia in patients with hereditary haemorrhagic telangiectasia: the Belgian Registry based on 30 patients. *Eur J Gastroenterol Hepatol*. 2010;22:1253-1259.

12. Mavrakis A, Demetris A, Ochoa ER, et al. Hereditary hemorrhagic telangiectasia of the liver complicated by ischemic bile duct necrosis and sepsis: case report and review of the literature. *Dig Dis Sci*. 2010;55:2113-2117.

13. Gaujoux S, Bucau M, Ronot M, et al. Liver resection in patients with hepatic hereditary hemorrhagic telangiectasia. *Dig Surg*. 2013;30:410-414.

14. Blewitt RW, Brown CM, Wyatt JI. The pathology of acute hepatic disintegration in hereditary haemorrhagic telangiectasia. *Histopathology*. 2003;42:265-269.

15. Ogren M, Bergqvist D, Bjorck M, et al. Portal vein thrombosis: prevalence, patient characteristics and lifetime risk. A population study based on 23,796 consecutive autopsies. *World J Gastroenterol*. 2006;12:2115-2119.

16. Diaz LA, Idalsoaga F, Cannistra M, et al. High prevalence of hepatic steatosis and vascular thrombosis in COVID-19: a systematic review and meta-analysis of autopsy data. *World J Gastroenterol*. 2020;26:7693-7706.

17. Verheij J, Schouten JN, Komuta M, et al. Histological features in western patients with idiopathic non-cirrhotic portal hypertension. *Histopathology*. 2013;62:1083-1091.

18. Almouradi T, Co P, Riles W, et al. Isolated hepatic artery thrombosis leading to multiple liver infarcts in a non-transplant patient. *Am J Case Rep*. 2014;15:382-387.

19. Gollackner B, Sedivy R, Rockenschaub S, et al. Increased apoptosis of hepatocytes in vascular occlusion after orthotopic liver transplantation. *Transpl Int*. 2000;13:49-53.

20. Liu TC, Nguyen TT, Torbenson MS. Concurrent increase in mitosis and apoptosis: a histological pattern of hepatic arterial flow abnormalities in post-transplant liver biopsies. *Mod Pathol*. 2012;25(12):1594-1598.

21. Darbari DS, Kple-Faget P, Kwagyan J, et al. Circumstances of death in adult sickle cell disease patients. *Am J Hematol*. 2006;81:858-863.

22. Perronne V, Roberts-Harewood M, Bachir D, et al. Patterns of mortality in sickle cell disease in adults in France and England. *Hematol J*. 2002;3:56-60.

23. Kakar S, Batts KP, Poterucha JJ, et al. Histologic changes mimicking biliary disease in liver biopsies with venous outflow impairment. *Mod Pathol*. 2004;17:874-878.

24. Bosch DE, Koro K, Richards E, et al. Validation of a congestive hepatic fibrosis scoring system. *Am J Surg Pathol*. 2019;43:766-772.

25. Balazs M. Sinusoidal dilatation of the liver in patients on oral contraceptives. Electron microscopical study of 14 cases. *Exp Pathol*. 1988;35:231-237.

26. Jacobi AM, Feist E, Rudolph B, et al. Sinusoidal dilatation: a rare side effect of azathioprine. *Ann Rheum Dis*. 2004;63:1702-1703.

27. Laffon A, Moreno A, Gutierrez-Bucero A, et al. Hepatic sinusoidal dilatation in rheumatoid arthritis. *J Clin Gastroenterol*. 1989;11:653-657.

28. Saadoun D, Cazals-Hatem D, Denninger MH, et al. Association of idiopathic hepatic sinusoidal dilatation with the immunological features of the antiphospholipid syndrome. *Gut*. 2004;53:1516-1519.

29. Durant C, Martin J, Hervier B, et al. Takayasu arteritis associated with hepatic sinusoidal dilatation. *Ann Hepatol*. 2011;10:559-561.

30. Curciarello J, Castelletto R, Barbero R, et al. Hepatic sinusoidal dilatation associated to giant lymph node hyperplasia (Castleman's): a new case in a patient with periorbital xanthelasmas and history of celiac disease. *J Clin Gastroenterol*. 1998;27:76-78.

31. Bruguera M, Aranguibel F, Ros E, et al. Incidence and clinical significance of sinusoidal dilatation in liver biopsies. *Gastroenterology.* 1978;75:474-478.

32. Kakar S, Kamath PS, Burgart LJ. Sinusoidal dilatation and congestion in liver biopsy: is it always due to venous outflow impairment? *Arch Pathol Lab Med.* 2004;128:901-904.

33. Bruguera M, Caballero T, Carreras E, et al. Hepatic sinusoidal dilatation in Hodgkin's disease. *Liver.* 1987;7:76-80.

34. Aoyagi T, Mori I, Ueyama Y, et al. Sinusoidal dilatation of the liver as a paraneoplastic manifestation of renal cell carcinoma. *Hum Pathol.* 1989;20:1193-1197.

35. Scoazec JY, Marche C, Girard PM, et al. Peliosis hepatis and sinusoidal dilation during infection by the human immunodeficiency virus (HIV). An ultrastructural study. *Am J Pathol.* 1988;131:38-47.

36. de Araujo MS, Gerard F, Chossegros P, et al. Vascular hepatotoxicity related to heroin addiction. *Virchows Arch A Pathol Anat Histopathol.* 1990;417:497-503.

37. de Kerguenec C, Hillaire S, Molinie V, et al. Hepatic manifestations of hemophagocytic syndrome: a study of 30 cases. *Am J Gastroenterol.* 2001;96:852-857.

38. Albuquerque A, Cardoso H, Lopes J, et al. Familial occurrence of nodular regenerative hyperplasia of the liver. *Am J Gastroenterol.* 2013;108:150-151.

39. Musumba CO. Review article: the association between nodular regenerative hyperplasia, inflammatory bowel disease and thiopurine therapy. *Aliment Pharmacol Ther.* 2013;38:1025-1037.

40. Cotte L, Benet T, Billioud C, et al. The role of nucleoside and nucleotide analogues in nodular regenerative hyperplasia in HIV-infected patients: a case control study. *J Hepatol.* 2011;54:489-496.

41. Wicherts DA, de Haas RJ, Sebagh M, et al. Regenerative nodular hyperplasia of the liver related to chemotherapy: impact on outcome of liver surgery for colorectal metastases. *Ann Surg Oncol.* 2011;18:659-669.

42. Malamut G, Ziol M, Suarez F, et al. Nodular regenerative hyperplasia: the main liver disease in patients with primary hypogammaglobulinemia and hepatic abnormalities. *J Hepatol.* 2008;48:74-82.

43. Fuss IJ, Friend J, Yang Z, et al. Nodular regenerative hyperplasia in common variable immunodeficiency. *J Clin Immunol.* 2013;33:748-758.

44. Agrawal M, Rahmani R, Nakkala K, et al. Hepatoportal sclerosis (obliterative portal venopathy) and nodular regenerative hyperplasia in a patient with myasthenia gravis: a case report and review of the published work. *Hepatol Res.* 2013;43:999-1003.

45. Ebert EC, Hagspiel KD. Gastrointestinal and hepatic manifestations of rheumatoid arthritis. *Dig Dis Sci.* 2011;56:295-302.

46. Leung VK, Loke TK, Luk IS, et al. Nodular regenerative hyperplasia of the liver associated with systemic lupus erythematosus: three cases. *Hong Kong Med J.* 2009;15:139-142.

47. Hussain N, Feld JJ, Kleiner DE, et al. Hepatic abnormalities in patients with chronic granulomatous disease. *Hepatology.* 2007;45:675-683.

48. Austin A, Campbell E, Lane P, et al. Nodular regenerative hyperplasia of the liver and coeliac disease: potential role of IgA anticardiolipin antibody. *Gut.* 2004;53:1032-1034.

49. Al-Hamoudi WK, Pasieka JL, Urbanski SJ, et al. Hepatic nodular regenerative hyperplasia in a patient with advanced carcinoid tumor. *Eur J Gastroenterol Hepatol.* 2009;21:1083-1085.

50. Hubscher SG. What is the long-term outcome of the liver allograft? *J Hepatol.* 2011;55:702-717.

51. Devarbhavi H, Abraham S, Kamath PS. Significance of nodular regenerative hyperplasia occurring de novo following liver transplantation. *Liver Transpl.* 2007;13:1552-1556.

52. Gane E, Portmann B, Saxena R, et al. Nodular regenerative hyperplasia of the liver graft after liver transplantation. *Hepatology.* 1994;20:88-94.

53. Tsokos M, Erbersdobler A. Pathology of peliosis. *Forensic Sci Int.* 2005;149:25-33.

54. Bull LN. Hereditary forms of intrahepatic cholestasis. *Curr Opin Genet Dev.* 2002;12:336-342.

55. Aagenaes O. Hereditary cholestasis with lymphoedema (Aagenaes syndrome, cholestasis-lymphoedema syndrome). New cases and follow-up from infancy to adult age. *Scand J Gastroenterol.* 1998;33:335-345.

56. Drivdal M, Trydal T, Hagve TA, et al. Prognosis, with evaluation of general biochemistry, of liver disease in lymphoedema cholestasis syndrome 1 (LCS1/Aagenaes syndrome). *Scand J Gastroenterol.* 2006;41:465-471.

57. Torbenson MS. Hamartomas and malformations of the liver. *Semin Diagn Pathol.* 2019;36:39-47.

58. Viveiros A, Reiterer M, Schaefer B, et al. CCBE1 mutation causing sclerosing cholangitis: expanding the spectrum of lymphedema-cholestasis syndrome. *Hepatology.* 2017;66:286-288.

59. Terayama N, Terada T, Hoso M, et al. Partial nodular transformation of the liver with portal vein thrombosis. A report of two autopsy cases. *J Clin Gastroenterol.* 1995;20:71-76.

60. Tsui WM, So KT. Partial nodular transformation of liver in a child. *Histopathology.* 1993;22:594-596.

61. Wanless IR, Lentz JS, Roberts EA. Partial nodular transformation of liver in an adult with persistent ductus venosus. Review with hypothesis on pathogenesis. *Arch Pathol Lab Med.* 1985;109:427-432.

62. Edmondson HA. *Tumors of the Liver and Intrahepatic Bile Ducts.* Vol 2. Armed Forces Institute of Pathology; 1958.

63. Ibarrola C, Castellano VM, Colina F. Focal hyperplastic hepatocellular nodules in hepatic venous outflow obstruction: a clinicopathological study of four patients and 24 nodules. *Histopathology.* 2004;44:172-179.

64. Cazals-Hatem D, Vilgrain V, Genin P, et al. Arterial and portal circulation and parenchymal changes in Budd-Chiari syndrome: a study in 17 explanted livers. *Hepatology.* 2003;37:510-519.

65. Choi JY, Lee HC, Yim JH, et al. Focal nodular hyperplasia or focal nodular hyperplasia-like lesions of the liver: a special emphasis on diagnosis. *J Gastroenterol Hepatol.* 2011;26:1004-1009.

66. Singhi AD, Maklouf HR, Mehrotra AK, et al. Segmental atrophy of the liver: a distinctive pseudotumor of the liver with variable histologic appearances. *Am J Surg Pathol.* 2011;35:364-371.

67. Torbenson M, Yasir S, Anders R, et al. Regenerative hepatic pseudotumor: a new pseudotumor of the liver. *Hum Pathol.* 2020;99:43-52.

68. Sempoux C, Paradis V, Komuta M, et al. Hepatocellular nodules expressing markers of hepatocellular adenomas in Budd-Chiari syndrome and other rare hepatic vascular disorders. *J Hepatol.* 2015;63:1173-1180.

14

TRANSPLANT PATHOLOGY

DONOR LIVER EVALUATION

- Macrovesicular steatosis: report out to the nearest 10%.
- Inflammation: report out portal and lobular inflammation separately as minimal, mild, moderate, or marked; minimal and mild inflammation are common and inconsequential.
- Necrosis: report out to nearest 10%, indicating zonation and distribution (focal, diffuse, etc.). Focal areas of subcapsular necrosis can sometimes be targeted for biopsy, wherein the histologic findings will not be representative of the liver as a whole.
- Fibrosis: report out the ordinary fibrosis stage using trichrome stains on permanent sections.
- Any other abnormal finings, such as granulomas, excess iron, etc.

Biopsies of the donor liver are often performed to determine the suitability of the liver for transplant. Remember that histologic findings are not the only factors that go into making the decision on suitability. Other important factors include the age of the donor, cause of death, warm ischemia time, and status of the recipient. When evaluating a donor liver biopsy, the histologic features that you should include in the report are the amount of fat, inflammation, necrosis, and fibrosis, as well as any other unusual findings.

Fat evaluation is best performed on hematoxylin-eosin (H&E) stains. Oil red O or Sudan black stain on frozen sections can be used, but there is a tendency to overcall the amount of fat on these stains because even normal livers can have abundant staining (Figure 14.1). The amount of macrovesicular steatosis is used to determine suitability for transplant, as allografts with less than 30% fat perform similarly to allografts with no fat, while those with more than 60% fat have an increased risk of primary graft nonfunction. Allografts with fat levels between 30% and 60% are used on a case-by-case basis. Livers with moderate macrovesicular steatosis are also associated with a higher risk for post-reperfusion syndrome (hemodynamic instability, asystole, or the need to start the infusion of vasopressors

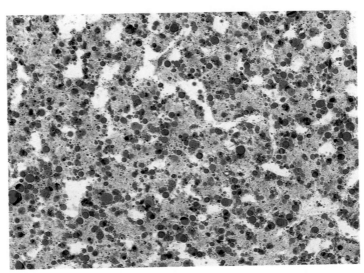

FIGURE 14.1   **Oil red O stain on normal liver.** This donor liver has abundant small droplet fat on oil red O stain. The small droplet fat is not included in the macrovesicular fat analysis of a potential donor liver. No steatosis was evident on hematoxylin-eosin (H&E) staining in this case.

immediately following graft reperfusion). For example, one study found an 8% frequency of reperfusion-associated cardiac arrest in patients who received grafts with moderate macrovesicular steatosis versus 1% for those with mild macrovesicular steatosis.[1]

Smaller droplets of fat within hepatocytes (Figure 14.2) are variably called *microvesicular steatosis* or *small droplet fat* or *intermediate droplet fat* or *small droplet macrovesicular steatosis*; this type of fat is currently thought to not have as strong an influence on the outcome as large droplet fat. Several studies found an effect on graft or patient outcomes,[2-4] but other studies, including one with nearly 12,000 allografts, found that the grafts with microvesicular steatosis performed similarly to those grafts without any fat.[5] In many donor livers, microvesicular steatosis (not the pattern, but at the individual cell level) coexists with macrovesicular steatosis, although their relative amounts correlate only poorly.[6] Based on our current understanding, it is the macrovesicular steatosis that should be scored for clinical care. If you or your clinical colleagues prefer to also report out the intermediate droplet fat/microvesicular steatosis, it can be included separately in the pathology report.

Fat is typically scored as none/less than 5%, 5% to 30%, 31% to 60%, and >60%. The reproducibility for classifying macrovesicular steatosis into these categories is excellent, even on frozen section. Occasional outlier studies have come to the opposite conclusion, but the center mass of the published data, as well as the enormous world-wide experience, all support the value of donor liver biopsies for estimating fat and evaluating graft suitability. For example, one landmark study showed that the rate of primary

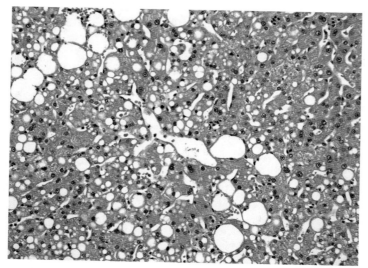

FIGURE 14.2 **Small droplet fat, hematoxylin-eosin (H&E) staining.** In this implant liver biopsy, only the macrovesicular component is scored; I estimate this image shows 5% to 10%. The smaller droplet fat is not scored. If you want to score the smaller droplet fat, it can be reported out separately.

nonfunction dropped from 8.5% to 1.4% after introducing frozen-section examination of potential donor livers.[7] Pretransplant biopsies of living donors can also identify fatty liver disease as well as unanticipated chronic hepatitis and fibrosis.[8]

Minimal to mild chronic portal inflammation is both nonspecific and common in potential donor liver biopsies, and typically does not impact graft suitability, but if the portal inflammation is mild and diffuse or focally moderate or greater in intensity, then the donor may have an undiagnosed chronic hepatitis. Necrosis, if present in donor biopsies, typically involves the zone 3 hepatocytes. Necrotic hepatocytes may still retain their normal size and sometimes even their nuclei, but the hepatocyte cytoplasm becomes distinctly oncocytic. Surgeons will sometimes target specific lesions visible on the liver surface; sections can then show marked necrosis that is not representative of the liver as a whole.

The frozen-section H&E stain may not pick up mild portal fibrosis but can identify more significant levels of fibrosis, including bridging fibrosis and cirrhosis. Trichrome stain are useful on permanent sections to establish the baseline fibrosis.

Iron stains are also commonly performed on permanent sections of the donor biopsy sample. There is relatively sparse data on the clinical relevance of iron positivity in donor liver specimens, but the findings to date suggest little or no impact on clinical outcomes.[8,9] For example, one study found iron in 49/284 (17%) of donor biopsies, which was occasionally at moderate levels, but did not impact survival outcomes.[8] Inadvertent transplantation of donor livers containing marked iron overload has also been reported,[10] but the number of cases is too small to draw strong conclusions about the posttransplant course. Likewise, the full range of outcomes has not been fully defined for cases where there is inadvertent transplant of livers with C282Y *HFE* mutations. Nonetheless, case reports have demonstrated that iron can accumulate rapidly in homozygotes,[11] or H63D/C282Y compound heterozygotes,[12] whereas in other cases, iron overloading does not manifest for several decades.[13]

PRESERVATION CHANGES IN THE ALLOGRAFT

Preservation changes can vary considerably in severity but typically include increased hepatocyte apoptosis (Figure 14.3; eFig. 14.1), minimal to focally mild portal and lobular lymphocytic inflammation (Figure 14.4), and scattered lobular Kupffer cell aggregates. Scattered ballooned hepatocytes may be present, along with mild cholestasis. Overall, the changes tend to be more pronounced in zone 3. Steatosis can be present and will reflect to some degree the amount of fat in the allograft at the time of donation, although it is typically lessened and, depending on the timing of the biopsy, can be absent. For examples, studies have shown that donor livers with moderate macrovesicular steatosis typically have the fat histologically cleared out of the liver within 7 days.[14]

In rare cases where the donor liver has marked steatosis, dying hepatocytes can release fat globules that stay in the hepatic cords and mimic dilated sinusoids (Figure 14.5).[15,16] In severe cases, this can lead to

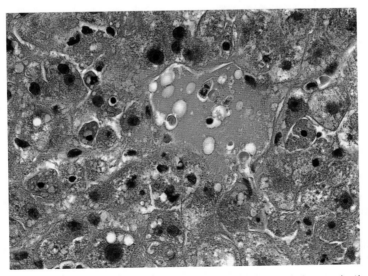

FIGURE 14.3 **Preservation changes.** Mild lobular spotty necrosis is seen in the zone 3 hepatocytes in this biopsy performed 3 days after transplant.

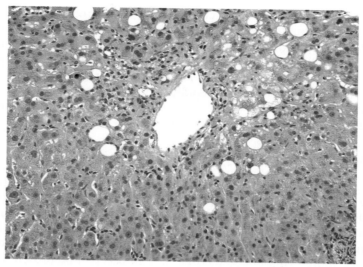

FIGURE 14.4 **Preservation changes.** There is mild zone 3 inflammation. There also is mild residual macrovesicular steatosis; the amount of fat diminished sharply from the implant biopsy and is now focal and mild.

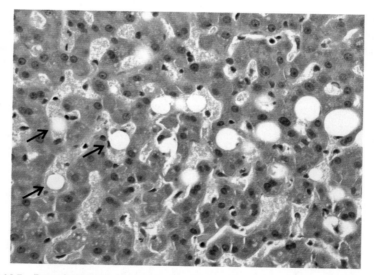

FIGURE 14.5 **Pseudopeliotic steatosis.** The fat has been released from hepatocytes and many of the droplets are in the sinusoids (*arrows*). This mild case did not lead to clinical symptoms.

sinusoidal obstruction[15] and the fat can even migrate to the lungs, causing pulmonary fat emboli.[16] The terms *lipopeliosis*[15] and *pseudopeliotic steatosis*[16] have been proposed for this finding in the liver, but it is so rarely encountered that neither have had a chance to catch on.

ACUTE CELLULAR REJECTION

- Most common in the first 3 months following transplant, but may occur anytime.
- Triggers may be evident, but in many cases, no inciting event is found. Frequent triggers include:
  - Reduced immunosuppression
  - Anything that upregulates the immune system
- Clinical findings
  - Often absent with mild/moderate rejection but can include fatigue, low-grade fevers, malaise; with severe rejection, there can be liver enlargement and liver tenderness.
  - Bile drainage from T tube (in patients who have them) can diminish or lose the normal deep gold or green color and become thin and pale.
- Biochemical findings: Alkaline-phosphatase-predominant elevations in liver enzyme levels.
- Definite diagnosis is made by biopsy.
  - Some centers will treat presumed rejections without biopsy when the clinical and biochemical findings are typical and there are no other likely causes based on clinical findings.
- Histologic features in typical acute cellular rejection include:
  - Portal inflammation
  - Bile duct lymphocytosis and injury
  - Endothelialitis
- Uncommon forms of acute cellular rejection include:
  - Lobular pattern
  - Central perivenulitis pattern
  - Plasma-cell-rich pattern

Definition

Acute cellular rejection is an immune-mediated, lymphocyte-based, inflammatory response to the allograft liver by the recipient's immune system. The Banff Working Group has proposed renaming acute cellular rejection as *T-cell-mediated rejection* (TCMR) because antibody-mediated rejection (AMR) is now recognized as a distinct clinicopathologic entity,[17] but most medical centers use the traditional terminology of acute cellular rejection. In this chapter, both terms will be used as synonyms.

Clinical Findings

The clinical findings with TCMR are generally mild and nonspecific, and many cases have no clinical findings, being identified by protocol evaluation of liver enzymes. More severe cases can present with right upper quadrant pain and graft tenderness. Most episodes of acute cellular rejection occur within the first several months following transplant, but they can also occur many years after transplant. At most medical centers, acute cellular rejection is rarely seen in the first few weeks after transplant. Some immune-suppression-sparing protocols, however, can have a higher frequency of acute cellular rejection early in the transplant time course, including rejection on day 7 biopsies. Recognized triggers for acute cellular rejection may include changes in immunosuppressive medications or anything that upregulates the immune system, such as an ascending cholangitis or enteric infection. Other less direct risk factors for acute cellular rejection include older donor age for the allograft, younger recipient age, and underlying autoimmune conditions such as primary sclerosing cholangitis (PSC) or autoimmune hepatitis.

Laboratory Findings

In most cases of acute cellular rejection, there are relatively abrupt increases in liver enzyme levels above baseline. The alkaline phosphatase levels will generally increase more than the aspartate transaminase (AST) and alanine transaminase (ALT) levels, but the AST and ALT levels may be increased as well.

Histologic Findings

The Banff Working Group has played an enormous role in defining and standardizing the histologic diagnosis of acute cellular rejection (Tables 14.1 and 14.2). Its publications are excellent and are an import-ant tool for surgical pathologists to stay current on important issues in

TABLE 14.1 Acute Cellular Rejection (T-Cell–Mediated Rejection)[18]	
Grade	Comment
Indeterminate	Portal and/or central perivenular inflammation that has no other likely cause, but the findings do not reach the full level of rejection.
Mild	Rejection type inflammation (including bile duct injury, endo-thelialitis) in less than half of portal tracts or perivenular areas. Inflammation is generally mild and does not lead to expansion of the portal tracts. There is no necrosis in cases that have a central perivenular pattern of rejection.
Moderate	Rejection type inflammation (including duct injury, endothelial-itis) in 50% or more of the portal tracts or perivenular areas. With portal-based rejection, the inflammation often expands the portal tracts. In cases of central perivenular rejection, there can be perivenular necrosis in a minority of zone 3 regions.
Severe	Similar to moderate rejection, but now with spillover of the portal inflammation into the periportal regions or perivenu-lar necrosis involving more than 50% of zone 3 regions.

Score	Comment
TABLE 14.2 Rejection Activity Index for Typical Acute Cellular Rejection[18]	
Portal inflammation	
1	Inflammation is mostly lymphocytic. Inflammation is present in less than 50% of portal tracts and does not lead to portal tract expansion.
2	Inflammation frequently expands the portal tracts and is mostly lymphocytic but may contain occasional lymphoblasts, neutrophils, and eosinophils. Note: also consider antibody-mediated rejection if eosinophils are prominent or if there is prominent portal tract edema or endothelial cell hypertrophy in the capillaries.
3	Inflammation is as in grade 2 but involves most of the portal tracts.
Bile duct injury	
1	Less than 50% of bile ducts are either cuffed or infiltrated by lymphocytes. The bile ducts show mild focal injury and mild reactive changes.
2	More than 50% of the bile ducts are either cuffed or infiltrated by lymphocytes. The ducts also show more than rare damage, but damage is present in less than 50% of ducts. Duct damage includes apoptotic cells, nuclear pleomorphism, and cytoplasmic vacuolization.
3	As in grade 2, but greater than 50% of ducts show damage.
Venous endothelialitis	
1	Endothelialitis is present in some portal tracts or central veins, but less than 50%. Endothelialitis can be subendothelial inflammation or lymphocytes attached to the luminal surface of the endothelial cells.
2	As for 1, but greater than 50% of portal/central veins show endothelialitis. There may be focal zone 3 confluent necrosis in less than 50% of perivenular areas.
3	As for 2, but there is zone 3 confluent necrosis in 50% or more of the perivenular areas.

transplant pathology. For example, the group's seminal 1997 paper on acute cellular rejection laid the foundation for our current and ongoing approach to the histologic diagnosis of rejection.[18]

The Banff Working Group has suggested that a biopsy should contain at least five portal tracts for adequacy and that at least two H&E levels should be examined.[18] Acute cellular rejection is fundamentally an inflammatory process and the key findings include portal lymphocytic inflammation, bile duct injury, and endotheliitis. The Banff classification requires that at least two out of three of these are present. The histologic findings can be reported out descriptively (Table 14.1) or with a formal scoring system (Table 14.2). A formal scoring system is mostly used to facilitate research.

When acute cellular rejection occurs within the first months following transplantation, essentially all cases will have portal lymphocytic inflammation and the vast majority will have bile duct injury. Endotheliitis is helpful when present but is often absent in milder episodes of acute cellular rejection. Episodes of rejection that occur later in the clinical course can have a typical pattern, but there are several additional patterns that can be seen (hepatitic, central perivenulitis, idiopathic hepatitis), which may have little or no bile duct injury.

PORTAL INFLAMMATION. The portal inflammation in acute cellular rejection is predominately lymphocytic but often includes a mild prominence in eosinophils (eFig. 14.2), as well as occasional plasma cells. The lymphocytes can be larger than normal, with somewhat more irregular nuclei, a subtle finding that is referred to as being "activated" (Figure 14.6). The inflammation is largely T cells and can range from mild to marked, with most cases on the milder end. Some degree of portal inflammation is present in the vast majority of cases of acute cellular rejection. In addition, acute cellular rejection will have some component of bile duct injury and/or endotheliitis.

BILE DUCT INJURY. The best evidence for active bile duct injury is bile duct lymphocytosis and/or apoptosis (Figures 14.7 and 14.8; eFigs. 14.3 and 14.4). Additional findings may include nuclear enlargement and "reactive changes,"

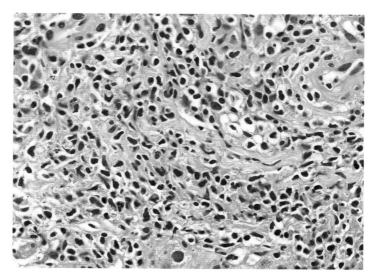

FIGURE 14.6 **Acute cellular rejection, activated portal inflammation.** The lymphocytes are activated; they are somewhat larger than normal and have irregular nuclei.

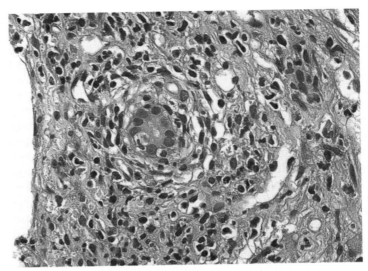

FIGURE 14.7 **Acute cellular rejection, bile duct injury.** The bile duct shows lymphocytosis and injury.

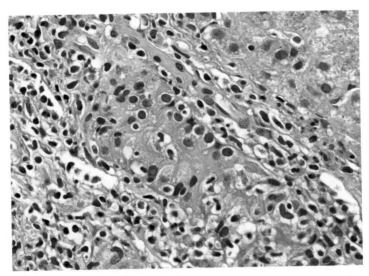

FIGURE 14.8 **Acute cellular rejection, bile duct injury.** The bile duct shows lymphocytosis and striking reactive changes.

wherein the cells lose their normal, orderly appearance. Of note, overemphasis on subtle changes may lead to overdiagnosis of acute cellular rejection, as milder bile duct reactive changes are highly nonspecific. In rare cases, the rejection can also affect the canals of Hering (eFigs. 14.5 and 14.6).

Bile duct lymphocytosis can also be seen as part of the inflammatory changes in several recurrent diseases, including hepatitis C, hepatitis B, and autoimmune hepatitis, but several observations can provide assistance in cases where you are struggling between rejection and recurrent disease. With recurrent disease, the bile duct injury is typically minimal, often equivocal, and almost always focal. Furthermore, it is usually associated with moderate or marked portal chronic inflammation. In contrast, mild acute cellular rejection often has only mild portal lymphocytic inflammation but clear and unequivocal bile duct injury. Furthermore, the bile duct injury in acute cellular rejection is more than focal in most cases: it is often patchy but is almost never limited to a single portal tract, outside the setting of protocol biopsies that happen to catch very early and mild cases of acute cellular rejection. Finally, the presence of other findings outside the portal tracts can lead to the right diagnosis, such as the presence of at least a mild lobular hepatitis in most cases of recurrent viral hepatitis or autoimmune hepatitis.

ENDOTHELIALITIS is diagnosed by identifying either portal veins or central veins that have lymphocytes adjacent to the endothelial cells or have lymphocytes that are within the lumen and adherent to the endothelial cells (Figure 14.9). The endothelial cells should also appear "different" than those in veins that are not affected by endothelialitis; the terms "reactive" and "injured" are often used to describe these affected endothelial cells. They can appear larger and have more hyperchromatic nuclei and may be lifted off of their basement membrane (Figure 14.10). Endothelialitis can be a very helpful finding, increasing the specificity of the diagnosis,[19]

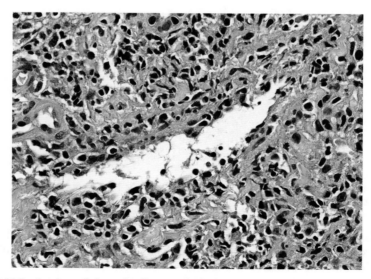

FIGURE 14.9 **Acute cellular rejection, endothelialitis.** Lymphocytosis and injury of the endothelium.

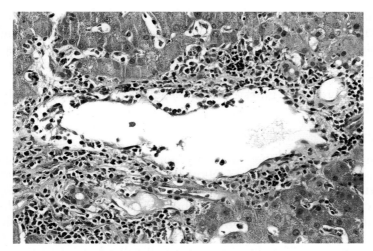

FIGURE 14.10 **Acute cellular rejection, endothelialitis.** The endothelium in this portal vein is inflamed and appears to be lifted off of the basement membrane.

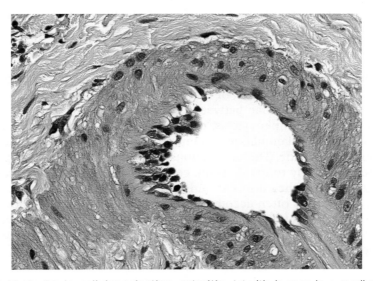

FIGURE 14.11 **Acute cellular rejection, arteritis.** Arteritis is seen in a medium-sized artery.

but it is not necessary for the diagnosis and is also easy to overcall; there should be clear endothelial reactive changes or injury to make the diagnosis (eFigs. 14.7-14.10). Acute cellular rejection can also rarely involve the hepatic arteries (Figure 14.11); such cases usually have coexisting AMR.[20]

Pathologists are often tempted into over-diagnosing endothelialitis because inflammatory cells are frequently near the portal vein, regardless of whether there is rejection. In addition, equivocal, nonspecific reactive endothelial changes are common in any biopsy with portal inflammation. Thus, to be diagnostically useful, the endothelial injury should not be equivocal. If you find a focus of equivocal endothelialitis, you can often take guidance from the rest of the biopsy—if there are no additional foci of endothelialitis, or if the other features of acute cellular rejection are not seen elsewhere in the biopsy, then the equivocal focus of endothelialitis is likely nonspecific.

Immunostain Findings

Immunostains are neither necessary nor specifically useful in making a diagnosis of acute cellular rejection. Immunostains find their main utility in ruling out other processes that may enter the differential diagnosis. In cases where the differential includes a lymphoproliferative disorder, immunophenotyping the lymphocytes may be helpful, as rejection has predominantly T-cell infiltrates, whereas most Epstein-Barr virus (EBV)-related lymphoproliferative disorders are B cell related. EBER and EBV-LMP stains are critical stains for identifying viral RNA and proteins, respectively. Immunostains are also useful to rule out cytomegalovirus (CMV) hepatitis. Immunostains for C4d are helpful if there are histologic or clinical findings concerning AMR

Differential for Acute Cellular Rejection

The differential for acute cellular rejection is typically drug-induced liver injury (DILI), viral infection, or recurrent disease. Of course, there can be areas of histologic overlap between rejection and DILI, such as the presence of bile duct lymphocytosis, but the overall pattern for acute cellular rejection (portal inflammation, duct injury, with or without endothelialitis) is reasonably specific. The medications used in the transplant population that are most likely to mimic acute cellular rejection are antibiotics, such as Augmentin, as they also can induce a portal-based pattern of inflammation, one that is often accompanied by bile duct injury. In these cases, however, the portal inflammation is more mixed than is typically seen with acute cellular rejection, including more neutrophils and sometimes more eosinophils.

An allergic type drug reaction can sometimes manifest with significant graft eosinophilia. Overall, commonly used medications for immunosuppression, such as tacrolimus and corticosteroids, do not cause eosinophilic type drug reactions, but allergic type drug reactions can occasionally be seen with other frequently used medication, such as antibiotics. In most cases, however, potential drug reactions will be idiosyncratic, will not have eosinophilia, and you will have to rely on other findings. The most useful guideline is to think of DILI when the histologic patterns are unusual for rejection or when the clinical setting is a poor fit. As one example, a biopsy that shows substantial and aggressive bile duct injury but has only mild portal chronic inflammation with no endothelialitis is somewhat unusual for acute cellular rejection and should prompt the differential of a drug reaction. As another example, a biopsy that shows marked lobular cholestasis with minimal portal chronic inflammation and only focal bile duct reactive changes does not fit well for acute cellular rejection and should prompt a differential that includes a drug reaction. Finally, EBV hepatitis will be in the differential in some cases, and an in situ hybridization for EBV (EBER) is a valuable tool.

At times, the differential may also include recurrent viral hepatitis. For patients who underwent transplant for chronic hepatitis C virus (HCV) infection, recurrent disease was almost universal historically (typically within the 3-9 months of transplant), but this has changed dramatically, with medications now reducing the recurrence rate to less than 1%. Overall, the patterns of injury seen in recurrent hepatitis C vary depending on the time after transplant, and the findings are discussed in more detail in the section Recurrent Hepatitis C. It is often noted that recurrent hepatitis C and rejection can have some histologic overlap. For example, it is well known that hepatitis C in individuals who have not undergone transplant can lead to bile duct injury and endothelialitis. While these points are true, it should not obscure the larger truth—in general, there are sufficient dissimilarities between the injury patterns in recurrent hepatitis C and rejection that a diagnosis of one or the other can be confidently made in most cases. Part of the challenge is simply that of experience—it can be hard to feel confident if you do not see very many liver transplant biopsies. In these cases, judicious use of consultant pathologists can very helpful both in specific case management and in refining your skills in this area. One of the common diagnostic pitfalls is to focus on a single criterion rather than the overall pattern. As one example, focal minimal duct injury, in a biopsy that shows otherwise typical changes of hepatitis C, should be called hepatitis C and not rejection. Other patterns of recurrent disease are discussed separately in the following sections.

OTHER PATTERNS OF ACUTE CELLULAR REJECTION

Lobular Based Rejection

Some cases of typical acute cellular rejection can have minimal or focally mild lobular hepatitis. In a few settings, however, lobular hepatitis can be more striking, and sometimes hepatitis can event dominate the histologic findings, with only mild and nonspecific portal tract changes. Risk factors are not always identified in cases with a lobular pattern of rejection, but when a triggering event is identified or suspected, the two most common risk factors tend to be pediatric transplant patients and adults who completely stop taking their antirejection medications, going from full immunosuppression to no immunosuppression. The biopsy findings may represent an early pattern that would evolve, if untreated, to a more typical rejection pattern, as some cases will also have conventional acute cellular rejection changes in the portal tracts.

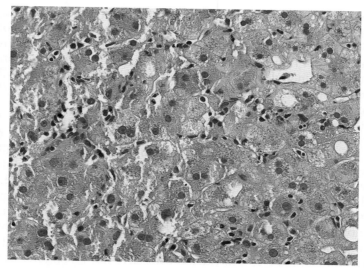

FIGURE 14.12 **Acute cellular rejection, lobular variant.** The lobules show a hepatitic pattern of rejection.

The lobules show mild to patchy moderate lymphocytic hepatitis (Figure 14.12). The lobular inflammation can be associated with active liver injury, such as scattered apoptotic bodies and mild Kupffer cell hyperplasia, or can show a sinusoidal pattern with relatively little evidence for hepatic injury.[21] In some cases, the sinusoidal endothelial cells can show focal injury.[22] The portal tract findings can range from the typical features of acute cellular rejection[21] to showing mild nonspecific lymphocytic inflammation with no endothelialitis and no or minimal duct injury. In some cases, a hepatitic pattern of rejection precedes the development of chronic rejection.[23] The differential for the lobular pattern of acute cellular rejection includes recurrent viral hepatitis, EBV hepatitis, and a drug reaction.

Central Perivenulitis

Central perivenulitis is an important injury pattern to recognize. The frequency is not well defined, but one study reported a frequency of 28%.[24] This frequency is probably higher than that seen at many centers and may reflect differences in patient populations, clinical treatment protocols, or histologic definition.

In cases with central perivenulitis, the lobules will have mild loss of zone 3 hepatocytes, usually with mild lymphocytic/lymphoplasmacytic inflammation in the areas of hepatocyte loss (Figure 14.13; eFig. 14.11). Extravasated red blood cells can also be seen in the zone 3 regions that have loss of hepatocytes. The endothelium of the central veins do not have the typical features of endothelialitis in most cases, and often appears essentially normal. Many times, the central perivenulitis pattern will be accompanied by more typical changes of acute cellular rejection in the portal

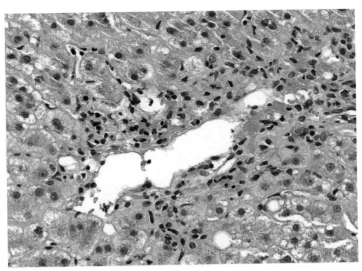

FIGURE 14.13 **Central perivenulitis.** The zone 3 region shows mild chronic inflammation with mild hepatocyte dropout.

tracts; in other cases, the central perivenulitis pattern will be an isolated finding. Isolated central perivenulitis is more common in later allograft biopsies. This pattern of rejection is less common than typical acute cellular rejection but appears to respond to antirejection therapy.[25] Central perivenulitis is often seen again on repeat biopsies of the same allograft if there are episodes of recurrent rejection. In some cases, this pattern of injury can lead to central vein fibrosis and is also associated with an increased risk for subsequent ductopenia.[24]

Chronic Hepatitis Pattern

In this pattern, the biopsy shows chronic portal inflammation with no or minimal bile duct injury and no endothelialitis. The term *idiopathic posttransplant hepatitis* is also used to describe this pattern of injury. The chronic inflammation in the portal tract is typically mild to focally moderate (Figure 14.14). The inflammatory cells are predominately lymphocytic, but in some cases, plasma cells can be mildly prominent. Mild interface activity may be present, especially in those portal tracts with moderate portal chronic inflammation. This pattern is only recognizable after recurrent diseases (such as autoimmune hepatitis or primary biliary cirrhosis/cholangitis [PBC], chronic viral hepatitis [including hepatitis E virus (HEV)], and DILI) have been excluded. If the patient underwent transplant for fulminant hepatitis A, then chronic hepatitis A should also be excluded.[26,27]

This pattern of injury is likely multifactorial and some cases can be associated with fibrosis progression,[28,29] so efforts to identify a cause are important. Some of these cases likely represent, or at least have a

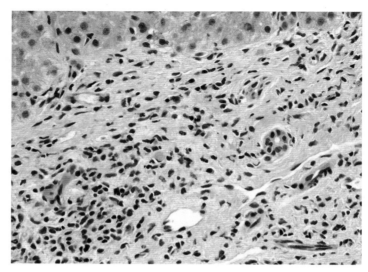

FIGURE 14.14 **Idiopathic posttransplant hepatitis.** A mild nonspecific portal hepatitis was seen in the biopsy from an individual who underwent transplant 15 years earlier for biliary atresia.

component of, chronic AMR (cAMR; please see separate section below). Some patients will also have elevated autoantibody levels, without other features of autoimmune hepatitis.[30,31] In those cases in which no cause can be identified, chronic idiopathic posttransplant hepatitis can benefit from optimized immunosuppression,[31] especially if there is an associated central perivenulitis. Molecular studies also suggest this pattern of injury is similar to rejection at the gene expression level.[32]

Plasma-Cell-Rich Rejection and De Novo Autoimmune Hepatitis

Occasional biopsies are performed to rule out rejection and show a plasma-cell-rich pattern of inflammation in the portal tracts or the central veins (Figure 14.15). If the biopsy shows other typical findings of acute cellular rejection, such as bile duct injury or venulitis, then the findings are most consistent with acute cellular rejection. In many cases of acute cellular rejection, the plasma cell numbers increase roughly in proportion to the severity of the rejection,[33] whereas in other cases the plasma cells are disproportionately numerous for the overall amount of inflammation. The reason(s) why some rejection infiltrates have more plasma cells is unclear, but presumably represents underlying genetic predispositions to autoimmune-type phenomenon. One study found that increased numbers of plasma cells in the native liver was associated with the subsequent risk for plasma-cell-rich rejection.[34] In this study, native livers were examined by randomly selecting five portal tracts with dense inflammation. The livers at highest risk were those with greater than 30% plasma cells in at least one portal tract.[34]

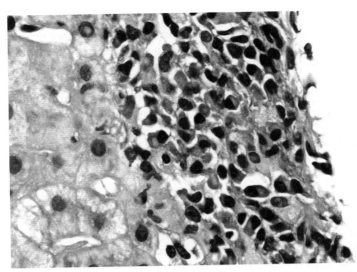

FIGURE 14.15 **Plasma-cell-rich rejection.** There was striking plasma-cell-rich inflammation in this case of rejection.

There is a separate group of cases that have a plasma-cell-rich pattern of inflammation but lack the classic features of acute cellular rejection, such as bile duct injury and endothelialitis. This pattern is sometimes called de novo *autoimmune hepatitis*; this term is not used consistently however,[35] so you have to read papers that use this term carefully in order to understand what the authors mean. In general, the term de novo autoimmune hepatitis is used in the following setting: (1) the patient did not have autoimmune hepatitis as an underlying liver disease (if so, the term *recurrent autoimmune hepatitis* would be used), (2) the clinical and histologic findings do not fit for typical acute cellular rejection, (3) the patient tests positive for autoantibodies, and (4) the allograft shows immune-mediated injury that contains at least a mild prominence in portal plasma cells. The diagnosis is significantly strengthened with a fifth finding: an unexplained lobular hepatitis. A central perivenulitis pattern of injury is typically classified as a variant of acute cellular rejection.

This group of patients may have preceding or subsequent biopsies that show more typical patterns of rejection. They often have serum autoantibody positivity, but at low titers.[36] This pattern of rejection responds to corticosteroids but can be difficult to manage and can lead to graft failure.[34,36] Anecdotally, there seems to be significant center-to-center variability in the frequency of this pattern of rejection.

Therapies for typical acute cellular rejection versus de novo autoimmune hepatitis are similar but not identical,[35] and clinical management often has to be guided by response to therapy. Other clues include clinical and laboratory findings. Recurrent/de novo autoimmune hepatitis typically occurs more than 2 years after transplant, whereas most plasma-cell-rich rejection cases occur within the first 2 years.[36] In addition, autoantibody titers are often negative or low in plasma-cell-rich rejection, in contrast to de novo or recurrent autoimmune hepatitis, where they are often high. Serum IgG levels are typically elevated in de novo/recurrent autoimmune hepatitis and not in plasma-cell-rich acute cellular rejection. Also, of note, many cases of plasma-cell–rich rejection are associated with prior episodes of more typical acute cellular rejection or with current subtherapeutic levels of immunosuppression.

ANTIBODY-MEDIATED REJECTION

These Four Features Are Needed for a Definite Diagnosis of AMR

1. Positive serum donor-specific antibodies (DSAs)
2. Histologic findings that are consistent with AMR
3. Diffuse C4d staining in microvasculature
4. Reasonable exclusion of other causes of graft dysfunction

AMR occurs when circulating antibodies to donor antigens are associated with graft injury. Of note, the presence of DSAs alone does not clearly predict the development of AMR. Nonetheless, the diagnosis can only be made with confidence when DSAs are present. In addition, the diagnosis requires clinical or laboratory evidence of graft dysfunction, histologic features consistent with AMR, compatible C4d staining, and reasonable exclusion of other potential causes for the graft dysfunction.

Clinical Findings

AMR occurs in a "primary" form in allograft recipients who have preformed ABO antibodies and develop hyperacute rejection. Other preformed antibodies that can play a role in AMR include lymphocytoxic antibodies and antiendothelial antibodies. This pattern is very rare. In contrast to hyperacute rejection in other allograft organs, which can occur within minutes after organ reperfusion, hyperacute rejection in the liver can be delayed by several hours or days. In cases of primary AMR, the graft shows early and often substantial graft dysfunction, usually within the first several days after transplant. The secondary form, where de novo antibodies develop after transplant, can be associated with both acute cellular rejection and chronic rejection.[37]

In certain cases, specific targets for AMR have been identified; in these relatively rare cases, the donor liver expresses normal liver proteins that are lacking in the recipient, either due to polymorphisms such as with glutathione-S-transferase T1 (GSTT1)[38,39] or due to inherited genetic diseases such as those involving the bile salt export proteins.[40] In time, the recipient's immune system recognizes these proteins as foreign and this can elicit an AMR. These cases often have features of de novo autoimmune hepatitis because they can have a hepatitic pattern of injury that is sometimes plasma cell rich, but they are discussed here because they may also have C4d staining in the portal tracts[41] and when they do appear to have an element of AMR.

Histologic Findings

In primary AMR ("hyperacute rejection"), the endothelium is the primary target and the liver shows endothelial injury, microvascular thrombi, variable sinusoidal dilatation, and congestion. Neutrophils can be prominent in the portal tracts and sinusoids. There can be substantial hemorrhagic liver necrosis. The histologic findings can overlap with ischemia and severe preservation injury, so these possibilities need to be excluded. In addition, the histologic findings need to be correlated with the presence of preformed donor antibodies to confidently make the diagnosis.

In acute AMR, the histologic findings can be roughly divided into early changes, those that can occur within the first weeks or few months after liver transplant, and later changes. The earliest changes can resemble preservation injury, with zone 3 hepatocyte ballooning, lobular spotty necrosis, and cholestasis.[37,42] Later changes can be more striking and can mimic biliary obstruction with portal tract edema, ductular proliferation (Figure 14.16), and portal neutrophilia.[37,43,44] In most cases, however, the findings are mild and may show mostly subtle dilatation

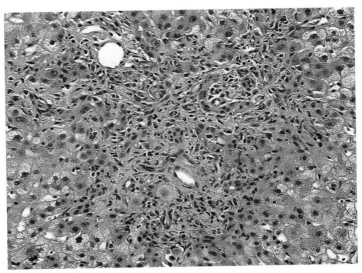

FIGURE 14.16 **Antibody-mediated rejection, portal tract changes.** The portal tracts show ductular proliferation and mixed inflammation that resembled downstream obstructive biliary tract disease.

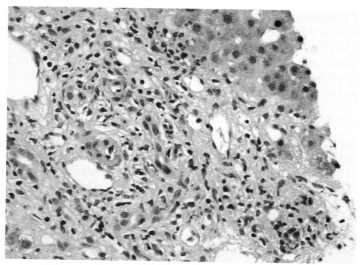

FIGURE 14.17 **Antibody-mediated rejection, portal tract changes.** The portal tracts show mild inflammation and mild capillary dilatation.

of the capillaries in the portal tracts with margination of neutrophils, lymphocytes, or eosinophils (Figure 14.17). The sinusoids can show varying degrees of neutrophilia in some cases. The lobules often show cholestasis. Eventually, untreated AMR can cause thrombosis of portal veins and hepatic arteries, leading to ischemic necrosis of bile ducts and hepatic parenchyma.

Immunostain Findings

Staining for C4d is important in making the diagnosis of AMR, as positive staining helps confirm a diagnosis of AMR in the setting of DSAs, clinical graft dysfunction that is unexplained by other processes, and a biopsy that shows active injury compatible with AMR. C4d staining can be seen in the portal tracts, in the zone 1 sinusoids, and in combined patterns. As a general rule of thumb, immunostaining in cases of AMR tends to be stronger in the portal veins and capillaries/stroma of the portal tracts than in the sinusoids and central veins (Figure 14.18); staining of sinusoids and central veins is not necessary for the diagnosis and can be nonspecific.[45] To support a diagnosis of AMR, most cases will show staining involving >50% of the portal microvasculature endothelium in more than 10% of the portal tracts.[17]

Also, of importance, C4d staining can be seen in a large proportion of allograft liver biopsies that have no evidence for AMR. In these cases, the C4d staining tends to be more focal, but in some cases, there can be overlap with the levels seen in AMR. Thus, it bears reemphasis that the diagnosis of AMR is not based solely on C4d staining and should be made when

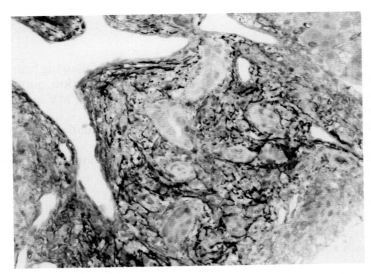

FIGURE 14.18 **Antibody-mediated rejection, C4d staining.** The portal tract stroma stains with C4d; same case as preceding image.

(1) DSAs are present, (2) there is clinical or laboratory evidence of graft dysfunction, (3) the liver biopsy features are consistent with AMR, and (4) the biopsy shows compatible C4d staining.

Chronic Antibody-Mediated Rejection

The management of patients with positive serum DSA but without biochemical liver dysfunction can be challenging. Some but not all these patients will have worse long-term outcomes. To better determine which of these patients are at risk for poor outcomes, studies have examined the histologic findings (mostly from protocol biopsies) and identified a subset of patients with worse outcomes whose biopsies show a histologic pattern of injury called cAMR. A diagnosis of cAMR requires recently positive serum DSA, histologic evidence of both lymphocytic portal inflammation and fibrosis, and reasonable exclusion of other causes of mild chronic hepatitis.[46]

The histologic findings are generally mild and may include mild lymphocytic portal inflammation, mild interface activity, portal venopathy, and portal and/or sinusoidal fibrosis. Histologically, there is significant overlap with the idiopathic chronic hepatitis pattern of injury; the distinction is made by the presence of DSAs, lack of response to optimization of immunosuppression, and exclusion of other potential causes. C4d staining is negative in the majority of cases with cAMR, but when the result is positive, it further supports the diagnosis (using the same criteria as for acute AMR).[46] For research studies, these findings can be combined using an equation to create a cAMR score, which can predict clinical outcomes.[46,47] For clinical care, it is sufficient to suggest the diagnosis in your differential, when appropriate.

CHRONIC REJECTION

- Usually not seen until >6 months to many years following transplant.
- Risk factors include multiple prior episodes of rejection, poor adherence to immunosuppression regiments, and prior CMV infection of allograft.
- Clinical findings are nonspecific; there may be jaundice in end-stage cases.
- Biochemical findings: alkaline-phosphatase-predominant elevations in liver enzyme levels; may be cholestatic.
- Definite diagnosis is made by biopsy.
- Histologic features in chronic rejection include:
  - Bile duct atrophy
  - Bile duct loss
  - Foam cell arteriopathy

Clinical and Laboratory Findings

Chronic rejection most commonly manifests as chronic cholestasis in an individual with no evidence of obstructive biliary tract disease, drug reactions, or other explanation for the cholestasis. Imaging studies may show fewer small branches of the intrahepatic biliary tree ("pruning"). In keeping with the biliary injury, the alkaline phosphatase level is chronically elevated. There may be mild chronic AST and ALT level elevations as well, but the predominant enzyme level elevation is alkaline phosphatase. Recognized risk factors for chronic rejection include prior acute cellular rejection episodes, particularly if they were refractory to treatment. Inadequate immunosuppression or treatment with immune activators, such as interferon, also increases the risk for chronic rejection.

Histologic Findings

The histologic criterion for a diagnosis of chronic rejection is any one of the following[48]: (1) senescence changes in >50% of bile ducts, with or without bile duct loss; (2) bile duct loss in >50% of bile ducts; or (3) foam cell obliterative arteriopathy.

Bile duct changes are the main findings in biopsy specimens. The earliest histologic changes are typically senescence/atrophic changes of the bile ducts. These atrophic bile ducts may have smaller diameters than expected for the size of the portal tract, and the epithelium tends to be more eosinophilic and flattened than normal biliary epithelium (Figure 14.19). The nuclei can almost look dysplastic, with irregular membranes, hyperchromasia, nuclear enlargement, and uneven nuclear spacing. When evaluating loss of bile ducts remember that bile ducts may not be apparent on H&E staining in a small proportion of portal

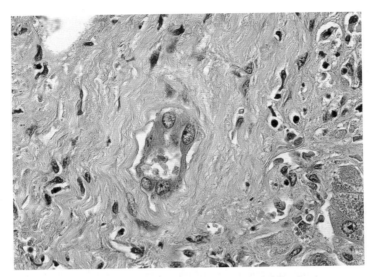

FIGURE 14.19 **Chronic rejection, senescent changes in a bile duct.**

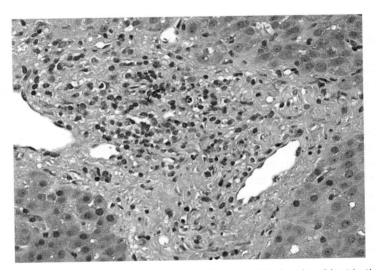

FIGURE 14.20 **Chronic rejection, loss of bile duct.** No bile duct is evident in the portal tract in this case of chronic rejection.

tracts in normal liver specimens, so the diagnosis of chronic rejection is made with most confidence when at least half of the portal tracts are missing a bile duct (Figure 14.20; eFig. 14.12). A cytokeratin immunostain can help confirm bile duct loss (Figure 14.21). Essentially all cases will show intermediate hepatocytes on CK7 stain and most have periportal copper deposition. The portal tracts typically have sparse to patchy mild lymphocytic inflammation. Bile ductular proliferation is

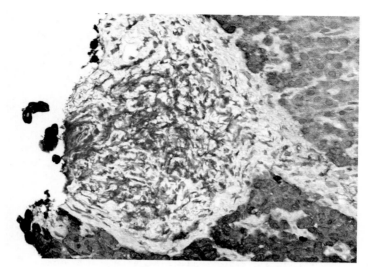

FIGURE 14.21 **Chronic rejection, loss of bile ducts.** A cytokeratin AE1/3 immunostain confirms the loss of the bile duct in this portal tract.

not a feature of chronic rejection. Portal fibrosis is also uncommon and should prompt evaluation of the extrahepatic biliary tree to rule out obstruction.

The lobules in chronic rejection may show cholestasis, as well as central perivenulitis with drop out of the hepatocytes immediately adjacent to the central vein. In some cases, the zone 3 regions can also become fibrotic.

Foam cell arteriopathy is most often seen in allograft livers explanted for graft failure and is only rarely seen on biopsy specimens; this is because the medium- and large-sized hepatic arteries that are mainly affected by foam cell arteriopathy are not sampled in typical needle biopsy cores. Foam cell arteriopathy shows obliteration or substantial narrowing of the arterial lumen, which is caused by marked thickening of the intima by numerous foamy macrophages (Figure 14.22; eFig. 14.13).

Differential

The diagnosis of chronic rejection can only be made on biopsy specimens if obstructive biliary tract disease has been excluded. For example, chronic biliary anastomotic strictures can also lead to ductopenia. For individuals who undergo transplant for PBC or PSC, the differential also includes recurrent disease (discussed later); the distinction is made by correlation with imaging findings to help exclude PSC and by looking for other histologic findings that would suggest PSC or PBC. For example, recurrent PSC often has bile ductular proliferation, whereas chronic rejection does not. Likewise, recurrent PBC typically has mild to patchy moderate portal chronic inflammation, whereas the portal

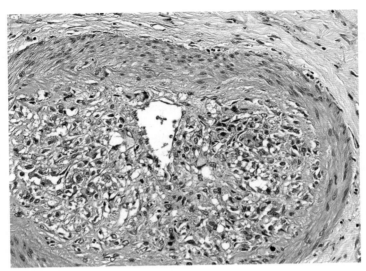

FIGURE 14.22 **Chronic rejection, foam cell change.** A large artery shows significant intimal proliferation with foam cells.

inflammation in chronic rejection is typically sparse. As noted earlier, portal fibrosis suggests alternative diagnoses to chronic rejection.

BILIARY OBSTRUCTION

Clinical Findings and Laboratory Findings

Fundamentally, the clinical, imaging, and laboratory findings in posttransplant obstruction are identical to those in patients who did not undergo transplant. Most bile duct strictures are located at the anastomotic site. The clinical and laboratory findings range in severity, but cases typically present with a cholestatic pattern of injury, including elevations in alkaline phosphatase and bilirubin levels.

Histologic Findings

The histologic findings are identical to those in nontransplanted livers. The biopsies can show varying amounts of portal edema, bile ductular proliferation, and portal neutrophilia in early stages of acute obstruction. The portal edema tends to be less prominent in later cases, but ductular proliferation and mixed portal inflammation are typically still present. In later cases, there can be ductopenia, fibro-obliterative duct lesions, and portal fibrosis.

Differential

There are several disease processes that can mimic some aspects of biliary obstruction (Table 14.3). For example, marked hepatitis from any cause can elicit a brisk bile ductular reaction. As another example, AMR can have

TABLE 14.3 Differential for Bile Ductular Proliferation in Posttransplant Biopsies

Cause	Comment
Anastomotic or other mechanical cause of obstruction	Seen most commonly in the first 3 months after transplant, but can also be seen many years out.
Marked acute hepatitis from any cause	An example would be a marked idiosyncratic drug reaction.
Cholestatic hepatitis C	Some cases of recurrent chronic hepatitis C are cholestatic but lack the full features of fibrosing cholestatic hepatitis C.
Fibrosing cholestatic hepatitis C	Correlate with other clinical and histologic findings to make the diagnosis (see text).
Antibody-mediated rejection	Correlate with other clinical and histologic findings to make the diagnosis (see text).
Small-for-size graft	Correlate with other clinical and histologic findings to make the diagnosis (see text).
Recurrent primary sclerosing cholangitis	Correlate with other clinical and histologic findings to make the diagnosis (see text).
Vascular outflow obstruction (eg, thrombus)	These cases will also have marked zone 3 congestion and other findings of vascular outflow disease.

bile ductular proliferation that mimics biliary obstruction. In most cases, other changes in the biopsy will clarify the diagnosis, but the final diagnosis requires correlation with radiographic studies of the biliary tree. The imaging findings are important but do not supplant the biopsy findings–positive correlation reinforces the diagnosis of obstructive disease, but negative imaging findings also have to be carefully weighed against the biopsy findings, as the imaging findings can sometimes be falsely negative due to technical or interpretive issues.

HEPATIC ARTERY INSUFFICIENCY

Clinical and Laboratory Findings

Hepatic artery problems include anastomotic stenosis as well as thrombosis; they occur most commonly within the first 3 months after transplant. The median posttransplant time for hepatic artery thrombosis is 7 days, with a range from 1 to 18 days.[49] The frequency of early hepatic artery thrombosis is 8% in children and 3% in adults.[49] Risk factors include transplants from a CMV-seropositive donor to a CMV-seronegative recipient, transplants with a prolonged operation time, retransplantation, unusual arterial anatomy, and transplant centers with low volume.[49] Early clinical findings can be nonspecific, with mild to moderate elevations in serum AST and ALT levels. Imaging findings can show stenosis or thrombosis of the hepatic artery.

Histologic Findings

The histologic findings are usefully considered as falling into two broad categories: changes that occur very early and those that occur later on. In cases of early hepatic artery thrombosis (Figure 14.23), the biopsy shows increased hepatocellular spotty necrosis without significant inflammation; the increased apoptosis results from ischemia. Zonation of the apoptosis has been reported in some[50,51] but not all studies.[52] The lobules can also show increased hepatocellular mitotic figures as the liver regenerates (Figure 14.24).[52] These increased mitotic figures can be an important clue, but some cases will only have moderate lobular spotty necrosis. The reason is unclear why some cases have increased mitoses while others do not; it may be related to the time interval from arterial flow problems to the time of the biopsy, or to the severity of the arterial flow changes, or to other variables such as donor age. Arteritis due to AMR can also be a rare cause of similar changes (lobular spotty necrosis without lobular inflammation).[52] Later changes (weeks, months) may include a range of findings, from coagulative necrosis (eFig. 14.14), to zone 3 hepatocyte dropout, to bile duct injury with a ductular reaction.[53,54]

Differential Diagnoses

The differential for spotty lobular necrosis without significant inflammation includes predominately recurrent hepatitis C, for individuals

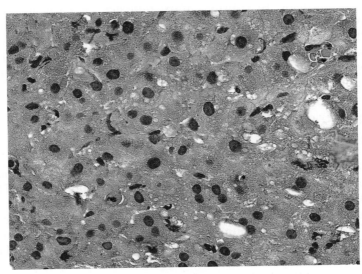

FIGURE 14.23 **Early changes in hepatic arterial thrombosis.** The lobules show increased hepatocyte apoptosis and increased numbers of mitotic figures.

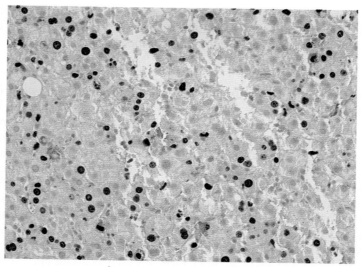

FIGURE 14.24 Early changes in hepatic arterial thrombosis. An immunostain for Ki67 highlights the brisk proliferate rate.

transplanted for hepatitis C, and preservation changes. If mitotic figures are also mildly prominent, the findings favor arterial flow abnormalities. Preservation injury can also show lobular apoptosis and increased mitotic activity, but the clinical course separates out most cases, as preservation changes are usually seen on protocol biopsies or on biopsies performed on return to the operating room for known problems, such as a bile leak. In contrast, most biopsies for early hepatic arterial flow problems are performed in the setting of a sudden and unexplained increase in AST and ALT enzyme levels. Preservation changes also commonly include mild lobular cholestasis, some swelling of zone 3 hepatocytes, and often minimal to mild patchy lobular inflammation with Kupffer cell hyperplasia.

OTHER VASCULAR PROBLEMS

Small-for-Size Graft

In some cases, a liver allograft can be sufficiently small that it has difficulty handling the blood flow from the recipient's portal vein. This can be particularly challenging in living-related donor transplants and in reduced liver transplants, especially when the graft volume is less than 30% of the native liver volume or less than 0.8% of the recipient's body weight.[55] Patients can present with cholestasis, coagulopathy, and ascites. Graft survival is improved by reducing portal vein pressure.[56]

Histologically, the hyperperfusion can lead to a series of changes within the liver.[55] Early changes include prominent portal veins and zone 1 sinusoidal dilatation, along with hemorrhage into the portal tract connective tissue. These findings, however, are more common in the larger portal tracts and may not be sampled in peripheral liver biopsies. Other findings are nonspecific and include mild lobular cholestasis and mild zone 3 fatty change. Some portal tracts can also show a mild bile ductular reaction. In severe cases, there may be arterial vasospasm or thrombosis, leading to necrosis of the larger-sized bile ducts in the liver hilum. Bile leaks, abscesses, and parenchymal infarcts can then develop.

In less severe cases, additional findings may include nodular regenerative hyperplasia and a low-grade persistent ductular reaction that can mimic biliary obstruction.[55] Of note, in many cases, there may be a clinically mild disease that results from small-for-size graft, but the problem is known to the clinical team before the biopsy and is seen incidentally as mild changes in the background when biopsies are performed for other indications, such as ruling out acute cellular rejection.

Congestive Hepatopathy Due to Piggyback Graft

The donor liver can be transplanted using a method that preserves the recipient's vena cava, wherein the donor's inferior vena cava is attached directly or "piggybacked" to the recipient's vena cava. Up to 8% of patients transplanted with this method will develop significant ascites.[48] The liver biopsies in these cases show patchy zone 3 sinusoidal dilatation (Figure 14.25) and areas of hepatocyte dropout. The hepatic arteries can also be atrophic or inapparent, and there can be mild patchy bile ductular proliferation (Figure 14.26).

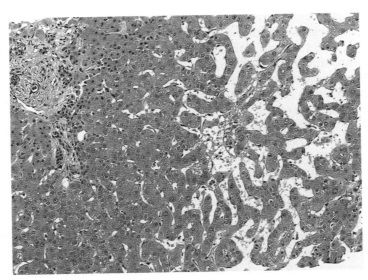

FIGURE 14.25 **Piggyback changes.** The lobules show sinusoidal dilation.

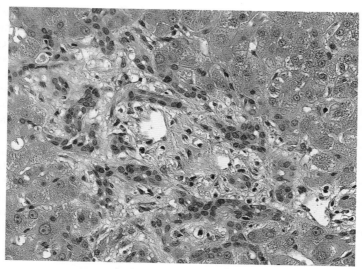

FIGURE 14.26 **Piggyback changes.** The portal tracts show mild patchy bile ductular proliferation.

OPPORTUNISTIC VIRAL INFECTIONS

The most commonly encountered viral infection after liver transplant, at least in biopsies of the liver, is CMV. Hepatocytes, endothelial cells, and bile ducts can all be infected. The histologic findings in CMV infection can be very mild and nonspecific, ranging from small foci of lobular lymphocytic inflammation (Figure 14.27) to small clusters of sinusoidal neutrophils. Of note, small clusters of sinusoidal neutrophils, also called mini-microabscesses, are neither sensitive nor specific for CMV infection and in most cases are idiopathic.[57] In some cases, there will be no viral cytopathic affect and no inflammation and the infection is only picked up by immunostains (Figure 14.28).

Other viral infections that may occur after transplant include herpes simplex virus and adenovirus infections. In both cases, there can be well-demarcated areas of azonal necrosis, a finding called *punched-out necrosis*. Viral inclusions can sometime be seen in viable hepatocytes at the edge of the necrosis, but they are often hard to see on H&E staining. In other cases, there can be severe panlobular necrosis with few viable hepatocytes. Immunostains are important in confirming the diagnosis of viral infection.

Hepatitis E Virus

HEV can cause both an acute and a chronic hepatitis pattern in immunosuppressed patients, including those with liver allografts. The two most common patterns of injury are that of an "idiopathic posttransplant hepatitis"[58-60] or an unexplained cholestatic hepatitis. Rapid fibrosis

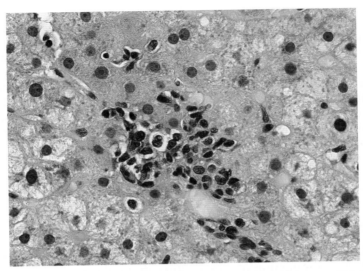

FIGURE 14.27 **Cytomegalovirus (CMV) infection, small microabscesses.** This CMV hepatitis was associated with small lobular aggregates of neutrophils, or microabscesses.

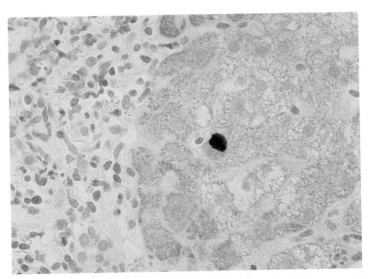

FIGURE 14.28 **Cytomegalovirus (CMV) infection with no tissue reaction.** In this image, a CMV-infected hepatocyte was identified only on immunostain. No viral cytopathic affect or inflammatory reaction was seen on H&E.

progression has been reported[58] but is not common. Most infected individuals will not have a clearly identifiable exposure risk, and a high index of suspicion is currently the best way to identify chronic HEV infections. For example, individuals with unexplained hepatitis should be tested for HEV infection.

Human Herpesvirus

Human herpesvirus 6 (HHV6) can be rarely seen after transplant, where it can cause a hepatitic pattern of injury[61] and rarely a giant cell hepatitis pattern of injury.[62] Infection can be de novo or more commonly results from reactivation. One study reported that HHV6 infection potentially explained 39% of cases of graft hepatitis of undetermined cause; they also reported that most cases of HHV6 hepatitis had a nonspecific lobular hepatitic pattern that was typically mild to moderate, but 4 of 10 cases had also had a portal-based hepatitic pattern with zone 1 necrosis (Figure 14.29).[63] Rarely, HHV6 can be integrated into the donor liver DNA and, when activated after liver transplant, leads to high viral loads, severe disease, and death.[64]

RECURRENT HEPATITIS C

HCV historically recurred in almost all liver allografts following transplant, but with the introduction of direct-acting antiviral agents (DAAs), the frequency of recurrence has dropped to less than 1% and is essentially seen only when patients cannot tolerate or are noncompliant with DAA medications. DAAs can be used either before or after the liver transplant. There initially was some concern about using DAA in patients with hepatocellular carcinoma (HCC), as early studies suggested DAAs might enhance the aggressiveness of HCC, but subsequent and larger studies have not confirmed this risk.[65]

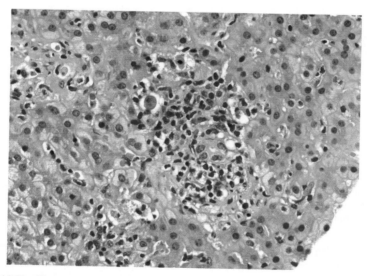

FIGURE 14.29 **Human herpesvirus 6 (HHV6) hepatitis.** The biopsy showed mild portal and lobular hepatitis. In several portal tracts, there was accentuation of apoptosis in zone 1 hepatocytes.

Clinical Findings and Laboratory Findings

Without pretransplant treatment with DAA, hepatitis C reinfects the liver allograft within a few hours, from virions that are circulating in the recipient blood. Nonetheless, there is generally a lag of weeks to months before the recurrent hepatitis C is associated with a biochemical and histologic hepatitis. When this happens, the liver enzyme levels suddenly increase, which may prompt a liver biopsy to distinguish acute cellular rejection from recurrent hepatitis C. This increase in liver enzyme levels is not associated with an increase in viral replication but instead reflects the onset of an immune response.

Histologic Findings

The histologic findings in recurrent HCV infection will vary considerably depending on the time since transplant. The earliest histologic changes are lobular spotty necrosis in the absence of significant inflammation (Figure 14.30; eFig. 14.15).[66,67] This pattern is typically associated with the first increase in AST and ALT levels, which tends to occur in the first weeks to months after transplant. In later biopsies, the lobular apoptosis will diminish and there will be increased but generally still mild lobular lymphocytic inflammation. The portal tracts will also develop chronic inflammation that is typically mild to moderate in grade. Overall, the histologic findings at this point are essentially identical to those seen in individuals with chronic HCV infection who did not undergo transplant.[66,68]

Historically, two patterns could be seen that reflected more severe cases of recurrent HCV infection: cholestatic HCV and fibrosing cholestatic HCV. Fibrosing cholestatic HCV is associated with high viral loads, typically

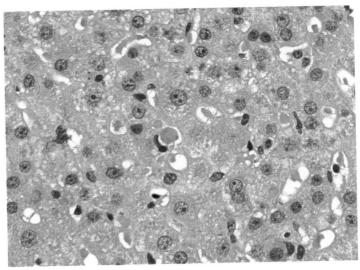

FIGURE 14.30 **Early recurrent hepatitis C.** The lobules show mild spotty necrosis with no significant inflammation.

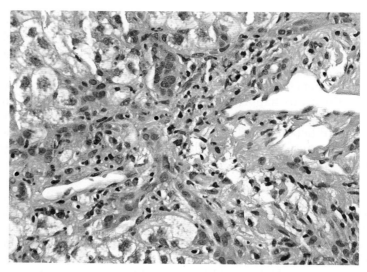

FIGURE 14.31 **Fibrosing cholestatic hepatitis C, portal tract changes.** The portal tracts show mild bile ductular proliferation.

greater than 30 million copies per milliliter[66]; this pattern of injury has virtually disappeared with the availability of DAAs. Some cases can have lower viral levels, but they are still generally above 10 million copies per milliliter. The predominant portal finding is ductular proliferation that mimics biliary obstruction (Figure 14.31), and obstruction should be ruled out in all cases by imaging studies. The portal tracts also show mild lymphocytic inflammation and occasionally neutrophilic inflammation. The lobules show moderate to marked cholestasis with hepatocyte swelling (Figure 14.32) and pericellular fibrosis. The lobular fibrosis most commonly has a zone 1 pattern of pericellular/periportal fibrosis (Figure 14.33), but a zone 3 pericellular pattern of fibrosis, or both, may be seen. There can be rapid fibrosis progression.

Cholestatic HCV is associated with lobular cholestasis, yet lacks the features of fibrosing cholestatic hepatitis; these cases typically show equivocal to mild hepatocyte swelling and patchy but definite ductular proliferation, with the overall findings falling between those of typical recurrent HCV and fibrosing cholestatic HCV. The differential for this pattern typically includes a drug reaction and sometimes biliary obstruction. This pattern of HCV infection tends to have more rapid fibrosis progression than recurrent cases of HCV infection without cholestasis.

OTHER RECURRENT DISEASES

Recurrent Hepatitis B

The histologic findings in recurrent hepatitis B are similar to those described for recurrent HCV infection. Ground glass hepatocytes take many decades to develop, so they will not be seen at the time of viral recurrence. The diagnosis

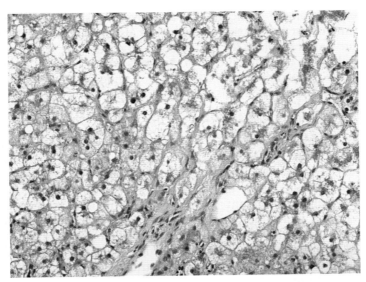

FIGURE 14.32 **Fibrosing cholestatic hepatitis C.** Marked lobular swelling is seen in this case.

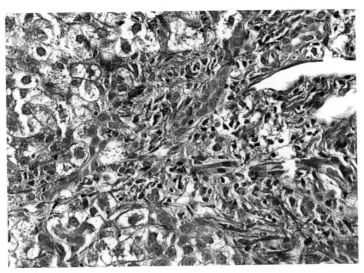

FIGURE 14.33 **Fibrosing cholestatic hepatitis C, zone 1 pericellular fibrosis.** A trichrome stain shows fibrosis extending into zone 1.

can be supported with immunostains for hepatitis B surface antigen (HBsAg) or hepatitis B core antigen (HBcAg).

Alcoholic Liver Disease

The frequency of recurrent alcoholic liver disease varies considerably in the literature, but is generally around 30% to 45%.[69,70] Overall, alcoholic liver disease is a good indication for transplant when measured by graft and patient outcomes.[69,71] Alcohol use after liver transplant, however, has a negative impact on patient survival, which is also true for those individuals who underwent transplant for nonalcoholic liver disease.[70] A diagnosis of active alcohol use is made on clinical grounds. Histologically, the findings are the same as in individuals who did not undergo transplant, ranging from steatosis to steatohepatitis.

Nonalcoholic Liver Disease

Nonalcoholic fatty liver disease (NAFLD) commonly recurs in the first 5 years after liver transplant.[72] The incidence of recurrence increases steadily with the length of follow-up and approaches 100%.[73] Recurrent NAFLD is associated with the metabolic syndrome[74] as well as steroid use as an immunosuppressant.[72] Other risk factors include steatosis in the donor liver and tacrolimus therapy.[75] NAFLD, including steatohepatitis, can recur histologically yet have normal liver enzyme levels.[74] Fibrosis can develop, but current data suggests that cardiovascular disease is the major risk for morbidity and mortality after liver transplant for patients with the metabolic syndrome.

Allograft steatosis and steatohepatitis can also develop de novo in individuals who did not undergo transplant for NAFLD. In some cases, the steatosis is associated with glucocorticoid therapy for control of rejection. The allograft in individuals who underwent transplant for cystic fibrosis or *ATP8B1* (FIC) deficiency can also develop de novo steatohepatitis, which sometimes can be severe.[76] Portal vein thrombosis can also lead to hepatic steatosis (Figure 14.34). Interestingly, de novo fatty liver disease is more likely to resolve over time (23%), when compared

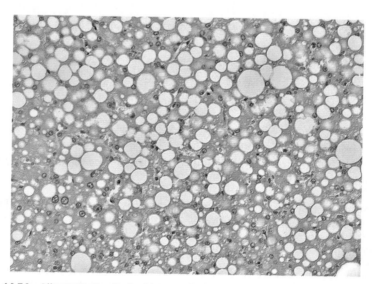

FIGURE 14.34 **Allograft steatosis.** Macrovesicular steatosis developed after a portal vein thrombosis in this liver allograft.

with recurrent fatty liver disease from the metabolic syndrome (0%); this indicates that at least in some cases, they represent different disease pathways.[11]

Primary Sclerosing Cholangitis

PSC recurs following liver transplantation in approximately 20% to 30% of individuals. The median time to a diagnosis of recurrent PSC is approximately 5 years, with a range from 0.5 years to greater than 10 years after transplant.[77,78] A colectomy before or at the time of transplant can be protective against recurrent PSC.[78]

The histologic findings on biopsies from allograft livers with recurrent PSC are fundamentally the same as those seen in patients who did not undergo transplant,[48] although one study has reported there can be more lobular hepatitis in recurrent disease, when compared with native disease.[79] The hilar bile ducts (usually not sampled on biopsy) can also show more lymphocytic cholangitis.[79] The differential for recurrent PSC includes biliary obstruction or bile duct strictures from surgical or other mechanical causes. There are no histologic findings, including onion-skin fibrosis or fibro-obliterative duct lesions, that allow reliable separation of these two possibilities.[48] Thus, imaging studies are important in supporting a final diagnosis of recurrent PSC and should show nonanastomotic biliary strictures and other radiographic findings of PSC. Strictures that occur within the first 90 days are more likely to be procedure related. Chronic rejection can also be in the differential if ductopenia is present. Chronic rejection generally does not have a ductular reaction in the portal tracts, whereas recurrent PSC typically does, at least focally. In contrast to recurrent PSC, chronic rejection can be associated with central perivenulitis, mild zone 3 lobular cholestasis, and mild perivenular fibrosis. Portal fibrosis, on the other hand, can be seen in recurrent PSC but is not a typical feature of chronic rejection. The clinical history can also be helpful, such as a history of suboptimal immunosuppression or prior episodes of acute cellular rejection.

Primary Biliary Cirrhosis/Cholangitis

PBC recurs in approximately 10% to 30% of individuals following liver transplant.[80] The average time to recurrence varies among studies but is generally between 3 and 6 years. PBC can also recur late, in some cases developing after more than 10 years of disease-free follow-up.[80] The histologic findings in allograft livers with recurrent PBC are fundamentally the same as those in patients who did not undergo transplant.[48,81] To make the diagnosis with confidence, serum antimitochondrial antibody (AMA) should be positive, there should be a firm diagnosis of PBC in the native liver, and there should be compatible histologic findings in the liver allograft. Florid duct lesions, when present, are very helpful (Figure 14.35), but in many cases the histologic findings will be those of a chronic portal-based hepatitis. Granulomas may also be seen. In some cases, the bile ducts

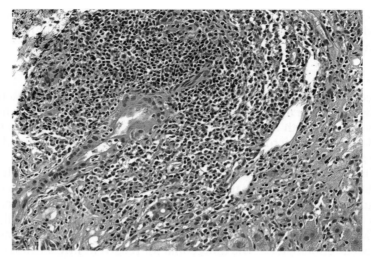

FIGURE 14.35 **Recurrent primary biliary cirrhosis/cholangitis (PBC).** This allograft liver biopsy shows a dense cuff of lymphocytic inflammation surrounding a medium-sized bile duct. There are also bile duct lymphocytosis and reactive changes.

will show lymphocytosis and reactive changes similar to that seen in PBC in native livers. Occasionally, patients who underwent transplant for PBC can have recurrent disease that resembles autoimmune hepatitis clinically, serologically, and histologically. In other cases, the recurrent disease will have overlapping features that fall between those of autoimmune hepatitis and PBC.[82] Such cases are probably best managed as autoimmune hepatitis, as they can quickly develop advanced fibrosis including cirrhosis.[82] In contrast, the rate of fibrosis in PBC is more indolent.

De novo PBC in the allograft is defined as clinical, serologic, and histologic features of PBC in the liver allograft, without a history of PBC as the underlying liver disease. The frequency is very low, and the explanted liver should also be re-examined to look for features of under-diagnosed PBC.

Autoimmune Hepatitis

Autoimmune hepatitis recurs in approximately 20% to 30% of liver transplant patients, but the numbers vary widely depending on diagnostic criteria and the length of follow-up. Centers that perform late protocol biopsies pick up more cases of mildly active recurrent autoimmune hepatitis. Overall, the average time to recurrence is similar to that of PSC and PBC, mostly falling within the 3- to 5-year range. Because the inflammation is attacking the allograft liver, the disease is often called *alloimmune hepatitis.*

The diagnosis of recurrent autoimmune hepatitis in the liver transplant recipient is made essentially the same way as that in individuals who did not undergo transplant.[48] Drug effects and acute and chronic viral hepatitis have to be reasonably excluded. After that, the biopsy should show chronic hepatitis, positive autoantibodies that are typically greater than 1:160 (antinuclear antibodies, anti-smooth muscle antibodies, or anti-liver-kidney microsome antibodies), and an increased serum gamma globulin fraction. Of note, however, increased autoantibody titers alone do not establish the diagnosis of autoimmune hepatitis, even when high. Serum autoantibody titers are also not useful for determining disease activity.

The portal inflammation in recurrent autoimmune hepatitis is typically mild to moderate and occasionally will have well-formed lymphoid aggregates. Interface activity is variable and generally correlates with the amount of portal inflammation. Plasma cells are typically at least mildly prominent. The lobules show mild to moderate hepatitis, and there can be patchy hepatocyte regenerative rosettes, especially in the setting of significant lobular injury. Cholestatic rosettes can be seen if the hepatitis is accompanied by cholestasis, which is usually seen only with moderate to severe lobular hepatitis. Lobular plasma cells, when present, are also helpful in making the diagnosis. When considering the possibility of de novo autoimmune hepatitis, it can be informative to reexamine the explanted livers; at least in some of these cases, there will be mild but convincing features of an underlying autoimmune hepatitis that was missed because the clinical findings at the time of transplant pointed toward a different underlying liver disease.

Plasma-cell–rich acute cellular rejection is also commonly in the differential. In most cases, plasma-cell–rich rejection is associated with other typical findings of acute cellular rejection and the degree of plasmacytosis will correlate with the severity of the rejection.[33] Serologic findings are also helpful, as plasma-cell–rich rejection will generally have low titer or absent autoantibodies.[36]

OTHER FINDINGS

Glycogenic Hepatopathy

Steroids are an important component of antirejection therapy. Steroids can cause temporary accumulation of glycogen in hepatocytes, leading to hepatocyte swelling and increased serum AST and ALT levels. When treating acute cellular rejection, follow-up biopsies are sometimes performed if serum studies fail to show the anticipated reduction in liver enzyme levels after treatment of acute cellular rejection with steroids. In some of these cases, the main finding in the follow-up biopsy will be that of glycogenic hepatopathy, with moderate to rarely marked hepatocyte swelling from glycogen accumulation (Figure 14.36). The histologic findings resolve rapidly with tapering of the steroids.

Drug-Induced Liver Injury

Drug reactions after liver transplant are often difficult to recognize because of the many medications that may be used and because other injury processes in the differential can show similar histologic findings,

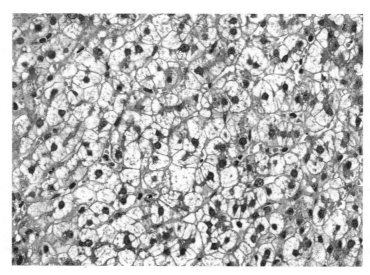

FIGURE 14.36 Glycogenic hepatopathy, steroid induced. After steroid-based therapy for acute cellular rejection, the hepatic enzyme levels remained elevated. A biopsy showed resolution of the rejection, but pale swollen hepatocytes of glycogenic hepatopathy.

including acute cellular rejection and recurrent disease. DILI is usually recognized when there are biopsy findings or clinical findings that do not fit well for rejection or for recurrent disease. One example would be a biopsy that shows moderate portal and lobular eosinophilia with mild portal lymphocytic inflammation and only equivocal duct injury. While rejection would be in the differential, the overall findings would be atypical for acute cellular rejection and should raise the possibility of a drug reaction. Another example is an injury pattern of bland lobular cholestasis without significant lobular or portal inflammation and no evidence of bile duct obstruction. This pattern should also suggest a drug reaction. Still another example would be portal-based inflammatory injury that also shows bile duct injury but has more neutrophils than seen in rejection (a pattern that would suggest antibiotic DILI, such as Augmentin). There are many other potential examples, but all share in common the principle that histologic and/or clinical findings are atypical for rejection or recurrent disease.

GRAFT-VERSUS-HOST DISEASE

Definition

Graft-versus-host disease (GVHD) is an inflammatory disease of the liver that occurs after allogenic bone marrow transplant, when engrafted donor immune cells recognize and attack the recipient's liver.

Clinical Findings

After bone marrow transplant, GVHD usually manifests as injury primarily to the gut, liver, and skin. The symptoms will vary depending on the pattern of GVHD injury. In most cases, liver GVHD is accompanied by skin or gut GVHD. While rare cases of isolated (or relatively isolated) liver GVHD have been reported,[83] a diagnosis of isolated hepatic GVHD should be made with caution.

Laboratory Findings

The laboratory findings in GVHD most commonly show a cholestatic pattern of injury with elevations in alkaline phosphatase and bilirubin levels.

Histologic Findings

The bile ducts are the main target of injury in GVHD and show apoptosis and reactive changes (Figure 14.37; eFig. 14.16). The degree of bile duct injury can be mild and patchy in early cases. Portal inflammation is typically sparse, but episodes of GVHD that occur at later time points are more likely to have portal inflammation.[84]

There tends to be less bile duct lymphocytosis than that seen with acute cellular rejection, and bile duct injury is the main criterion for the diagnosis. In fact, convincing lymphocytosis is not seen in about half of cases.[84] The bile duct injury manifests as apoptosis of cholangiocytes, as well as irregularly shaped and spaced cholangiocytes; sometimes there can be reactive atypia that even suggests dysplasia. Bile ductular proliferation is typically absent. The lobules can show cholestasis but generally will not show significant hepatitis. A small proportion of patients, however, can

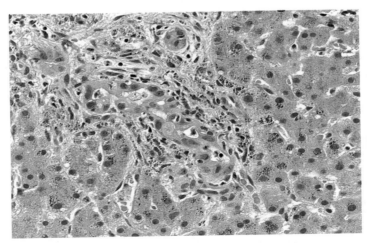

FIGURE 14.37 **Graft-versus-host disease, bile duct injury.** The bile duct shows apoptosis and reactive changes.

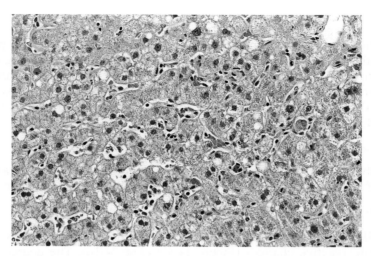

FIGURE 14.38 **Graft-versus-host disease (GVHD), hepatitic variant.** After donor lymphocyte infusion, this biopsy showed mild lobular hepatitis and mild hepatocyte apoptosis, consistent with mild hepatitic variant of GVHD.

have a hepatic pattern of injury, with moderate to severe lobular hepatitis[84]; this pattern is especially common in patients who had sharp reductions in immunosuppression or had recent donor lymphocyte infusions (Figure 14.38).[85]

ENGRAFTMENT SYNDROME

Engraftment syndrome typically occurs within 96 hours of engraftment and is thought to result from the release of cytokines by recently engrafted cells. Clinical findings typically include fever, erythematous rash, rapid weight, and reduction of serum albumin levels. Pulmonary symptoms can also develop. Histologically, the findings can mimic veno-occlusive disease because there can be marked sinusoidal congestion (Figure 14.39). However, no sinusoidal injury or extravasation of red blood cells into the spaces of Disse is seen. The time course and clinical findings usually can help separate these two entities.

POSTTRANSPLANT LYMHOPROLIFERATIVE DISORDER

Posttransplant lymphoproliferative disorders (PTLDs) are typically EBV-driven and are usually B cell in nature. However, about 10% of PTLD cases are negative for EBV[86] and rare cases of PTLDs can be of T-cell or natural killer (NK)-cell origin.[86]

Histologically, the findings vary considerably, but typically there is moderate portal infiltrates, sometimes with distinct B-cell nodules. The lobules also show lymphocytic infiltrates; there can be some associated

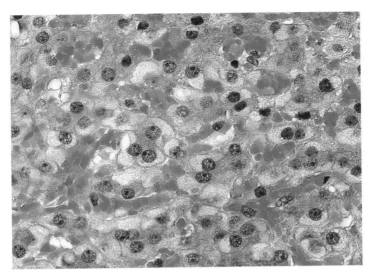

FIGURE 14.39 **Engraftment syndrome.** The liver biopsy shows marked congestive changes. No sinusoidal injury is seen.

hepatocyte injury, but often there is relatively little injury, given the amount of lobular infiltrates. Cytologically, the lymphocytes can appear "atypical," with larger nuclei and irregular nuclear contours. In many cases, however, the lymphocyte atypia is hard to appreciate and the best way to identify PTLDs is a high index of suspicion when there are unusual histologic or clinical findings. Some cases can show marked plasma cell infiltrates (eFig. 14.17).[87] Cases with unexplained hepatitis often benefit by an EBER stain to evaluate for PTLD, especially if the patient has moderate or heavy levels of immunosuppression. If there is extensive necrosis, then immunostains for EBV latent membrane protein may perform better than EBER. PTLDs are classified as per the current WHO system.

In some cases, a patient may have documented PTLD in a lymph node or other organ, but not in the liver. Biopsies of the liver in these cases show a variety of findings, ranging from acute cellular rejection, to recurrent disease, to mild nonspecific inflammatory changes.[88] The acute cellular rejection in these cases can still be successfully treated, even in the setting of PTLDs.

REFERENCES

1. Croome KP, Lee DD, Croome S, et al. The impact of postreperfusion syndrome during liver transplantation using livers with significant macrosteatosis. *Am J Transplant.* 2019;19:2550-2559.
2. Choi WT, Jen KY, Wang D, et al. Donor liver small droplet macrovesicular steatosis is associated with increased risk for recipient allograft rejection. *Am J Surg Pathol.* 2017;41:365-373.

3. Ferri F, Lai Q, Molinaro A, et al. Donor small-droplet macrovesicular steatosis affects liver transplant outcome in HCV-negative recipients. *Chin J Gastroenterol Hepatol.* 2019;2019:5862985.

4. Croome KP, Lee DD, Croome S, et al. Does donor allograft microsteatosis matter? Comparison of outcomes in liver transplantation with a propensity-matched cohort. *Liver Transplant.* 2019;25:1533-1540.

5. Dutkowski P, Schlegel A, Slankamenac K, et al. The use of fatty liver grafts in modern allocation systems: risk assessment by the balance of risk (BAR) score. *Ann Surg.* 2012;256:861-868; discussion 8-9.

6. Biesterfeld S, Knapp J, Bittinger F, et al. Frozen section diagnosis in donor liver biopsies: observer variation of semiquantitative and quantitative steatosis assessment. *Virchows Arch.* 2012;461:177-183.

7. Markin RS, Wisecarver JL, Radio SJ, et al. Frozen section evaluation of donor livers before transplantation. *Transplantation.* 1993;56:1403-1409.

8. Minervini MI, Ruppert K, Fontes P, et al. Liver biopsy findings from healthy potential living liver donors: reasons for disqualification, silent diseases and correlation with liver injury tests. *J Hepatol.* 2009;50:501-510.

9. Shaked O, Gonzalez A, Bahirwani R, et al. Donor hemosiderosis does not affect liver function and regeneration in the setting of living donor liver transplantation. *Am J Transplant.* 2014;14:216-220.

10. Pungpapong S, Krishna M, Abraham SC, et al. Clinicopathologic findings and outcomes of liver transplantation using grafts from donors with unrecognized and unusual diseases. *Liver Transpl.* 2006;12:310-315.

11. Dwyer JP, Sarwar S, Egan B, et al. Hepatic iron overload following liver transplantation of a C282y homozygous allograft: a case report and literature review. *Liver Int.* 2011;31:1589-1592.

12. Veitsman E, Pras E, Pappo O, et al. Hepatic iron overload following liver transplantation from a C282Y/H63D compound heterozygous donor. *Case Reports Hepatol.* 2018;2018:4298649.

13. Monino L, Reding R, Komuta M, et al. Metabolic iron disorder after liver transplant: hereditary hemochromatosis in a pediatric recipient of a pediatric donor with unknown HFE C282Y homozygous mutation. *Clin Res Hepatol Gastroenterol.* 2020;44:e129-e131.

14. Croome KP, Livingston D, Croome S, et al. Sequential protocol biopsies post-liver transplant from donors with moderate macrosteatosis: what happens to the fat? *Liver Transpl.* 2020;27:248-256.

15. Cha I, Bass N, Ferrell LD. Lipopeliosis. An immunohistochemical and clinicopathologic study of five cases. *Am J Surg Pathol.* 1994;18:789-795.

16. Bioulac-Sage P, Balabaud C, Ferrell L. Lipopeliosis revisited: should we keep the term? *Am J Surg Pathol.* 2002;26:134-135.

17. Demetris AJ, Bellamy C, Hübscher SG, et al. 2016 comprehensive update of the Banff working group on liver allograft pathology: introduction of antibody-mediated rejection. *Am J Transplant.* 2016;16:2816-2835.

18. Banff Working Group. Banff schema for grading liver allograft rejection: an international consensus document. *Hepatology* 1997;25:658-663.

19. Koo J, Wang HL. Acute, chronic, and humoral rejection: pathologic features under current immunosuppressive regimes. *Surg Pathol Clin.* 2018;11:431-452.

20. Stevenson HL, Prats MM, Isse K, et al. Isolated vascular "v" lesions in liver allografts: how to approach this unusual finding. *Am J Transplant.* 2018;18:1534-1543.

21. Siddiqui I, Selzner N, Hafezi-Bakhtiari S, et al. Infiltrative (sinusoidal) and hepatitic patterns of injury in acute cellular rejection in liver allograft with clinical implications. *Mod Pathol.* 2015;28:1275-1281.

22. Shi Y, Dong K, Zhang YG, et al. Sinusoidal endotheliitis as a histological parameter for diagnosing acute liver allograft rejection. *World J Gastroenterol.* 2017;23:792-799.

23. Quaglia AF, Del Vecchio Blanco G, Greaves R, et al. Development of ductopaenic liver allograft rejection includes a "hepatitic" phase prior to duct loss. *J Hepatol.* 2000;33:773-780.

24. Krasinskas AM, Demetris AJ, Poterucha JJ, et al. The prevalence and natural history of untreated isolated central perivenulitis in adult allograft livers. *Liver Transpl.* 2008;14:625-632.

25. Sundaram SS, Melin-Aldana H, Neighbors K, et al. Histologic characteristics of late cellular rejection, significance of centrilobular injury, and long-term outcome in pediatric liver transplant recipients. *Liver Transpl.* 2006;12:58-64.

26. Gane E, Sallie R, Saleh M, et al. Clinical recurrence of hepatitis A following liver transplantation for acute liver failure. *J Med Virol.* 1995;45:35-39.

27. Eisenbach C, Longerich T, Fickenscher H, et al. Recurrence of clinically significant hepatitis A following liver transplantation for fulminant hepatitis A. *J Clin Virol.* 2006;35:109-112.

28. Syn WK, Nightingale P, Gunson B, et al. Natural history of unexplained chronic hepatitis after liver transplantation. *Liver Transpl.* 2007;13:984-989.

29. Seyam M, Neuberger JM, Gunson BK, et al. Cirrhosis after orthotopic liver transplantation in the absence of primary disease recurrence. *Liver Transpl.* 2007;13:966-974.

30. Evans HM, Kelly DA, McKiernan PJ, et al. Progressive histological damage in liver allografts following pediatric liver transplantation. *Hepatology.* 2006;43:1109-1117.

31. Miyagawa-Hayashino A, Haga H, Egawa H, et al. Idiopathic post-transplantation hepatitis following living donor liver transplantation, and significance of autoantibody titre for outcome. *Transpl Int.* 2009;22:303-312.

32. Londono MC, Souza LN, Lozano JJ, et al. Molecular profiling of subclinical inflammatory lesions in long-term surviving adult liver transplant recipients. *J Hepatol.* 2018;69:626-634.

33. Alexander J, Chu W, Swanson PE, et al. The significance of plasma cell infiltrate in acute cellular rejection of liver allografts. *Hum Pathol.* 2012;43:1645-1650.

34. Ward SC, Schiano TD, Thung SN, et al. Plasma cell hepatitis in hepatitis C virus patients post-liver transplantation: case-control study showing poor outcome and predictive features in the liver explant. *Liver Transpl.* 2009;15:1826-1833.

35. Stirnimann G, Ebadi M, Czaja AJ, et al. Recurrent and de novo autoimmune hepatitis. *Liver Transpl.* 2019;25:152-166.

36. Fiel MI, Agarwal K, Stanca C, et al. Posttransplant plasma cell hepatitis (de novo autoimmune hepatitis) is a variant of rejection and may lead to a negative outcome in patients with hepatitis C virus. *Liver Transpl.* 2008;14:861-871.

37. Hubscher SG. Antibody-mediated rejection in the liver allograft. *Curr Opin Organ Transplant.* 2012;17:280-286.

38. Aguilera I, Sousa JM, Gavilan F, et al. Glutathione S-transferase T1 genetic mismatch is a risk factor for de novo immune hepatitis in liver transplantation. *Transplant Proc.* 2005;37:3968-3969.

39. Aguilera I, Wichmann I, Sousa JM, et al. Antibodies against glutathione S-transferase T1 (GSTT1) in patients with de novo immune hepatitis following liver transplantation. *Clin Exp Immunol.* 2001;126:535-539.

40. Keitel V, Burdelski M, Vojnisek Z, et al. De novo bile salt transporter antibodies as a possible cause of recurrent graft failure after liver transplantation: a novel mechanism of cholestasis. *Hepatology.* 2009;50:510-517.

41. Aguilera I, Sousa JM, Gavilan F, et al. Complement component 4d immunostaining in liver allografts of patients with de novo immune hepatitis. *Liver Transpl.* 2011;17:779-788.

42. Kozlowski T, Andreoni K, Schmitz J, et al. Sinusoidal C4d deposits in liver allografts indicate an antibody-mediated response: diagnostic considerations in the evaluation of liver allografts. *Liver Transpl.* 2012;18:641-658.

43. Demetris AJ, Nakamura K, Yagihashi A, et al. A clinicopathological study of human liver allograft recipients harboring preformed IgG lymphocytotoxic antibodies. *Hepatology.* 1992;16:671-681.

44. Hubscher SG. Transplantation pathology. *Semin Liver Dis.* 2009;29:74-90.

45. Neil DAH, Bellamy CO, Smith M, et al. Global quality assessment of liver allograft C4d staining during acute antibody-mediated rejection in formalin-fixed, paraffin-embedded tissue. *Hum Pathol.* 2018;73:144-155.

46. O'Leary JG, Cai J, Freeman R, et al. Proposed diagnostic criteria for chronic antibody-mediated rejection in liver allografts. *Am J Transplant.* 2016;16:603-614.

47. O'Leary JG, Smith C, Cai J, et al. Chronic AMR in liver transplant: validation of the 1-year cAMR score's ability to determine long-term outcome. *Transplantation.* 2017;101:2062-2070.

48. Demetris AJ, Adeyi O, Bellamy CO, et al. Liver biopsy interpretation for causes of late liver allograft dysfunction. *Hepatology.* 2006;44:489-501.

49. Bekker J, Ploem S, de Jong KP. Early hepatic artery thrombosis after liver transplantation: a systematic review of the incidence, outcome and risk factors. *Am J Transplant.* 2009;9:746-757.

50. Sedivy R, Gollackner B, Casati B, et al. Apoptotic hepatocytes in rejection and vascular occlusion in liver allograft specimens. *Histopathology.* 1998;32:503-507.

51. Gollackner B, Sedivy R, Rockenschaub S, et al. Increased apoptosis of hepatocytes in vascular occlusion after orthotopic liver transplantation. *Transpl Int.* 2000;13:49-53.

52. Liu TC, Nguyen TT, Torbenson MS. Concurrent increase in mitosis and apoptosis: a histological pattern of hepatic arterial flow abnormalities in post-transplant liver biopsies. *Mod Pathol.* 2012;25:1594-1598.

53. Valente JF, Alonso MH, Weber FL, et al. Late hepatic artery thrombosis in liver allograft recipients is associated with intrahepatic biliary necrosis. *Transplantation.* 1996;61:61-65.

54. Adeyi O, Fischer SE, Guindi M. Liver allograft pathology: approach to interpretation of needle biopsies with clinicopathological correlation. *J Clin Pathol.* 2010;63:47-74.

55. Demetris AJ, Kelly DM, Eghtesad B, et al. Pathophysiologic observations and histopathologic recognition of the portal hyperperfusion or small-for-size syndrome. *Am J Surg Pathol.* 2006;30:986-993.

56. Miyagi S, Shono Y, Tokodai K, et al. Risks of living donor liver transplantation using small-for-size grafts. *Transplant Proc.* 2020;52:1825-1828.

57. MacDonald GA, Greenson JK, DelBuono EA, et al. Mini-microabscess syndrome in liver transplant recipients. *Hepatology.* 1997;26:192-197.

58. Schlosser B, Stein A, Neuhaus R, et al. Liver transplant from a donor with occult HEV infection induced chronic hepatitis and cirrhosis in the recipient. *J Hepatol.* 2012;56:500-502.

59. Pischke S, Suneetha PV, Baechlein C, et al. Hepatitis E virus infection as a cause of graft hepatitis in liver transplant recipients. *Liver Transpl.* 2010;16:74-82.

60. Kamar N, Selves J, Mansuy JM, et al. Hepatitis E virus and chronic hepatitis in organ-transplant recipients. *N Engl J Med.* 2008;358:811-817.

61. Phan TL, Lautenschlager I, Razonable RR, et al. HHV-6 in liver transplantation: a literature review. *Liver Int.* 2018;38:210-223.

62. Potenza L, Luppi M, Barozzi P, et al. HHV-6A in syncytial giant-cell hepatitis. *N Engl J Med.* 2008;359:593-602.

63. Buyse S, Roque-Afonso AM, Vaghefi P, et al. Acute hepatitis with periportal confluent necrosis associated with human herpesvirus 6 infection in liver transplant patients. *Am J Clin Pathol*. 2013;140:403-409.

64. Bonnafous P, Marlet J, Bouvet D, et al. Fatal outcome after reactivation of inherited chromosomally integrated HHV-6A (iciHHV-6A) transmitted through liver transplantation. *Am J Transplant*. 2018;18:1548-1551.

65. Tse CS, Yang JD, Mousa OY, et al. Direct-acting antiviral therapy in liver transplant patients with hepatocellular carcinoma and hepatitis C. *Transplant Direct*. 2021;7:e635.

66. Demetris AJ. Evolution of hepatitis C virus in liver allografts. *Liver Transplant*. 2009;15(suppl 2):S35-S41.

67. Saxena R, Crawford JM, Navarro VJ, et al. Utilization of acidophil bodies in the diagnosis of recurrent hepatitis C infection after orthotopic liver transplantation. *Mod Pathol*. 2002;15:897-903.

68. Greenson JK, Svoboda-Newman SM, Merion RM, et al. Histologic progression of recurrent hepatitis C in liver transplant allografts. *Am J Surg Pathol*. 1996;20:731-738.

69. Bjornsson E, Olsson J, Rydell A, et al. Long-term follow-up of patients with alcoholic liver disease after liver transplantation in Sweden: impact of structured management on recidivism. *Scand J Gastroenterol*. 2005;40:206-216.

70. Faure S, Herrero A, Jung B, et al. Excessive alcohol consumption after liver transplantation impacts on long-term survival, whatever the primary indication. *J Hepatol*. 2012;57:306-312.

71. Bellamy CO, DiMartini AM, Ruppert K, et al. Liver transplantation for alcoholic cirrhosis: long term follow-up and impact of disease recurrence. *Transplantation*. 2001;72:619-626.

72. Dureja P, Mellinger J, Agni R, et al. NAFLD recurrence in liver transplant recipients. *Transplantation*. 2011;91:684-689.

73. Contos MJ, Cales W, Sterling RK, et al. Development of nonalcoholic fatty liver disease after orthotopic liver transplantation for cryptogenic cirrhosis. *Liver Transpl*. 2001;7:363-373.

74. Malik SM, Devera ME, Fontes P, et al. Recurrent disease following liver transplantation for nonalcoholic steatohepatitis cirrhosis. *Liver Transpl*. 2009;15:1843-1851.

75. Dumortier J, Giostra E, Belbouab S, et al. Non-alcoholic fatty liver disease in liver transplant recipients: another story of "seed and soil". *Am J Gastroenterol*. 2010;105:613-620.

76. Miyagawa-Hayashino A, Egawa H, Yorifuji T, et al. Allograft steatohepatitis in progressive familial intrahepatic cholestasis type 1 after living donor liver transplantation. *Liver Transpl*. 2009;15:610-618.

77. Alexander J, Lord JD, Yeh MM, et al. Risk factors for recurrence of primary sclerosing cholangitis after liver transplantation. *Liver Transpl*. 2008;14:245-251.

78. Alabraba E, Nightingale P, Gunson B, et al. A re-evaluation of the risk factors for the recurrence of primary sclerosing cholangitis in liver allografts. *Liver Transpl*. 2009;15:330-340.

79. Miyagawa-Hayashino A, Egawa H, Yoshizawa A, et al. Frequent overlap of active hepatitis in recurrent primary sclerosing cholangitis after living-donor liver transplantation relates to its rapidly progressive course. *Hum Pathol*. 2011;42:1329-1336.

80. Silveira MG, Talwalkar JA, Lindor KD, et al. Recurrent primary biliary cirrhosis after liver transplantation. *Am J Transplant*. 2010;10:720-726.

81. Hubscher SG, Elias E, Buckels JA, et al. Primary biliary cirrhosis. Histological evidence of disease recurrence after liver transplantation. *J Hepatol*. 1993;18:173-184.

82. Hytiroglou P, Gutierrez JA, Freni M, et al. Recurrence of primary biliary cirrhosis and development of autoimmune hepatitis after liver transplant: a blind histologic study. *Hepatol Res*. 2009;39:577-584.

83. Yeh KH, Hsieh HC, Tang JL, et al. Severe isolated acute hepatic graft-versus-host disease with vanishing bile duct syndrome. *Bone Marrow Transplant.* 1994;14:319-321.

84. Quaglia A, Duarte R, Patch D, et al. Histopathology of graft versus host disease of the liver. *Histopathology.* 2007;50:727-738.

85. Akpek G, Boitnott JK, Lee LA, et al. Hepatitic variant of graft-versus-host disease after donor lymphocyte infusion. *Blood.* 2002;100:3903-3907.

86. Nalesnik MA. The diverse pathology of post-transplant lymphoproliferative disorders: the importance of a standardized approach. *Transpl Infect Dis.* 2001;3:88-96.

87. Vishnu P, Jiang L, Cortese C, et al. Plasmacytoma-like posttransplant lymphoproliferative disorder following orthotopic liver transplantation: a case report. *Transplant Proc.* 2011;43:2806-2809.

88. Randhawa P, Blakolmer K, Kashyap R, et al. Allograft liver biopsy in patients with Epstein-Barr virus-associated posttransplant lymphoproliferative disease. *Am J Surg Pathol.* 2001;25:324-330.

15

IRON OVERLOAD IN THE LIVER

OVERVIEW

Over the past several decades, molecular and epidemiological studies have dramatically changed our understanding of the causes and significance of iron accumulation in the liver. There are many excellent review articles on the molecular biology and the clinical management of iron overload in the liver, which are readily found on PubMed and to which the reader is referred to for full molecular biology details. Instead, this chapter is focused on the surgical pathology of iron overload. These findings, however, make more sense when key aspects of iron metabolism are understood, so some of the most important features are reviewed below.

NORMAL IRON METABOLISM

Iron is important in a number of metabolic processes but can be toxic to cells at high levels, so the body tightly regulates iron levels in order to balance the need for iron but avoid toxicity. Toxicity results from reactive oxygen species that bind to and react with proteins, in particular cysteine, leading to protein cross-linking and oxidation. DNA adducts are also formed, and there can be peroxidation damage to the phospholipids of the inner bilayer of the cell membrane. Cell death driven by lipid peroxidation has been called *ferroptosis*.

The normal adult body contains a total of 3 to 5 g of iron (for comparison, a US nickel weighs 5 g). A total of 20 mg of iron is needed each day for normal physiological functions, but the majority of this daily need is met through extracting and reappropriating iron from damaged red blood cells. The remaining iron that is needed is absorbed in the small intestine from dietary sources. Interestingly, there are no physiological ways to excrete iron, so whatever iron is absorbed in the blood has to be either used or stored. Thus, the physiological mechanisms of iron regulation focus tightly on controlling absorption of iron from the small intestine. There are many proteins and cells involved in iron metabolism, but the major ones are shown in Table 15.1 as a quick reference. They work as an integrated network to regulate iron absorption and to regulate blood and cellular levels of iron.

TABLE 15.1 Important Proteins and Cells That Play a Role in Iron Metabolism	
Protein or Cells	Notes
Protein	
DMT-1	Dimetal transporter-1. Transports iron from the gut lumen to the enterocyte cytoplasm.
Ferritin	This protein has an enormous capacity to bind iron and is a major physiological storage form of iron.
Ferroportin	Transports iron out of cells (principally enterocytes and macrophages, also hepatocytes) into the bloodstream.
Hemojuvelin	Interacts with important signaling pathways (BMP, SMAD) that have hepcidin as a downstream target. Without hemojuvelin, these signaling pathways do not active hepcidin gene synthesis in a normal fashion.
Transferrin	Protein that transports iron once it is in blood.
HFE	Protein that is similar to MHC class I proteins. Mutations are the most common cause of genetic hemochromatosis. Interacts with transferrin receptor 1 and regulates hepcidin levels.
Cells	
Enterocytes	Absorption and short-term storage of iron.
Hepatocytes	Major producer of ferritin and hepcidin. Major organ for storage of iron in the form of ferritin.
Macrophages	Main recycler of old/damage red blood cells. Important storage site for iron in the form of ferritin.
Other	
Hemosiderin	Abnormal deposits of iron

Iron Absorption

Most iron is absorbed in the duodenum and the proximal jejunum. Dietary heme iron is disassociated from globin and then taken up by the enterocytes. Dietary nonheme iron requires additional steps, and has to be first reduced from a ferric to a ferrous state, before it can be transported into the cytoplasm of enterocytes by a protein called DMT-1. Once iron is within the enterocyte cytoplasm, it can be transported out of the enterocyte into the blood via the protein ferroportin, with some help from additional proteins such as ceruloplasmin and hephaestin. Once in the blood, iron is bound by transferrin (Figure 15.1). On the other hand, if the body has sufficient iron stores, then the iron remains within the cytoplasm of the enterocytes, and is not transported into the blood; this

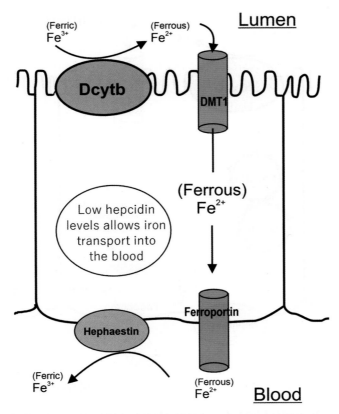

FIGURE 15.1 **Diagram of iron absorption when the body needs iron.** Low hepcidin levels allow iron to be transported from enterocytes into the blood.

results from high levels of hepcidin that degrade ferroportin. When the enterocyte eventually dies, the iron will be lost within the fecal stream, preventing iron overload (Figure 15.2).

In healthy individuals, there is more transferrin protein than iron within the blood, with about 30% of the transferrin molecules saturated with iron. If blood iron levels increase, the excess transferrin protein serves as a reservoir that can quickly sop up the excess iron to prevent toxicity.

Iron Storage

Hepatocytes and macrophages serve as major storage depots of iron, with iron incorporated into ferritin molecules for storage. Ferritin can hold up to 4500 atoms of iron per ferritin protein complex. Ferritin is typically not visible on Perls Prussian Blue stain, but occasionally is seen as a diffuse blue-blush in the cytoplasm of hepatocytes (Figure 15.3). The iron in ferritin is readily available to meet physiological needs. On the

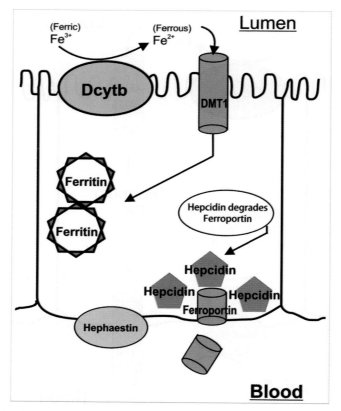

FIGURE 15.2 **Diagram of iron absorption when the body does not need iron.** When blood iron levels are adequate, increased hepcidin levels degrade ferroportin, blocking transfer of blood from enterocytes into the blood.

other hand, if ferritin levels are excessive over a sufficiently long period of time, hemosiderin deposits can develop. Hemosiderin is composed of iron along with degraded ferritin and small amounts of other proteins. On hematoxylin and eosin (H&E) stain, hemosiderin is a granular, golden brown cytoplasmic deposit (Figure 15.4). In contrast to the iron stored as ferritin, the iron in hemosiderin deposits is not readily available for biological needs.

In sum, two important iron reservoirs are used to keep blood iron levels at physiologically correct levels: (1) a short-term reservoir of iron stored within enterocytes and (2) a longer-term reservoir of iron stored as ferritin, principally in hepatocytes and macrophages. If both reservoirs are unable to meet the demands for iron, then anemia develops; on the other hand, if iron control mechanisms are dysregulated (eg, if key proteins are mutated), or if there is excess exogenous iron intake (eg, transfusions), then iron overload can develop.

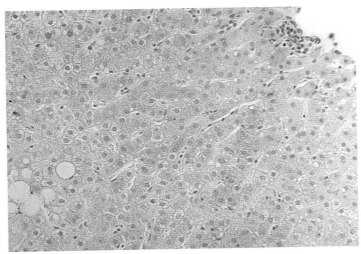

FIGURE 15.3 **Perls iron stain with ferritin blush.** Ferritin is seen as a subtle, pale, blue blush in the hepatocyte cytoplasm.

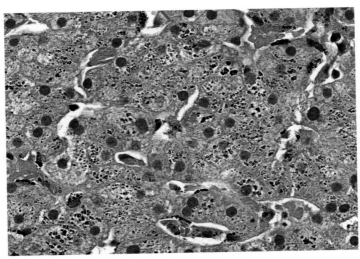

FIGURE 15.4 **Hemosiderin on hematoxylin and eosin (H&E).** Iron deposits are seen as brown granules in the hepatocyte cytoplasm. The granules can vary in color from golden brown to more of a chocolate brown.

Iron Release From Stores in the Enterocytes, Liver, and Macrophages

Hepcidin is the major controller of iron metabolism[1,2]: when iron levels are adequate, it functions by blocking the release of iron stored in hepatocytes, macrophages, and enterocytes, keeping it from entering the blood

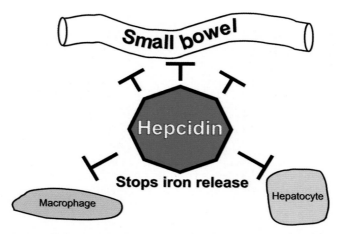

FIGURE 15.5 **Hepcidin serves as the central regulator of iron metabolism.** Hepcidin blocks release of iron from hepatocytes and macrophages and blocks iron absorption from the gut.

(Figure 15.5). When serum hepcidin levels are lowered, more iron is absorbed from the gut and more iron is released into the blood from stores in hepatocytes and macrophages. Hepcidin (encoded by the gene *HAMP*) is produced by hepatocytes[3] and biliary epithelium.[4] Hepcidin is also an acute phase reactant, and hepcidin levels are elevated in many inflammatory and infectious conditions; this is thought to lower blood iron levels in situations where the body is facing an infection, as iron is needed by many infectious organisms. In sum, hepcidin's main physiological role is to lower blood iron levels, which it does by blocking the transfer of iron from enterocytes into the blood and by blocking the release of iron stores from the liver and macrophages into the blood; hepcidin accomplishes these two tasks by degrading ferroportin, the protein that exports iron out of cells into the blood.[5]

Mutations in Iron-Related Genes

Hepcidin dysregulation plays a central role in all known causes of hemochromatosis.[1] In fact, mutations that lead to hemochromatosis all function by decreasing hepcidin production or impairing hepcidin function, including mutations in *HFE*, *HAMP*, *HJV*, and *TfR2*.[6] Key features of these diseases are summarized in Table 15.2. The abnormally low levels of hepcidin, or the impairment in hepcidin function, that result from these mutations gradually lead to excess iron absorption and eventually to iron deposition in the liver and other organs. Interestingly, to date, most reported mutations lead to loss of hepcidin function. Rare mutations, however, have been described that increase hepcidin function, leading to severe congenital refractory anemia.[7] Increased expression of hepcidin (with subsequent development of anemia) has also been reported in a hepatic adenoma.[8]

TABLE 15.2   Summary of Genetic Iron Diseases Involving the Liver

Disease (Other Designations)	Gene (Protein)	Inheritance	Primary Ethnicity	Onset	Principal Iron Location
HFE hemochromatosis (hemochromatosis type 1)	HFE	Recessive	Northern European	Late	Hepatocytes > Kupffer cells
Juvenile hemochromatosis (hemochromatosis type 2A)	HFE2 (also known as HJV)	Recessive	European	Early	Hepatocytes > Kupffer cells
Juvenile hemochromatosis (hemochromatosis type 2B)	HAMP (hepcidin)	Recessive	European	Early	Hepatocytes > Kupffer cells
TFR2 hemochromatosis (hemochromatosis type 3)	TfR2	Recessive	European Asian	Late	Hepatocytes > Kupffer cells
Ferroportin disease (ferropotin disease type A; hemochromatosis type 4)	SLC40A1 (ferroportin, loss of function mutation)	Dominant	Pan-ethnic	Late	Kupffer cells > hepatocytes
Ferroportin hemochromatosis (ferroportin disease type B)	SLC40A1 (ferroportin, activating mutation)	Dominant	Pan-ethnic	Late	Hepatocytes > Kupffer cells
DMT1 hemochromatosis	SCL11A2 (DMT-1)	Recessive	European	Early	Hepatocytes > Kupffer cells
Hypotransferrinemia	Tf (transferrin)	Recessive	European Asian	Early	Kupffer cells > hepatocytes
Hypoceruloplasminemia	CP (ceruloplasmin)	Recessive	European Asian	Late	Hepatocyte > Kupffer cells

Interestingly, hepatic adenomas occurring in individuals with type 1a glycogen storage disease are also associated with anemia that resolves after the adenoma is resected,[9] implying hepcidin overexpression by the adenomas. In contrast, hepatocellular carcinomas tend to have suppressed levels of hepcidin expression.[10]

IRON BLOOD TESTING

Serum testing for iron-related disease is common, and it can be helpful to understand the most common tests and what they mean. Broad interpretation of patterns is shown in Table 15.3.

IRON. This test measures the amount of iron in the serum. Most iron in the blood is bound to transferrin.

FERRITIN. Ferritin is the main storage form of iron in the body, being present in abundance in hepatocytes and macrophages. A small amount of ferritin will escape from these sources and enter the blood. The amount of ferritin that escapes into the blood is proportional to and a good measure of the total amount of body iron stores. Thus, ferritin will be low if there is anemia and high if there is excess body iron stores. Ferritin is an important screening test for iron overload. Of note, however, ferritin is an acute phase reactant and can also be elevated with fatty liver disease or other inflammatory conditions of the liver. Thus, ferritin levels are typically measured on at least two separate occasions. Also, mildly elevated ferritin levels in the setting of a normal transferrin saturation usually indicates that there is no iron overload and the ferritin elevations are likely part of an acute phase response to other illness.

TRANSFERRIN. Transferrin is the main protein that transports iron in the blood. Transferrin levels can decrease during inflammatory processes (the opposite of an acute phase reactant), and levels also depend on nutritional status and liver synthetic function.

TOTAL IRON-BINDING CAPACITY (TIBC). This tests the total amount of iron that can be bound by proteins in the blood. Since transferrin is the major protein that binds iron in blood, the results will be similar to those that directly measure transferrin levels.

UNSATURATED TIBC. This test measures the amount of transferrin that is in the blood, but not bound to iron.

TRANSFERRIN SATURATION (ALSO CALLED TRANSFERRIN SATURATION INDEX). This is the ratio of the total iron divided by the TIBC. In normal health, about 30% of the transferrin is saturated with iron. Levels above 45% commonly trigger additional clinical workup. Transferrin saturation (how much iron is in the blood) is elevated before ferritin levels (reflecting total body iron stores) in the early clinical course of HFE-hemochromatosis, other genetic causes of hemochromatosis, and secondary iron overload.

TABLE 15.3 Patterns in Blood Testing for Iron-Related Disease

Disease	Hemoglobin	Blood iron[b]	Ferritin[c]	Transferrin	TIBC	Transferrin Saturation[c]
Typical normal[a]	13.5-17.5 g/dL	10-30 nmol/L	15-300 µg/L	2-3.5 mg/L	240-450 µg/dL	24%-45%
HFE hemochromatosis	Normal	High	High	Normal to slightly low	Normal to slightly low	High
Ferroportin disease	Normal to low	Low to normal	High	Limited data	Limited data	Low
Iron deficiency anemia	Low	Low (normal in early disease)	Low	High	High	Low
Secondary iron overload[d]	Variable, depending on cause	Normal to high	High	Slightly low to normal to slightly high	Normal to slightly low	High
Chronic illnesses such as chronic viral hepatitis, alcoholic hepatitis, metabolic syndrome	Normal to low	Low	Normal to high; when high does not exceed 3× normal	Normal to low	Normal to low	Normal to low

[a]These are approximate normal ranges; each laboratory will have its own normal range.
[b]Serum iron is best interpreted with other blood work, since it can be highly variable depending on diet, inflammation, infection, etc.
[c]Serum ferritin and transferrin saturation are the main tests used to screen for iron overload disease.
[d]There can be a fair amount of variability in the test results, depending on the specific type of underlying disease leading to the secondary iron overload; the most common pattern is shown.

DETECTION OF IRON IN THE LIVER

Iron Stains

The major histochemical stain used to detect iron in the liver is Perls Prussian Blue, a stain named after Max Perls, a German pathologist. The history of the Perls iron stain actually starts in 1704, when Heinrich Diesbach (a color maker) and Johann Konrad Dippel (a physician) developed a dark blue pigment that they called "Berliner blau." This color looked great and so was used for uniforms in the Prussian army, where it became widely known as "Prussian blue." A century plus later, in 1847, Rudolph Virchow used this same basic dye method to examine areas of hemorrhage by light microscopy and found hemosiderin stained blue. About 20 years later, this method was improved by Max Perls, who also showed that hemosiderin could be detected in a variety of tissues.

The basic chemistry of Perls Prussian Blue is that iron in the ferric state will react with hydrochloric acid to form ferric ferrocyanide, an insoluble blue compound (Prussian Blue) that is well visualized on light microscopy. The distribution and density of blue staining correlates well, but not perfectly, with tissue iron concentrations. The stain is not sensitive enough to detect very low levels of iron but is easy to perform and reproducible. The basic staining patterns are as follows.

FERRITIN. Normally no ferritin will be seen. However, in cases of elevated serum ferritin levels, ferritin may be seen as a light, diffuse, blue-blush within the hepatocyte or Kupffer cell cytoplasm (Figure 15.3).

HEMOSIDERIN. Hemosiderin is seen as brown, granular cytoplasmic deposits on H&E stains and as bright blue granular deposits on iron stain. Residual brown granular material is often seen on iron stain and represents lipofuscin in most cases (Figure 15.6).

Iron Grading Systems

Many iron grading systems have been proposed over the years. They vary in their approach, but all attempt to provide semiquantitative data on the extent of iron accumulation. Some systems are based on the zonation of iron distribution, some on the lowest magnification that discernible granules can be seen, and some on the percent of hepatocytes positive for iron. Is one system clearly the best? Probably not. I personally use a schema (Table 15.4) based on the percent of hepatocytes positive for iron, similar to that described by LeSage et al.[11] This simple-to-use classification system provides sufficient clinical information for patient care, but there are many reasonable alternatives if you prefer a different approach. A modified Scheuer system (shown in Table 15.5) is also a very useful and popular system.[12] If a grading system is employed, separate numbers should be given for hepatocellular and the Kupffer cell iron.

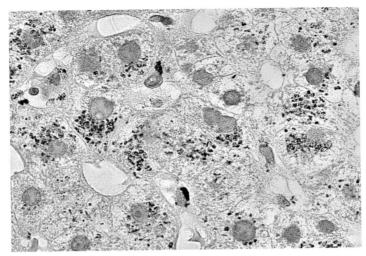

FIGURE 15.6 **Perls iron stain.** The residual brown-black pigment in the hepatocyte cell cytoplasm is lipofuscin.

TABLE 15.4	Simple Scoring System for Iron in the Liver		
Grade	Description	Hepatocytes	Lobular Kupffer Cells
0	None	None	None
1	Minimal	<5%	<5%
2	Mild	5%-30%	5%-30%
3	Moderate	31%-60%	31%-60%
4	Marked	>60%	>60%

Note: For studies, it is helpful to record the zonal pattern of iron and whether the distribution is homogeneous; endothelial iron and portal macrophage iron is scored separately.

TABLE 15.5	Modified Scheuer Grading System for Iron in the Liver
Grade	Description
0	Iron granules absent or Iron granules barely seen at 400×
1	Iron granules resolved at 250×
2	Iron granules resolved at 100×
3	Iron granules resolved at 25×
4	Iron deposits resolved at 10× or iron deposits visible without magnification

Remember that using a numerical system does not make a diagnostic pathology report more scientific, nor does it make it more accurate, since the numbers act essentially as synonyms for words. A numerical system is important in research studies, on the other hand, as it allows statistical comparison of groups.

Quantitative Measurement of Hepatic Iron Concentrations

Hepatic iron concentrations measured in fresh liver tissues are equivalent to those measured in paraffin-embedded tissues.[13] Thus, paraffin-embedded tissues are preferred because it allows direct visualization of the tissue and assures the tissue is representative. This prevents submission of tissue that is largely composed of collapsed/fibrotic stroma or a nodule that is either unusually high or low in stainable iron, compared to the rest of the tissue.

The normal adult liver has between 10 and 36 μmol iron/g dry weight of liver. As a frame of reference, excess iron accumulation can be classified as mild (up to 150 μmol iron/g dry weight of liver), moderate (151-300), or marked (>301).[14]

Hepatic Iron Index

Historically, the hepatic iron index was calculated as an aide to interpreting quantitative tissue iron levels. The hepatic iron index adjusts the total iron concentration for age, based on the observation that hepatic iron concentrations increase steadily with age in individuals with genetic hemochromatosis, but not in individuals with "secondary" iron overload. A hepatic iron index greater than 1.9 was interpreted as consistent with genetic hemochromatosis. Given the advances in understanding the causes of hemochromatosis, and the readily available genetic testing for *HFE* mutations, the diagnostic role for the hepatic iron index is largely gone. Quantitative iron levels are still useful in managing individuals on iron depletion therapy, regardless of the underlying cause of disease, and many laboratories provide the hepatic iron index when doing quantitative iron levels, so the formula is shown below for interest. The value of 55.846 represents the atomic weight of iron. The normal range is less than 1.

$$\frac{\text{μg of iron per gram dry weight of liver}/55.846}{\text{patient's age in years}}$$

Noninvasive Measurements of Hepatic Iron

Magnetic resonance–based imaging studies have advanced to the point that they can reasonably assess iron accumulation and can also distinguish hepatic from reticuloendothelial iron deposits. For this reason, magnetic resonance imaging (MRI) has established for itself a role in measuring iron in the liver. Liver biopsies continue to be important in determining iron levels and also provide additional information on the fibrosis stage and other concomitant disease processes.

HISTOLOGICAL FINDINGS IN IRON OVERLOAD

Up-Front Stains

Many but not all medical centers do an up-front iron stain on all medical liver biopsies.

To date, practices are based on local preferences, as there are no data to determine the relative value (vs costs) of up-front iron stains. While iron stains in general can be very helpful, there are some situations where an iron stain is probably not necessary as an up-front stain, such as in the transplant setting where a liver biopsy is obtained to rule out rejection. In the nontransplant setting, an alternative to obtaining up-front iron stains is to perform iron stains only when pigment is visible on H&E, in order to confirm the diagnosis of iron overload, determine the iron distribution pattern, and grade the amount of iron deposition. This approach would likely miss some cases of mild iron deposition, but in most of these cases, the iron deposition is secondary and of no clinical significance. In this approach, additional clinical findings could also be used to trigger obtaining an iron stain, such as significantly elevated serum ferritin levels (>1000) or transferrin saturation levels that are >45%. Other clinical findings that could prompt an iron stain include unexplained heart disease or gonadal dysfunction.

Iron in Hepatocytes

In genetic hemochromatosis, iron classically accumulates first within zone 1 hepatocytes, and a clear gradient in the amount of iron can often be seen between zone 1 and zone 3 hepatocytes, even with advanced iron accumulation (Figure 15.7). In addition, the iron distribution within individual cells often clusters around the bile canaliculi (Figure 15.8). Both of these patterns, however, can be seen in nongenetic conditions, and a diagnosis of genetic hemochromatosis should not be based on recognizing these patterns alone. Instead, it seems most likely that the zone 1-predominant pattern of iron deposition reflects dysregulation of hepcidin, which can be either through mutations or through reduced hepcidin production from other causes. Over time, injury and death of hepatocytes will lead to a redistribution of some amount of iron into Kupffer cells and portal macrophages. In practice, even mild hepatocellular iron is often accompanied by mild Kupffer cell iron.

Iron in Bile Ducts

Iron can also be deposited in the epithelium of the bile duct proper (Figure 15.9). At times, this finding has been interpreted as being highly suggestive

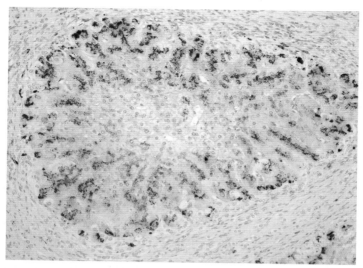

FIGURE 15.7 **Perls iron stain, zone 1 pattern.** A zonal pattern of iron deposition is still evident in this case of *HFE*-associated cirrhosis.

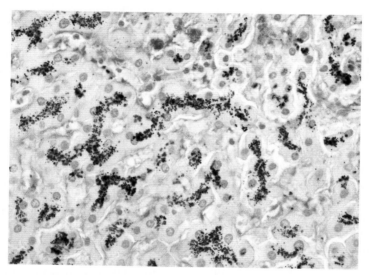

FIGURE 15.8 **Perls iron stain, pericanalicular staining.** A pericanalicular pattern of iron deposition is seen in this case of *HFE*-associated hemochromatosis.

or even diagnostic of *HFE* genetic hemochromatosis. Caution is warranted, however, as this finding can also be seen when there is marked iron overload from nongenetic causes. In addition, iron is commonly seen in proliferating bile ductules in areas of subacute parenchymal collapse in cirrhotic or noncirrhotic livers (Figure 15.10). This finding is not uncommon and has no association with hemochromatosis.

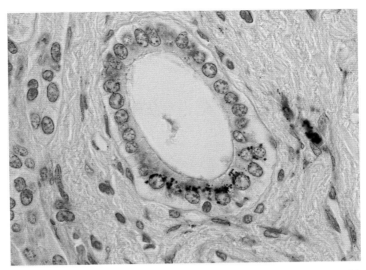

FIGURE 15.9 **Perls iron stain, bile duct.** Patchy bile duct epithelial iron deposition is seen.

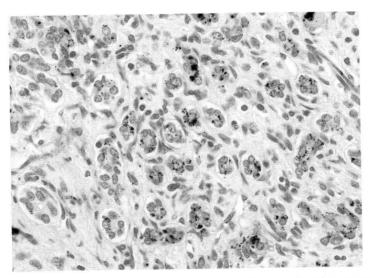

FIGURE 15.10 **Perls iron stain, bile ductules.** The proliferating ductules are positive on Perls stain in this case of marked acute hepatitis with parenchymal collapse.

Iron in Kupffer Cells

When the liver shows iron overload that results from transfusion-dependent anemias or other nongenetic causes, iron is classically first deposited in Kupffer cells and then, with time, there is involvement of the hepatocytes, although, in practice, most cases show a mixed hepatocellular and Kupffer cell pattern of iron deposition.

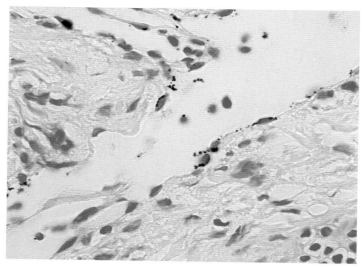

FIGURE 15.11 **Perls iron stain, endothelial cells.** In this liver biopsy, iron was only present in the endothelial cells.

Iron Staining of Endothelium

In some cases, iron is deposited either exclusively in portal endothelial cells (Figure 15.11) or in a combination of endothelial cells, hepatocytes, and Kupffer cells. There has been no specific linkage between endothelial iron accumulation and any disease process or genetic mutation, but it would not be surprising if this changes in the future. Only a few studies have looked at the biology or significance of endothelial iron deposits. In one study, endothelial iron positivity was linked to decreased interferon response in individuals with chronic hepatitis C infection.[15]

Iron-Positive Staining in Hepatocyte Nuclei

In rare cases, a Perls iron stain can be positive within nuclear pseudoinclusion of hepatocytes (Figure 15.12). The significance of this finding is unclear, in particular if it is a focal finding limited to one or two hepatocytes. Larger patches of nuclear staining have been reported in the setting of neuroferitinopathy.[16]

GENETIC VERSUS SECONDARY CAUSES OF IRON OVERLOAD

Once iron overload is identified in a patient, determining the role of genetic changes versus secondary causes is based primarily on clinical findings, laboratory testing, and genetic testing. Imaging findings also can be helpful, as iron deposits in the spleen and bone marrow are common in secondary causes of iron overload but are not present in most cases of

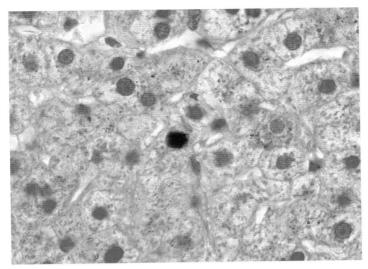

FIGURE 15.12 **Perls iron stain, hepatocyte nuclear pseudoinclusions.** A rare nuclear pseudoinclusion was positive on Perls iron stain in this biopsy performed for staging and grading of known chronic viral hepatitis.

hemochromatosis. In cases with ambiguous findings, histological changes can help guide the classification process by determining the location and amount of iron deposition within the liver, identifying concomitant liver diseases, and assessing fibrosis.

In the majority of genetic causes of iron overload, iron is deposited primarily in hepatocytes and shows a zone 1-predominant pattern. In contrast, in the majority of secondary causes of iron overload, iron is primarily found within Kupffer cells and has a zone 3 predominance. These patterns are broadly true and can help guide thinking. On the other hand, in cases with marked iron overload, from either genetic or nongenetic causes, these patterns can diminish or be lost because there is substantial iron redistribution over time.

When Should Pathologists Suggest Additional Testing to Rule Out Genetic Hemochromatosis?

When iron deposits are present in a liver biopsy, it can be helpful to have some guidelines to follow, as to when it would be reasonable to suggest additional testing to evaluate for possible genetic causes of iron overload. There currently are no well-established guidelines, at least none driven by data and none published by professional liver pathology societies, but there are several guiding principles that are derived from practical experience and the published literature. These principles depend on several key factors, which should be available in essentially every case: the patient's age, the amount of iron seen on the biopsy, and whether or not there

TABLE 15.6 Testing for Genetic Iron Overload	
Iron Grade on Perls Iron Stain	**Other Findings**
Mild	Only if patient is young (eg, younger than 40 y), noncirrhotic, and there is no other chronic liver disease on biopsy, such as chronic hepatitis or fatty liver disease
Moderate	All noncirrhotic livers of any age
Marked	All ages, all fibrosis stages. Alcohol-related cirrhosis is a possible exception

These guidelines only apply for cases when there is no other explanation for iron overload, such as multiple transfusions.

is advanced liver fibrosis. These principles are summarized below and in Table 15.6, using as the starting point the amount of iron seen in the liver biopsy specimen on a Perls iron stain.

MILD HEPATOCELLULAR IRON. Overall, this is by far the most common amount of iron seen in biopsy specimens and is the least specific. Additional genetic testing can be suggested if the patient is youngish (younger than 40 years), the liver is noncirrhotic, and there is no other chronic liver disease on biopsy, such as chronic hepatitis or fatty liver disease

MODERATE HEPATOCELLULAR IRON. This degree of iron is less common than mild iron, but is not rare either. For purposes of these guidelines, the moderate iron deposition should be diffuse, with most of the periportal regions showing moderate hepatocellular iron accumulation (Figure 15.13). In this setting, genetic testing can be suggested for patients of any age when the livers are noncirrhotic, even if there is another active liver disease such as fatty liver disease.

MARKED HEPATOCELLULAR IRON. When iron is marked and diffuse, testing can be suggested when there is no known risk factor(s) for secondary iron overload, such as transfusion-dependent anemia. This includes patients of any age, livers with known underlying chronic diseases, and livers with any degrees of fibrosis, including cirrhosis. Alcohol-related cirrhosis may be an exception, but data are limited.

KUPFFER CELL–PREDOMINANT IRON ACCUMULATION. This pattern is most often a result of secondary iron deposition, but testing for ferroportin disease should be considered when individuals have elevated ferritin levels but normal or low transferrin saturation levels. Patients should also be tested if there is a family history of iron overload liver disease (or of unexplained elevated liver enzymes), because such a history suggests an autosomal

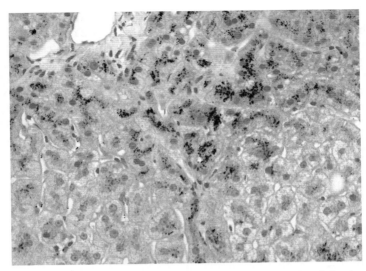

FIGURE 15.13 **Too much iron.** This biopsy of a young man with mildly elevated liver enzymes showed no significant inflammation and no fibrosis, but there was patchy moderate hepatocellular iron deposition, warranting follow-up laboratory and possible genetic testing for iron overload disease.

dominant pattern of inheritance. At the histological levels, the iron deposition can be mild to marked. The iron deposition should be predominantly in Kupffer cell, but some hepatocellular iron can also be seen.

HFE HEMOCHROMATOSIS

Genetics

HFE mutations were first linked to hereditary hemochromatosis in 1996.[17] Since that time, over 35 mutations have been reported,[18] but C282Y and H63D mutations are the most important, both numerically and clinically. Overall, C282Y mutations account for 80% to 90% of genetic hemochromatosis cases. Of the remaining cases, 60% are explained by H63D homozygous mutations.[19,20] H63D heterozygous mutations and other *HFE* mutations, such as S65C, have also been linked to iron accumulation.[19] Data from numerous studies suggest H63D heterozygous mutations and S65C mutations do not lead to clinical hemochromatosis by themselves, but they can contribute to excess iron deposits if individuals have additional mutations in iron metabolism genes.

C282Y mutations are strongly associated with northern European genetic ancestry.[18] H63D mutations also have a higher frequency in Caucasian populations, but have a wider ethnic distribution,[21,22] while S65C mutations are most common in populations from Brittany, France.[23]

Individuals with C282Y mutations have a higher risk for iron accumulation than those with H63D mutations. Likewise, C282Y homozygotes have greater risk for iron accumulation than do C282Y heterozygotes. Nonetheless, there is great phenotypic variation, even for individuals who are homozygous for C282Y mutations. For example, one major population-based study from Australia followed 203 individuals who were homozygous for C282Y mutations for 12 years. During this time, 28% of men and 1% of women developed iron overload–related diseases.[24] A similar study followed C282Y/H63D compound heterozygote individuals over the same 12-year interval and found that only 1/82 men and none of 95 women developed iron related disease.[25] The striking phenotypic variation is likely related to gender, environmental factors, dietary composition, and other genetic polymorphisms.[25]

Clinical Presentation

Clinical presentation is striking for its variety. The classic presentation of cirrhosis, diabetes, and bronze skin, that so many of us learned in medical school, is now very uncommon because of earlier diagnosis. In many cases, individuals can present with vague findings of fatigue and bone and joint pain. Another common presentation is mild liver enzyme elevations or iron blood work abnormalities identified while being evaluated for other conditions. Presentations later in the disease course can include varying combinations of endocrine dysfunctions, for example, adrenal insufficiency or diabetes mellitus, cirrhosis, heart failure, or joint disease.

Clinical Indications for Liver Biopsy in Individuals With HFE Mutations

In many patients, a diagnosis of *HFE* mutations is made by genetic testing and a diagnosis of iron overload by blood work and/or imaging findings. Liver biopsy now plays a role mostly in determining fibrosis, in particular if noninvasive markers of fibrosis give results that do not fit well with clinical findings. For example, guidelines from the Europe Association for the Study of the Liver (EASL) recommend liver biopsies in patients who have homozygous C282Y mutations, in order to stage the liver fibrosis, when serum ferritin levels are above 1000 μg/L, or there is elevated aspartate aminotransferase (AST) levels, hepatomegaly, or age older than 40 years. American Association for the Study of Liver Diseases (AASLD) guideline are similar, recommending liver biopsies to stage fibrosis in patients who have homozygous C282Y mutations, or in patients who have compound heterozygous C282Y/H63D mutations, when ferritin is >1000 μg/L or there are elevated serum levels of AST or alanine aminotransferase (ALT).

Histological Findings

The degree of iron overload can vary considerably but classically shows heaviest deposition in zone 1 hepatocytes (Figure 15.14). The iron is readily seen on H&E stain in cases with moderate or greater iron deposition

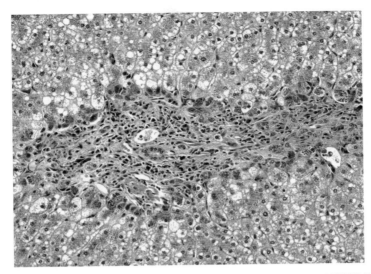

FIGURE 15.14   **HFE hemochromatosis.** In this patient with homozygous C282Y *HFE* mutations, a zone 1 pattern of iron deposition can be seen.

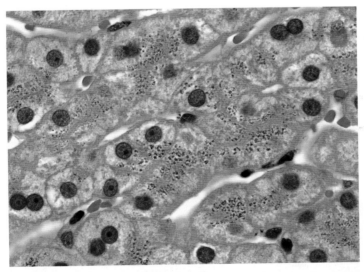

FIGURE 15.15   **HFE hemochromatosis.** Iron is visible on hematoxylin and eosin (H&E) and shows a pericanalicular staining pattern, from a patient with homozygous C282Y *HFE* mutations.

(Figure 15.15), as well as many cases with mild iron deposition. The iron typically shows a pericanalicular deposition pattern within individual hepatocytes (Figures 15.15 and 15.16), and there can be iron accumulation within cholangiocytes in cases of moderate to severe iron overload (Figure 15.17). Over time, there can be redistribution of iron into the Kupffer cells as well.

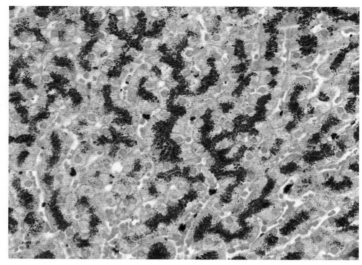

FIGURE 15.16 **HFE hemochromatosis, Perls iron stain.** There is marked diffuse iron deposition, but a pericanaliuclar staining pattern is still evident, from a patient with homozygous C282Y *HFE* mutations.

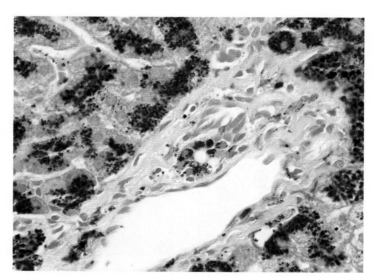

FIGURE 15.17 **HFE hemochromatosis, Perls iron stain.** Iron can be seen in the bile ducts (same case as preceding image).

Links Between *HFE* Mutations and Other Chronic Diseases

For individuals with *HFE* mutations, other chronic liver diseases can affect iron overload risk. Likewise, *HFE* mutations have been linked to disease severity in other chronic liver diseases, such as chronic hepatitis C or fatty liver disease. Furthermore, some etiologies of cirrhosis, such as alpha-1-antitrypsin deficiency or cryptogenic cirrhosis, can be enriched for *HFE* mutations and show marked iron accumulation.[26]

For the major causes of chronic liver diseases, such as chronic viral hepatitis and fatty liver disease, numerous studies have examined the relationship between disease severity (grade and stage) and the presence of tissue iron accumulation and/or the presence of *HFE* mutations. The evidence in general supports an overall association between more severe disease and the presence of excess iron in the liver, although many studies could not identify an association. These negative studies highlight the difficulty of identifying a modest affect from within the very complex setting of clinical studies, where the challenge is to control for all of the factors that can influence iron status as well as fibrosis progression.

RARE CAUSES OF GENETIC HEOCHROMATOSIS

Hemojuvelin Mutations (Usually Children/Young Adults)

There are two subtypes of juvenile hemochromatosis based on the mutated gene, *HFE2* (encodes hemojuvelin) and *HAMP* (encodes hepcidin). In contrast to *HFE* mutations, the general population has a very low frequency of *HFE2* and *HAMP* mutations. Hemojuvelin-related iron disease is rare but is still the most common cause of juvenile hemochromatosis.[27,28] In contrast to *HFE*-related disease, hemojuvelin disease typically presents with impotence or amenorrhea and not with liver or joint disease. Cardiomyopathy is also common at presentation.[29] The hepatocytes can show marked iron overload, with initial sparing of the Kupffer cells. The disease typically runs a severe clinical course and can be rapidly progressive,[2] with cirrhosis at young ages in up to 40% of affected persons.[30]

Transferrin Receptor Gene 2 (Usually Adults/Late Onset, But Broad Range)

This form of genetic iron overload is rare in Western populations. Mutations have also been reported in other populations including Africa[31] and Iran,[32] but the overall epidemiology is unclear. Patients have variable clinical courses, with some but not all individuals having significant hepatocellular iron accumulation. Cirrhosis can develop in patients in their 20s.[33] In many cases, however, the disease is mild and the amount of iron deposition is less than that seen with HFE hemochromatosis. Also, of note, polymorphisms in *TRF2* are common in the general asymptomatic adult population, where they can lead to mild increases in blood iron levels without overt iron overload disease.[34]

DMT-1 Mutations (Usually Older Children)

Mutations in the *SLC11A2* gene are a very rare cause of genetic iron over-load, and clinical and histological data are limited.[35] Children present with severe microcytic anemia. Ferritin levels can be low, or only mildly elevated, even when there is significant iron overload. Iron accumulation is primarily in hepatocytes and can be severe,[36] but biopsies can be negative for iron in very young children.

Ferritin Mutations (Hyperferritinemia)

Ferritin is a protein composed of two subunits: *FTL* encodes the light chain and *FTH* encodes the heavy chain. With both mutations, patients present with high serum ferritin levels, but low transferrin saturation levels. However, only patients with *FTL* mutations develop hereditary hyperferritinemia cataract syndrome and hereditary neuroferritinopathy. Liver biopsies show no or scant iron deposition, but hepatocyte nuclei can stain positive on Perls iron.[37,38] In contrast, *FTH* mutations lead to iron accumulates in hepatocytes.[39]

Transferrin Mutations

TF mutations are a rare cause of genetic hemochromatosis, with an autosomal recessive inheritance pattern.[40-43] Patients who have homozygous mutations develop iron overload, while heterozygous mutations only lead to iron overload if the patient has an additional mutation in genes involving iron metabolism, such as *HFE*.[44] Patients who have homozygous mutations present in childhood with severe hypochromic, microcytic anemia and blood testing shows high serum iron, high serum ferritin, but low TIBC and very low or absent transferrin levels. Histologically, the liver shows marked hepatic iron overload.[45]

Ceruloplasmin Mutations

CP (encodes ceruloplasmin) mutations are a rare cause of genetic hemochromatosis. Patients typically present later in life with diabetes and neurological symptoms, including ataxia and dementia, but there is a wide age range at initial presentation, from teenagers to elderly.[46,47] Younger patients often present with anemia, mild elevations in liver enzymes, and serum iron test abnormalities, including elevated ferritin levels, but low iron transferrin saturation.[48,49] Patients develop iron deposits in the liver, brain, and pancreas islet cells. Within the liver, iron deposits are seen mostly in hepatocytes, and there can be a pan-lobular pattern.[50-54]

More to Come

There remains a subset of hepatic iron overload cases that do not appear to have the mutations described above. For example, in a study from

Brazil, one-third of cases with marked iron overload did not have the typical mutations discussed above.[55] Similarly, iron overload in Africa is now recognized to be not exclusively diet-related, suggesting an unrecognized genetic component.[56]

NONHEPATOCELLULAR GENETIC OVERLOAD DISEASE

Ferroportin Disease and Ferroportin-Associated Hemochromatosis

- Ferroportin mutations have an autosomal dominant pattern of inheritance
- Most patients present as adults
- One gene, *SLC40A1*, but two distinct mutational and disease patterns[57,58]
  - Loss of function mutations: *Ferroportin disease*, with Kupffer cell–predominant iron deposits and mild disease. In these cases, blood testing shows elevated serum ferritin levels but normal or minimally elevated transferrin saturation levels. Transferrin saturation levels, however, can be elevated as the disease progresses
  - Gain of function mutations: *Ferroportin-associated hemochromatosis*, with hepatocellular and Kupffer cell iron accumulation that resembles *HFE*-related hemochromatosis histologically and clinically

Ferroportin Disease

GENE MUTATIONS. The ferroportin protein is encoded by *SLC40A1*. Mutations can lead to either loss of function or gain of function, resulting in distinctly different outcomes and histological patterns.[57,58] Overall, loss of function mutations are more common and lead to *ferroportin disease* (sometimes called ferroportin disease type A), with generally mild iron overloading, an indolent clinical course, and Kupffer cell–predominant iron deposits on histology. In contrast, gain of function mutations lead to *ferroportin-associated hemochromatosis* (sometimes called ferroportin disease type B), which can have a disease course more similar to *HFE* hemochromatosis.

CLINICAL PRESENTATION FOR FERROPORTIN DISEASE. Patients with ferroportin disease commonly present as adults with mild anemia, mildly elevated liver enzymes, and sometimes with a family history of liver disease. Ferroportin disease also stands out from other causes of genetic hemochromatosis by its dominant inheritance pattern.[2] Nonetheless, the disease is often underdiagnosed because it can have a mild clinical course, so a family history is often not evident. At the laboratory level, a key finding is high ferritin levels but low serum transferrin saturation levels. By way of contrast, *HFE* hemochromatosis has both high ferritin and transferrin saturation levels. Transferrin saturation levels in ferroportin disease may become elevated, but not until much later in the disease course. Other rare diseases can show a similar pattern of blood testing, with high ferritin levels but low transferrin saturation levels (aceruloplasminemia, ferritin mutations), but they do not have the Kupffer cell–predominant pattern of iron deposition that is typical for ferroprotein disease. Imaging can also separate ferroportin disease from aceruloplasminemia, since siderosis of the liver and spleen is seen in ferroportin disease and not aceruloplasminemia.

Histologically, iron deposits in Kupffer cells predominate over that of hepatocytes in ferroportin disease (Figures 15.18 and 15.19), while hepatocellular iron is heavier than Kupffer cell iron in ferroportin-associated hemochromatosis.[59] Ferroportin disease can also have small sideronecrotic foci composed of iron-laden macrophages in small clumps within the lobules. Clinically both types have milder disease than those with *HFE* mutations, but ferroportin-associated hemochromatosis can lead to iron accumulation that resembles that seen with HFE-associated hemochromatosis. Ferroportin-associated hemochromatosis can also lead to iron deposits in the heart and the pancreatic islet cells, leading to cardiac arrhythmias and to diabetes.

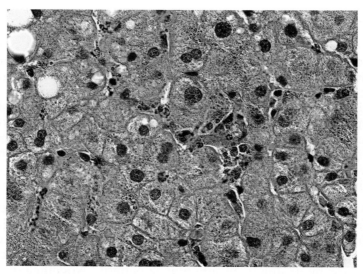

FIGURE 15.18 **Ferroportin disease.** The iron is deposited predominately in the Kupffer cells.

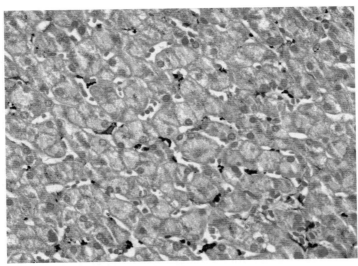

FIGURE 15.19 **Ferroportin disease, iron stain.** The iron is deposited exclusively in Kupffer cells.

NEONATAL HEMOCHROMATOSIS

Neonatal hemochromatosis is broadly classified as a severe liver disease of the neonate accompanied by extrahepatic deposits of iron. Despite the term "hemochromatosis" in neonatal hemochromatosis, this disease is fundamentally different than the other iron-related diseases discussed previously. Cottier first described this disease in 1957, reporting newborn siblings with advanced liver fibrosis and iron deposited in hepatocytes, the pancreas, thyroid, and myocardium, but without iron deposits in the spleen (which is common in secondary iron overload).[60] Subsequent studies have found that the majority of neonatal hemochromatosis cases result from an alloimmune gestational disease, wherein maternal antibodies cross the placenta and attack the fetal liver in utero.[61] The target antigen on hepatocytes has not been clearly identified, but it is presumed to be on the cell surface. The mothers often have other serum autoantibodies, such as antinuclear antibodies (ANA), which are positive in about 50% of cases.[62] On the other hand, there is no association with autoimmune hepatitis or other autoimmune diseases in the mother.

Many cases of neonatal hemochromatosis manifest as late second-term or third-term fetal loss, because the fetus did not survive the massive liver injury. Fetuses commonly show intrauterine growth retardation, oligohydramnios, and hydrops. Newborns typically present with massive liver failure at birth, or within the first few days of life, leading to hypoglycemia and coagulopathy. Despite the often massive liver injury, serum AST and ALT levels can be normal or only mildly elevated. Serum alpha fetoprotein (AFP) levels, on the other hand, are elevated in most cases, typically being greater than 100,000 ng/mL and can be as high as 800,000 ng/mL (the healthy neonate has values less than 80,000 ng/mL). For newborns, the placenta may show hydrops on gross examination[62] and, on histological examination, show chronic villitis and intervillitis, but usually without vasculopathy, deciduitis, or chorioamniotis.[62]

On biopsy of the liver (or on postmortem examination of the liver), the histology can range from massive liver necrosis with almost no residual hepatocytes, to a severely damaged liver with regenerative nodules that gives the liver a cirrhotic appearance. The residual hepatocytes are often cholestatic (Figure 15.20) and may show giant cell transformation. Inflammatory changes are commonly mild. Iron stains show hepatocellular iron accumulation, with course granules of iron that are qualitatively similar to that seen in adult hemochromatosis (Figure 15.21), while the Kupffer cells generally have little iron accumulation. Fibrosis is mild or absent in specimens obtained soon after disease onset, but more advanced fibrosis can be seen in later cases, including cirrhosis. In many of these later cases, the lobules can also show diffuse pericellular fibrosis.

The hepatocytes typically show moderate to marked iron accumulation, but the iron can be quite patchy and can be entirely negative in some areas. In addition, you may not see much iron in cases where most of the hepatocytes are necrotic. In general, specimens that are examined early in the disease course have more iron and no or mild fibrosis, while later specimens can have only mild iron and advanced fibrosis.[62] Kupffer cells generally have no or mild iron accumulation.

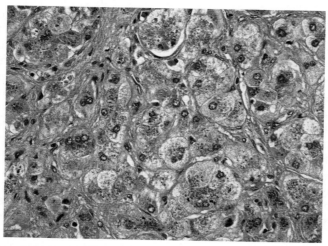

FIGURE 15.20 **Neonatal hemochromatosis.** This patient received a liver transplant, and the explanted liver showed submassive liver necrosis with regenerative nodules. The surviving hepatocytes were swollen and cholestatic.

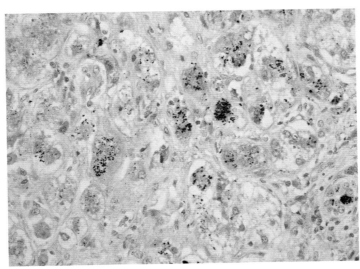

FIGURE 15.21 **Neonatal hemochromatosis, Perls iron.** An iron stain showed moderate patchy hepatocellular iron deposition; same case as preceding image.

Of note, *extrahepatic* iron deposits are important to confidently make this diagnosis. The best places to look for iron are (in approximate order): acini of the pancreas, thyroid follicles, renal tubules, myocardium, minor salivary glands, and other epithelium (Brunner glands, stomach, thymus, trachea, etc).[63] While this list is helpful, there can be a lot of heterogeneity in the patterns of iron deposition, so sampling multiple organs may be needed. Lip biopsies can be helpful clinically and are often performed because of ease of access, but biopsies are only informative when they are positive. Biopsies can be falsely negative because of heterogeneity in iron deposition,[62] or if they do not go deep enough to adequately sample the minor salivary glands. The bone marrow and spleen generally do not have increased iron.

The prognosis is poor unless the disease is recognized quickly. Treatment revolves around supportive care and removing the maternal antibody through plasmapharesis. For those children who do survive, there does not appear to be any significant clinical sequelae. If an infant is affected by this disease, there is about a 90% chance that subsequent pregnancies in the mother will be likewise affected, regardless of the father of the baby, so this is an important disease to diagnose.[64] Once the disease is recognized, it can be completely prevented in subsequent pregnancies by giving the mother IV IgG from about the 18th week of gestation until delivery.

Differential

Following massive necrosis from any cause, there can be extensive bile ductular proliferation, and these proliferating bile ductules often have mild

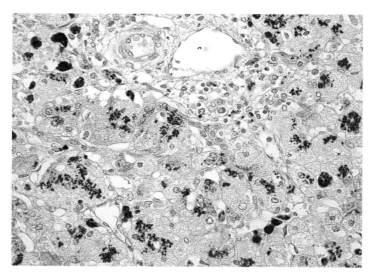

FIGURE 15.22 **GRACILE syndrome, Perls iron.** There is marked hepatocellular iron overload.

hemosiderin on Perls iron stain. This pattern, however, is nonspecific, whereas iron in hepatocytes as well as extrahepatic organs would suggest neonatal hemochromatosis.

There are several other rare causes of massive liver necrosis in neonates that can resemble neonatal hemochromatosis histologically, with extensive hepatocyte necrosis, inflammation, cholestasis, and some of them with hepatocellular iron deposits. These include primarily rare genetic diseases, such as the mitochondrial cytopathies and the related GRACILE syndrome, which can have massive liver injury, advanced fibrosis, and elevated serum iron studies. In mitochondrial cytopathies, iron stains in the liver and extrahepatic tissues are negative,[65] but there can be massive iron deposits with the GRACILE syndrome, which stands for Growth Retardation, Amino aciduria, Cholestasis, Iron overload, Lactic acidosis, and Early death. This syndrome is caused by is caused by mutations in the *BCS1L* gene, which encodes a mitochondrial protein, and mutations lead to defects in mitochondrial complex III. The syndrome is enriched in persons of Finnish heritage.[66,67] Like cases of neonatal hemochromatosis, there can be massive liver injury, often with death in the first week of life, and massive hepatocyte iron deposits (Figure 15.22). The eponymous clinical findings will typically lead to the correct diagnosis. Extrahepatic iron would also be unusual for the GRACILE syndrome.

IRON OVERLOAD IN DIFFERENT SETTINGS

Cirrhotic Livers

Cirrhosis from many different causes can have iron deposits in the hepatocytes and Kupffer cells. In a classic study, Ludwig et al studied iron levels in 447 liver explants.[68] Iron stains were positive in 100% of hereditary hemochromatosis cases, 65% of cases of cryptogenic cirrhosis, 63% of alcohol cirrhosis cases, 65% of chronic hepatitis B cases, 56% of alpha-1-antitrypsin deficiency cases, 43% of chronic hepatitis C cases, 10% of PBC cases, and 7% of primary sclerosing cholangitis cases. In this same study, the number of cases with a marked iron overload, as defined by a hepatic iron index of greater than 1.9, were as follows: hereditary hemochromatosis (100%), alpha-1-antitrypsin deficiency (28%), cryptogenic cirrhosis (19%), alcohol cirrhosis (14%), chronic hepatitis B cirrhosis (18%), chronic hepatitis C cirrhosis (7%), PBC (1%), and primary sclerosing cholangitis (1%). An important take home message from these data is that 20% or more of cirrhotic livers from alpha-1-antitrypsin deficiency or cryptogenic cirrhotic livers can have marked iron overload, with hepatic iron indexes greater than 1.9. Another important observation is that biliary cirrhosis is only rarely associated with iron overload.

Iron in the Explanted Liver

Iron in the explanted liver can be clinically relevant. For example, patients with significant hepatic iron accumulation have decreased survival following transplantation, regardless of whether they have *HFE* mutations.[69] Fenton et al reported a set of cases with marked iron accumulation in the liver and heart, but without *HFE* mutations. This cohort of cases had cardiac iron deposits and significant heart failure.[70] Others have also reported that non–*HFE*-related cardiac iron overload can occur in the liver transplant population when the liver graft has severe iron overload.[71]

IRON IN DONOR LIVER BIOPSIES

There are relatively little data on the clinical relevance of iron positivity in donor livers. In one interesting study, iron was found in 49/284 (17%) of donor biopsies and was occasionally at moderate levels, but overall did not impact survival outcomes.[72] Another study of living donors found increased iron in 8% of liver biopsies.[73] A third study looked at the significance of donor iron in terms of subsequent fibrosis progression in individuals transplanted for chronic HCV.[74] They found a modest link between increased pretransplant iron content, female gender, and risk for fibrosis progression.

Inadvertent transplantation of donor livers with C282Y homozygous mutations have been reported.[75,76] While the number of cases is too small to draw conclusions on how this effects the posttransplant course, iron continues to accumulate within the liver allograft.[76] This topic is further discussed in Chapter 14.

IRON IN LIVER BIOPSIES WITH CHRONIC VIRAL HEPATITIS

When biopsies are performed to stage and grade chronic HCV, iron deposits are seen on Perls iron stains in approximately 30% of cases, with a range of 5% to 48% of cases, depending on the study.[77] This wide range in the frequency of iron positivity reflects differences in gender, viral genotypes, and the proportion of cirrhotic livers in the different study cohorts.

Histologically, the iron deposit can include both hepatocellular as well as Kupffer cell iron, and many times involves both compartments.[77] In the majority of cases, the iron deposits are mild, occasionally moderate, and only very rarely severe.

What do the iron/*HFE* mutations mean for the patient in this setting? A large body of literature has investigated the significance of these questions, albeit with substantially mixed results on whether there is an increased risk for fibrosis progression with either *HFE* mutations or with increased iron on Perls iron stain without *HFE* mutations. A reasonable way to synthesize the findings is as follows[78]: (1) individuals with chronic HCV do not have an increased risk for *HFE* mutations; (2) individuals with HFE mutations have on average more iron than those without mutations, but iron accumulation in heterozygotes is generally mild; (3) *HFE* mutations may modestly increase the rate of fibrosis progression; many but not all studies have found that *HFE* mutations are associated with higher fibrosis stage; (4) overall, C282Y alleles have a stronger risk for fibrosis progression than H63D alleles; (5) when an individual has a long history of chronic HCV infection, the risk of advanced fibrosis or cirrhosis is high regardless of *HFE* mutational status and the effect of *HFE* mutations are harder to discern; (6) for patients with iron accumulation but without *HFE* mutations, a significant risk for fibrosis progression is not evident, unless the iron deposition is severe. The results of iron studies in the setting of chronic hepatitis B are broadly similar to that discussed for chronic hepatitis C: iron is present in about a third of biopsy specimens; deposits are mainly mild and are associated with higher stages of fibrosis but not *HFE* mutational status.[78]

Iron in Nonalcoholic Fatty Liver Disease

Hepatic iron deposition in nonalcoholic fatty liver disease (NAFLD) is common, with approximately 30% to 40% of liver biopsies showing iron accumulation. As with chronic viral hepatitis, in most cases, the siderosis is mild and involves either or both of the hepatocyte and Kupffer cell compartments.[79] Minimal or mild iron accumulation is typical, while moderate iron accumulation is uncommon and marked iron accumulation is rare. The frequency of iron deposition is higher in livers with advanced fibrosis, but in most cases, the iron levels remain mild, and they do not appear to be a major driver of fibrogenesis in most cases.[80-82]

Iron Overload in Alcohol-Related Liver Disease

Alcohol inhibits the activity of hepcidin, so chronic alcoholic liver disease is commonly associated with iron accumulation. *HFE* heterozygous mutations can further increase the likelihood of liver iron deposition in this population but does not appear to strongly influence the degree of fibrosis, the histological degree of alcoholic liver disease activity, or the clinical course.[83,84]

IRON AND LIVER CARCINOMA

Individuals with *HFE* hemochromatosis and marked iron accumulation have an increased risk for hepatocellular carcinoma. The vast majority of carcinomas develop in livers with cirrhosis, but rare carcinomas in non-cirrhotic livers have been reported.[85,86] The risk for carcinoma was previously estimated to be as high as 200 fold, but more recent data suggest a lower, but still elevated, risk.[87] In terms of frequency, studies of explanted cirrhotic livers indicate that 15% of all liver explants for *HFE* hemochromatosis will have a hepatocellular carcinoma, which is similar to that for cirrhosis from chronic hepatitis C (15%) and hepatitis B (17%).[88] Precursor lesions include iron-free foci.

Most liver carcinomas in genetic hemochromatosis are hepatocellular carcinomas, but intrahepatic cholangiocarcinomas have also been reported.[89,90] Rare hepatocellular carcinomas occurring in individuals with secondary iron overload have also been reported.[91] In fact, if there is significant iron accumulation in cirrhotic livers from any etiology, there is a mild but statistically significant increased risk for hepatocellular carcinoma.[88]

ACQUIRED IRON OVERLOAD

Secondary iron overload tends to show an exclusively or predominantly Kupffer cell pattern of iron deposition early on (Figure 15.23), but a mixed pattern is commonly seen as iron overloading progresses, and in time, there may be substantial hepatocellular iron accumulation (Figure 15.24).

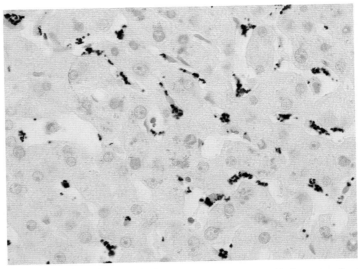

FIGURE 15.23 **Perls iron stain, Kupffer cell.** In this case of chronic congestive heart failure, iron deposits are seen primarily in Kupffer cells.

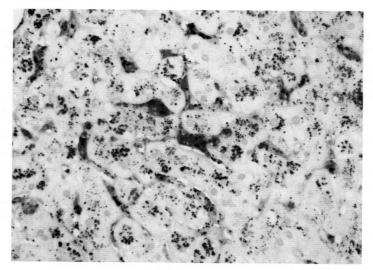

FIGURE 15.24 **Perls iron stain, mixed hepatocellular and Kupffer cell.** In this case of end-stage renal disease and transfusion-dependent anemia, marked iron deposits are present in both the Kupffer cells and hepatocytes.

Transfusion-Dependent Anemias

Iron deposition is frequently found in liver biopsies of patients with various hematological disorders, including sickle cell disease and thalassemia. Other common causes of secondary iron overload include transfusion-dependent anemia, renal dialysis (Figure 15.24), and bone marrow transplants. In cases of early siderosis from any of these causes, the iron is deposited primarily in the Kupffer cells and/or portal macrophages. Over time, iron is also seen in hepatocytes and can reach very high levels.

Sideroblastic Anemia

Sideroblastic anemia is a heterogeneous group of disorders that can be acquired, hereditary, or idiopathic and is defined by the presence of both anemia and ringed sideroblasts in the bone marrow. The most common inherited cause is from mutation in *ALAS2*, leading to an X-linked sideroblastic anemia. The sideroblast is an erythroid precursor (a nucleated erythroblast) that has granules of iron in the cytoplasm, often with granules that surround the nucleus. The ringed sideroblast pattern results from deposition of iron in mitochondria and is found in the bone marrow, but not the liver. Instead, the liver may have marked hepatocellular iron accumulation, which can show a zone 1-predominant pattern of staining (Figures 15.25 and 15.26).

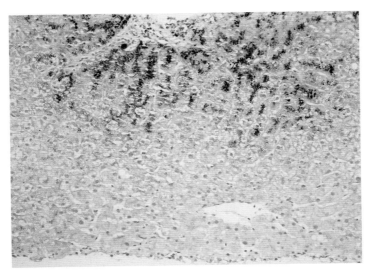

FIGURE 15.25 **Sideroblastic anemia, Perls iron stain.** The iron shows a zone 1 pattern of distribution.

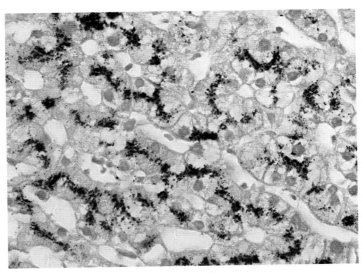

FIGURE 15.26 **Sideroblastic anemia, Perls iron stain.** At higher power, iron is seen within hepatocytes.

Glucose-6-Phosphatase Dehydrogenase Deficiency

Glucose-6-phosphatase dehydrogenase is an enzyme important in red blood cell synthesis. Mutations lead to an X-linked, recessive disorder (seen only in males) that is characterized by hemolytic anemia when patients are exposed to various triggers, such as infection, chemicals, or

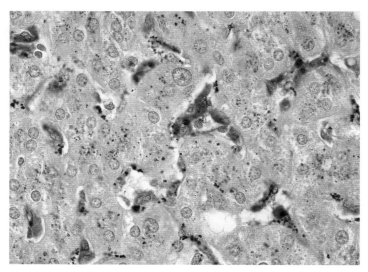

FIGURE 15.27 **Glucose-6-phosphatase dehydrogenase, Perls iron stain.** There is mixed hepatocellular and Kupffer cell iron deposition.

other substances. Rare cases can also present as neonatal cholestasis.[92] Liver biopsies in adults show predominantly Kupffer cell iron accumulation, but there can be hepatocellular iron deposition too (Figure 15.27).

PORPHYRIA CUTANEA TARDA

Porphyria cutanea tarda is a mixed group of acquired and genetic diseases that lead to deficiencies in the enzyme uroporphyrinogen decarboxylase, which is important in normal heme synthesis; the disease is sporadic in about 80% of cases and inherited in 20% (mutations in *UROD*). Clinical disease manifests as blistering after exposure to sunlight and hyperpigmentation. Disease can be precipitated by chronic hepatitis C infection or alcohol use, and it is also associated with *HFE* gene mutations.

The histological findings in porphyria cutanea tarda vary based on the precipitating factors, whether it be chronic hepatitis C, alcohol, etc. Mild macrovesicular steatosis is found in 80% of cases.[93] Significant iron deposition is more common in cases without *UROD* mutations and can be severe, leading to liver cirrhosis. Early on, iron accumulation is seen in the periportal hepatocytes[94] as well as portal macrophages. In the lobules, there can be small granuloma-like aggregates of pigment and iron-laden macrophages.[95] The hepatocytes may also contain needle-shaped, birefringent crystals that are very subtle and nearly impossible to see on H&E stains; they are typically sparse and often found only after spending a lot of time with your oil immersion lens,[93] and even then it can be hard to be certain that what you do find is not some sort of artifact. One study reported the crystals could be highlighted by Fontana stains and that crystals also have autofluorescent properties.[93] Of note, the crystals are water soluble so are best found using

38. Mancuso M, Davidzon G, Kurlan RM, et al. Hereditary ferritinopathy: a novel mutation, its cellular pathology, and pathogenetic insights. *J Neuropathol Exp Neurol.* 2005;64:280-294.

39. Kato J, Fujikawa K, Kanda M, et al. A mutation, in the iron-responsive element of H ferritin mRNA, causing autosomal dominant iron overload. *Am J Hum Genet.* 2001;69:191-197.

40. Knisely AS, Gelbart T, Beutler E. Molecular characterization of a third case of human atransferrinemia. *Blood.* 2004;104:2607.

41. Beutler E, Gelbart T, Lee P, et al. Molecular characterization of a case of atransferrinemia. *Blood.* 2000;96:4071-4074.

42. Aslan D, Crain K, Beutler E. A new case of human atransferrinemia with a previously undescribed mutation in the transferrin gene. *Acta Haematol.* 2007;118:244-247.

43. Athiyarath R, Arora N, Fuster F, et al. Two novel missense mutations in iron transport protein transferrin causing hypochromic microcytic anaemia and haemosiderosis: molecular characterization and structural implications. *Br J Haematol.* 2013;163:404-407.

44. Beaumont-Epinette MP, Delobel JB, Ropert M, et al. Hereditary hypotransferrinemia can lead to elevated transferrin saturation and, when associated to HFE or HAMP mutations, to iron overload. *Blood Cells Mol Dis.* 2015;54:151-154.

45. Hamill RL, Woods JC, Cook BA. Congenital atransferrinemia. A case report and review of the literature. *Am J Clin Pathol.* 1991;96:215-218.

46. Harris ZL, Takahashi Y, Miyajima H, et al. Aceruloplasminemia: molecular characterization of this disorder of iron metabolism. *Proc Natl Acad Sci USA.* 1995;92:2539-2543.

47. Yoshida K, Furihata K, Takeda S, et al. A mutation in the ceruloplasmin gene is associated with systemic hemosiderosis in humans. *Nat Genet.* 1995;9:267-272.

48. Meral Gunes A, Sezgin Evim M, Baytan B, et al. Aceruloplasminemia in a Turkish adolescent with a novel mutation of ceruloplasmin gene: the first diagnosed case from Turkey. *J Pediatr Hematol Oncol.* 2014;36:e423-e425.

49. Doyle A, Rusli F, Bhathal P. Aceruloplasminaemia: a rare but important cause of iron overload. *BMJ Case Rep.* 2015;2015:bcr2014207541.

50. Kono S, Suzuki H, Takahashi K, et al. Hepatic iron overload associated with a decreased serum ceruloplasmin level in a novel clinical type of aceruloplasminemia. *Gastroenterology.* 2006;131:240-245.

51. Rusticeanu M, Zimmer V, Schleithoff L, et al. Novel ceruloplasmin mutation causing aceruloplasminemia with hepatic iron overload and diabetes without neurological symptoms. *Clin Genet.* 2014;85:300-301.

52. Bethlehem C, van Harten B, Hoogendoorn M. Central nervous system involvement in a rare genetic iron overload disorder. *Neth J Med.* 2010;68:316-318.

53. Hofmann WP, Welsch C, Takahashi Y, et al. Identification and in silico characterization of a novel compound heterozygosity associated with hereditary aceruloplasminemia. *Scand J Gastroenterol.* 2007;42:1088-1094.

54. Perez-Aguilar F, Burguera JA, Benlloch S, et al. Aceruloplasminemia in an asymptomatic patient with a new mutation. Diagnosis and family genetic analysis. *J Hepatol.* 2005;42:947-949.

55. Bittencourt PL, Marin ML, Couto CA, et al. Analysis of HFE and non-HFE gene mutations in Brazilian patients with hemochromatosis. *Clinics (Sao Paulo).* 2009;64:837-841.

56. Gordeuk VR. African iron overload. *Semin Hematol.* 2002;39:263-269.

57. Montosi G, Donovan A, Totaro A, et al. Autosomal-dominant hemochromatosis is associated with a mutation in the ferroportin (SLC11A3) gene. *J Clin Invest.* 2001;108:619-623.

58. Njajou OT, Vaessen N, Joosse M, et al. A mutation in SLC11A3 is associated with autosomal dominant hemochromatosis. *Nat Genet.* 2001;28:213-214.

59. Girelli D, De Domenico I, Bozzini C, et al. Clinical, pathological, and molecular correlates in ferroportin disease: a study of two novel mutations. *J Hepatol.* 2008;49:664-671.
60. Cottier H. A hemochromatosis similar disease in newborn. *Schweiz Med Wochenschr.* 1957;87:39-43.
61. Whitington PF. Gestational alloimmune liver disease and neonatal hemochromatosis. *Semin Liver Dis.* 2012;32:325-332.
62. Collardeau-Frachon S, Heissat S, Bouvier R, et al. French retrospective multicentric study of neonatal hemochromatosis: importance of autopsy and autoimmune maternal manifestations. *Pediatr Dev Pathol.* 2012;15:450-470.
63. Whitington PF. Neonatal hemochromatosis: a congenital alloimmune hepatitis. *Semin Liver Dis.* 2007;27:243-250.
64. Lopriore E, Mearin ML, Oepkes D, et al. Neonatal hemochromatosis: management, outcome, and prevention. *Prenat Diagn.* 2013;33:1221-1225.
65. Pronicka E, Weglewska-Jurkiewicz A, Taybert J, et al. Post mortem identification of deoxyguanosine kinase (DGUOK) gene mutations combined with impaired glucose homeostasis and iron overload features in four infants with severe progressive liver failure. *J Appl Genet.* 2011;52:61-66.
66. Fellman V. The GRACILE syndrome, a neonatal lethal metabolic disorder with iron overload. *Blood Cells Mol Dis.* 2002;29:444-450.
67. Visapaa I, Fellman V, Vesa J, et al. GRACILE syndrome, a lethal metabolic disorder with iron overload, is caused by a point mutation in BCS1L. *Am J Hum Genet.* 2002;71:863-876.
68. Ludwig J, Hashimoto E, Porayko MK, et al. Hemosiderosis in cirrhosis: a study of 447 native livers. *Gastroenterology.* 1997;112:882-888.
69. Kowdley KV, Brandhagen DJ, Gish RG, et al. Survival after liver transplantation in patients with hepatic iron overload: the national hemochromatosis transplant registry. *Gastroenterology.* 2005;129:494-503.
70. Fenton H, Torbenson M, Vivekanandan P, et al. Marked iron in liver explants in the absence of major hereditary hemochromatosis gene defects: a risk factor for cardiac failure. *Transplantation.* 2009;87:1256-1260.
71. O'Glasser AY, Scott DL, Corless CL, et al. Hepatic and cardiac iron overload among patients with end-stage liver disease referred for liver transplantation. *Clin Transplant.* 2010;24:643-651.
72. Minervini MI, Ruppert K, Fontes P, et al. Liver biopsy findings from healthy potential living liver donors: reasons for disqualification, silent diseases and correlation with liver injury tests. *J Hepatol.* 2009;50:501-510.
73. Ryan CK, Johnson LA, Germin BI, et al. One hundred consecutive hepatic biopsies in the workup of living donors for right lobe liver transplantation. *Liver Transpl.* 2002;8:1114-1122.
74. Toniutto P, Fabris C, Bortolotti N, et al. Evaluation of donor hepatic iron concentration as a factor of early fibrotic progression after liver transplantation. *J Hepatol.* 2004;41:307-311.
75. Pungpapong S, Krishna M, Abraham SC, et al. Clinicopathologic findings and outcomes of liver transplantation using grafts from donors with unrecognized and unusual diseases. *Liver Transpl.* 2006;12:310-315.
76. Dwyer JP, Sarwar S, Egan B, et al. Hepatic iron overload following liver transplantation of a C282y homozygous allograft: a case report and literature review. *Liver Int.* 2011;31:1589-1592.
77. Torbenson M. Iron in the liver: a review for surgical pathologists. *Adv Anat Pathol.* 2011;18:306-317.
78. Martinelli AL, Filho AB, Franco RF, et al. Liver iron deposits in hepatitis B patients: association with severity of liver disease but not with hemochromatosis gene mutations. *J Gastroenterol Hepatol.* 2004;19:1036-1041.

79. Buzzetti E, Petta S, Manuguerra R, et al. Evaluating the association of serum ferritin and hepatic iron with disease severity in non-alcoholic fatty liver disease. *Liver Int.* 2019;39:1325-1334.

80. Chitturi S, Weltman M, Farrell GC, et al. HFE mutations, hepatic iron, and fibrosis: ethnic-specific association of NASH with C282Y but not with fibrotic severity. *Hepatology.* 2002;36:142-149.

81. Zamin I Jr, Mattos AA, Mattos AZ, et al. Prevalence of the hemochromatosis gene mutation in patients with nonalcoholic steatohepatitis and correlation with degree of liver fibrosis. *Arq Gastroenterol.* 2006;43:224-228.

82. Nelson JE, Wilson L, Brunt EM, et al. Relationship between the pattern of hepatic iron deposition and histological severity in nonalcoholic fatty liver disease. *Hepatology.* 2011;53:448-457.

83. Costa-Matos L, Batista P, Monteiro N, et al. Hfe mutations and iron overload in patients with alcoholic liver disease. *Arq Gastroenterol.* 2013;50:35-41.

84. Gleeson D, Evans S, Bradley M, et al. HFE genotypes in decompensated alcoholic liver disease: phenotypic expression and comparison with heavy drinking and with normal controls. *Am J Gastroenterol.* 2006;101:304-310.

85. Britto MR, Thomas LA, Balaratnam N, et al. Hepatocellular carcinoma arising in non-cirrhotic liver in genetic haemochromatosis. *Scand J Gastroenterol.* 2000;35:889-893.

86. von Delius S, Lersch C, Schulte-Frohlinde E, et al. Hepatocellular carcinoma associated with hereditary hemochromatosis occurring in non-cirrhotic liver. *Z Gastroenterol.* 2006;44:39-42.

87. Kowdley KV. Iron, hemochromatosis, and hepatocellular carcinoma. *Gastroenterology.* 2004;127:S79-S86.

88. Ko C, Siddaiah N, Berger J, et al. Prevalence of hepatic iron overload and association with hepatocellular cancer in end-stage liver disease: results from the National Hemochromatosis Transplant Registry. *Liver Int.* 2007;27:1394-1401.

89. Morcos M, Dubois S, Bralet MP, et al. Primary liver carcinoma in genetic hemochromatosis reveals a broad histologic spectrum. *Am J Clin Pathol.* 2001;116:738-743.

90. Nkontchou G, Tran Van Nhieu J, Ziol M, et al. Peripheral intrahepatic cholangiocarcinoma occurring in patients without cirrhosis or chronic bile duct diseases: epidemiology and histopathology of distant nontumoral liver in 57 White patients. *Eur J Gastroenterol Hepatol.* 2013;25:94-98.

91. Chung H, Kudo M, Kawasaki T, et al. Hepatocellular carcinoma associated with secondary haemochromatosis in non-cirrhotic liver: a case report. *Hepatol Res.* 2003;26:254-258.

92. Mizukawa B, George A, Pushkaran S, et al. Cooperating G6PD mutations associated with severe neonatal hyperbilirubinemia and cholestasis. *Pediatr Blood Cancer.* 2011;56:840-842.

93. Cortes JM, Oliva H, Paradinas FJ, et al. The pathology of the liver in porphyria cutanea tarda. *Histopathology.* 1980;4:471-485.

94. Campo E, Bruguera M, Rodes J. Are there diagnostic histologic features of porphyria cutanea tarda in liver biopsy specimens? *Liver.* 1990;10:185-190.

95. Lefkowitch JH, Grossman ME. Hepatic pathology in porphyria cutanea tarda. *Liver.* 1983;3:19-29.

96. Barton JC, Lee PL, West C, et al. Iron overload and prolonged ingestion of iron supplements: clinical features and mutation analysis of hemochromatosis-associated genes in four cases. *Am J Hematol.* 2006;81:760-767.

97. De Matos LD, Azevedo LF, Vieira ML, et al. The use of exogenous iron by professional cyclists pervades abdominal organs but not the heart. *Int J Cardiol.* 2013;167:2341-2343.

16

GENETIC DISEASES OF THE LIVER

OVERVIEW OF GENETIC DISEASES

Genetic diseases that have significant involvement of the liver can manifest with a variety of clinical and histological findings. In some cases, the histological findings are fairly specific for a given genetic disease, while in other cases, the liver will show a nonspecific pattern of injury. In general, most of the genetic diseases in this chapter manifest as an abnormal accumulation of material in cytoplasm of the hepatocytes or Kupffer cells. Genetic iron overload disease, genetic biliary tract disease, and genetic vascular diseases are discussed separately in their respective chapters.

ALPHA-1-ANTITRYPSIN DEFICIENCY

Definition and Mechanism

Alpha-1-antitrypsin deficiency is an autosomal recessive disease. The alpha-1-antitrypsin gene, *SERPINA1*, is codominant with each allele contributing 50% of the total protein in the blood. There are numerous gene polymorphisms (over 100), but only a few are disease-causing. Patients can be tested for mutant alleles either by Pi typing or by sequencing. When testing by Pi typing, the normal allele is called M, and the most common disease-causing alleles are Z and S. The phenotypes MS and MZ typically are not disease-associated, while SZ, SS, and ZZ all can cause liver disease, with ZZ causing the worst disease. Intrahepatic globules can be seen in hepatocytes in cases of homozygosity, compound heterozygosity, and heterozygosity. Globules in the setting of MS disease, however, are most likely to be seen when other concomitant liver diseases are present.[1-3] The Z and S alleles are enriched in ethnic groups from northern Europe but have been reported worldwide. Rare alleles, called Mmalton and Mdurate, can also cause liver disease with classic intrahepatocellular inclusions. In contrast, the rare null phenotype does not lead to liver inclusions or liver disease but can cause lung disease.

Clinical

The presentation of patients with clinical liver disease tends to fall into several different patterns. The first pattern is neonates and infants with cholestatic liver disease. Overall, only about 10% of all individuals with homozygous alleles for alpha-1-antitrypsin deficiency will present with disease in childhood.[4] A subset of these cases progress to fibrosis in childhood, but most recover and have minimal or no liver disease by adult years. The risk factors for presentation as a child are still unclear.

The second major group of cases is adults with known alpha-1-antitrypsin disease who are biopsied because of concern for concomitant liver disease or to stage fibrosis. Males are more likely to have advanced liver fibrosis. Fatty liver disease or other chronic liver disease also increases the risk for fibrosis progression.

A third group of cases, the largest overall for liver biopsy specimens, is when the biopsy is performed to evaluate for some other disease, and the biopsy also shows globules of alpha-1-antitrypsin protein. Most of these cases represent heterozygous mutations.

The presence of globules in the liver is not used to define alpha-1-antitrypsin deficiency per se. Instead, a diagnosis of deficiency is made based on serum levels. In fact, most liver biopsy specimens with the unexpected finding of alpha-1-antitrypsin globules in hepatocytes do not have alpha-1-antitrypsin deficiency. Most of these are livers with heterozygous mutations (MZ or MS), and the globules are incidental in patients who do not have a true deficiency and typically do not have clinical lung or liver disease. On the other hand, heterozygous mutations may contribute to fibrosis progression in patients with chronic hepatitis, fatty liver, or other diseases where the hepatocytes are the primary target of injury, while fibrosis in the setting of chronic biliary disease appears to be less affected.[5,6] Livers with heterozygous mutations may also be suitable for transplantation,[7] although data is limited.

Pathology

The periportal hepatocytes show eosinophilic, round-to-oval inclusions on hematoxylin and eosin (H&E) stain (Figure 16.1). On trichrome stain, the globules are bright red in color and often have a thin rim of blue (Figure 16.2). The inclusions are found in the hepatocytes and can be somewhat patchy early in the disease course, with many periportal hepatocytes not affected. With more severe diseases, the hepatocytes in all the zones can be affected, but a zone 1 predominance is still evident in most cases. Infants less than 3 months of age often completely lack the globules and can present with a neonatal cholestasis pattern of injury. In these young individuals, the H&E, periodic acid-Schiff (PAS) with diastase treatment (PASD), and immunostains are often not informative and the diagnosis is made by serological or genetic testing. In cases of the null phenotype, an extremely rare form of disease with mutations that prevent any protein production, the biopsies will completely lack the typical intrahepatic PASD-positive globules and individuals generally do not have liver disease. In cases of cryptogenic cirrhosis, the presence of alpha-1-antitrypsin globules on PASD stain do not necessarily indicate the patient has cirrhosis from alpha-1-antitrypsin deficiency, especially when they are sparse, so correlation with serum studies and clinical findings is important.

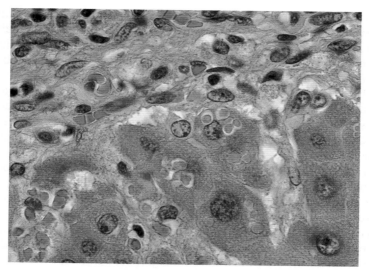

FIGURE 16.1 **Alpha-1-antitrypsin deficiency, hematoxylin and eosin (H&E) stain.** Hepatocytes show distinctive round, eosinophilic globules.

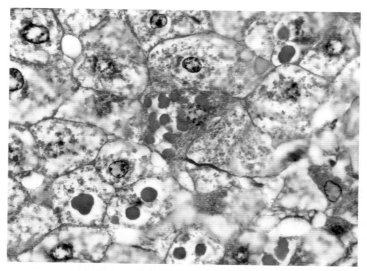

FIGURE 16.2 **Alpha-1-antitrypsin deficiency, Trichrome stain.** On trichrome stain, the globules are bright red and have a thin rim of blue.

Differential

The most common mimic of globules of alpha-1-antitrypsin deficiency are megamitochondria. The location can be a helpful clue, as megamitochondria tends to be randomly distributed, while alpha-1-antitrypsin globules will have a periportal predominance. Special stains can help in difficult cases, including a phosphotungstic acid–hematoxylin stain (PTAH) for megamitochondria and a PASD for alpha-1-antitrypsin globules. Other uncommon mimics include hepatocellular globules that can be seen with chronic congestive liver disease. These tend to have a zone 3 distribution and can be either PASD-positive or negative; they can also be positive on alpha-1-antitrypsin immunostain[8] but are a reactive change that is not associated with *SERPINA1* mutations.

Special Stains

PASD is the classic stain for identifying the accumulation of alpha-1-antitrypsin proteins in hepatocytes; PASD stains highlight the alpha-1-antitrypsin proteins as bright magenta globules (Figure 16.3; eFigs. 16.1 and 16.2). If the stain is over-digested, however, a false negative can result. The globules can be somewhat patchy in early disease, so multiple portal areas should be examined. Interestingly, the globules can also be somewhat patchy in cirrhotic livers and, once again, it is important to check the whole section and not simply spot-check a few areas. An immunostain for alpha-1-antitrypsin can also be helpful but tends to have high background (Figure 16.4); the larger globules tend to stain at their periphery, with weaker staining in the middle. As noted previously, infants less than 3 months of age often lack globules, in which case PASD stains and immunostains can be negative.

WILSON DISEASE

Definition and Mechanism

Wilson disease is caused by mutations in the gene *ATPB7*, which leads to copper accumulation in affected individuals. *ATPB7* encodes an ATPase called copper-transporting ATPase 2 that both transports copper into the bile for

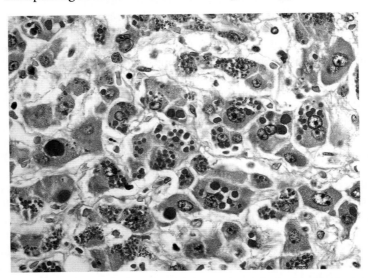

FIGURE 16.3 **Alpha-1-antitrypsin deficiency, periodic acid-Schiff with diastase (PASD) stain.** The globules are stained with a strong magenta color.

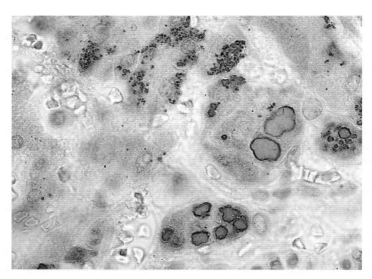

FIGURE 16.4 **Alpha-1-antitrypsin deficiency, immunostain.** The globules are high-lighted by immunostaining. Note how the large globules often stain only as a rim of positivity around the globules. The background liver often stains a muddy brown, so distinctive round structures are needed to make the diagnosis if you use this stain.

excretion and also helps incorporate copper into ceruloplasmin. Since bile is the main route for copper excretion, defects in copper-transporting ATPase 2 leads to a marked reduction in the amount of copper excreted into the bile, with retention of copper in the hepatocytes. Mutations also lead to increased copper in the blood that is not bound to ceruloplasmin. This free copper can then precipitate in different organs, such as the brain, eyes, and kidneys.

Overall, 90% of individuals with a clinical diagnosis of Wilson disease will have a mutation detected with full sequencing of the *ATPB7* gene. The remaining 10% presumably have mutations in other genes that affect the same metabolic pathway. Wilson disease is autosomal recessively inherited, with an estimated carrier frequency of 1 in 100 individuals. Because of the relatively high carrier frequency, there can be kindreds with successive generations that are affected by Wilson disease, despite the recessive inheritance pattern.[9] Heterozygotes may have mild biochemical abnormalities in copper metabolism, but they have no clinical disease in most cases. Over 500 mutations have been reported in the *ATPB7* gene, of which approximately 379 are thought to be disease-causing. Genetic testing for clinical diagnosis is difficult because of the large number of mutations and because not all mutations are disease-causing.[10] Once a mutation is identified in an individual with copper overload, however, focused genetic testing can be very helpful for screening the extended family. There are hot-spot mutations that tend to correlate with ethnicity, which can also help focus the genetic screens for probands. For example, H1096Q is present in about 50% of Caucasians with Wilson disease, but is rare in Chinese, who tend to have the R778L mutation.

Clinical

The current approach for diagnosing Wilson disease incorporates clinical, radiological, serological, laboratory, and histological findings. To help integrate these findings, scoring method have been developed. For examination, in the method below, a score of ≥4 is considered highly likely to be Wilson disease, a score of 2 or 3 is probably Wilson disease, and a score of 0 or 1 is unlikely to be Wilson disease.[11,12]

- *Kayser-Fleischer rings:*
  - Absent: 0 points
  - Present: 2 points
- *Typical brain MRI or typical clinical neuropsychiatric symptoms*
  - Absent: 0 points
  - Present: 2 points
- *Serum ceruloplasmin (mg/dL)*
  - >21: 0 points
  - 10 to 20: 1 point
  - >20: 2 points
- *Coombs negative hemolytic anemia plus high serum copper*
  - Absent: 0 points
  - Present: 1 point
- *24-hour urine copper excretion (μg/24 hours) OR after penicillamine treatment (μg/24 hours)*
  - <100 (24-hour urine copper): 0 points OR <1500 (24-hour urine copper after penicillamine): 0 points
  - 100 to 200: 1 point OR 1500 to 2500: 1 point
  - >200: 2 points OR >2500: 2 points
- *Quantitative copper on liver tissue (μg/g dry)*
  - < 50: −1 points
  - 50 to 100: 0 points
  - 100 to 250: 1 point
  - > 250: 2 points
- *Rhodanine copper stain (only if quant copper not available)*
  - Absent: 0 points
  - Present: 1 point
- *ATP7B mutations known to be disease-causing*
  - No mutations: 0 points
  - 1 mutation: 1 point
  - 1 mutation on each chromosome: 4 points

Most individuals present between the ages of 5 and 35 years, but individuals can present as young as 3 years of age and as late as 80 years of age.[13] Clinical presentations vary considerably but tend to fall into broad categories of neurological symptoms and/or liver disease. Liver disease often is the main finding in younger individuals, while neurological disease at presentation increases in frequency with increasing age. In terms of liver disease, presentation patterns include acute hepatitis, chronic unexplained elevation in liver enzymes, and cryptogenic cirrhosis.

The main sites of copper accumulation are the liver and the basal ganglia, but the eyes, kidneys, and heart can also be affected. Eye disease manifests as copper deposits in the cornea, which are called *Kayser-Fleischer rings*. Kayser-Fleischer rings are seen in two-third of individuals with Wilson disease but are present in almost all persons with neurological or psychiatric symptoms, and about 50% of those with liver predominant disease. While Kayser-Fleischer are often considered pathognomonic, there are a variety of mimics that can lead to a false positive eye examination.[14] Important laboratory findings for diagnosing Wilson disease include a low-serum ceruloplasmin and an elevated 24-hour urine copper. Because ceruloplasmin is an acute phase reactant, levels can be normal or even mildly elevated if individuals with Wilson disease also have significant active ongoing liver inflammation. Estrogens also increase ceruloplasmin levels, and levels can be normal in Wilson disease during pregnancy or with oral contraceptive pills. Twenty-four-hour urine copper studies are also helpful but can be falsely elevated in individuals with marked inflammatory liver disease from many different causes. Gender affects the disease course, with women more commonly having liver disease than men.[15]

Histological Findings

As an overview, the histological findings are variable but tend to fall into several broad categories. In terms of clinical clues, an increased suspicion of Wilson disease is useful when (1) young patients have unexplained chronic liver disease; (2) young or middle-aged individuals have both liver and neurological disease; and (3) young individuals present with acute liver failure. Histological clues that raise suspicion for Wilson disease include fatty liver disease in normoweight, younger individuals; or an acute unexplained hepatitis injury pattern in a young individual; or cryptogenic cirrhosis in a young or middle-aged adult.

The most common liver injury patterns associated with Wilson disease are considered below. Glycogenated nuclei and nuclear pleomorphism can be seen in any of these patterns but are more common with advanced liver disease. Of note, glycogenated nuclei lack both sensitivity and specificity for Wilson disease, so are not an important histological feature.

"ALMOST NORMAL" LIVER PATTERN. The biopsy shows minimal nonspecific findings (eFig. 16.3) with minimal lymphocytic inflammation, minimal to absent macrovesicular steatosis, and often scattered glycogenated hepatocyte nuclei. This pattern can be seen in patients who are biopsied because they have a family member with known Wilson disease in order to stage fibrosis or for quantitative copper analysis.

ACUTE HEPATITIS PATTERN. The acute hepatitis pattern can manifest histologically as marked portal and lobular inflammation with hepatocyte necrosis. Plasma cells and interface activity can be prominent and the histological findings can mimic autoimmune hepatitis. Preexisting fibrosis can also be present. Girls are more likely to present with fulminant liver failure than boys.[16]

FATTY LIVER DISEASE PATTERN. The biopsy shows macrovesicular steatosis that can vary from mild to marked (Figure 16.5). Mallory bodies and balloon cells may be present and the H&E findings can be essentially identical to fatty liver disease from the metabolic syndrome.

CRYPTOGENIC FIBROSIS/CIRRHOSIS PATTERN. The biopsies show advanced fibrosis or established cirrhosis with minimal or mild septal and portal chronic inflammation. Lobular cholestasis can be seen, but most cases have little or no ongoing lobular inflammation. Steatosis can also be present. Ballooned hepatocytes and Mallory hyaline can be prominent in a subset of cases. Giant cell transformation of hepatocytes can also be occasionally seen, especially in the setting of cholestasis. If there is sufficient copper accumulation, granular reddish-brown deposits can be seen in periportal hepatocytes (Figure 16.6).

Copper Stains

The rhodanine copper stain is most commonly used to identify copper deposition in hepatocytes and shows a red-brown granular staining (Figure 16.7; eFig. 16.4). For optimal sensitivity, sections for the rhodanine stain should be 10 microns in thickness; thinner sections significantly reduce the stain's sensitivity. The Timm silver sulfide stain is also reported to work well[17] but is not widely used. If the Timm method is used, a longer (24-hour) deparaffinization time has been

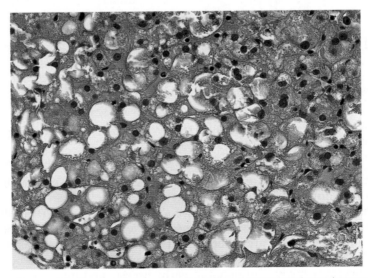

FIGURE 16.5 **Wilson disease, steatosis pattern.** The liver biopsy showed macrovesicular steatosis in a normoweight young individual.

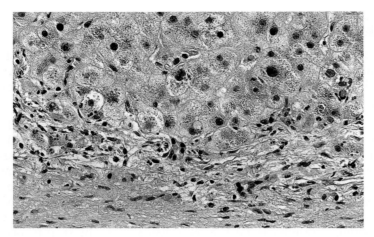

FIGURE 16.6 **Wilson disease, cryptogenic cirrhosis pattern.** In this case of cryptogenic cirrhosis, a clue to the diagnosis of Wilson's disease was the reddish-brown and granular deposits in the hepatocytes at the edges of the cirrhotic nodules.

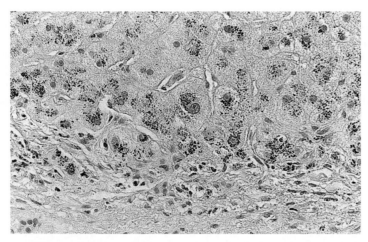

FIGURE 16.7 **Wilson disease, Rhodanine stain.** A Rhodanine stain shows abundant copper deposition (same case as preceding image).

recommended.[18] Orcein and Victoria blue stains detect copper-binding protein and not copper itself.

Positive copper stains tend to have a zone 1 distribution,[19] but the copper deposition can be panlobular. A negative copper stain should be interpreted cautiously if there are other clinical or laboratory findings that strongly suggest Wilson disease. This is because the increased copper in the cytoplasm of hepatocytes is finely distributed in early disease, and may not be evident on rhodanine or other copper stains. Over time, the copper accumulates in larger granules within the lysosomes of hepatocytes, and it is this copper that is identified on rhodanine stain. If a case is negative for copper by rhodanine or other special stains, but clinical concern for Wilson disease remains, then submitting the tissue for quantitative copper analysis can be helpful.

Positive copper stains also have to be interpreted in the context of other laboratory and histological findings, as chronic cholestasis from any cause can lead to copper accumulation, if the cholestasis is of long enough duration (typically months to years). Livers with advanced fibrosis (bridging fibrosis and cirrhosis) can also show nonspecific copper staining within hepatocytes.

Another potential pitfall to avoid when interpreting the copper stain is mistaking lipofuscin pigment for copper staining, as the staining quality of a lightly stained rhodanine can sometimes mimic lipofuscin. If in doubt, the location of the pigment can be helpful (periportal for copper vs pericentral for lipofuscin), as well as a Fontana-Masson stain (positive in lipofuscin).

Quantitative Copper

The results for quantitative copper analysis are essentially the same whether performed on fresh liver tissue or paraffin-embedded tissue. There is no absolute cut-off that can be used for diagnosis in isolation from the clinical and histological findings, as discussed earlier. Historically, a cut-off of greater than 250 µg copper/g dry weight tissue was thought to be specific for Wilson disease, but that cut-off was based on a very small number of cases (less than 10) and subsequent studies have shown that cut-off is too high, missing many cases.[11,20]

OTHER COPPER OVERLOAD DISEASES

There are a number of inherited copper overload diseases outside of Wilson disease. All of these diseases are rare but include Indian childhood cirrhosis, Tyrolean infantile cirrhosis, and idiopathic copper toxiocosis. Patients with these diseases develop cirrhosis, often very rapidly, and cirrhosis is usually present at first diagnosis. For this reason, the precirrhotic histological findings are poorly understood. The livers have marked copper accumulation but genetic testing shows no mutations in the *ATPB7* gene. The histology for all of these three conditions is similar and idiopathic copper toxiocosis is described in more detail as a representative histology.

Individuals with idiopathic copper toxiocosis have normal ceruloplasmin levels, in contrast to Wilson disease. Most cases present before the age of 2 with histories of progressive lethargy, increased infections, and hepatomegaly. A second peak of patient presentation is seen around 5 years of age, and rare cases can be diagnosed as late as 10 years of age.[21] The etiology remains unclear, but there may be both environmental and genetic risk factors.[21,22] Essentially, all cases to date have been diagnosed at the cirrhotic stage and the cirrhosis pattern is typically that of tiny cirrhotic nodules. The hepatocytes show marked reactive changes with abundant Mallory hyaline and scattered acidophil bodies.[22] Inflammation tends to be mild but can be composed of both lymphocytes and neutrophils. Cholestasis can be prominent. A subset of cases has been described as having significant fibrosis of the central veins. In addition to the micronodular pattern of cirrhosis, marked pericellular fibrosis can also be seen on trichrome stain.

GLYCOGEN STORAGE DISEASES

There are many glycogen storage diseases that present as abnormal accumulations of glucose within the hepatocytes.[23,24] These include primarily types Ia/b, IIIa/b, VI, IX, and XI. The injury patterns in glycogen storage diseases tend to be either steatosis or glycogenosis or mixed patterns with both glycogenosis and steatosis (Table 16.1). PAS stains can show abundant glycogen accumulation, but this finding is not specific, as even normal hepatocytes can have abundant glycogen. Thus, the best approach is based on combining the H&E findings with the clinical history to suggest a diagnosis of a glycogen storage disease.

Common clinical findings at presentation for many of the different subtypes of glycogen storage disease include hepatomegaly, hypoglycemia, short stature, and recurrent infections. On the other hand, glycogen storage disease types II and IV are typically not associated with hypoglycemia. The glycogen storage diseases most likely to be associated with liver fibrosis are types III and IV, but fibrosis can also be seen in types I and IX.[25]

In many cases, a precise diagnosis of the subtype of glycogen storage disease cannot be reliably made on the basis of clinical findings and or histology alone. Instead, additional biochemical assays or sequencing are needed to precisely classify the type of glycogen storage disease.[24]

Glycogen Storage Disease Type 0

Patients present with fasting hypoglycemia and hepatomegaly, usually in the first year of life. The hepatocytes typically show macrovesicular steatosis with no glycogenosis. In fact, PAS stains can show diminished glycogen.

Glycogen Storage Disease Type Ia/b

Individuals present with hypoglycemia and hepatomegaly, typically in the first year of life. A subset of individuals with type Ib glycogen storage disease will also have severe neutropenia and can develop inflammatory bowel disease that resembles ulcerative colitis or Crohn disease.[26,27] Short stature is present in most individuals. The liver shows mixed glycogenosis and macrovesicular steatosis (Figure 16.8). The hepatocytes can show prominent glycogenated nuclei.[25] Steatosis is often more prominent in younger individuals. Fibrosis can rarely be present. Hepatic adenomas can develop, often right around the time of puberty but can also be found at younger ages. Most are of the inflammatory subtype and they can have beta-catenin activation, with a risk for malignant transformation.[28] The hepatic adenomas can also be associated with anemia that resolves after the adenoma is resected.[29]

TABLE 16.1 Glycogen Storage Diseases That Affect the Liver

Type	Gene	Protein	Main Liver Findings	Other Liver Findings
0	GYS2	Glycogen synthetase	Steatosis	
1a	G6PC	Glucose-6-phosphatase	Steatosis glycogenosis	Hepatic adenoma with risk of malignant transformation
1b	SLC37A4	Glucose-6-phosphate translocase	Steatosis glycogenosis	Hepatic adenoma with risk of malignant transformation
II	GAA	Acid alpha-glucosidase (also called acid maltase)	Cytoplasmic vacuoles	
IIIa/b	AGL	Amylo-1-6 glucosidase	Steatosis Glycogenosis	Fibrosis, can progress to cirrhosis Hepatic adenoma with risk of malignant transformation
IV	GBE1	1,4-Alpha-glucan branching enzyme 1	Hepatocyte inclusions that resemble ground-glass change	Fibrosis, can progress to cirrhosis
VI	PYGL	Liver phosphorylase	Steatosis Glycogenosis	Hepatic adenoma with risk of malignant transformation
IX	PHKA1 PHKA2 PHKB PHKG2	Liver phosphorylase kinase	Steatosis Glycogenosis	Fibrosis, can progress to cirrhosis
XI	SLC2A2	GLUT 2 transporter	Glycogenosis	

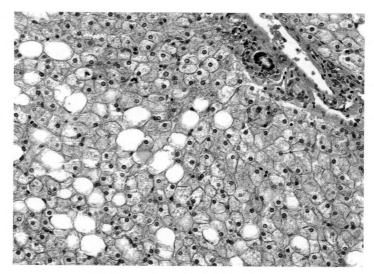

FIGURE 16.8 **Glycogen storage disease type I.** The liver shows predominately macrovesicular steatosis with a subtle glycogenosis.

Glycogen Storage Disease Type II

This form is also known as *Pompe disease* or *acid maltase deficiency*. Glycogen storage disease type II was the first type of glycogen storage disease to be recognized by the medical community and was identified by J.C. Pompe in 1932. The disease can present in infancy or in later childhood or in adults. The infantile form presents with "floppy baby syndrome" with muscle weakness, an enlarged tongue, and marked cardiomegaly. Later presentations can also involve muscle weakness, which may include the respiratory muscles, leading to difficulty breathing or impaired coughing. Biopsies of the liver show marked glycogenosis. Fibrosis is typically absent.

Glycogen Storage Disease Type III

This form most commonly affects both the liver and the muscle (80% of cases, type IIIa), but may also affect the liver only (type IIIb). Individuals typically present with hepatomegaly, hypoglycemia, and short stature. Muscle symptoms are variable but can dominate the clinical findings in adults with type IIIa disease. Biopsies show marked hepatocellular glycogenosis (Figure 16.9). Fibrosis is often present and can progress to cirrhosis (Figure 16.10). Cirrhotic livers are further at risk for hepatocellular carcinoma (Figure 16.11).

Glycogen Storage Disease Type IV

This form is also known as *Andersen disease, Brancher deficiency*, and *amylopectinosis*. Affected children are typically normal at birth but present later with failure to thrive and hepatomegaly. Hypoglycemia is uncommon. A subset of individuals has the classic hepatic form and commonly develop

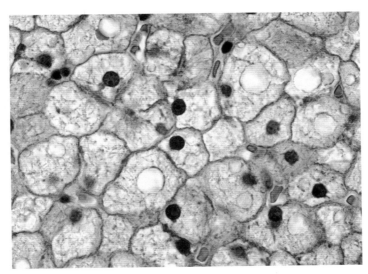

FIGURE 16.9 **Glycogen storage disease type III.** The liver shows marked glycogenosis with enlarged hepatocytes showing cytoplasmic clearing as a result of glycogen accumulation.

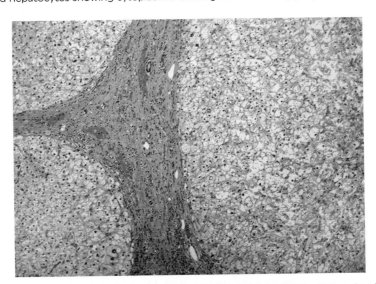

FIGURE 16.10 **Glycogen storage disease type III.** Established cirrhosis has developed in this individual.

cirrhosis in early childhood (often by age 5), while others can have a non-progressive form of the disease that does not lead to fibrosis.

Biopsies show hepatocellular ground-glass type inclusions (Figure 16.12) and chronic hepatitis B infection, as well as drug-induced glycogen pseudoground-glass changes, should be excluded. The inclusions are PAS-positive and are completely or partially diastase resistant (because the inclusions are composed of amylopectin-like material and not typical glycogen), but this will depend somewhat on how aggressively the slide is digested.

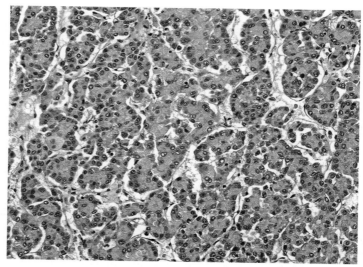

FIGURE 16.11 **Glycogen storage disease type III.** Hepatocellular carcinomas can develop in cirrhotic livers with glycogen storage disease type III, as seen in this case.

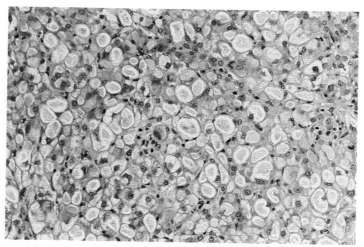

FIGURE 16.12 **Glycogen storage disease type IV.** The hepatocytes show cytoplasmic inclusions that resemble the ground-glass change of hepatitis B or drug effect.

Glycogen Storage Disease Type VI

This form is also known as *Hers disease*. Affected individuals can present with failure to thrive, hepatomegaly, and hypoglycemia, but the clinical course is typically benign with symptom remission as children mature. Biopsies show glycogenosis with lesser degrees of steatosis. Patients can develop various hepatocellular nodular lesions including focal nodular hyperplasia and hepatic adenomas. Malignant transformation of the hepatic adenomas can occur, even at young ages.

Glycogen Storage Disease Type IX

Affected individuals may present with hypoglycemia, hepatomegaly, and failure to thrive in the first year of life, but the disease course tends to be benign with most symptoms resolving by adulthood. The hepatocytes can show marked glycogenosis (Figure 16.13). The glycogen is diastase sensitive, but occasional cells can accumulate material that is resistant to digestion (Figure 16.14). A subset of cases can develop fibrosis or cirrhosis (Figure 16.15).

Glycogen Storage Disease Type XI

This form is also known as *Fanconi-Bickel syndrome*. Affected individuals present with hypoglycemia as well as postprandial hyperglycemia. Individuals are typically short, have a "moon" face, and have fat deposits in their shoulders and abdomen. The kidneys are also involved, and there can be severe proximal tubular dysfunction leading to the development of rickets. Liver biopsy shows a mixed picture of both macrovesicular steatosis and glycogenosis.

Lafora Disease

Lafora disease is an autosomal recessively inherited disease where mutations lead to insufficiently branched glycogen molecules. The glycogen

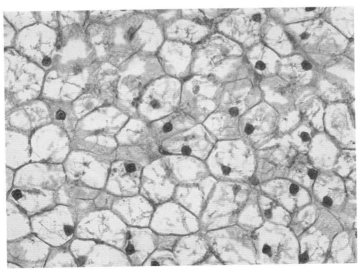

FIGURE 16.13 **Glycogen storage disease type IX.** The hepatocytes show marked glycogenosis.

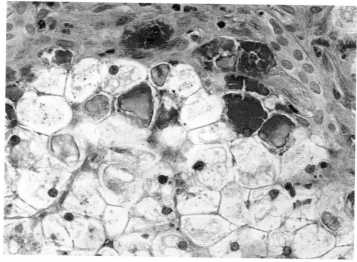

FIGURE 16.14 **Glycogen storage disease type IX, PASD stain.** The glycogen in the hepatocytes will digest with diastase treatment, but occasional cells can be seen with material resistant to digestion.

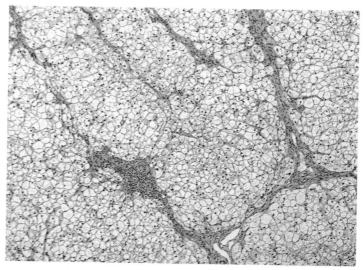

FIGURE 16.15 **Glycogen storage disease type IX.** A subset of cases can develop advanced fibrosis.

then becomes poorly soluble and precipitates out as polyglucosan bodies. These bodies accumulate in hepatocytes and can resemble the inclusions in type IV glycogen storage disease on H&E stains. Clinically, Lafora disease presents in late childhood, is accompanied by epilepsy, and is usually fatal.

UREA CYCLE DEFECTS

Clinical Findings

Nitrogen is a by-product of protein metabolism, and the urea cycle converts nitrogen into urea so that it can be safely excreted in the urine. When there are mutations that impair the urea cycle, nitrogen in the form of ammonia can accumulate in tissues and blood. Mutations are relatively rare in the population but mainly affect six genes (Table 16.2).

Most cases either present in the neonate or childhood period, although increasing numbers of adult cases with mild disease are being reported, likely because of improved testing. In the neonate period, urea cycle defects may account for some cases of sudden infant death syndrome. Other presentations include lethargy, vomiting, and irritability, along with seizures in the first few days of life. Childhood presentations can vary but may include avoidance of meat, hyperactivity with self-injury behavior, lethargy or vomiting after high-protein meals. Adult presentations often include substantial components of neurological or psychiatric abnormalities.

TABLE 16.2 Genes Involved in Urea Cycle Inborn Errors of Metabolism

Gene Name	Gene	Disease	Main Laboratory Finding
Arginase	ARG1	Arginase deficiency (also known as argininemia)	Increased arginine
Argininosuccinase acid lyase	ASL	Argininosuccinase acid lyase deficiency (also known as argininosuccinic aciduria)	Increased citrulline, and argininosuccinic acid
Argininosuccinic acid synthetase	ASS1	Argininosuccinic acid synthetase deficiency (also known as citrullinemia)	Increased citrulline
Carbamoyl phosphate synthetase I	CPS1	Carbamoyl phosphate synthetase I deficiency	Increased ammonia
N-acetylglutamate synthetase	NAGS	N-acetylglutamate synthase deficiency	Increased ammonia
Ornithine transcarbamylase	OTC	Ornithine transcarbamylase deficiency	Increased ornithine, uracil, orotic acid

Histological Findings

Liver biopsies show a range of findings but typically show some glycogen accumulation. The glycogen accumulation can be very mild, and there can be subtle changes of nodular regenerative hyperplasia (Figures 16.16 and 16.17). In other cases, the glycogen accumulation can be marked (Figure 16.18), often accompanied by prominent megamitochondria and glycogenated nuclei (Figure 16.19). For example, one study found marked liver glycogen accumulation in 8 of 11 children with urea cycle defects, including those with ornithine transcarbamylase deficiency, argininosuccinate lyase deficiency, and carbamoyl phosphate synthetase deficiency.[30] The histological findings are similar to glycogenic hepatopathy, but the clinical settings are distinctively different. The histological findings in adults have not been well described but include varying degrees of glycogen accumulation and steatosis. Inflammatory changes are generally mild, but there can be advanced fibrosis or cirrhosis.

MUCOPOLYSACCHARIDE DISEASE

Mutations in pathways involving mucopolysaccharide metabolism can lead to accumulation of excess mucopolysaccharides in the liver and other tissues. Most of these inborn errors of metabolism are inherited as autosomal recessive diseases, or rarely as X-linked diseases. The major disorders are Hunter syndrome, Hurler syndrome, Morquio syndrome, Sanfilippo syndrome, and Maroteaux-Lamy syndrome. They can all have liver involvement, with the liver biopsies showing a range of findings. Some

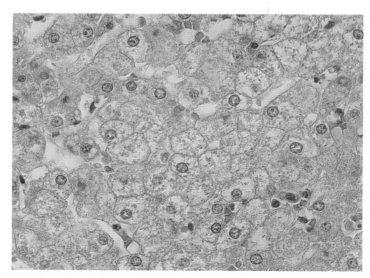

FIGURE 16.16 **Urea cycle defects, carbamoyl phosphate synthetase I deficiency.** The hepatocytes show only a very mild and subtle glycogenosis.

FIGURE 16.17 **Urea cycle defects, carbamoyl phosphate synthetase I deficiency.** At low power, the liver shows subtle changes of nodular regenerative hyperplasia (same case as preceding image).

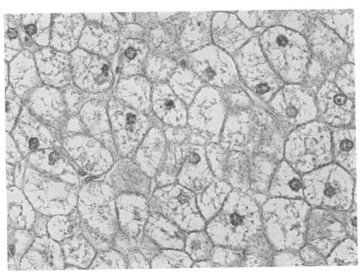

FIGURE 16.18 **Argininosuccinate lyase deficiency.** The hepatocytes show marked cytoplasmic glycogenosis.

cases can show rarified cytoplasm that resembles glycogenosis but will be PAS-negative. Other cases will have numerous medium-sized and small-sized cytoplasmic vacuoles in hepatocytes and Kupffer cells (Figure 16.20). In most cases, the excess mucopolysaccharides are removed by routine processing for histology, but some may have residual mucopolysaccharides

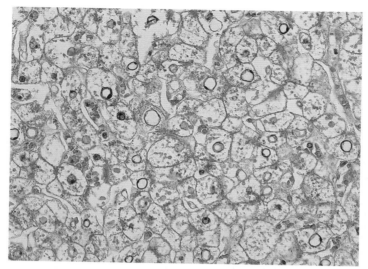

FIGURE 16.19 **Arginase deficiency**. The hepatocytes show marked glycogenosis with many glycogenated nuclei.

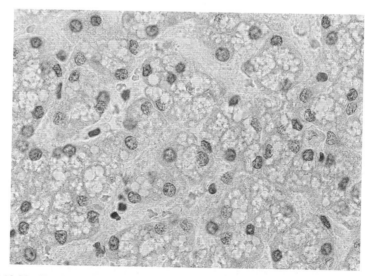

FIGURE 16.20 **Hunter syndrome**. The hepatocyte cytoplasm is distended by numerous small- and medium-sized vacuoles.

that can be highlighted by colloidal iron stains. For patients in which a potential mucopolysaccharide disease is suspected prior to the biopsy, special fixatives can help preserve the mucopolysaccharides, including adding a 10% solution of acetyl trimethylammonium bromide to the formalin fixative. Oil Red O stains on frozen sections are not helpful.

INBORN ERRORS OF AMINO ACID METABOLISM

There is an extensive list of genetic diseases that impair normal amino acid metabolism. Most of these diseases are autosomal recessively inherited and most present in the early years of life. Many have liver disease but not all will show abnormal accumulation of metabolic products on histological examination. One illustrative example is lysinuric protein intolerance.

Lysinuric protein intolerance is autosomal recessively inherited. Mutations in *SLC7A7* lead to abnormal metabolism of the amino acids ornithine, arginine, and lysine, with excess urine secretion.[31] These amino acids are also poorly absorbed in the gut, leading to abnormally low-serum levels. The reduced levels of these amino acids lead to impairments in the urea cycle, leading in turn to difficulty processing meals that are high in protein. Most infants present at the time of weaning with the introduction of foods higher in protein. Affected children can show failure to thrive and irritability, with enlarged livers and spleens. Another clue can be elevated serum ferritin and lactate dehydrogenase levels.

The biopsy findings are usually very mild and nonspecific, with no significant inflammation, fatty change, or biliary tract disease. Early in the disease course, the biopsies can show very subtle glycogenosis as well as prominent megamitochondria (Figure 16.21). Discrete foci of glycogen accumulation that affect aggregates of several hundred hepatocytes (glycogen storing foci) have also been reported.[32] This finding, however, is not specific and can be seen in many other disease settings. Fibrosis is not evident early in the disease course but can develop if the disease is not

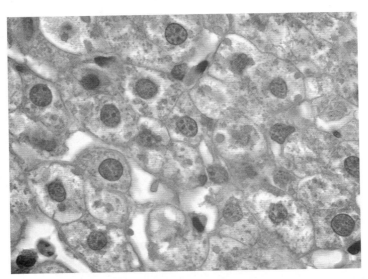

FIGURE 16.21 **Lysinuric protein intolerance.** The liver is almost normal but careful examination shows very mild glycogenosis in the hepatocytes along with prominent megamitochondria.

diagnosed and treated by dietary modifications. Microvesicular steatosis can be seen on thick sections prepared for electron microscopy,[32] later biopsy findings can also include macrovesicular steatosis.[33]

PRADER-WILLI DISEASE

Prader-Willi disease is caused by deletions of a variable set of paternally inherited genes on chromosome 15. Interestingly, one of the most important genes affected is *SNORD116* which does not code for a protein but instead a noncoding RNA. Affected individuals have persistent feelings of hunger despite adequate food intake, and the hyperphagia leads to the metabolic syndrome with obesity and insulin resistance.[34,35] Infants with Prader-Willi disease can be significantly underweight, but severe obesity is common in older children and adults. The biopsy findings show the typical changes of fatty liver disease, with macrovesicular steatosis (Figure 16.22). Rare cases of hepatic adenomas have been reported.[36]

GLUCOSE-6-PHOSPHATASE DEHYDROGENASE DEFICIENCY

Glucose-6-phosphatase dehydrogenase deficiency is inherited in an X-linked recessive fashion. The enzyme glucose-6-phosphatase dehydrogenase is important in red blood cell synthesis and mutations lead to hemolytic anemia. The anemia is often triggered by exposure to infection, chemicals, or other substances. Symptoms are only seen in males and typically are related to hemolytic crises. The most common findings are increased iron deposits in the Kupffer cells and hepatocytes (Figures 16.23 and 16.24). Rare cases, however, can present as neonatal cholestasis.[37]

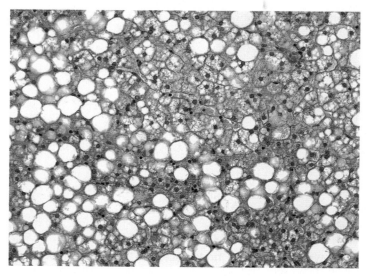

FIGURE 16.22 **Prader Willi.** The liver biopsy shows moderate macrovesicular steatosis.

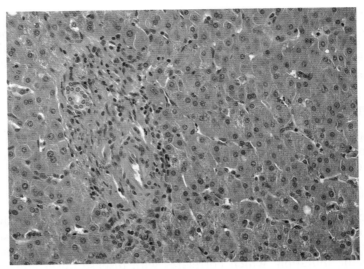

FIGURE 16.23 **Glucose-6-phosphatase dehydrogenase deficiency.** The liver biopsy is almost normal, other than for increased iron (see next image).

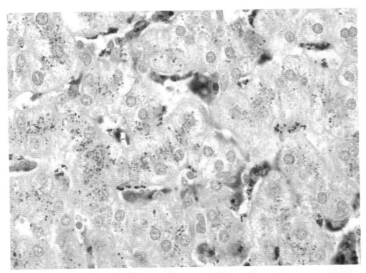

FIGURE 16.24 **Glucose-6-phosphatase dehydrogenase deficiency.** An iron stain shows iron deposits in both Kupffer cells and hepatocytes.

ERYTHROPOIETIC PROTOPORPHYRIA

Erythropoietic protoporphyria typically presents with photosensitivity in young children. The enzyme ferrochelatase is defective and leads to impaired heme synthesis, with the inability to insert iron into protoporphyrin, leading to excess protoporphyrin accumulation in the liver. Liver disease typically does not develop until the teenage years or later. On liver biopsy, the hepatocytes show dense dark brown deposits in the bile canaliculi and in the Kupffer cells (Figure 16.25). On polarization, the protoporphyrin deposits tend to have a red-to-orange birefringence and often demonstrate a Maltese cross pattern (Figure 16.26).

DISORDERS OF LIPID METABOLISM

There are numerous disorders of lipid metabolism, some of which lead to abnormal deposits of material in the liver. While still rare, the most common are Gaucher disease and Nieman-Pick disease.

Gaucher Disease

Gaucher disease occurs most often in individuals who are of Ashkenazi Jewish descent and results from mutations in the beta-glucosidase gene, *GBA*. The disease has been further subclassified into three types based on the specific mutation, which correlates with disease onset and progression. Serum alkaline phosphatase levels and serum angiotensin-converting enzyme (ACE) levels are often elevated. On the liver biopsy, the typical Gaucher cells show large, amphophilic, and striated deposits in the Kupffer cell (Figure 16.27).

Niemann-Pick Disease

Niemann-Pick disease (also called *sphingomyelin-cholesterol lipidosis*) is caused by mutations in the *SMPD1* gene (types A and B) or *NPC1* or

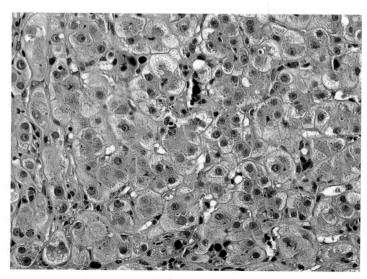

FIGURE 16.25 **Erythropoietic protoporphyria.** The hepatocytes show marked dense dark brown deposits in the bile canaliculi and Kupffer cells.

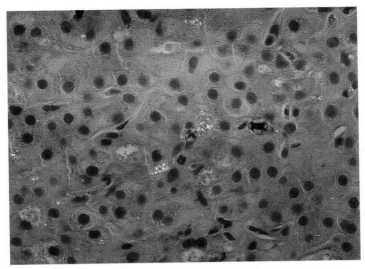

FIGURE 16.26 **Erythropoietic protoporphyria**. With polarization, scattered orange protoporphyrin deposits are seen, some with Maltese cross patterns.

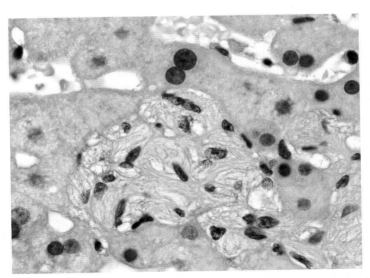

FIGURE 16.27 **Gauche disease**. The Kupffer cell is filled with amphophilic and striated deposits that are sometimes referred to as "tissue paper–like."

NPC2 gene (type C). These mutations lead to sphingomyelin deposits in the central nervous system, liver, spleen, and bone marrow. Type A is the most common (80%-90% of cases) and has the worst prognosis, with most cases leading to death by 2 years. Liver biopsies show foamy appearing macrophages, often present in small but discrete clumps in the sinusoids (Figure 16.28).

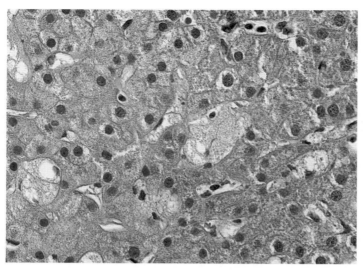

FIGURE 16.28 **Niemann-Pick disease.** Clumps of foamy appearing Kupffer cells are present in the lobules.

Tangier Disease

Tangier disease is a cholesterol ester disease named after Tangier Island, Virginia, where the disease was first discovered. The disease is caused by mutations in *ABCA1*, leading to diminished or absent levels of high-density lipoproteins. The lack of high-density lipoproteins then leads to cholesterol ester deposits in a number of different organs, the most common being the peripheral nerves and the reticuloendothelial system, including the liver, spleen, lymph nodes, and tonsils. In the liver, Kupffer cell changes are the main findings, with Kupffer cells enlarged by abundant, foamy cytoplasm (Figure 16.29).

Lysosomal Acid Lipase Deficiency

Lysosomal acid lipase deficiency (LALD) is caused by mutations in the *LIPA* gene. Clinical liver disease develops in patients with heterozygous mutations; liver disease in heterozygous patients has not been well delineated. With homozygous mutations, the decreased or absent lysosomal acid lipase activity leads to deposits of cholesteryl esters in the reticuloendothelial system including the liver, spleen, and macrophages. The clinical severity of the disease reflects the degree of residual gene activity. The severe form of LALD was historically known as *Wolman disease* and presents in infants with failure to thrive, vomiting, malabsorption, diarrhea, steatorrhea, and hepatosplenomegaly; the clinical course is severe, with a median age at death of about 4 months.[38] In contrast, patients that have some residual enzyme activity can present at older ages, from childhood to adults. In older patients, the clinical findings are usually mild and nonspecific, but patients commonly have hepatosplenomegaly.

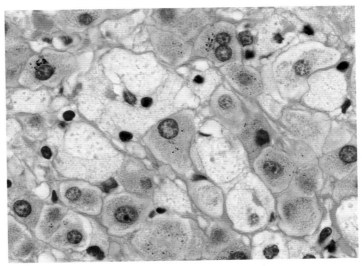

FIGURE 16.29 **Tangier disease.** The Kupffer cells enlarged by abundant, foamy cytoplasm.

On biopsy, the Kupffer cells and portal macrophages are enlarged by foamy cytoplasm. The foamy macrophages can be seen throughout the lobules and sometimes form small clusters in the sinusoids.[39] The hepatocytes show microvesicular steatosis but may also have admixed intermediate-sized droplets of fat and often large-sized droplets of fat (Figure 16.30). The fatty changes are diffuse and show no strong zonal pattern.[40] Cholesteryl ester crystals show a bright silver birefringence under polarized light, when using frozen sections.[39] The livers can become fibrotic[41] and some cases will progress to cirrhosis.[39]

DISORDERS OF MITOCHONDRIA

Mitochondria function depends on both nuclear-encoded genes as well as mitochondrial-encoded genes. Mitochondria diseases that result from mutations in nuclear-encoded genes are autosomal-inherited, while diseases deriving from defects in mitochondrial DNA are either de novo or exclusively maternally inherited, since the vast majority of mitochondrial DNA is maternally inherited. A subset of the mitochondrial diseases involves the liver. Many different mutations have been described, although all are very rare. As a general rule, most mutations can be classified by whether they impair mitochondrial function by defects in a single protein (most cases) or whether they lead to depletions in total mitochondrial DNA (a subset of about 10% of all mitochondrial cytopathies). Diseases caused by mutations in single proteins often lead to impairment in the mitochondrial respiratory chain and can present clinically with liver failure. Neurological symptoms are often present but other organs can also be involved, with eye

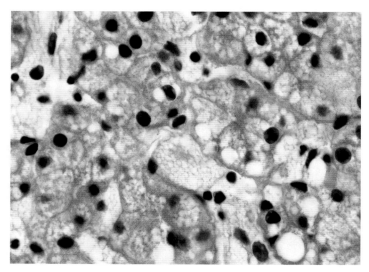

FIGURE 16.30 **Lysosomal acid lipase deficiency.** The hepatocytes and Kupffer cells show microvesicular steatosis. Occasional hepatocytes have larger droplets of fat.

disease, deafness, and intestinal pseudo-obstruction.[42] The disease spectrum is very wide and varies from death in the early years of life to a wide range of often confusing medical signs and symptoms. Charles Darwin, for example often suffered from debilitating health problems, which are now thought, at least by some authors, to have been possibly caused by a mitochondrial cytopathy called "mitochondrial encephalomyopathy, lactic acidosis, and stroke-like episodes" or MELAS syndrome.[43]

The rarity of the mitochondrial diseases involving the liver makes it difficult for large series to be put together, so most descriptions are from small numbers of cases. In addition, most cases are from patients with severe disease, so the histological findings in patients with mild liver disease are not well understood.

Overall, the liver biopsies tend to show steatosis that can have a prominent microvesicuclar steatosis component (Figures 16.31 and 16.32), along with hepatocyte ballooning and variable cholestasis.[44-46] Bile ductular proliferation can also be seen, in particular, if there is cholestasis. Hepatocellular iron deposition has also been reported,[45,46] and can sometimes be a dominant finding; of these, the GRACILE (growth retardation, aminoaciduria, cholestasis, iron overload, lactacidosis, and early death) syndrome is discussed and illustrated in Chapter 15, on iron overload disease. Fibrosis can develop and can progress rapidly, with some cases showing micronodular cirrhosis by 6 months of age.[46]

In the mitochondrial DNA depletion syndromes, the liver can show subacute necrosis with replacement of hepatocytes by proliferating bile ductules.[47] There can be patches of hepatocytes with oncocytic cytoplasmic

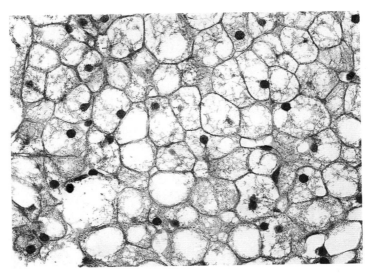

FIGURE 16.31 **Mitochondrial cytopathy.** The diffuse microvesicular steatosis in this case resembles glycogenosis, but the fine droplets of fat can be seen with careful examination.

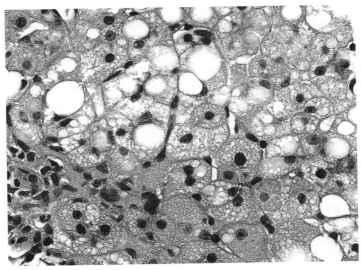

FIGURE 16.32 **Mitochondrial cytopathy.** Mixed micro- and macrovesicular steatosis can be seen in this case.

changes (Figure 16.33) or distinct tumor-like nodules in noncirrhotic livers, with the nodules showing steatosis and having adenoma-like appearances.[44] Other cases may show advanced fibrosis or established cirrhosis with mild fatty changes and mild nonspecific inflammation. Hepatocellular carcinomas can develop in the setting of cirrhosis.[45]

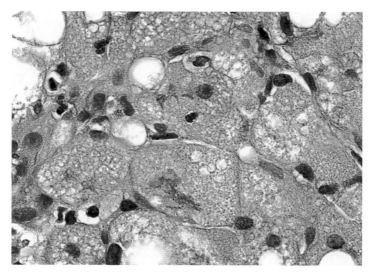

FIGURE 16.33   **Mitochondrial cytopathy.** Some hepatocytes show striking oncocytosis.

SHORT TELOMERE SYNDROME

Short telomere syndromes are a diverse group of diseases that all lead to accelerated aging. The shortened telomeres result from mutations in various genes, such as *TERT, TERC,* and *DCK1.* The shortened telomeres affect primarily those organs that have a lot of cell cycling, such as the skin, bone marrow, lungs, gastrointestinal tract, and liver; clinical presentation often results from signs and symptoms of aplastic anemia, idiopathic pulmonary fibrosis, and cryptogenic liver disease.[48] The liver biopsy findings are not well described and what has been described is not very specific, so the best clue to the diagnosis is typically a patient with a history of unexplained lung and liver disease; some of these patients may also have unexplained anemia. In addition, some families may have "genetic anticipation", where the lung or liver disease develops at an earlier age in the patient than it did in their parents or grandparents.

The histological findings can vary from massive necrosis without significant inflammation to cryptogenic cirrhosis.[49] Inflammation is generally mild and nonspecific, including patchy portal chronic inflammation and mild patchy lobular hepatitis, especially when there is clinical disease involving the gut.[50] In addition, the portal veins may be atrophic or absent (Figure 16.34).[49] In response to the altered portal blood flow, the lobules may become arterialized (Figure 16.35) and show nodular regenerative hyperplasia.[49,51] Fibrosis can develop, with portal fibrosis and thin delicate bridging fibrosis (Figure 16.36); some cases progress to cirrhosis.[48,52] Large cell change can also be seen[53] but is not a specific finding. Of course, patients may also have fatty liver disease or other concomitant acute or chronic diseases and those findings can dominate the histological findings.

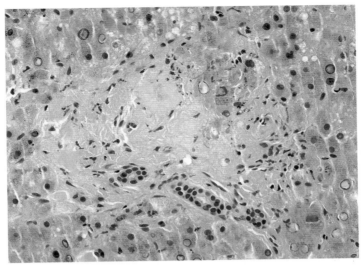

FIGURE 16.34 **Telomere shortening syndrome, portal veins.** The portal tracts show loss of portal veins, sometimes with a small fibrous plug where the vein should be.

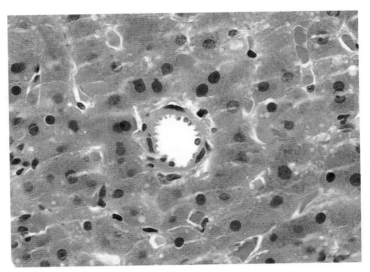

FIGURE 16.35 **Telomere shortening syndrome, lobules.** An isolated artery is seen in the lobules.

TURNER SYNDROME

Turner syndrome is caused by monosomy X (karyotype 45X), in which female patients are missing all or portions of one copy of the X chromosome. Affected individuals often have a classic phenotype of short stature, broad chest, webbed neck, and low-set ears, but there is a wide

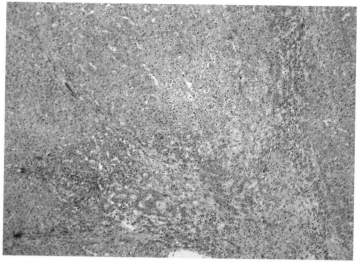

FIGURE 16.36 **Telomere shortening syndrome, incomplete septal cirrhosis**. On trichrome stain, the biopsy shows thin delicate and sometimes, incomplete fibrous bridges.

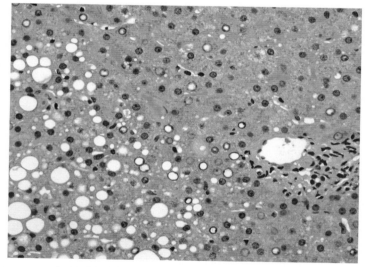

FIGURE 16.37 **Turner syndrome.** Mild macrovesicular steatosis is seen.

range of phenotypes, and some individuals have less obvious physical examination findings.

Turner syndrome is associated with a number of medical conditions, the classic being gonadal dysfunction with sterility. Many individuals will also have abnormal liver enzyme levels. Biopsies in most cases show steatosis (Figure 16.37) or steatohepatitis, but a subset can also have abnormal vasculature.[54,55] The portal veins can be atrophic or absent. The livers can show nodular regenerative hyperplasia as well as focal nodular hyperplasia, including multiple lesions. Patchy bile ductular proliferation that resembles biliary obstruction can also be seen. Some individuals will develop cirrhosis.[54] In cases with cirrhosis, it is often unclear if the fatty liver disease or the vascular abnormalities, or both, are the driving force leading to cirrhosis.

REFERENCES

1. Millward-Sadler GH. Alpha-1-antitrypsin deficiency and liver disease. *Acta Med Port.* 1981;(suppl 2):91-102.
2. Kelly JK, Taylor TV, Milford-Ward A. Alpha-1-antitrypsin Pi S phenotype and liver cell inclusion bodies in alcoholic hepatitis. *J Clin Pathol.* 1979;32:706-709.
3. Gourley MF, Gourley GR, Gilbert EF, et al. Alpha 1-antitrypsin deficiency and the PiMS phenotype: case report and literature review. *J Pediatr Gastroenterol Nutr.* 1989;8:116-121.
4. Arroyo M, Crawford JM. Hepatitic inherited metabolic disorders. *Semin Diagn Pathol.* 2006;23:182-189.
5. Cacciottolo TM, Gelson WT, Maguire G, et al. Pi*Z heterozygous alpha-1 antitrypsin states accelerate parenchymal but not biliary cirrhosis. *Eur J Gastroenterol Hepatol.* 2014;26:412-417.
6. Schaefer B, Mandorfer M, Viveiros A, et al. Heterozygosity for the alpha-1-antitrypsin Z allele in cirrhosis is associated with more advanced disease. *Liver Transpl.* 2018;24:744-751.
7. Doshi SD, Wood L, Abt PL, et al. Outcomes of living-donor liver transplantation using grafts heterozygous for alpha-1 antitrypsin gene mutations. *Transplantation.* 2019;103:1175-1180.
8. Buglioni A, Wu TT, Mounajjed T. Immunohistochemical and ultrastructural features of hepatocellular cytoplasmic globules in venous outflow impairment. *Am J Clin Pathol.* 2019;152:563-569.
9. Bennett JT, Schwarz KB, Swanson PD, et al. An exceptional family with three consecutive generations affected by Wilson disease. *JIMD Rep.* 2013;10:1-4.
10. Bennett J, Hahn SH. Clinical molecular diagnosis of Wilson disease. *Semin Liver Dis.* 2011;31:233-238.
11. Yang X, Tang XP, Zhang YH, et al. Prospective evaluation of the diagnostic accuracy of hepatic copper content, as determined using the entire core of a liver biopsy sample. *Hepatology.* 2015;62:1731-1741.
12. Ferenci P. Whom and how to screen for Wilson disease. *Expert Rev Gastroenterol Hepatol.* 2014;8:513-520.
13. Rosencrantz R, Schilsky M. Wilson disease: pathogenesis and clinical considerations in diagnosis and treatment. *Semin Liver Dis.* 2011;31:245-259.
14. Suvarna JC. Kayser-Fleischer ring. *J Postgrad Med.* 2008;54:238-240.
15. Litwin T, Gromadzka G, Czlonkowska A. Gender differences in Wilson's disease. *J Neurol Sci.* 2012;312:31-35.
16. Markiewicz-Kijewska M, Szymczak M, Ismail H, et al. Liver transplantation for fulminant Wilson's disease in children. *Ann Transplant.* 2008;13:28-31.
17. Pilloni L, Lecca S, Van Eyken P, et al. Value of histochemical stains for copper in the diagnosis of Wilson's disease. *Histopathology.* 1998;33:28-33.
18. Nemolato S, Serra S, Saccani S, et al. Deparaffination time: a crucial point in histochemical detection of tissue copper. *Eur J Histochem.* 2008;52:175-178.

19. Faa G, Nurchi V, Demelia L, et al. Uneven hepatic copper distribution in Wilson's disease. *J Hepatol.* 1995;22:303-308.

20. Ferenci P, Steindl-Munda P, Vogel W, et al. Diagnostic value of quantitative hepatic copper determination in patients with Wilson's Disease. *Clin Gastroenterol Hepatol.* 2005;3:811-818.

21. Muller T, Muller W, Feichtinger H. Idiopathic copper toxicosis. *Am J Clin Nutr.* 1998;67:1082S-1086S.

22. Muller T, Schafer H, Rodeck B, et al. Familial clustering of infantile cirrhosis in Northern Germany: a clue to the etiology of idiopathic copper toxicosis. *J Pediatr.* 1999;135:189-196.

23. McAdams AJ, Hug G, Bove KE. Glycogen storage disease, types I to X: criteria for morphologic diagnosis. *Hum Pathol.* 1974;5:463-487.

24. Jevon GP, Finegold MJ. Reliability of histological criteria in glycogen storage disease of the liver. *Pediatr Pathol.* 1994;14:709-721.

25. Gogus S, Kocak N, Ciliv G, et al. Histologic features of the liver in type Ia glycogen storage disease: comparative study between different age groups and consecutive biopsies. *Pediatr Dev Pathol.* 2002;5:299-304.

26. Yamaguchi T, Ihara K, Matsumoto T, et al. Inflammatory bowel disease-like colitis in glycogen storage disease type 1b. *Inflamm Bowel Dis.* 2001;7:128-132.

27. Couper R, Kapelushnik J, Griffiths AM. Neutrophil dysfunction in glycogen storage disease Ib: association with Crohn's-like colitis. *Gastroenterology.* 1991;100:549-554.

28. Torbenson M. Hepatic adenomas: classification, controversies, and consensus. *Surg Pathol Clin.* 2018;11:351-366.

29. Wang DQ, Carreras CT, Fiske LM, et al. Characterization and pathogenesis of anemia in glycogen storage disease type Ia and Ib. *Genet Med.* 2012;14:795-799.

30. Miles L, Heubi JE, Bove KE. Hepatocyte glycogen accumulation in patients undergoing dietary management of urea cycle defects mimics storage disease. *J Pediatr Gastroenterol Nutr.* 2005;40:471-476.

31. Sperandeo MP, Andria G, Sebastio G. Lysinuric protein intolerance: update and extended mutation analysis of the SLC7A7 gene. *Hum Mutat.* 2008;29:14-21.

32. Shinawi M, Dietzen DJ, White FV, et al. Early-onset hepatic fibrosis in lysinuric protein intolerance. *J Pediatr Gastroenterol Nutr.* 2011;53:695-698.

33. McManus DT, Moore R, Hill CM, et al. Necropsy findings in lysinuric protein intolerance. *J Clin Pathol.* 1996;49:345-347.

34. Haqq AM, Muehlbauer MJ, Newgard CB, et al. The metabolic phenotype of Prader-Willi syndrome (PWS) in childhood: heightened insulin sensitivity relative to body mass index. *J Clin Endocrinol Metab.* 2011;96:E225-E232.

35. Brambilla P, Crino A, Bedogni G, et al. Metabolic syndrome in children with Prader-Willi syndrome: the effect of obesity. *Nutr Metab Cardiovasc Dis.* 2011;21:269-276.

36. Takayasu H, Motoi T, Kanamori Y, et al. Two case reports of childhood liver cell adenomas harboring beta-catenin abnormalities. *Hum Pathol.* 2002;33:852-855.

37. Mizukawa B, George A, Pushkaran S, et al. Cooperating G6PD mutations associated with severe neonatal hyperbilirubinemia and cholestasis. *Pediatr Blood Cancer.* 2011;56:840-842.

38. Jones SA, Valayannopoulos V, Schneider E, et al. Rapid progression and mortality of lysosomal acid lipase deficiency presenting in infants. *Genet Med.* 2016;18:452-458.

39. Bernstein DL, Hulkova H, Bialer MG, et al. Cholesteryl ester storage disease: review of the findings in 135 reported patients with an underdiagnosed disease. *J Hepatol* 2013;58:1230-1243.

40. Hulkova H, Elleder M. Distinctive histopathological features that support a diagnosis of cholesterol ester storage disease in liver biopsy specimens. *Histopathology*. 2012;60:1107-1113.

41. Vij M, Bachina P. Liver histology in cholesteryl ester storage disease. *Indian J Pathol Microbiol*. 2018;61:302-304.

42. Oztas E, Ozin Y, Onder F, et al. Chronic intestinal pseudo-obstruction and neurological manifestations in early adulthood: considering MNGIE syndrome in differential diagnosis. *J Gastrointestin Liver Dis*. 2010;19:195-197.

43. Hayman J. Charles Darwin's mitochondria. *Genetics*. 2013;194:21-25.

44. Teraoka M, Yokoyama Y, Ichimura K, et al. Fatal neonatal mitochondrial cytopathy with disseminated fatty nodules in the liver. *Pediatr Int*. 2003;45:570-573.

45. Scheers I, Bachy V, Stephenne X, et al. Risk of hepatocellular carcinoma in liver mitochondrial respiratory chain disorders. *J Pediatr*. 2005;146:414-417.

46. Bioulac-Sage P, Parrot-Roulaud F, Mazat JP, et al. Fatal neonatal liver failure and mitochondrial cytopathy (oxidative phosphorylation deficiency): a light and electron microscopic study of the liver. *Hepatology*. 1993;18:839-846.

47. Pronicki M, Piekutowska-Abramczuk D, Rokicki D, et al. Histopathological liver findings in patients with hepatocerebral mitochondrial depletion syndrome with defined molecular basis. *Pol J Pathol*. 2018;69:292-298.

48. Alder JK, Chen JJ, Lancaster L, et al. Short telomeres are a risk factor for idiopathic pulmonary fibrosis. *Proc Natl Acad Sci U S A*. 2008;105:13051-13056.

49. Calado RT, Regal JA, Kleiner DE, et al. A spectrum of severe familial liver disorders associate with telomerase mutations. *PLoS One*. 2009;4:e7926.

50. Jonassaint NL, Guo N, Califano JA, et al. The gastrointestinal manifestations of telomere-mediated disease. *Aging Cell*. 2013;12(2):319-323.

51. Kapuria D, Ben-Yakov G, Ortolano R, et al. The spectrum of hepatic involvement in patients with telomere disease. *Hepatology*. 2019;69:2579-2585.

52. Speckmann C, Sahoo SS, Rizzi M, et al. Clinical and molecular heterogeneity of RTEL1 deficiency. *Front Immunol*. 2017;8:449.

53. Johnson SM, McGinty KA, Hayashi PH, et al. Large cell change in a small liver: a histological clue to short telomere syndromes? *Hepatology*. 2020;72(6):2231-2234.

54. Roulot D, Degott C, Chazouilleres O, et al. Vascular involvement of the liver in Turner's syndrome. *Hepatology*. 2004;39:239-247.

55. Roulot D. Liver involvement in Turner syndrome. *Liver Int*. 2013;33:24-30.

17

LIVER DISEASE IN SYSTEMIC CONDITIONS

In this chapter, we discuss systemic conditions that lead to liver pathology. In many of these cases, biopsies are performed for elevated liver enzyme levels, hepatomegaly, or abnormal imaging findings in patients with known systemic conditions, such as celiac disease or cystic fibrosis. In other cases, the biopsy may provide the first evidence for a systemic disease. Some systemic conditions are discussed separately in other chapters, such as sarcoidosis and granulomatous infections in Chapter 7 and sickle cell anemia and congestive hepatopathy from heart failure in Chapter 13.

AMYLOID

Liver biopsies are avoided in individuals with known amyloidosis because of the risk for bleeding, but amyloidosis can be a difficult clinical diagnosis and new diagnoses of amyloid continue to be made on liver biopsies. Most cases of amyloidosis in the liver are associated with plasma cell dyscrasias, but amyloid deposits can be associated with a wide range of inflammatory and inherited conditions.

Amyloid in the liver looks the same as it does elsewhere—paucicellular deposits of pink-to-amphophilic material. The amyloid deposits can be striking and associated with significant hepatocyte atrophy or can be mild, subtle, and easily missed. In some cases, the amyloid is seen exclusively or predominately in the small arterioles (Figure 17.1; eFigs. 17.1-17.3). Amyloid can be deposited in the sinusoids (Figure 17.2), the portal tract stroma, or the hepatic arteries (Figure 17.3). Most cases have mixed deposits, but sinusoidal deposition is the most common pattern. In most cases, the specific type of amyloid cannot be determined by the hematoxylin-eosin (H&E) staining findings and amyloid deposits are further subtyped, when clinically needed, by immunostains or by laser microdissection and mass spectrometry on formalin-fixed, paraffin-embedded tissues[1]; the latter method has advantages of greater accuracy, the ability to identify rare and novel subtypes of

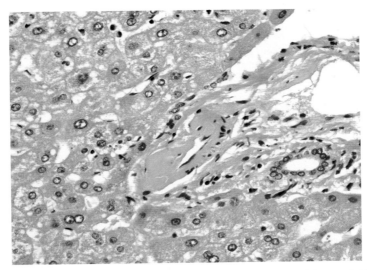

FIGURE 17.1 **Amyloid, subtle finding.** In this case of fibrinogen alpha amyloidosis, the amyloid deposits were subtle and limited to the vessels.

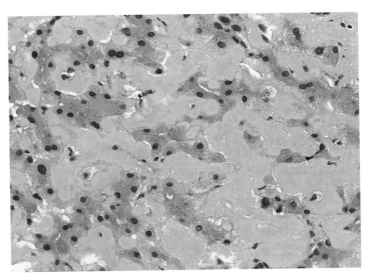

FIGURE 17.2 **Amyloid, sinusoids.** The hepatic sinusoids are filled with amyloid.

amyloidosis, and being less expensive than a large panel of immunostains. Nonetheless, immunostains can also be helpful and can identify the type of amyloid in many cases.

Leukocyte Chemotactic Factor 2 Amyloid

Leukocyte chemotactic factor 2 (LECT2) amyloidosis was historically called globular amyloid[2] and is caused by mutations in *LECT2*. Clinically,

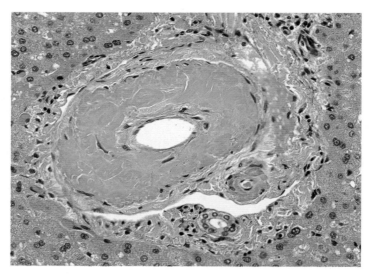

FIGURE 17.3 **Amyloid, vessels.** The hepatic artery is markedly thickened because of amyloid deposition.

LECT2 amyloidosis can cause renal disease[3] and is rarely associated with portal hypertension,[4] but in most cases, it does not lead to a clinically significant liver disease; when seen on liver biopsy, LECT2 amyloidosis is typically an incidental finding.[5] LECT amyloid also involves the spleen, adrenal glands, and lungs, but typically not the heart.[6] LECT2 amyloidosis is most common in persons of Hispanic descent, with a frequency of 3% based on autopsy studies.[6] LECT2 amyloid appears to also be enriched in several other populations, including Native Americans, First Nations persons of Canada, and Punjabis.

LECT2 amyloid is histologically distinctive (Figure 17.4), showing round, globular inclusions that are primarily located in the hepatocytes and sometimes found as extracellular, sinusoidal deposits.[2,7] The globules can show laminations in some cases. The amyloid tends to be located in zone 3 and occasionally can be associated with focal areas of more typical amyloid deposits in the sinusoids and vessels. Of note, in some cases the globular amyloid tends to be less congophilic on Congo red, with only faint birefringence on polarization. Immunostains for Lect 2 protein can confirm the diagnosis (Figure 17.5).[7]

Stains and Other Ancillary Studies

A Congo red stain is necessary to confirm the diagnosis of amyloid. By routine light microscopy, the amyloid deposits should demonstrate a distinctive, red-orange color termed "congophilia" (Figure 17.6). Polarization will then demonstrate "apple-green" birefringence (Figure 17.7). You may have to polarize in a dark room to optimally see the birefringence. Removing all the other light filters on your microscope can also help visualize the birefringence.

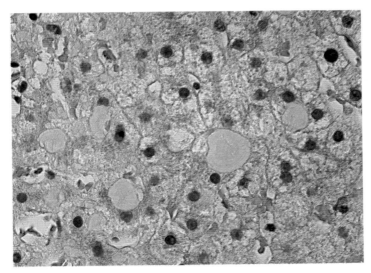

FIGURE 17.4 **Globular amyloid**. The pale round intracellular inclusions represent globular amyloid.

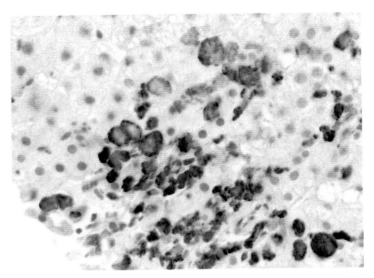

FIGURE 17.5 **Globular amyloid, Lect 2 immunostain**. The amyloid is strongly positive.

Even in the best of cases, the "apple-green" color tends to be somewhat pale and patchy. As an important diagnostic pitfall, the normal collagen in portal tracts will also polarize; the lack of congophilia in normal portal tracts on routine light microscopy, however, allows separation from true amyloid. Also, normal collagen tends to polarize with a bright, silvery white (Figure 17.8) and lacks the yellow-green of true amyloid.

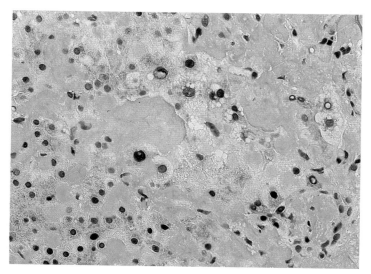

FIGURE 17.6 **Amyloid, Congo red stain.** This image, from the case as shown in Figure 17.2, shows the extracellular material is congophilic.

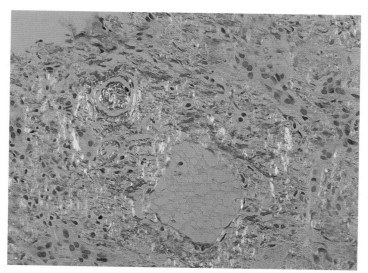

FIGURE 17.7 **Amyloid, Congo red stain with polarization.** Apple-green birefringence is seen.

Amyloid-like Material That Is Congo Red Negative

TECHNICAL CONSIDERATIONS. The first step is to repeat the Congo red staining, making sure the slide was cut to the appropriate thickness (10 μm instead of the usual 4 μm for light microscopy). Polarization is best done in a very dark room; turning off all the microscope light filters can also be very helpful.

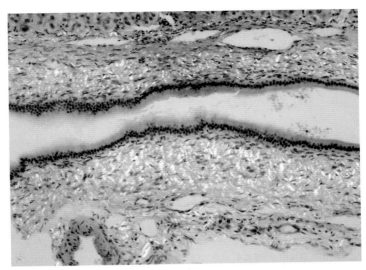

FIGURE 17.8 **Normal portal tract, Congo red stain with polarization.** The normal collagen shows a silvery white birefringence.

WALDENSTRÖM MACROGLOBULINEMIA. If the Congo red stain result is still negative, then consider the possibility of Waldenström macroglobulinemia, which is associated with deposits of IgM heavy chains. The deposits in Waldenström macroglobulinemia can closely resemble amyloid but are Congo red negative.[8] Deposits are kappa light chain restricted (if they are lambda restricted, classical amyloid disease is more likely).

LIGHT CHAIN DEPOSITION DISEASE. Light chain deposition disease is another diagnosis to consider when extracellular deposits resemble amyloid on H&E staining (Figure 17.9) but are Congo red negative. Light chain deposition disease is typically associated with renal disease, but sometimes liver disease can be the first clinical manifestation. The deposits tend to be diffuse and heavy, with a strong sinusoidal pattern, but are Congo red negative.[9] They still have a β-sheet pattern at the ultrastructural level, but like the deposits in Waldenström macroglobulinemia, they lack the congophilic staining and birefringence on Congo red stain.

FIBRONECTIN. Fibronectin can rarely be deposited as amyloidlike material in the liver (Figure 17.10). The deposits are dense, eosinophilic, and sinusoidal, leading to hepatocyte atrophy.[10] Data is too limited to know the organ distribution or the clinical correlates.

CYSTIC FIBROSIS

Clinical, Laboratory, and Imaging Findings

Cystic fibrosis is the most common inherited disease in Caucasians, with a frequency of 1 in 3000 live births. The disease is caused by mutations in *CFTR*, with the most common mutation being ΔF508. The CFTR protein

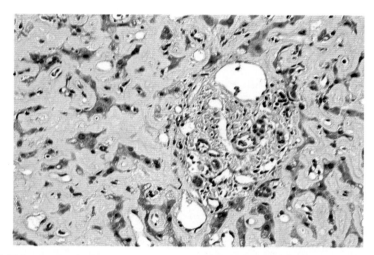

FIGURE 17.9 **Light chain disease**. The striking extracellular deposits in light chain disease closely resemble amyloid but are Congo red negative.

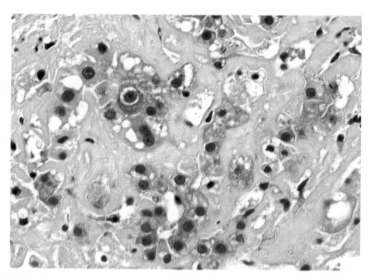

FIGURE 17.10 **Fibrinogen deposition disease**. The fibrinogen deposits are striking but are Congo red negative.

is a glycoprotein located at the apical end of secretory cells that facilitates chloride transport from cells into the lumens of various anatomic structures. Mutations lead to thick viscous secretions in the airways, intestine, pancreas, and biliary tree. In rare cases, the diagnosis is first suggested by liver pathologic findings.[11]

Aspartate transaminase (AST), alanine transaminase (ALT), and γ-glutamyltransferase (GGT) levels are mildly elevated, typically less than 2.5 times the upper limit of normal. Transient enzyme elevations are common in the first 3 months of life (approximately 50% of cases) but typically resolve.[12] Persistent enzyme level elevations, however, often develop in those aged 10 years and older, affecting approximately 40% of older children and young adults.[12]

Other findings include biliary strictures, both intrahepatic and extrahepatic. By magnetic resonance cholangiopancreatography (MRCP), biliary pathology is seen in almost all patients with clinical liver disease and half of those without clinical liver disease. The imaging findings include bile duct dilatation, focal strictures, narrowed areas, and beading caused by alternating areas of stricture and dilatation.[13] The extrahepatic strictures often involve the common bile duct as a result of pancreatic disease. A microgallbladder is present in about one-fourth of cases and cholelithiasis develops in 10%.

Hepatomegaly, elevated liver enzyme levels, splenomegaly, and esophageal varices were historically the most common clinical indications for liver biopsy in order to establish the presence of advanced fibrosis,[14] but noninvasive markers of liver fibrosis have reduced that need. Instead, biopsies are now most often performed to rule out potential concomitant liver diseases.

Histologic Findings

In general, liver biopsies reveal pathology in the majority of patients with cystic fibrosis (approximately 80%). Not surprisingly, pathology is more common in cases with abnormal liver enzyme levels.[12,15] The portal tracts can show a pattern of mild chronic biliary tract obstruction, with patchy bile ductular proliferation (Figure 17.11) and nonspecific portal chronic inflammation. The portal inflammation is typically minimal to mild and

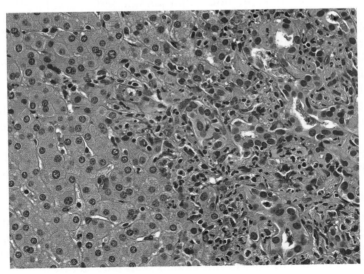

FIGURE 17.11 **Cystic fibrosis.** Bile ductular proliferation is seen.

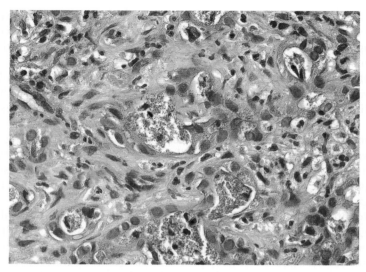

FIGURE 17.12 **Cystic fibrosis.** Granular, eosinophilic secretions are present in the bile ducts.

composed of admixed lymphocytes and neutrophils. In some cases, especially with more advanced fibrosis, the bile ductular proliferation can be brisk.[12] Inspissated secretions in the bile ducts are rarely seen (Figure 17.12), being present in approximately 5% of cases,[14] and are patchy when present.

The portal tracts can also show loss of the portal veins in some cases. When there is portal vein loss, the liver parenchyma can also demonstrate changes of nodular regenerative hyperplasia. Nodular regenerative hyperplasia has been reported by only a few groups, but it may be an underappreciated aspect of the pathology of cystic fibrosis.[16,17] Nodular regenerative hyperplasia can be associated with portal hypertension despite the lack of significant fibrosis.

The most common finding in the hepatic lobules is macrovesicular steatosis (Figure 17.13). At least some degree of fatty change is seen in approximately 65% of cases, with moderate or severe fatty change in 30% of cases.[12,14] Fatty liver disease also commonly develops in liver allografts after liver transplant.[18] The etiology of the fatty liver disease is unclear, and its role in fibrosis progression is also unknown. In most cases, the fibrosis appears to be driven by the biliary pathology and not the steatosis. In keeping with this observation, steatohepatitis is less common than steatosis.

Fibrosis

In most cases, fibrosis begins in late childhood and teenage years, but rarely infants and young children can have rapid fibrosis progression, especially those with meconium ileus.[12] Overall, moderate or severe fibrosis is seen in approximately 40% to 60% of individuals with persistently abnormal liver

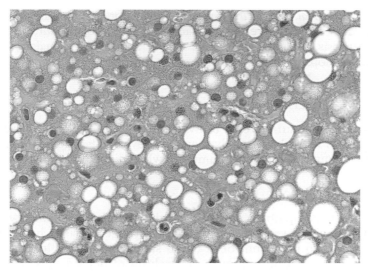

FIGURE 17.13 **Cystic fibrosis.** This biopsy showed macrovesicular steatosis as the primary finding.

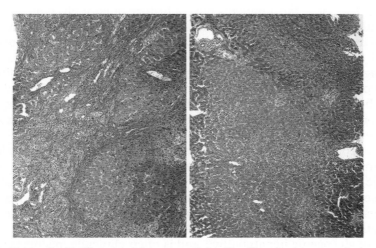

FIGURE 17.14 **Cystic fibrosis, trichrome stain.** The fibrosis shows marked variation. One core shows extensive fibrosis and appears cirrhotic, while another core from the same biopsy procedure shows only very mild portal fibrosis.

enzyme levels, representing about 10% to 20% of all individuals with cystic fibrosis.[12,14] Of note, advanced fibrosis can sometimes be seen even if liver enzyme levels are normal, or near normal.[19]

Early fibrosis is portal based and often associated with portal tract changes of biliary obstruction. The fibrosis can be patchy, with marked fibrosis in one part of the biopsy and minimal or absent in other parts (Figure 17.14), a pattern called *focal biliary cirrhosis* in the cystic fibrosis literature. The fibrosis in later cases can be more diffuse, with extensive bridging fibrosis or established cirrhosis, but even here, there can be an element of patchiness, with areas of the biopsy that appear relativelyless fibrotic.

DIABETES MELLITUS

There are three main patterns of liver injury seen in liver biopsies of diabetic patients with abnormal liver enzyme levels. Glycogenic hepatopathy and fatty change are the most common, while diabetic sclerosis is rare.

Glycogenic Hepatopathy

Glycogenic hepatopathy is a distinctive clinicopathologic entity where the normal balance between glycogenesis and glycogenolysis in hepatocytes is disrupted due to poor control of blood sugar levels. This leads to excess glycogen accumulation within the cytoplasm of hepatocytes. The classic triad of clinical findings is a history of poorly controlled blood sugar levels, elevated liver enzyme levels, and hepatomegaly.

CLINICAL FINDINGS. Most patients have a history of poor glycemic control in the setting of type I diabetes mellitus. Glycogenic hepatopathy can also be part of the Mauriac syndrome. This syndrome results from very poorly controlled type I diabetes and includes growth retardation, delayed puberty, cushingoid features, and hypercholesterolemia. These clinical findings are accompanied by hepatomegaly, abnormal liver enzyme levels, and glycogenic hepatopathy on liver biopsy. The Mauriac syndrome is only rarely seen today because of improved diagnosis and care of type I diabetes, but glycogenic hepatopathy is still seen on a regular basis.

Glycogenic hepatopathy is universally accompanied by elevated transaminase levels and hepatomegaly. In some cases, the patient's hepatic enzyme levels can exceed 10 times the upper limit of normal.[20] The enzymes levels may fluctuate considerably over time, reflecting periods of better and worse control of blood sugar levels.[21] In all cases, the livers' synthetic function is well preserved. Ascites is a rare but dramatic presentation of glycogenic hepatopathy[20] and is often clinically misinterpreted as evidence for advanced liver disease. The ascites, however, results not from fibrosis but from compression of the sinusoids by the rapidly expanded hepatocyte cytoplasm, and the ascites resolves with adequate control of blood sugar.[20,22] Also of note, both fatty liver disease and glycogenic hepatopathy can appear echogenic on ultrasound evaluation,[22,23] so individuals may have a working clinical diagnosis of fatty liver disease at the time of liver biopsy. The hepatomegaly and abnormal liver enzyme levels associated with glycogenic hepatopathy will improve with glycemic control.[24,25] In addition, the histologic findings resolve with proper blood sugar level control.[26]

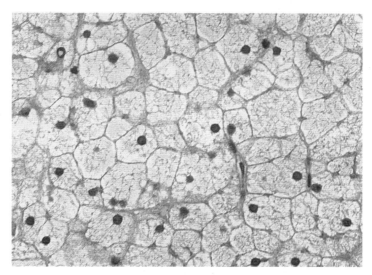

FIGURE 17.15 **Glycogenic hepatopathy.** The biopsy is from a young child with brittle diabetes mellitus and enzyme level elevations in the 400 IU/L range. The hepatocytes are distended and have clear cytoplasm because of glycogen accumulation.

HISTOLOGIC FINDINGS The hepatocytes have abundant pale cytoplasm, often with accentuation of the cell membranes (Figure 17.15; eFig. 17.4). This distinctive histologic finding, along with a history of poorly controlled diabetes, is usually sufficient to make a diagnosis of glycogenic hepatopathy. If preferred, a periodic acid-Schiff (PAS) stain can be used to highlight the glycogen within the cytoplasm of hepatocytes, and the stain will disappear after digestion with diastase. Remember, however, that even normal livers will have abundant PAS positivity (Figure 17.16) and a diagnosis of glycogenic hepatopathy requires the typical H&E findings and an appropriate clinical setting.

The differential for the glycogenic hepatopathy pattern of injury includes short-term, high-dose steroid therapy, which can also lead to glycogenic hepatopathy.[27] In fact, the clinical presentation after high-dose steroid therapy (hepatomegaly and elevated transaminases levels), as well as the histologic findings, can be very similar, although generally less striking than the changes of glycogenic hepatopathy from poorly controlled diabetes mellitus (Figure 17.17). While counterintuitive, the differential also includes anorexia nervosa.[28,29] Glycogenic hepatopathy can also be induced by poorly controlled blood sugar levels in type II diabetic patients.[22] Finally, the differential includes dumping syndrome secondary to fundoplication for gastroesophageal reflux disease[30] and intake of excess insulin as a suicide attempt.[31]

In the setting of the metabolic syndrome and ordinary fatty liver disease, mild patchy glycogenosis is common and associated with insulin resistance; its major significance is that the glycogen-rich hepatocytes can mimic balloon cells.[32]

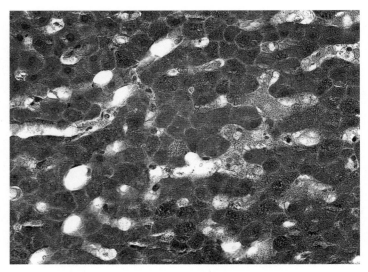

FIGURE 17.16 **Normal liver, periodic acid-Schiff (PAS) stain.** The normal liver has abundant glycogen.

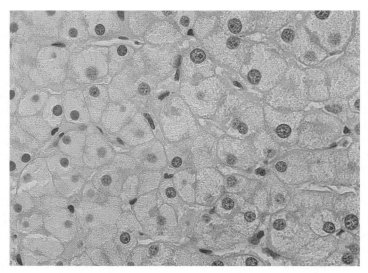

FIGURE 17.17 **Glycogenic hepatopathy, steroid induced.** The hepatocytes are swollen and filled with glycogen.

In this setting, the glycogenosis is seen in patches of hepatocytes, often with a zone 3 distribution, and not as a diffuse finding like is seen with glycogenic hepatopathy. The histologic changes in glycogen storage disease and urea cycle defects can also be similar to glycogenic hepatopathy, but at the practical level, the clinical situations are sufficiently different that there is little difficulty in separating these two diagnoses.

Macrovesicular Steatosis

In type I diabetic patients who have hepatomegaly, glycogenic hepatopathy is the most frequent histologic finding, but fatty liver disease is also common. For example, in one study of 99 children with diabetes and hepatomegaly, glycogen accumulation was the most common cause of hepatomegaly, with moderate glycogen accumulation in 22% of cases and marked glycogen accumulation in 19% of cases.[33] Fatty liver, however, was also present in nearly half of all cases. While the fatty change was usually mild, it appeared to explain the hepatomegaly in 8% of the children.[33]

Diabetic Hepatosclerosis

Diabetic hepatosclerosis occurs in patients with long-standing diabetes mellitus.[34] Affected individuals often have extensive histories of diabetes-related microangiopathic complications that involve multiple organs, suggesting that hepatosclerosis is a microangiopathic disease of the liver. Autopsy studies have found a frequency that ranges from 2% to 12% in diabetic patients.[30,35] Liver enzyme level elevations typically show an alkaline phosphatase predominance, which can be striking.[34,36]

Liver biopsy specimens show dense sinusoidal fibrosis, even though the livers are typically not cirrhotic (Figure 17.18). Trichrome stains highlight the striking sinusoidal fibrosis (Figure 17.19). Earlier cases have also been reported, where the fibrosis is less striking. Overall, fibrosis progression appears to be slow.[36] Other findings include lobular cholestasis,

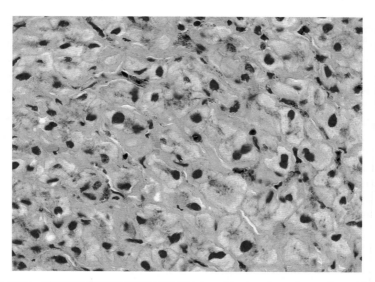

FIGURE 17.18 **Diabetic hepatosclerosis.** The hepatocytes show dense sinusoidal deposits of extracellular material. Some cases can raise the differential of amyloid or light chain deposition disease.

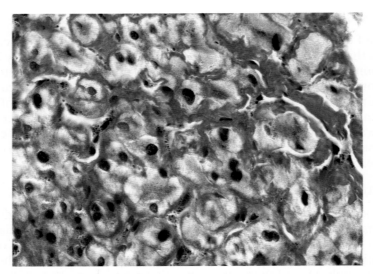

FIGURE 17.19 **Diabetic hepatosclerosis, trichrome.** Strong diffuse sinusoidal fibrosis is seen.

without features of large duct obstruction; in some cases the cholestasis can be severe.[37] Hepatosclerosis is typically an independent finding that is not accompanied by fatty liver disease or glycogenic hepatopathy.

HYPERTENSION, SYSTEMIC

Systemic hypertension-related changes are most evident in the larger vessels and thus are more commonly seen in resection or autopsy specimens, compared with biopsies. In some individuals with long-standing hypertension, however, the smaller arteries seen in percutaneous liver biopsies can show significant intimal thickening and hyalinosis (Figure 17.20; eFig. 17.5); the risk for these changes increases if patients also have diabetes mellitus.[38] The hyalinosis can resemble amyloidosis, so Congo red stains can be helpful. Mild, patchy bile ductular proliferation is common, even in cases with no obstruction, and may represent low-grade bile duct ischemia.

Malignant hypertension (typically with pressures above 180/120 mm Hg) can lead to liver injury from ischemia. There is bland zone 3 necrosis with little or no inflammation.

ENDOCRINE DISORDERS

Hypopituitary Disease

Hypopituitary disease can be part of inherited syndromes or secondary to parenchymal loss, for example, following pituitary surgery. In

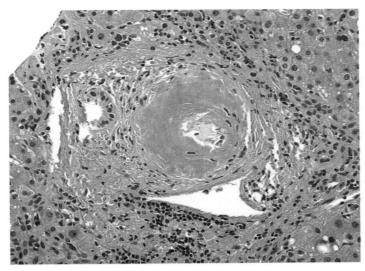

FIGURE 17.20 **Systemic hypertension.** The biopsy is from an individual with severe systemic hypertension.

children, hypopituitary disease can be seen in the setting of septo-optic dysplasia, a syndrome with congenital hypoplasia of the optic nerve, absence of septum pellucidum, and hypopituitarism. The histologic findings can range from mild and bland lobular cholestasis to neonatal hepatitis with abundant giant cells.[39] The reason for the cholestasis and giant cell changes in infants with panhypopituitarism is not completely understood, but may result from lack of growth hormone or cortisol. Fibrosis is generally absent or mild. Many of the cases will also have bile duct hypoplasia.[39]

In adults, most cases of hypopituitary disease result from head trauma or develop following pituitary surgery. The most common pattern of liver injury is fatty liver disease, which may include steatosis or steatohepatitis; this pattern is especially common if patients have growth hormone deficiency. The fatty liver disease may progress to cirrhosis.[40,41]

Thyroid Disease

Hypothyroid disease can be associated with bland lobular cholestasis and mild elevations in liver enzyme levels. In general, liver biopsies are not obtained in this setting unless the thyroid disease was not clinically apparent or is seen incidentally when biopsies are performed for other indications. An exception is hypothyroidism in infants and children, which can lead to cholestatic liver disease in the form of neonatal hepatitis and may be biopsied to rule out other pediatric cholestatic liver diseases. Hypothyroidism has also been associated with fatty liver disease,[42] although it remains unclear if hypothyroidism primarily increases the risk in individuals who already have the metabolic syndrome or if it can independently lead to macrovesicular steatosis.

HEMATOLOGIC DISORDERS

Hemophagocytic Lymphohistiocytosis

TERMINOLOGY AND RISK FACTORS. The term *hemophagocytic lymphohistiocytosis* has now largely replaced what used to be called the *hemophagocytic syndrome*. After the renaming, hemophagocytic lymphohistiocytosis was divided, at least for a while, into primary (genetic) forms and secondary forms. This new terminology, however, was still unsatisfactory for some nomenclature mavens, who now prefer the terms *hemophagocytic lymphohistiocytosis disease* (genetic form, early onset) and *hemophagocytic lymphohistiocytosis syndrome* (nongenetic form, usually later onset).

In any case, the disease has stayed the same. There is an early-onset form that occurs primarily in infants and children younger than 2 years (mostly younger than 3 months), who may have a number of different mutations, including in *PRF1*, *UNC13D*, *STX11*, and *STXBP2*. These mutations lead to an excessive activation of macrophages in response to various stimuli, often infections, leading to cytokine storms that can cause death if untreated. Hemophagocytic lymphohistiocytosis in children can also be associated with other genetic immune deficiencies, such as X-linked lymphoproliferative disease or chronic granulomatous disease. Children are also at risk if they have various rheumatologic disorders, including systemic juvenile idiopathic arthritis (formerly called Still disease) and juvenile rheumatoid arthritis. In children with rheumatologic disorders, the hemophagocytic lymphohistiocytosis syndrome is usually called the *macrophage activation syndrome*, but it is still the same disease.

In adults, there is a strong association with malignant lymphomas (about 50% of cases, usually non-Hodgkin lymphoma), various chronic infections (about 25% of cases), and various autoimmune/rheumatologic conditions (about 10% of cases). In addition, adult patients with the hemophagocytic lymphohistiocytosis syndrome often have additional sources of immunosuppression, usually HIV infection, malignancies, or medications.

CLINICAL FINDINGS Patients present with hepatosplenomegaly and fevers (>38.5°C), often a prolonged history of fevers. Further workup typically shows cytopenias that usually affect at least two of the three cell lineages, that is, red blood cells, white blood cells, or platelets. Serum ferritin levels are high (>500 µg/L) as part of the acute inflammatory response. In general, high serum ferritin levels are more informative in children than adults, as adults can have several other potential causes. Triglyceride levels are typically elevated, with fasting triglyceride level >265 mg/dL, and most patients have hypofibrinogenemia (<150 mg/dL). Patients have elevated soluble CD25 levels. Natural killer (NK) cell activity is low or absent. Liver enzyme levels are elevated in up to 90% of cases and show an alkaline phosphate predominant pattern. A common clinical approach to establish the diagnosis requires five of eight of the following abnormal findings: splenomegaly, fevers, cytopenias, high ferritin levels, high triglyceride levels, high CD25 levels, low or absent NK activity, and hemophagocytosis in the liver, bone marrow, spleen, or lymph nodes.

HISTOLOGIC FINDINGS The histologic manifestation is primarily that of sinusoidal Kupffer cell hyperplasia with hemophagocytosis (Figure 17.21). In milder cases, the liver histology changes are mostly Kupffer cell hyperplasia with only equivocal hemophagocytosis. Of note, a final diagnosis of the hemophagocytic lymphohistiocytosis syndrome/disease requires clinical findings (five of eight features, as discussed earlier), as the liver injury pattern of sinusoidal Kupffer cell hyperplasia with hemophagocytosis is also common in a variety of systemic infectious conditions that do not have other clinical features of hemophagocytic lymphohistiocytosis syndrome, although they share common risk factors (infections and medications in immunosuppressed patients).

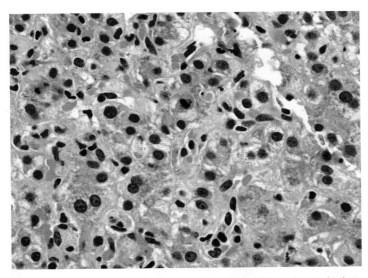

FIGURE 17.21 **Hemophagocytic lymphohistiocytosis.** There is marked Kupffer cell hyperplasia and erythrophagocytosis in a young teenager with a genetic autoimmune condition.

General Pattern of Reactive Kupffer Cell Hyperplasia With Hemophagocytosis

This pattern of injury is rare but more common in immunosuppressed persons (Figure 17.22). In patients with HIV infection, for example, up to 8% of liver biopsies show sinusoidal Kupffer cell hyperplasia with hemophagocytosis.[43] Other common causes that systemically activate macrophages, including within the liver, include infections (most frequent), malignancies, autoimmune conditions, or drug effects (Table 17.1). Most infectious causes are viral related, such as cytomegalovirus (CMV) or Epstein-Barr virus (EBV), although in immunosuppressed patients, bacterial or parasitic causes have an increased frequency.

Liver biopsies show diffuse Kupffer cell hyperplasia with erythrophagocytosis (often patchy and subtle) as the main pattern of injury. There is generally little or no portal inflammation, no cholestatic liver disease, and no fatty liver disease. Importantly, the histologic findings of Kupffer cell hyperplasia and erythrophagocytosis can show substantial overlap between cases of true hemophagocytic lymphohistiocytosis syndrome/disease and the general reactive pattern discussed here, so a final diagnosis requires correlation with the clinical findings.

The findings can be subtle and challenging to identify at the lower end of the spectrum, or at least can be subjective. In these cases, CD68 can be used to highlight the Kupffer cell hyperplasia and will also sometimes highlight the erythrophagocytosis, as the red blood cells will be nonstaining and will stand out in negative relief. An immunostain for GLUT1 can

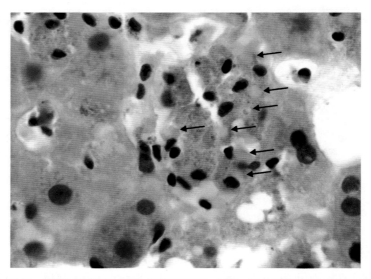

FIGURE 17.22 **Mild Kupffer cell hyperplasia with hemophagocytosis.** This case appeared to be viral related and shows a cluster of pigmented macrophages with phagocytosed red blood cells. The red cells (*arrows*) stand out against the pigmented cytoplasm.

TABLE 17.1 Causes of Kupffer Cell Hyperplasia and Hemophagocytosis	
Causes	Examples
Viral infections	CMV
	EBV
	HHV8
	Varicella zoster
Bacterial infections	*Mycobacterium tuberculosis*
	Escherichia coli
	Shigella
	Nocardiosis
	Coxiella burnetii (Q fever)
Autoimmune conditions/inflammatory disorders	Rheumatoid arthritis
	Ankylosing spondylitis
	Dermatomyositis
	Sarcoidosis
	CVID
	Crohn disease
	Castleman disease
Drug-induced liver injury	
Malignancies	Usually lymphomas

CMV, cytomegalovirus; CVID, common variable immunodeficiency; EBV, Epstein-Barr virus; HHV8, human herpesvirus 8.

occasionally be helpful, as it will stain the red blood cells in the macrophage cytoplasm.

Mild sinusoidal dilatation is common and can occasionally be striking. In contrast to vascular outflow disease, however, the sinusoids are both dilated and stuffed with Kupffer cells. Typically, there is little or no lobular inflammation and minimal or mild portal inflammation, unless there is a preexisting underlying liver disease. Correlation with other histologic findings is important. For example, Kupffer cell hyperplasia is common with cholestatic liver disease or acute hepatitis from any cause, but in these settings, Kupffer cell hyperplasia is secondary and not the main finding. Likewise, Kupffer cell hyperplasia can be prominent in some cases of steatohepatitis.

Langerhans Histiocytosis

Langerhans histiocytosis is a rare systemic disease that frequently involves the liver. About half of the cases are associated with BRAF^{V600E} mutations, which can be used to guide therapy.[44] While more common in young children, patients can present at essentially any age. The biliary tree is frequently involved and individuals may present with features of chronic biliary tract disease. Imaging studies may suggest primary sclerosing cholangitis. On liver biopsy, the Langerhans cells can be seen surrounding and infiltrating the bile ducts, sometimes leading to destructive cholangitic lesions. In other cases, the Langerhans cells can form discrete mass lesions, while a third pattern is that of small clusters of cells in the lobules and portal tracts that mimic granulomas (Figure 17.23). The Langerhans cells are commonly accompanied by a mixture of other inflammatory cells, frequently with a mild eosinophilia; the mild eosinophilia can be an important diagnostic clue. The Langerhans cells are positive for CD1a, S100, and langerin (Figures 17.24 and 17.25).

Rosai-Dorfman Disease

Rosai-Dorfman disease is a rare histiocytic disorder of unknown cause that is more common in children than adults. The disease is also known as *sinus histiocytosis with massive lymphadenopathy*. All genders are equally affected and the disease is most common in immunocompetent individuals. Patients present with systemic symptoms of fever and leukocytosis and are often anemic. Besides lymph nodes, the skin and upper respiratory tract are the most common organs involved, but essentially any organ can be affected. The disease can resolve spontaneously, although cases of systemic disease leading to death have also been reported.

Rosai-Dorfman disease can rarely present as a mass lesion in the liver[45] or as hepatitic-like infiltrates in the lobules, but most commonly shows predominately portal tract disease. On biopsy, the portal tracts

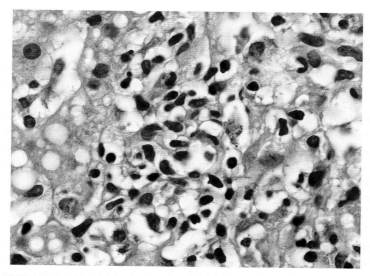

FIGURE 17.23 **Langerhans cell disease.** This case of Langerhans cell disease shows numerous clusters of Langerhans cells that resembled small lobular and portal tract granulomas.

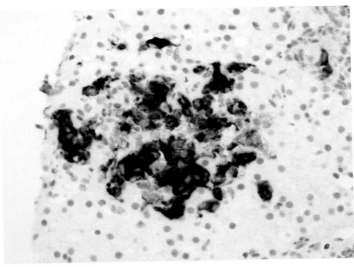

FIGURE 17.24 **Langerhans cell disease, CD1a.** The Langerhans cells are strongly CD1a positive. Same case as the preceding image.

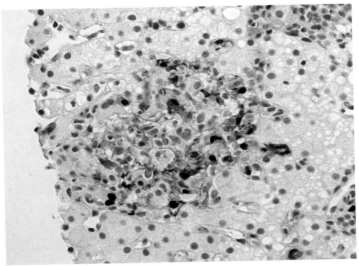

FIGURE 17.25 **Langerhans cell disease, S100.** The Langerhans cells are S100 positive. Same case as the preceding image.

are expanded by a histiocytic infiltrate (Figure 17.26), often admixed with smaller numbers of lymphocytes, plasma cells, and eosinophils. Cytologically, the histiocytes have moderate to abundant amounts of pale, eosinophilic cytoplasm (Figure 17.27). There may be mild nuclear irregularities. There can be bile duct damage, and in many cases, the portal vein is not clearly evident in the affected portal tracts. In some cases, the inflammation has been reported as granulomatous.[45] The abnormal

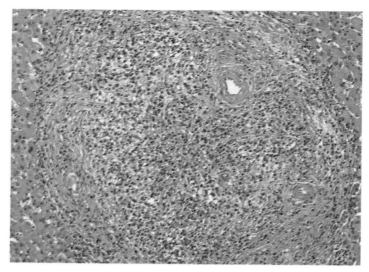

FIGURE 17.26 **Rosai-Dorfman disease**. The portal tract is expanded by a dense infiltrate of histiocytes and inflammatory cells. The bile duct and portal vein are not present.

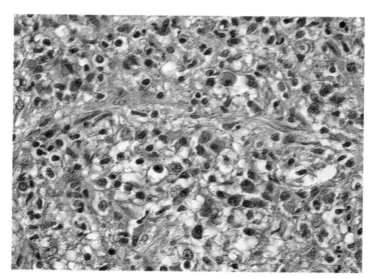

FIGURE 17.27 **Rosai-Dorfman disease**. On higher magnification, the histiocytes have moderate amounts of pale eosinophilic cytoplasm.

histiocyte population in Rosai-Dorfman disease will stain strongly with S100 (Figure 17.28) and CD68, while immunostains for CD1a are negative.

Crystal-Storing Histiocytosis

Crystal-storing histiocytosis is very rare, and most cases are associated with multiple myeloma, lymphoplasmablastic lymphoma, or monoclonal gammopathy of undetermined significance.[46] The Kupffer cells are distended

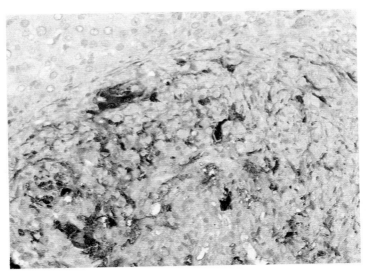

FIGURE 17.28 **Rosai-Dorfman disease.** The histiocytes are strongly S100 positive.

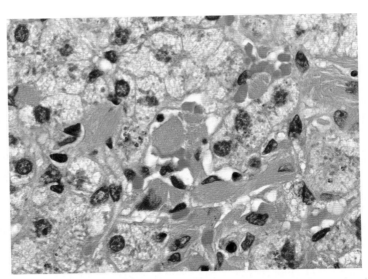

FIGURE 17.29 **Crystal-storing histiocytosis.** The Kupffer cells have dense, chunky, eosinophilic cytoplasm with faint striations.

by the accumulation of pink, chunky inclusions (Figure 17.29); sometimes, the cytoplasmic inclusions can show striations. These inclusions represent kappa immunoglobulin light chain in most cases that are associated with hematologic disorders (Figure 17.30). Rarely, similar findings have been reported with clofazimine, cysteine, or silica exposure.[46] The crystal-storing histiocytes can involve multiple organs including the bone marrow, lymph nodes, spleen, and kidney.[46]

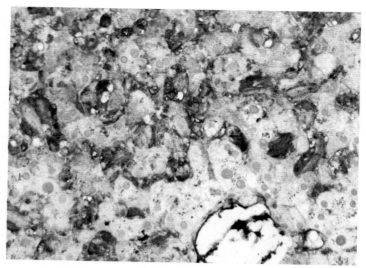

FIGURE 17.30 **Crystal-storing histiocytosis, IgG kappa.** The Kupffer cells are strongly positive.

Mast Cell Disease

Patients with systemic mastocytosis tend to cluster into two groups: children who often have self-limited disease and adults in whom mastocytosis can lead to death.[47] Most cases have *KIT* mutations, with D816V being the most common. Liver disease is usually not dominant in the clinical presentation, but systemic mastocytosis can involve the liver, leading to hepatomegaly and liver enzyme elevations, often with an alkaline phosphatase predominance.[48] Uncommon presentations include liver failure.[49] Patients can also present with portal hypertension and splenomegaly that mimics cirrhosis.

Histologically, mast cells can be located in the portal tracts and the sinusoids. When mast cells are visible on H&E stain, they typically show moderately abundant, pale to clear cytoplasm. The nuclei are round to oval and have small nucleoli (Figure 17.31). There often is a mild eosinophilia associated with the mast cell infiltrates (Figure 17.32). The mast cells are brought out by immunostains for CKIT (Figure 17.33), mast cell tryptase, and CD25.

The injury patterns are variable but tend to cluster into one of these three patterns: almost normal liver/minimal nonspecific changes, biliary tract obstructive disease pattern, or vascular changes. In some patients, cirrhosis can develop.[50] The diagnosis can be almost impossible to make on H&E stain in cases that are nearly normal or have only minimal nonspecific changes, except for in retrospect when a diagnosis is made elsewhere and prior specimens are reexamined by immunostains.

The biliary pattern can also be easily overlooked, with attention drawn to the bile duct injury, bile ductular proliferation, and portal fibrosis

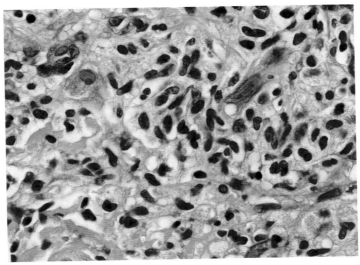

FIGURE 17.31 **Mast cell disease.** The mast cells have abundant clear cytoplasm and oval nuclei.

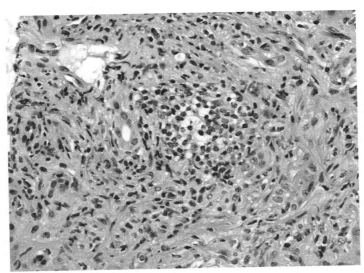

FIGURE 17.32 **Mast cell disease.** At low power, the mast cell infiltrates are associated with a mild eosinophilia.

that resembles primary sclerosing cholangitis or other causes of large bile duct obstruction.[51-53] The mast cells in this pattern can be subtle, but one clue can be more duct injury than that is typical for large duct obstruction.

In some cases, the vascular changes can be striking and may include varying degrees of portal venopathy, nodular regenerative hyperplasia, and veno-occlusive disease.[54]

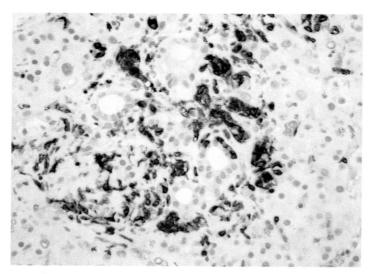

FIGURE 17.33 **Mast cell disease, CKIT.** The mast cells are strongly positive on the CKIT immunostain.

INFLAMMATION OF THE GUT

Celiac Disease

Approximately 30% of individuals with celiac disease will have elevated transaminase levels at the time of diagnosis.[55] On the other hand, about 5% of individuals with unexplained liver enzyme elevation levels will be subsequently diagnosed with celiac disease.[55] Transaminases average about 60 IU/L for ALT and 50 IU/L for AST, but occasionally can be in the several hundreds.[56] In most cases (approximately 90%), liver enzyme levels will normalize following the introduction of a gluten-free diet, although the normalization often takes several months and may take up to a year. Also of note, about 4% of individuals with celiac disease will have mild elevations in their antinuclear antibody (ANA) levels and 9% have mild elevations of smooth muscle antibody levels.[57]

The histology of celiac disease is typically very mild and consists of nonspecific portal and lobular lymphocytic inflammation, often with some mild fatty change (Table 17.2). It is often unclear if the fatty change is from a coexisting metabolic syndrome or is directly related to celiac disease. Nonetheless, some authors recommend testing for celiac disease as part of the workup for unexplained liver steatosis.[62] Portal venopathy and nodular regenerative hyperplasia have also been described in patients with celiac disease.[60,63] In general, the mild inflammatory changes of celiac disease are not associated with fibrosis. Advanced fibrosis or cirrhosis can be seen but results from coexisting inflammatory diseases including primary biliary cirrhosis/cholangitis (PBC), primary sclerosing cholangitis, or autoimmune hepatitis.

TABLE 17.2	**Major Patterns in Celiac Disease**

Normal or near-normal appearing liver[58]
Mild nonspecific inflammation[58]
Chronic portal and lobular inflammation[58]
PSC/PBC/autoimmune hepatitis[59]
Nodular regenerative hyperplasia[60]
Acute hepatitis with extensive necrosis[61]
Inactive cirrhosis

PBC, primary biliary cholangitis; PSC, primary sclerosing cholangitis.

PBC, primary sclerosing cholangitis, and autoimmune hepatitis can be seen in individuals with celiac disease. Their frequency in biopsy specimens of patients with celiac disease varies enormously depending on local treatment practices, ranging from a few percentage of cases[58] to almost two-thirds of cases.[59] Meta-analysis and large epidemiologic studies support an increased risk for PBC and autoimmune hepatitis in individuals with celiac disease,[56] but a true risk for primary sclerosing cholangitis is less clear and co-occurrence may be by chance. Because of the link between celiac disease and PBC, patients with newly diagnosed PBC can benefit from celiac disease testing.[56] The diagnostic findings for PBC, primary sclerosing cholangitis, and autoimmune hepatitis are the same in patients with celiac disease as those in patients without celiac disease.[59] Small bowel bacterial overgrowth from diabetes or from anatomic anomalies, etc. can also lead to mild inflammatory changes in the liver that are similar to those seen in celiac disease.

Crohn Disease

Liver enzyme levels are elevated in 10% to 20% of patients with Crohn disease[64,65] and can be persistent or intermittent, but tend to be mild.

In most cases, biopsies are performed for one of these three reasons: an increase in liver enzyme levels above the baseline, clinical concern for primary sclerosing cholangitis, or in patients who are undergoing other abdominal procedures, such as cholecystectomy. Isolated epithelioid granulomas can be seen in any of these settings, but a true granulomatous hepatitis would be unusual and suggest an alternative diagnosis such as infection or drug-induced liver injury.

In cases where biopsies are performed to evaluate an increase in enzyme levels above baseline, the findings can range from a cholestatic pattern of injury to a hepatitic pattern of injury and the diagnostic approach is largely similar to biopsies in patients without Crohn disease. If the patient is under active immunomodulatory therapy, the biopsy should be carefully examined for CMV infection and other opportunistic infections. If there is significant lobular or portal lymphocytosis, then you should carefully evaluate the biopsy for EBV infection and lymphoproliferative disorders. Drug reactions, including hepatocyte pseudoground glass change, can also occur. In other cases, biopsies may show mild nonspecific portal and minimal lobular inflammation; the inflammation often results from intestinal Crohn disease, with increased mucosal permeability leading to increased antigens in the portal circulation and secondary mild liver inflammation. Mild fatty change may also be seen. Primary sclerosing cholangitis develops in about 2% of patients with Crohn disease; the diagnosis is made in the usual way, looking for bile ductular proliferation, mixed inflammation, and portal-based fibrosis. In biopsies performed while doing other medical procedures, the findings are typically minimal when patients do not have elevated liver enzyme levels.

Common Variable Immunodeficiency

Common variable immunodeficiency (CVID) involves the liver in 10% to 20% of patients, at least when assessed by liver enzyme level elevations.[66]

On biopsy, the histologic findings can be thought of as falling into four main categories, and any given case may have any or all of these findings. The most common finding is mild nonspecific portal and lobular lymphocytic inflammation (Figure 17.34), typically reflecting coexisting inflammation of the small bowel.[67-69] Secondly, granulomas are present in about 40% of cases. The granulomas can be found in both the portal tracts and the lobules and are typically small and epithelioid.[67,70,71] The granulomas do not show necrosis and acid-fast bacteria (AFB) and Grocott-Gomori methenamine silver (GMS) stains are negative. In most cases, they

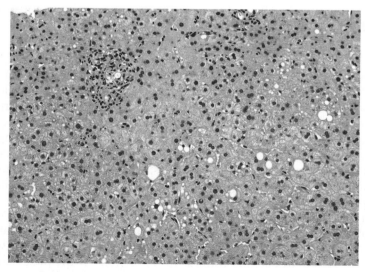

FIGURE 17.34 **Common variable immunodeficiency.** This case shows mild nonspecific lobular inflammation and minimal macrovesicular steatosis.

lack the fibrosis that is typical of sarcoidosis. As a third pattern, mild macrovesicular steatosis is common. Fourthly, many cases show mild nodular regenerative hyperplasia and some patients will develop portal hypertension.[72-74] Nodular regenerative hyperplasia can develop after liver transplant, suggesting the liver is responding to systemic factors.[75] Finally, mild portal fibrosis[67] or delicate pericellular fibrosis[76] is common, but advanced fibrosis suggests an additional disease process. For example, a small subset of patients will develop typical features of PBC.[76]

PREGNANCY

Hyperemesis Gravidarum

Hyperemesis gravidarum is defined by intractable nausea and vomiting that often leads to hospitalization; patients have dehydration, ketosis, and weight loss of at least 5%.[77] Liver enzyme levels are typically elevated, with ALT levels greater than AST levels. ALT levels are typically 2 to 10 times the upper limit of normal, but rarely can exceed 1000 IU/L.[78] However, if ALT levels are greater than 10× normal or if there is jaundice, other causes of hepatitis should be carefully excluded. Enzyme levels, even when high, return to normal when the vomiting resolves.[78] The pathology has not been well described because biopsies are not part of patient management (Table 17.3).

TABLE 17.3 Pregnancy-Associated Liver Disease

Disease	Trimester	Frequency	Major Findings
Hyperemesis gravidarum	First	1%	Elevated liver enzyme levels, ALT > AST
			Histology: not well described
Intrahepatic cholestasis of pregnancy	Second or third	1%–16%, strong regional variation	Pruritus, high ALT levels
			Histology: bland lobular cholestasis
Preeclampsia/ eclampsia	Third	7%	Hypertension with proteinuria with or without HELLP syndrome
			Histology: periportal hemorrhage and fibrin deposition
Acute fatty liver of pregnancy	Third	<1%	Nausea, vomiting, abdominal pain. Hypertension in 50%.
			Histology: microvesicular steatosis

ALT, alanine transaminase; AST, aspartate transaminase; HELLP syndrome, hemolysis, elevated liver enzyme levels, and low platelets.

Intrahepatic Cholestasis of Pregnancy

Intrahepatic cholestasis of pregnancy is the most common liver disease seen in pregnant women. A typical presentation is pruritus in the second or third trimester. The pruritus is often worse at night and has a predilection for the soles of the feet and the palms of the hands. Bilirubin levels are elevated, as are the ALT levels. The pruritus and elevated liver enzyme levels will normalize after delivery. There are significant regional variations in the frequency of intrahepatic cholestasis of pregnancy, ranging from approximately 1% to 6% in the United States to 12% to 18% in Chile, correlating with ethnicity.[79] The risk for intrahepatic cholestasis of pregnancy is also higher with twin pregnancies.

The symptoms improve with ursodeoxycholic acid treatment and resolve with delivery. There is an important caveat, however, as intrahepatic cholestasis of pregnancy can be associated with underlying liver diseases including chronic hepatitis C, gallstones, and PBC.[80] There also is an association with pancreatitis.[80] Thus, patients with a diagnosis of intrahepatic cholestasis of pregnancy should have a careful workup for underlying diseases. Another large group of patients at risk for intrahepatic cholestasis of pregnancy includes those with mutations in genes that code for proteins involved in bile acid secretion and bile acid detoxification.[81,82] These genes include *ABCB4*, *ABCB11*, *ATP8B1*, and *FXR*. Environmental and dietary factors also appear to play a role. For example, a reduction in the prevalence of intrahepatic cholestasis of pregnancy in Chile correlated with increased levels of selenium in the diet.[83]

Biopsies are only rarely performed, as they are generally not needed for diagnosis or management, but they show bland lobular cholestasis with bile in the hepatocyte cytoplasm and bile canaliculi. Changes of biliary obstruction are not seen unless there are associated biliary stones. Despite the elevated ALT levels, there is no more than minimal portal chronic inflammation or mild lobular spotty necrosis.[84,85] Fibrosis is not a feature.

There can be associated changes in the placenta, with thickened, glassy amniotic basement membranes. The chorionic villi can be small for gestational age, with dense fibrotic stroma and increased syncytial knots.[86]

Preeclampsia/Eclampsia With HELLP Syndrome

Preeclampsia is typically defined as de novo hypertension developing after the 20th week of pregnancy, with a blood pressure of >140/90 mm Hg, plus the presence of proteinuria. A small group of patients, however, lack the proteinuria and are diagnosed when there is new onset pulmonary edema, visual symptoms, elevated liver enzyme levels 2× greater than the baseline, or thrombocytopenia. Risk factors include a family history of preeclampsia, the presence of antiphospholipid antibodies, hypertension, diabetes, BMI >35, twin pregnancy, and maternal age >40 years. If the patient develops seizures, then the findings are classified as eclampsia.

Overall, about 30% of women with preeclampsia will have elevated liver enzyme levels and a subset of these patients will develop a severe form of the disease called the HELLP syndrome (hemolysis, elevated liver enzyme levels, and low platelets). Occasional patients with the HELLP syndrome may lack the typical hypertension and proteinuria of preeclampsia. The presentation of the HELLP syndrome varies widely but usually develops in the third trimester and often includes abdominal pain, as well as nausea, vomiting, and malaise. Interestingly, up to 30% of cases can present post partum.

The liver biopsy shows zone 1 hemorrhage accompanied by fibrin deposition (Figure 17.35) in both preeclampsia and the HELLP syndrome.[87,88] Microvesicular steatosis can be seen in about a quarter of cases on H&E stain[88,89] and in essentially all cases with an oil red O stain.[89] In more severe cases, areas of the liver may undergo infarction. Rarely, there may be substantial subcapsular hemorrhage with the formation of a hematoma. These areas of hemorrhage and/or necrosis can also rarely lead to spontaneous rupture of the liver.

Acute Fatty Liver of Pregnancy

Acute fatty liver of pregnancy is rare, with a frequency of approximately 1 per 20,000 deliveries. Patients present between the 30th and 38th week of pregnancy. As with preeclampsia, however, some patients develop the disease (or at least are first diagnosed with disease) only after delivery. The frequency is higher with twins and reaches up to 7% with triplets. Clinical presentations are nonspecific, with nausea, vomiting, abdominal pain, anorexia, and often jaundice. Hypertension is present in about half of the cases and may be severe. Portal hypertension with ascites can

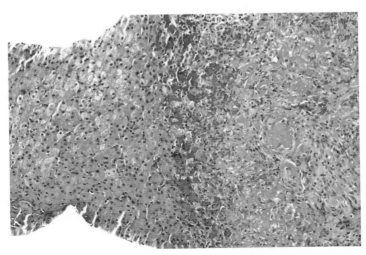

FIGURE 17.35 **Preeclampsia.** The liver biopsy shows striking zone 1 hemorrhage and fibrin deposition.

also develop. The portal hypertension can contribute to hepatic insufficiency, which, along with disseminated intravascular coagulation, can result in coagulation disorders. A low platelet count is common. Polyuria and polydipsia with diabetes is uncommon, but, if present, strongly suggests the diagnosis.[79] Rapid delivery is the treatment for fatty liver of pregnancy.

The cause remains unknown but acute fatty liver of pregnancy has been associated with inherited defects in β-oxidation of fatty acids. Reported mutations include the alpha subunit of long-chain 3-hyroxyacyl-CoA dehydrogenase, (*HADHA* gene) carnitine palmitoyltransferase I, and short- and medium-chain acyl-CoA dehydrogenase deficiency.[79] Genetic testing for mutations in the *HADHA* gene has been recommended in all babies born to a mother with acute fatty liver of pregnancy, as the baby can later develop liver-threatening metabolic crises.[79] The diagnosis was historically made, or at least confirmed, by liver biopsy, but currently the diagnosis is made using laboratory and clinical findings, such as the Swansea criteria.[90]

Histologically, the main finding is diffuse microvesicular steatosis.[91-93] Some but not all studies have reported relative zone 1 sparing by the microvesicular steatosis. Early in the course of the disease, the hepatocytes may demonstrate more cytoplasmic swelling and relatively less microvesicular steatosis.[93] Mild to moderate lobular cholestasis is seen in two-thirds of cases.[93] Lobular atrophy can manifest as close approximation of the portal tracts and central veins.[93] Acidophil bodies are present but not abundant. Small lobular Kupffer aggregates are seen in the majority of cases and can be prominent, representing foci of prior hepatocyte necrosis and subsequent cleanup.[93] Megamitochondria can be prominent.[92] Extramedullary hematopoiesis has been reported.[93] Several studies have reported a subset of cases with substantial lymphoplasmacytic lobular inflammation that mimicked viral hepatitis,[91,93,94] but it remains unclear if some of these reported cases may have had additional liver insults. Also of note, patients with acute fatty liver of pregnancy can develop eclampsia or the HELLP syndrome.[91,94,95]

Oil red O staining on frozen sections will highlight the microvesicular steatosis, but the H&E findings should be the basis for the diagnosis, as small- and intermediate-sized fat droplets on oil red O stain are common and nonspecific. The histologic findings reverse rapidly after delivery and largely disappear by 3 weeks, without scarring of the liver.

SEPSIS

Liver biopsy findings in patients who are septic can show a variety of changes, but most fall into three patterns: nonspecific portal and lobular inflammation, fatty change (Figure 17.36), or bland lobular cholestasis.[96] In some cases, varying degrees of all three of these patterns can be seen. The smaller branches of the portal veins may have small fibrin thrombi in patients with disseminated intravascular coagulation (DIC) (Figure 17.37).

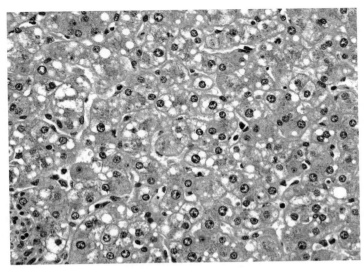

FIGURE 17.36 **Sepsis.** The lobules show mild azonal steatosis with intermediate-sized fat droplets; this pattern is common in sepsis.

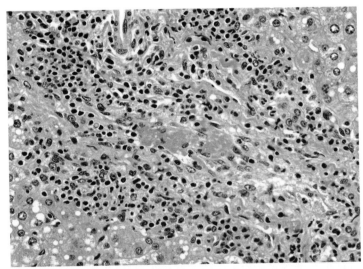

FIGURE 17.37 **Sepsis.** There is mild nonspecific portal inflammation, along with small fibrin thrombi.

In some cases of sepsis, the portal tracts may show a mild reactive bile ductular proliferation, without imaging evidence for biliary obstruction. Patients who are severely debilitated, and then become septic, often have an underlying severe cholestasis and some may also show a cholangitis lenta pattern, with bile plugs in the proliferating bile ductules, but this pattern reflects the severe underlying disease and not sepsis per se. If the patient is significantly hypotensive, the biopsy may also show ischemic changes with bland lobular necrosis that begins in zone 3 and extends to involve larger areas, depending on the severity of the hypotension.

THROMBOTIC THROMBOCYTOPENIC PURPURA

Thrombotic thrombocytopenic purpura is a clotting disorder that leads to the formation of extensive microscopic clots in different organ systems. The disease can be caused by autoantibodies to the enzyme *ADAMTS13*; these autoantibodies block normal cleavage of von Willebrand factor. Other causes include medications, bone marrow transplant, pregnancy, and paraneoplastic syndromes.

The pathology in thrombotic thrombocytopenic purpura is poorly described in the literature, but biopsies can show mild patchy sinusoidal congestion with, in some cases, marked lobular disarray, scattered hepatocyte apoptosis, and marked hepatocyte nuclear pleomorphism (Figure 17.38). These findings presumably reflect low-grade ischemia.

SYSTEMIC AUTOIMMUNE CONDITIONS

Mild increases in liver enzyme levels are common in many systemic autoimmune conditions, including systemic lupus erythematosus, rheumatoid arthritis, juvenile rheumatoid arthritis, and various connective tissue disorders. The enzyme level elevations can be persistent or intermittent and sometimes prompt liver biopsies.

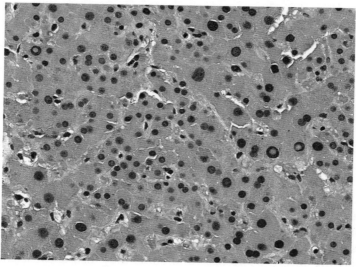

FIGURE 17.38 **Thrombotic thrombocytopenic purpura.** The lobules show marked hepatocyte disarray with nuclear anisocytosis.

The liver biopsies most commonly show a mild nonspecific lymphocytic hepatitis involving the portal tracts with minimal or mild lobular lymphocytic inflammation. There is an older term for this pattern, *reactive hepatitis*, but this term is not well defined and so usage varies; it is also not a satisfying diagnosis to many clinicians, so it is usually better to describe what you see in terms of the minimal inflammation and write a note explaining what it means. There is no evidence that the mild inflammatory changes in these cases lead to liver fibrosis. A drug effect can be particularly hard to exclude in cases that show only a mild nonspecific hepatitis, as many times patients will be taking numerous medications. In these cases, the best evidence comes not from histology but from identifying a temporal correlation between the onset of the liver enzyme level elevations and starting a new medication. Most drug-induced liver injuries that show a hepatitic pattern of injury occur within the first 6 weeks of starting the medication.

On the other hand, if there are more than mild inflammatory changes, or other changes such as biliary tract disease, fatty liver, cholestasis, or definite fibrosis, then a superimposed or coexisting liver disease is likely. True autoimmune hepatitis can be seen in these systemic autoimmune conditions, but it will look histologically like a typical autoimmune hepatitis and will be accompanied by positive serologic test results for ANA and/or anti-smooth muscle antibodies, as well as elevated serum IgG levels. Similarly, chronic biliary tract diseases may also co-occur by chance and should be diagnosed as per the usual features.

Other common patterns include mild fatty liver disease or nodular regenerative hyperplasia. Nodular regenerative hyperplasia typically has an alkaline-phosphatase-predominant pattern of liver enzyme level elevations and can be associated with portal hypertension. Although the precise cause of nodular regenerative hyperplasia in this setting is not clear, it is known to be associated with systemic autoimmune conditions.

REFERENCES

1. Rodriguez FJ, Gamez JD, Vrana JA, et al. Immunoglobulin derived depositions in the nervous system: novel mass spectrometry application for protein characterization in formalin-fixed tissues. *Lab Invest*. 2008;88:1024-1037.
2. Makhlouf HR, Goodman ZD. Globular hepatic amyloid: an early stage in the pathway of amyloid formation. A study of 20 new cases. *Am J Surg Pathol*. 2007;31:1615-1621.
3. Larsen CP, Kossmann RJ, Beggs ML, et al. Clinical, morphologic, and genetic features of renal leukocyte chemotactic factor 2 amyloidosis. *Kidney Int*. 2014;86:378-382.
4. Damlaj M, Amre R, Wong P, et al. Hepatic ALECT-2 amyloidosis causing portal hypertension and recurrent variceal bleeding: a case report and review of the literature. *Am J Clin Pathol*. 2014;141:288-291.
5. Bell PD, Huber AR, DeRoche TC. Along for the ride: intrahepatic cholangiocarcinoma with concomitant LECT2 amyloidosis. *Case Rep Pathol*. 2020;2020:8830763.
6. Larsen CP, Beggs ML, Wilson JD, et al. Prevalence and organ distribution of leukocyte chemotactic factor 2 amyloidosis (ALECT2) among decedents in New Mexico. *Amyloid*. 2016;23:119-123.

7. Chandan VS, Shah SS, Lam-Himlin DM, et al. Globular hepatic amyloid is highly sensitive and specific for LECT2 amyloidosis. *Am J Surg Pathol.* 2015;39:558-564.

8. Terada T, Hirata K, Hisada Y, et al. Obstructive jaundice caused by the deposition of amyloid-like substances in the extrahepatic and large intrahepatic bile ducts in a patient with multiple myeloma. *Histopathology.* 1994;24:485-487.

9. Mena-Duran A, Munoz Vicente E, Pareja Llorens G, et al. Liver failure caused by light chain deposition disease associated with multiple myeloma. *Intern Med.* 2012;51:773-776.

10. Yasir S, Rech KL, Chen ZE, et al. Amyloid-like Fibronectin deposits in the liver: a novel morphologic finding. *Am J Surg Pathol.* 2021;45:205-208.

11. Collardeau-Frachon S, Bouvier R, Le Gall C, et al. Unexpected diagnosis of cystic fibrosis at liver biopsy: a report of four pediatric cases. *Virchows Arch.* 2007;451:57-64.

12. Lindblad A, Glaumann H, Strandvik B. Natural history of liver disease in cystic fibrosis. *Hepatology.* 1999;30:1151-1158.

13. Moyer K, Balistreri W. Hepatobiliary disease in patients with cystic fibrosis. *Curr Opin Gastroenterol.* 2009;25:272-278.

14. Potter CJ, Fishbein M, Hammond S, et al. Can the histologic changes of cystic fibrosis-associated hepatobiliary disease be predicted by clinical criteria? *J Pediatr Gastroenterol Nutr.* 1997;25:32-36.

15. Strandvik B, Samuelson K. Fasting serum bile acid levels in relation to liver histopathology in cystic fibrosis. *Scand J Gastroenterol.* 1985;20:381-384.

16. Schwarzenberg SJ, Wielinski CL, Shamieh I, et al. Cystic fibrosis-associated colitis and fibrosing colonopathy. *J Pediatr.* 1995;127:565-570.

17. Witters P, Libbrecht L, Roskams T, et al. Noncirrhotic presinusoidal portal hypertension is common in cystic fibrosis-associated liver disease. *Hepatology.* 2011;53:1064-1065.

18. Cortes-Santiago N, Leung DH, Castro E, et al. Hepatic steatosis is prevalent following orthotopic liver transplantation in children with cystic fibrosis. *J Pediatr Gastroenterol Nutr.* 2019;68:96-103.

19. Hultcrantz R, Mengarelli S, Strandvik B. Morphological findings in the liver of children with cystic fibrosis: a light and electron microscopical study. *Hepatology.* 1986;6:881-889.

20. Torbenson M, Chen YY, Brunt E, et al. Glycogenic hepatopathy: an underrecognized hepatic complication of diabetes mellitus. *Am J Surg Pathol.* 2006;30:508-513.

21. van den Brand M, Elving LD, Drenth JP, et al. Glycogenic hepatopathy: a rare cause of elevated serum transaminases in diabetes mellitus. *Neth J Med.* 2009;67:394-396.

22. Chatila R, West AB. Hepatomegaly and abnormal liver tests due to glycogenosis in adults with diabetes. *Medicine (Baltimore).* 1996;75:327-333.

23. Carcione L, Lombardo F, Messina MF, et al. Liver glycogenosis as early manifestation in type 1 diabetes mellitus. *Diabetes Nutr Metab.* 2003;16:182-184.

24. Tomihira M, Kawasaki E, Nakajima H, et al. Intermittent and recurrent hepatomegaly due to glycogen storage in a patient with type 1 diabetes: genetic analysis of the liver glycogen phosphorylase gene (PYGL). *Diabetes Res Clin Pract.* 2004;65:175-182.

25. Olsson R, Wesslau C, William-Olsson T, et al. Elevated aminotransferases and alkaline phosphatases in unstable diabetes mellitus without ketoacidosis or hypoglycemia. *J Clin Gastroenterol.* 1989;11:541-545.

26. Fridell JA, Saxena R, Chalasani NP, et al. Complete reversal of glycogen hepatopathy with pancreas transplantation: two cases. *Transplantation.* 2007;83:84-86.

27. Iancu TC, Shiloh H, Dembo L. Hepatomegaly following short-term high-dose steroid therapy. *J Pediatr Gastroenterol Nutr.* 1986;5:41-46.

28. Kransdorf LN, Millstine D, Smith ML, et al. Hepatic glycogen deposition in a patient with anorexia nervosa and persistently abnormal transaminase levels. *Clin Res Hepatol Gastroenterol.* 2016;40:e15-e18.

29. Komuta M, Harada M, Ueno T, et al. Unusual accumulation of glycogen in liver parenchymal cells in a patient with anorexia nervosa. *Intern Med.* 1998;37:678-682.

30. Hudacko RM, Sciancalepore JP, Fyfe BS. Diabetic microangiopathy in the liver: an autopsy study of incidence and association with other diabetic complications. *Am J Clin Pathol.* 2009;132:494-499.

31. Fujisaki N, Kosaki Y, Nojima T, et al. Glycogenic hepatopathy following attempted suicide by long-acting insulin overdose in patient with type 1 diabetes. *J Am Coll Emerg Physicians Open.* 2020;1:1097-1100.

32. Allende DS, Gawrieh S, Cummings OW, et al. Glycogenosis is common in nonalcoholic fatty liver disease and is independently associated with ballooning, but lower steatosis and lower fibrosis. *Liver Int.* 2021;41(5):996-1011.

33. Lorenz G, Barenwald G. Histologic and electron-microscopic liver changes in diabetic children. *Acta Hepatogastroenterol (Stuttg).* 1979;26:435-438.

34. Harrison SA, Brunt EM, Goodman ZD, et al. Diabetic hepatosclerosis: diabetic microangiopathy of the liver. *Arch Pathol Lab Med.* 2006;130:27-32.

35. Chen G, Brunt EM. Diabetic hepatosclerosis: a 10-year autopsy series. *Liver Int.* 2009;29:1044-1050.

36. King RJ, Harrison L, Gilbey SG, et al. Diabetic hepatosclerosis: another diabetes microvascular complication? *Diabet Med.* 2016;33:e5-e7.

37. Nazzari E, Grillo F, Celiento T, et al. Diabetic hepatosclerosis presenting with severe cholestasis. *Diabetes Care.* 2013;36:e206.

38. Balakrishnan M, Garcia-Tsao G, Deng Y, et al. Hepatic arteriolosclerosis: a small-vessel complication of diabetes and hypertension. *Am J Surg Pathol.* 2015;39:1000-1009.

39. Torbenson M, Hart J, Westerhoff M, et al. Neonatal giant cell hepatitis: histological and etiological findings. *Am J Surg Pathol.* 2010;34:1498-1503.

40. Nishizawa H, Iguchi G, Murawaki A, et al. Nonalcoholic fatty liver disease in adult hypopituitary patients with GH deficiency and the impact of GH replacement therapy. *Eur J Endocrinol.* 2012;167:67-74.

41. Suzuki K, Kanamoto M, Hinohara H, et al. A case of hypopituitarism complicated by non-alcoholic steatohepatitis and severe pulmonary hypertension. *Am J Case Rep.* 2021;22:e928004.

42. Lonardo A, Mantovani A, Lugari S, et al. NAFLD in some common endocrine diseases: prevalence, pathophysiology, and principles of diagnosis and management. *Int J Mol Sci.* 2019;20(11):2841.

43. Prendki V, Stirnemann J, Lemoine M, et al. Prevalence and clinical significance of Kupffer cell hyperplasia with hemophagocytosis in liver biopsies. *Am J Surg Pathol.* 2011;35:337-345.

44. Selway JL, Harikumar PE, Chu A, et al. Genetic homogeneity of adult Langerhans cell histiocytosis lesions: insights from BRAF(V600E) mutations in adult populations. *Oncol Lett.* 2017;14:4449-4454.

45. Lauwers GY, Perez-Atayde A, Dorfman RF, et al. The digestive system manifestations of Rosai-Dorfman disease (sinus histiocytosis with massive lymphadenopathy): review of 11 cases. *Hum Pathol.* 2000;31:380-385.

46. Dogan S, Barnes L, Cruz-Vetrano WP. Crystal-storing histiocytosis: report of a case, review of the literature (80 cases) and a proposed classification. *Head Neck Pathol.* 2012;6:111-120.

47. Rouet A, Aouba A, Damaj G, et al. Mastocytosis among elderly patients: a multicenter retrospective French study on 53 patients. *Medicine (Baltimore).* 2016;95:e3901.

48. Yam LT, Chan CH, Li CY. Hepatic involvement in systemic mast cell disease. *Am J Med.* 1986;80:819-826.

49. Jiang ZG, Vardeh H, Evenson A. A case of cryptogenic liver failure. *Gastroenterology.* 2018;155:23-24 e1.

50. Horny HP, Kaiserling E, Campbell M, et al. Liver findings in generalized mastocytosis. A clinicopathologic study. *Cancer*. 1989;63:532-538.

51. Marbello L, Anghilieri M, Nosari A, et al. Aggressive systemic mastocytosis mimicking sclerosing cholangitis. *Haematologica*. 2004;89:ECR35.

52. Kyriakou D, Kouroumalis E, Konsolas J, et al. Systemic mastocytosis: a rare cause of noncirrhotic portal hypertension simulating autoimmune cholangitis--report of four cases. *Am J Gastroenterol*. 1998;93:106-108.

53. Safyan EL, Veerabagu MP, Swerdlow SH, et al. Intrahepatic cholestasis due to systemic mastocytosis: a case report and review of literature. *Am J Gastroenterol*. 1997;92:1197-1200.

54. Mican JM, Di Bisceglie AM, Fong TL, et al. Hepatic involvement in mastocytosis: clinicopathologic correlations in 41 cases. *Hepatology*. 1995;22:1163-1170.

55. Sainsbury A, Sanders DS, Ford AC. Meta-analysis: coeliac disease and hypertransaminasaemia. *Aliment Pharmacol Ther*. 2011;34:33-40.

56. Duggan JM, Duggan AE. Systematic review: the liver in coeliac disease. *Aliment Pharmacol Ther*. 2005;21:515-518.

57. da Rosa Utiyama SR, da Silva Kotze LM, Nisihara RM, et al. Spectrum of autoantibodies in celiac patients and relatives. *Dig Dis Sci*. 2001;46:2624-2630.

58. Jacobsen MB, Fausa O, Elgjo K, et al. Hepatic lesions in adult coeliac disease. *Scand J Gastroenterol*. 1990;25:656-662.

59. Mounajjed T, Oxentenko A, Shmidt E, et al. The liver in celiac disease: clinical manifestations, histologic features, and response to gluten-free diet in 30 patients. *Am J Clin Pathol*. 2011;136:128-137.

60. Riestra S, Dominguez F, Rodrigo L. Nodular regenerative hyperplasia of the liver in a patient with celiac disease. *J Clin Gastroenterol*. 2001;33:323-326.

61. Ojetti V, Fini L, Zileri Dal Verme L, et al. Acute cryptogenic liver failure in an untreated coeliac patient: a case report. *Eur J Gastroenterol Hepatol*. 2005;17:1119-1121.

62. Abenavoli L, Milic N, De Lorenzo A, et al. A pathogenetic link between non-alcoholic fatty liver disease and celiac disease. *Endocrine*. 2013;43:65-67.

63. Biecker E, Trebicka J, Fischer HP, et al. Portal hypertension and nodular regenerative hyperplasia in a patient with celiac disease. *Z Gastroenterol*. 2006;44:395-398.

64. Cappello M, Randazzo C, Bravata I, et al. Liver function test abnormalities in patients with inflammatory bowel diseases: a hospital-based survey. *Clin Med Insights Gastroenterol*. 2014;7:25-31.

65. Broome U, Glaumann H, Hellers G, et al. Liver disease in ulcerative colitis: an epidemiological and follow up study in the county of Stockholm. *Gut*. 1994;35:84-89.

66. Hermaszewski RA, Webster AD. Primary hypogammaglobulinaemia: a survey of clinical manifestations and complications. *Q J Med*. 1993;86:31-42.

67. Daniels JA, Torbenson M, Vivekanandan P, et al. Hepatitis in common variable immunodeficiency. *Hum Pathol*. 2009;40:484-488.

68. Ebrahimi Daryani N, Aghamohammadi A, Mousavi Mirkala MR, et al. Gastrointestinal complications in two patients with common variable immunodeficiency. *Iran J Allergy Asthma Immunol*. 2004;3:149-152.

69. Bjoro K, Haaland T, Skaug K, et al. The spectrum of hepatobiliary disease in primary hypogammaglobulinaemia. *J Intern Med*. 1999;245:517-524.

70. Ardeniz O, Cunningham-Rundles C. Granulomatous disease in common variable immunodeficiency. *Clin Immunol*. 2009;133:198-207.

71. Baron-Ruiz I, Martin-Mateos MA, Plaza-Martin AM, et al. Lymphoma as presentation of common variable immunodeficiency. *Allergol Immunopathol*. 2009;37:51-53.

72. Fuss IJ, Friend J, Yang Z, et al. Nodular regenerative hyperplasia in common variable immunodeficiency. *J Clin Immunol*. 2013;33:748-758.

73. Ward C, Lucas M, Piris J, et al. Abnormal liver function in common variable immunodeficiency disorders due to nodular regenerative hyperplasia. *Clin Exp Immunol.* 2008;153:331-337.

74. Malamut G, Ziol M, Suarez F, et al. Nodular regenerative hyperplasia: the main liver disease in patients with primary hypogammaglobulinemia and hepatic abnormalities. *J Hepatol.* 2008;48:74-82.

75. Hercun J, Parikh E, Kleiner DE, et al. Recurrent nodular regenerative hyperplasia post-liver transplantation in common variable immunodeficiency. *Hepatology.* 2021. doi:10.1002/hep.31775.

76. Crotty R, Taylor MS, Farmer JR, et al. Spectrum of hepatic manifestations of common variable immunodeficiency. *Am J Surg Pathol.* 2020;44:617-625.

77. Westbrook RH, Dusheiko G, Williamson C. Pregnancy and liver disease. *J Hepatol.* 2016;64:933-945.

78. Conchillo JM, Pijnenborg JM, Peeters P, et al. Liver enzyme elevation induced by hyperemesis gravidarum: aetiology, diagnosis and treatment. *Neth J Med.* 2002;60:374-378.

79. Bacq Y. Liver diseases unique to pregnancy: a 2010 update. *Clin Res Hepatol Gastroenterol.* 2011;35:182-193.

80. Ropponen A, Sund R, Riikonen S, et al. Intrahepatic cholestasis of pregnancy as an indicator of liver and biliary diseases: a population-based study. *Hepatology.* 2006;43:723-728.

81. van der Woerd WL, van Mil SW, Stapelbroek JM, et al. Familial cholestasis: progressive familial intrahepatic cholestasis, benign recurrent intrahepatic cholestasis and intrahepatic cholestasis of pregnancy. *Best Pract Res Clin Gastroenterol.* 2010;24:541-553.

82. Van Mil SW, Milona A, Dixon PH, et al. Functional variants of the central bile acid sensor FXR identified in intrahepatic cholestasis of pregnancy. *Gastroenterology.* 2007;133:507-516.

83. Reyes H, Baez ME, Gonzalez MC, et al. Selenium, zinc and copper plasma levels in intrahepatic cholestasis of pregnancy, in normal pregnancies and in healthy individuals, in Chile. *J Hepatol.* 2000;32:542-549.

84. Bacq Y, Sapey T, Brechot MC, et al. Intrahepatic cholestasis of pregnancy: a French prospective study. *Hepatology.* 1997;26:358-364.

85. Keitel V, Vogt C, Haussinger D, et al. Combined mutations of canalicular transporter proteins cause severe intrahepatic cholestasis of pregnancy. *Gastroenterology.* 2006;131:624-629.

86. Geenes VL, Lim YH, Bowman N, et al. A placental phenotype for intrahepatic cholestasis of pregnancy. *Placenta.* 2011;32:1026-1032.

87. Tsokos M, Longauer F, Kardosova V, et al. Maternal death in pregnancy from HELLP syndrome. A report of three medico-legal autopsy cases with special reference to distinctive histopathological alterations. *Int J Leg Med.* 2002;116:50-53.

88. Barton JR, Riely CA, Adamec TA, et al. Hepatic histopathologic condition does not correlate with laboratory abnormalities in HELLP syndrome (hemolysis, elevated liver enzymes, and low platelet count). *Am J Obstet Gynecol.* 1992;167:1538-1543.

89. Minakami H, Oka N, Sato T, et al. Preeclampsia: a microvesicular fat disease of the liver? *Am J Obstet Gynecol.* 1988;159:1043-1047.

90. Ch'ng CL, Morgan M, Hainsworth I, et al. Prospective study of liver dysfunction in pregnancy in Southwest Wales. *Gut.* 2002;51:876-880.

91. Burroughs AK, Seong NH, Dojcinov DM, et al. Idiopathic acute fatty liver of pregnancy in 12 patients. *Q J Med.* 1982;51:481-497.

92. Reyes H, Sandoval L, Wainstein A, et al. Acute fatty liver of pregnancy: a clinical study of 12 episodes in 11 patients. *Gut.* 1994;35:101-106.

93. Rolfes DB, Ishak KG. Acute fatty liver of pregnancy: a clinicopathologic study of 35 cases. *Hepatology.* 1985;5:1149-1158.

94. Riely CA, Latham PS, Romero R, et al. Acute fatty liver of pregnancy. A reassessment based on observations in nine patients. *Ann Intern Med*. 1987;106:703-706.

95. Treem WR, Shoup ME, Hale DE, et al. Acute fatty liver of pregnancy, hemolysis, elevated liver enzymes, and low platelets syndrome, and long chain 3-hydroxyacyl-coenzyme A dehydrogenase deficiency. *Am J Gastroenterol*. 1996;91:2293-2300.

96. Koskinas J, Gomatos IP, Tiniakos DG, et al. Liver histology in ICU patients dying from sepsis: a clinico-pathological study. *World J Gastroenterol*. 2008;14:1389-1393.

18

CRYPTOGENIC CIRRHOSIS

INTRODUCTION

A common challenge in liver pathology is to evaluate for possible causes of cirrhosis when clinical and serological findings have not established the etiology.[1] Much relevant information on cryptogenic cirrhosis is located in other chapters, but this chapter attempts to put it together in one convenient place. The emphasis is on a diagnostic approach, so epidemiology and genomic testing, while interesting, is beyond the scope of this chapter.

Identifying the cause of the cirrhosis has been an important challenge in surgical pathology for more than 100 years. Certainly, after major causes of cirrhosis, such as chronic hepatitis B and C and the metabolic syndrome, were identified, the number of cases of cryptogenic cirrhosis diminished substantially, but cryptogenic cirrhosis continues to be an important challenge today.

The most common known causes of cirrhosis are chronic viral hepatitis, steatohepatitis, and chronic biliary tract diseases, but there are many other less frequent causes (Table 18.1). As a general statement, the overall approach for cases of cryptogenic cirrhosis is to systematically rule out potential causes. As part of this, the histological findings are critical because they can identify likely causes and also help exclude causes. Children or young adults with cirrhosis, and no obvious cause by imaging or laboratory findings or histology, often benefit from sequencing to look for inherited causes of cirrhosis.

CRYPTOGENIC CIRRHOSIS

Cryptogenic Cirrhosis

- A liver that is cirrhotic by histology and has no identifiable cause based on clinical, laboratory, imaging, or histological findings.
- Diagnosis of exclusion; your job is to recognize possible causes of cirrhosis.

TABLE 18.1	Potential Causes of Cryptogenic Cirrhosis
Patient Population	Cause
Pediatric	Alpha-1-antitrypsin deficiency
	Bile salt deficiency disorders
	Congenital viral hepatitis
	Glycogen storage diseases
	Neonatal hemochromatosis
	Wilson disease
	Other rare genetic diseases
Teenage and young adults	Autoimmune hepatitis
	Bile salt deficiency disorders
	Congenital viral hepatitis B or C
	Cholesteryl Ester Storage Disease
	PSC
	Short telomere syndrome
	Wilson disease
Adults	Autoimmune hepatitis
	Alcohol-related disease
	Nonalcoholic fatty liver disease
	PBC
	Short telomere syndrome
	Viral hepatitis

PBC, primary biliary cholangitis; PSC, primary sclerosing cholangitis.

Definition

Cryptogenic cirrhosis is defined as a cirrhotic liver with no identifiable etiology that could reasonably explain the cirrhosis. Older terms include *nonspecific cirrhosis* and *inactive cirrhosis*, but the term cryptogenic cirrhosis is preferred. The context of usage is also important, as a liver can be clinically cryptogenic (but the histology not yet examined) or histologically cryptogenic (with incomplete or absent clinical or laboratory data). In this chapter, the focus is on histological changes, but a final diagnosis requires combining the clinical, laboratory, and histological findings.

Also, of note, liver cirrhosis can be assigned an etiology when a reasonable cause has been identified, even if it is not completely proven. This naturally leads to challenges, as there are no well-established criteria for the minimal findings needed to classify an etiology as "being a reasonably likely." For clinical care, the emphasis is on finding etiologies that might still be amenable to treatment, or would potentially impact the health of the patient or their family members; for this purpose ordinary, strict diagnostic criteria apply. For research purposes, etiological classification is often a bit looser.

Frequency

As previously noted, the frequency of cryptogenic cirrhosis has declined substantially over the past decades, as new causes of chronic liver disease have been identified; currently, the frequency of cryptogenic cirrhosis is about 10%.[2,3]

Natural History

The average age at diagnosis for cryptogenic cirrhosis is mid-60s. There is a mild enrichment for female gender (~60% women) versus other common causes of cirrhosis, such as chronic hepatitis C (~30% women).[4] Many patients have some but not all of the features of the metabolic syndrome.[4] The natural history of cryptogenic cirrhosis is broadly similar to that of cirrhosis from known causes, with a poor prognosis compared to patients without cirrhosis. One study found a high risk for hepatocellular carcinoma in cases of well-compensated cryptogenic cirrhosis (Child-Pugh class A) versus patients with known causes of cirrhosis.[4]

Histological Findings in Liver Transplants for Clinically Cryptogenic Cirrhosis

In patients transplanted with a clinical diagnosis of cryptogenic cirrhosis, histological examination of the explanted liver identifies a cause in 30% to 85% of cases.[5-9] Overall, fatty liver disease and autoimmune hepatitis are by far the most common causes in most studies of adult transplant patients (Table 18.2). Of note, the minimal criteria for establishing the cause based on histology are not well established, so there is a lot of heterogeneity in the results of these sorts of studies.

Outcomes After Liver Transplantation

Cryptogenic cirrhosis is generally thought to encompass a heterogeneous group of diseases and is not the end result of a single common disease process. Nevertheless, graft and patient survival after liver transplantation are similar to those cases transplanted for known diseases.[10,11]

Careful attention to the histological findings in the explanted liver is still important for clinical care, even though the patient has a new liver, as identifying potential causes can be relevant to disease recurrence, including autoimmune hepatitis, fatty liver disease, and chronic biliary tract disease. In cases where fatty liver disease is identified in the allograft liver, the differential includes recurrent fatty liver disease from the metabolic syndrome or alcohol use, as well as less common causes including FIC deficiency[12,13]

TABLE 18.2 **Histological Causes Identified in Adult Patients Transplanted With Clinically Cryptogenic Cirrhosis**

Cause	Frequency
Nonalcoholic steatohepatitis	15%-30%
Autoimmune hepatitis	5%-50%
Alcohol liver disease	5%
Vascular disease	5%
PSC or PBC	5%
Hemochromatosis	1%-5%
Occult viral hepatitis	1%-5%

Rare causes:
    Congenital hepatic fibrosis
    Sarcoidosis
    Other rare causes of biliary cirrhosis
    such as MDR3 deficiency
	<1%

MDR 3, multidrug resistance protein 3; PBC, primary biliary cholangitis; PSC, primary sclerosing cholangitis.

and cystic fibrosis.[14] The differential also includes de novo steatosis/steatohepatitis; in fact, denovo fatty liver disease develops in about 20% of patients transplanted for other known liver diseases.[15]

HISTOLOGICAL APPROACH FOR CLINICALLY CRYPTOGENIC CIRRHOSIS

General Approach to Cryptogenic Cirrhosis

A diagnosis of cryptogenic cirrhosis is by definition a diagnosis of exclusion, which requires full clinical and histological work-up in order to reasonably exclude recognizable causes. At the histological level, establishing a likely cause of the cirrhosis requires two key features (1) an appropriate degree of injury present in the liver and (2) findings compatible with the known natural history of the disease. For example, a diagnosis of alpha-1 antitrypsin deficiency as the cause of the cirrhosis would be inappropriate in a 20-year-old man with an MS phenotype and a few hepatocellular globules on periodic acid-Schiff with diastase (PASD); that is not the natural history of the disease, as the MS phenotype does not cause enough liver damage to be the sole cause of the cirrhosis. As another example, a 55-year-old woman with cirrhosis and a history of acute hepatitis C the year prior would not be classified as having hepatitis C virus (HCV) cirrhosis, even if she still has active HCV infection; the time interval is too short, inconsistent with the natural history of the disease. As a final example, a 70-year-old woman with cirrhosis and homozygous *HFE* C282Y mutations, who is untreated for iron overload yet has only mild iron deposition, did not develop cirrhosis because of hemochromatosis; that is not enough iron deposition to cause cirrhosis.

A reasonable way to think about the diagnostic approach is this: if the findings are not sufficient to establish an active disease process in a noncirrhotic liver, then they are insufficient to establish the *histological diagnosis* in a cirrhotic liver. Some diseases become "burned-out" over time (see below), but this should not lead to the conclusion that histological diagnostic standards can be lowered in accommodation. Instead, these cases typically have nonspecific histological findings and that is OK; the final diagnosis is established by clinical and laboratory findings and histology plays a supporting role, serving mostly by showing no findings inconsistent with the clinical/laboratory-based diagnosis and having no positive findings that would strongly suggest an alternative diagnosis.

CHALLENGES IN IDENTIFYING THE CAUSE OF CIRRHOSIS

Nonspecific Findings

Mild portal and septal chronic inflammation are common in cirrhotic livers and does not indicate the patient had a chronic hepatitis, such as viral hepatitis or autoimmune hepatitis, as the cause of the cirrhosis. Interface activity in isolation does not provide strong evidence for autoimmune hepatitis as the cause of the cirrhosis.

Minimal macrovesicular steatosis is common and does not indicate fatty liver disease was the cause of cirrhosis. Likewise, isolated ballooned cells or Mallory hyaline are insufficient evidence for establishing a diagnosis of cirrhosis from steatohepatitis. Several small studies have suggested the opposite, but the presence of minimal fat, balloon cells, and/or Mallory hyaline are insufficient to determine the cause of the cirrhosis. Also, of note, pericellular fibrosis does not indicate that steatohepatitis was the etiology of cirrhosis (Figure 18.1), since it is common in cirrhotic livers of many different etiologies; in addition, cirrhosis from burned-out steatohepatitis sometimes has no pericellular fibrosis (Figure 18.2).

This all makes sense, of course, but the challenge then becomes the minimal accepted criteria. For example, if a patient has a history of mild obesity but no other features of the metabolic syndrome, and the biopsy shows mild macrovesicular steatosis—is that constellation enough for a diagnosis of nonalcoholic fatty liver disease as the cause of the cirrhosis? What if the patient has been overweight/obese for only 3 years? You can think of many other combinations that all illustrate the problem of the minimal criteria needed for diagnosis. Currently, the best approach is holistic, wherein the histological findings, laboratory findings, and clinical findings are all interpreted together; this often does not happen in today's busy and sometimes fragmented health care system, and sometimes pathologists can feel some pressure to make a definite diagnosis at the time of sign-out. If

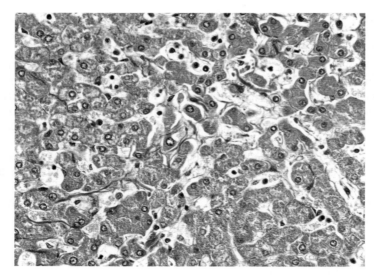

FIGURE 18.1 **Pericellular fibrosis.** This explanted liver is cirrhotic from chronic hepatitis B and the patient never had fatty liver disease.

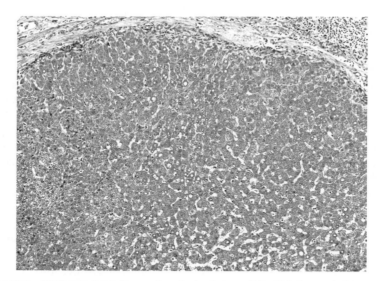

FIGURE 18.2 **Cirrhosis from burned-out steatohepatitis.** This image is from a section of an explanted liver and searching the entire trichrome-stained slide showed no pericellular fibrosis.

that can be done, great, go ahead and do it, but if the histological findings are not specific and you do not know the relevant clinical and laboratory findings, then its best to report out accurately what you see histologically, and provide a differential with relevant caveats, such as the histology findings being mild and nonspecific.

Contribution of Coexisting Diseases

In some cases, a patient with cirrhosis has two definite diseases of the liver based on histology and clinical/laboratory findings. While this is a different problem than having a case with minimal nonspecific histological changes, it requires some of the same skills in assessing potential roles for the cause of the cirrhosis. In general, the major disease process is defined as the one that is causing the most injury and is generally thought to be the driver of the cirrhosis. The second disease is often a cofactor. Common cofactors include *HFE* heterozygous mutations with mild to moderate iron deposition and *SERPIN1A* heterozygous mutations with a scattered PASD-positive globules in the lobules. Less common potential cofactors include heterozygous *ABCB4* or *MDR3* mutations, as well as keratin 8 mutations.[16,17]

It is often the case, when there are two histologically evident disease processes, that the disease activity for both is similar (usually minimal or mild). For example, a person may have cirrhosis and a history of unsuccessfully treated or untreated chronic HCV, plus significant alcohol use, and the biopsy shows both mildly active chronic hepatitis consistent with the HCV, plus mildly active steatohepatitis. In these types of cases, there is generally no reliable method to determine the relative contributions of each disease process to the cirrhosis, so it is usually best to just say so in a note in your pathology report.

Celiac disease has been studied for a potential relationship to cirrhosis for many years. These studies have shown that celiac disease is about twice as common in patients with cirrhosis, compared to the general population, regardless of the cause of cirrhosis.[18] However, the data best supports the conclusion that patients with chronic liver disease from many different etiologies have an increased risk for celiac disease, not that celiac disease is a cause of cirrhosis.

Burned-Out Disease

Several diseases can lose many or all of the typical histological findings once the liver becomes cirrhotic; this is particularly true for autoimmune hepatitis and for alcoholic and nonalcoholic fatty liver disease. This phenomenon is called "burned-out" disease. In these cases, the diagnosis is assigned based on clinical findings and the lack of any histological findings that (1) would be inconsistent with the clinical diagnosis and (2) show no findings to suggest a different etiology.

GENERAL PATTERNS OF CIRRHOSIS

Micronodular and Macronodular Cirrhosis

These gross-pathology-based patterns are no longer diagnostically useful but are reviewed here because they occasionally come up in medical discussions. Many years ago, cirrhosis was subclassified by the size of the nodules. The *micronodular pattern* had nodules that were less than 3 mm in greatest dimension on average, while the nodules in the *macronodular pattern* were greater than 3 mm on average. If no clear pattern predominated, then the term *mixed micro- and macronodular cirrhosis* was used. This classification system was in use at a time when the etiologies of most cases of cirrhosis were unknown and represented an early and historically important effort to understand the causes of cirrhosis. Today, however, cirrhosis is classified by etiology and not the size of the cirrhotic nodules. In addition, these patterns were found to be unstable over time, as micronodular patterns of cirrhosis can evolve to mixed and macronodular patterns.[19]

While there are many exceptions, retrospective studies have shown that the micronodular pattern of cirrhosis tended to correlate with alcoholic cirrhosis, alpha-1 antitrypsin deficiency, primary sclerosing cholangitis (PSC), primary biliary cholangitis (PBC), vascular disease, and hemochromatosis. On the other hand, macronodular cirrhosis generally correlated with chronic viral hepatitis B and C, autoimmune hepatitis, and Wilson disease, but also some cases of alcoholic liver disease and alpha-1 antitrypsin deficiency.[20]

Biliary Pattern of Cirrhosis

A biliary pattern of cirrhosis does not necessarily identify a specific etiology but can suggest further workup for biliary disease, or support a clinical diagnosis of chronic biliary tract disease. A precise definition for a biliary pattern of cirrhosis has not been developed, but the essential notion is that the histological findings suggest a chronic biliary tract disease. The histological findings are best thought of as a pattern, or a constellation of several possible individual findings, none of which are specific in isolation. The more individual findings are present, the greater the confidence in a likely diagnosis of chronic biliary disease. The constellation of findings includes these key changes: "halo-sign" or other evidence for significant cholate stasis, irregular cirrhotic nodules (sometimes likened to jigsaw puzzle pieces; this finding is not as robust as the others), onion-skin fibrosis, fibro-obliterative bile duct lesions, and bile duct loss (Figure 18.3). While bile ductular proliferation is an important part of the pattern of injury seen with acute and chronic biliary obstruction, this finding is nonspecific in cirrhotic livers (Figure 18.4), so is not part of the biliary pattern of cirrhosis. In fact, many cases of known biliary cirrhosis will have inconspicuous bile ductular proliferation, while cases of cirrhosis with significant ongoing inflammatory injury can have mildly prominent bile ductular proliferation even when the cirrhosis is not biliary-related.

Fibro-obliterative duct lesions are most commonly seen in cases of PSC but are not specific and are also found with other causes of chronic biliary obstructive disease (including ischemic strictures, biliary obstruction secondary to sarcoidosis,[21] chronic hepatolithiasis[22]), segmental cholangiectasia,[23] and MDR3 deficiency in adults.[24]

Granulomas and florid duct lesions are important parts of the pathology of PBC but are uncommon once the liver becomes cirrhotic (Figure 18.5). In fact, if a cirrhotic liver shows prominent florid duct lesions or

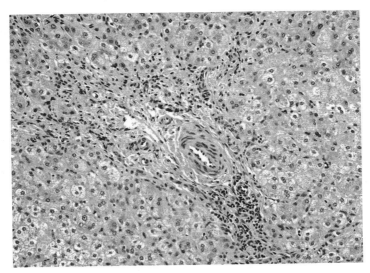

FIGURE 18.3 **Bile duct loss.** At least 50% of the portal tracts should be missing bile ducts. The smaller portal tracts will lose their bile ducts before the larger portal tracts.

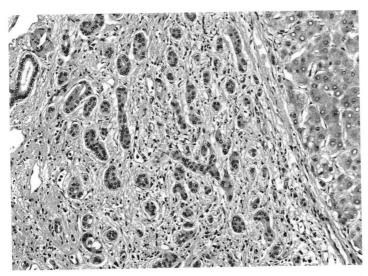

FIGURE 18.4 **Bile ductular proliferation.** This is a nonspecific finding in a cirrhotic liver; this patient was transplanted for chronic hepatitis C virus (HCV).

numerous granulomas, PBC is not the most likely diagnosis. Instead, drug-induced liver injury or infections superimposed on a cirrhotic liver is the most common cause of this PBC-mimicking pattern.

Copper deposition and abundant cytokeratin 7 (CK7)–positive intermediate hepatocytes are seen in nearly all cases of biliary cirrhosis. However, both stains are positive in many cases of cirrhosis from nonbiliary causes, so

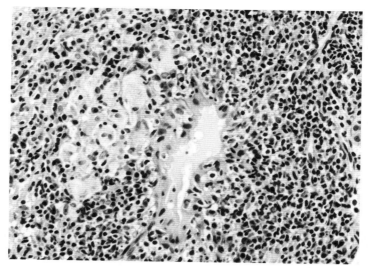

FIGURE 18.5 **Florid duct lesion, cirrhotic liver.** The patient was antimitochondrial anti-body (AMA)–negative, had a normal alkaline phosphatase, and cytokeratin 7 (CK7) and cop-per stains were negative, all suggesting the cirrhosis was not from primary biliary cholangitis (PBC), despite the florid duct lesion.

these stains are best interpreted in this manner: the lack of abundant CK7 positive intermediate hepatocytes and/or the lack of copper deposition in a cirrhotic liver suggests the cause of the cirrhosis is not biliary related.

PRACTICAL APPROACH

> **Practical Histological Classification System for Histological Findings**
>
> • Cirrhosis, no cause identified histologically
> • Cirrhosis, possible cause identified histologically
> • Cirrhosis, probable or definite cause identified histologically

When interpreting the histological findings in a cirrhotic liver, the con-stellation of findings can be usefully thought of as falling into three broad categories: no cause is identified; a possible cause of cirrhosis is identified; or a probable or definite cause of cirrhosis is identified. The next step is for the histological findings to be interpreted in the context of the clinical and laboratory findings. A final determination for the cause of the cirrhosis requires both steps (Table 18.3).

Cirrhosis, No Cause Identified Histologically

The livers in these cases typically show minimal to mild portal and sep-tal chronic inflammation. The lobules may show minimal hepatitis and or

TABLE 18.3 Final Classification for Cirrhosis, Assuming That Histology and Clinical and Laboratory Findings Are Congruent

Pathology Findings	Clinical/Laboratory Findings		
	Entirely nonspecific	Possible etiology	Definite or near definite etiology
Entirely nonspecific	Cryptogenic	Cryptogenic, but possible cause identified	Cause identified
Possible etiology	Cryptogenic, but possible cause identified	Cause identified	Cause identified
Definite or near definite etiology	Cause identified	Cause identified	Cause identified

minimal macrovesicular steatosis (less than 5%). There are no abnormal hepatocellular inclusions (such as hepatitis B virus [HBV] ground glass). There is no evidence for a biliary pattern of cirrhosis. PASD stains are negative. Iron stains show mild or less iron deposition.

For these cases, the final cause of cirrhosis is assigned based on laboratory and clinical findings, as long as the final clinical/laboratory-based diagnosis is compatible with the histological findings. For example, even if a patient has homozygous C282Y *HFE* mutations, the liver should show marked iron deposition (in an untreated patient) in order to establish a diagnosis of hemochromatosis as the cause of the cirrhosis.

Cirrhosis, Possible Cause Identified Histologically

The livers in these cases show changes that suggest a possible diagnosis. The most common example is livers with at least mild fat (>5%), suggesting either alcoholic or nonalcoholic fatty liver disease as the cause of the cirrhosis. Another example is a liver with mild portal and septal chronic inflammation but with a definite plasma cell enrichment, suggesting autoimmune hepatitis. Biliary patterns of cirrhosis also are within this category. Of course, correlation with laboratory and clinical findings is needed before determining the final cause of cirrhosis. Many cases where a potential cofactor is found histologically also fall into this category, such as finding PASD-positive globules (Figure 18.6).

Cirrhosis, Probable or Definite Cause Identified Histologically

Examples include cirrhosis from chronic hepatitis B, confirmed by positive immunostains, cirrhosis from genetic hemochromatosis or Wilson disease

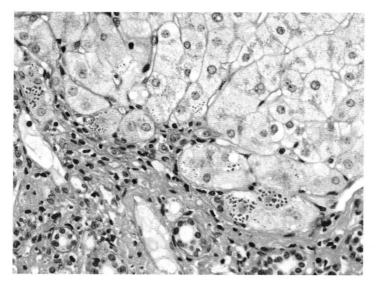

FIGURE 18.6 **Alpha-1 antitrypsin, periodic acid-Schiff with diastase (PASD).** This cirrhotic liver shows globules of alpha-1 antitrypsin protein. On further testing, the patient had an MZ Pi type and serum protein levels were normal.

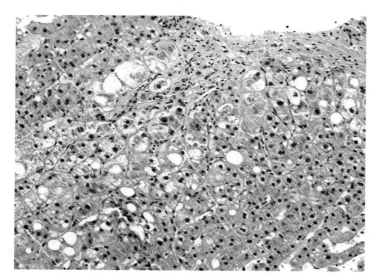

FIGURE 18.7 **Steatohepatitis.** This cirrhotic liver shows steatohepatitis and the patient had the metabolic syndrome.

(with marked iron and copper overload, respectively), or cirrhosis with ongoing active steatohepatitis (Figure 18.7). In this category, the final cause of cirrhosis still requires clinical correlation, but the histological findings identify a specific cause or likely cofactor for the cirrhosis.

REFERENCES

1. Torbenson MS, Arnold CA, Graham RP, et al. Identification of key challenges in liver pathology: data from a multicenter study of extramural consults. *Hum Pathol.* 2019;87:75-82.

2. Dehghani SM, Imanieh MH, Haghighat M, et al. Etiology and complications of liver cirrhosis in children: report of a single center from southern Iran. *Middle East J Dig Dis.* 2013;5:41-46.

3. Dalgic A, Ozcay F, Arslan G, et al. Living-related liver transplantation in pediatric patients. *Transplant Proc.* 2005;37:3133-3136.

4. Rinaldi L, Nascimbeni F, Giordano M, et al. Clinical features and natural history of cryptogenic cirrhosis compared to hepatitis C virus-related cirrhosis. *World J Gastroenterol.* 2017;23:1458-1468.

5. Alamo JM, Bernal C, Barrera L, et al. Liver transplantation in patients with cryptogenic cirrhosis: long-term follow-up. *Transplant Proc.* 2011;43:2230-2232.

6. Ayata G, Gordon FD, Lewis WD, et al. Cryptogenic cirrhosis: clinicopathologic findings at and after liver transplantation. *Hum Pathol.* 2002;33:1098-1104.

7. Duclos-Vallee JC, Yilmaz F, Johanet C, et al. Could post-liver transplantation course be helpful for the diagnosis of so called cryptogenic cirrhosis? *Clin Transplant.* 2005;19:591-599.

8. Tardu A, Karagul S, Yagci MA, et al. Histopathological examination of explanted liver after transplantation in patients with cryptogenic cirrhosis. *Transplant Proc.* 2015;47:1450-1452.

9. Nayak NC, Vasdev N, Saigal S, et al. End-stage nonalcoholic fatty liver disease: evaluation of pathomorphologic features and relationship to cryptogenic cirrhosis from study of explant livers in a living donor liver transplant program. *Hum Pathol.* 2010;41:425-430.

10. Thuluvath PJ, Hanish S, Savva Y. Liver transplantation in cryptogenic cirrhosis: outcome comparisons between NASH, alcoholic, and AIH cirrhosis. *Transplantation.* 2018;102:656-663.

11. Golabi P, Bush H, Stepanova M, et al. Liver transplantation (LT) for cryptogenic cirrhosis (CC) and nonalcoholic steatohepatitis (NASH) cirrhosis. Data from the Scientific Registry of Transplant Recipients (SRTR): 1994 to 2016. *Medicine (Baltimore).* 2018;97:e11518.

12. Lykavieris P, van Mil S, Cresteil D, et al. Progressive familial intrahepatic cholestasis type 1 and extrahepatic features: no catch-up of stature growth, exacerbation of diarrhea, and appearance of liver steatosis after liver transplantation. *J Hepatol.* 2003;39:447-452.

13. Miyagawa-Hayashino A, Egawa H, Yorifuji T, et al. Allograft steatohepatitis in progressive familial intrahepatic cholestasis type 1 after living donor liver transplantation. *Liver Transpl.* 2009;15:610-618.

14. Cortes-Santiago N, Leung DH, Castro E, et al. Hepatic steatosis is prevalent following orthotopic liver transplantation in children with cystic fibrosis. *J Pediatr Gastroenterol Nutr.* 2019;68:96-103.

15. Sutedja DS, Gow PJ, Hubscher SG, et al. Revealing the cause of cryptogenic cirrhosis by posttransplant liver biopsy. *Transplant Proc.* 2004;36:2334-2337.

16. Ku NO, Darling JM, Krams SM, et al. Keratin 8 and 18 mutations are risk factors for developing liver disease of multiple etiologies. *Proc Natl Acad Sci U S A.* 2003;100:6063-6068.

17. Halangk J, Berg T, Puhl G, et al. Keratin 8 Y54H and G62C mutations are not associated with liver disease. *J Med Genet.* 2004;41:e92.

18. Wakim-Fleming J, Pagadala MR, McCullough AJ, et al. Prevalence of celiac disease in cirrhosis and outcome of cirrhosis on a gluten free diet: a prospective study. *J Hepatol.* 2014;61:558-563.

19. Fauerholdt L, Schlichting P, Christensen E, et al. Conversion of micronodular cirrhosis into macronodular cirrhosis. *Hepatology.* 1983;3:928-931.

20. Anthony PP, Ishak KG, Nayak NC, et al. The morphology of cirrhosis. Recommendations on definition, nomenclature, and classification by a working group sponsored by the World Health Organization. *J Clin Pathol.* 1978;31:395-414.

21. Nakanuma Y, Kouda W, Harada K, et al. Hepatic sarcoidosis with vanishing bile duct syndrome, cirrhosis, and portal phlebosclerosis. Report of an autopsy case. *J Clin Gastroenterol.* 2001;32:181-184.

22. Nakanuma Y, Yamaguchi K, Ohta G, et al. Pathologic features of hepatolithiasis in Japan. *Hum Pathol.* 1988;19:1181-1186.

23. Zhao L, Hosseini M, Wilcox R, et al. Segmental cholangiectasia clinically worrisome for cholangiocarcinoma: comparison with recurrent pyogenic cholangitis. *Hum Pathol.* 2015;46:426-433.

24. Wendum D, Barbu V, Rosmorduc O, et al. Aspects of liver pathology in adult patients with MDR3/ABCB4 gene mutations. *Virchows Arch.* 2012;460:291-298.

19

BENIGN AND MALIGNANT PEDIATRIC TUMORS

VASCULAR MALFORMATION

Definition

Vascular malformations are nonneoplastic vascular mass lesions (pseudo-tumors) that result from a vascular shunt.

Clinical Findings

The clinical findings vary, but most patients are symptomatic at birth or within the first few weeks after birth.[1] Some patients present with cardiac or respiratory failure that results from hemodynamic compromise. Some patients may present with a bleeding diathesis from platelet sequestration and consumption (Kasabach-Merritt syndrome).

Histologic Findings

Vascular malformations of the liver can be diagnosed on imaging and are often not biopsied. When biopsied, there can be significant overlap with infantile hemangiomas on small samples, especially if only the periphery of the vascular malformation is sampled.

Vascular malformations tend to have large, central cystic spaces filled with blood, organizing thrombi, and fibrous tissue, all surrounded by a rim of proliferating, reactive, small-caliber blood vessels (which can mimic infantile hemangiomas). Occasional thick-walled, tortuous vessels can be seen in the center or periphery of the lesion. The edges of the lesion tend to be irregular and commonly have entrapped hepatocytes and/or portal tracts. Over time, the center of the lesion can become fibrotic, with large, thick-walled, and malformed vessels that are fibrotic (Figure 19.1) and sometimes completely replaced by fibrosis. The adjacent liver parenchyma shows reactive changes, with nodularity and fibrosis that can focally resemble focal nodular hyperplasia (FNH). The blood vessels in vascular malformations are GLUT-1 negative, or weakly positive, in contrast to much stronger and more diffuse staining seen in infantile hemangiomas.[1]

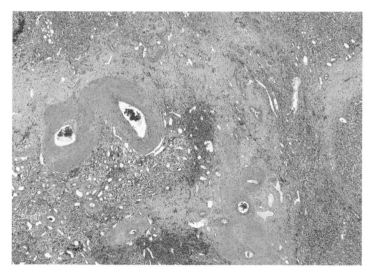

FIGURE 19.1 **Vascular malformation.** This vascular malformation shows thick-walled arteries, dense fibrosis, and nonspecific inflammation.

INFANTILE HEMANGIOMA

Definition

Infantile hemangiomas are benign vascular neoplasms of the pediatric liver. The older term *infantile hemangioendothelioma* has been replaced with *infantile hemangioma*. Additional terminology used by some authors include *diffuse neonatal hemangiomatosis* or *diffuse hemangiomatosis*, especially if there are numerous systemic hemangiomas, including cutaneous hemangiomas and/or hemangiomas elsewhere in the viscera.

Clinical Findings

Infantile hemangiomas are the most common vascular tumor of the liver in infants/toddlers, with about 90% of cases occurring before 6 months of age. However, rare cases are first identified in teenagers or adults. There is a female predominance of about 2:1. Most cases present with clinical symptoms (60%), although the symptoms tend to be nonspecific, such as failure to thrive or gastrointestinal problems. The hemangiomas show rapid postnatal growth (0-12 months), followed by slow involution (1-5 years). Infantile hemangiomas may be associated with congenital anomalies, but the anomalies are varied and show no clear patterns, ranging from extranumerary digits to hydrocephalus. In approximately 10% of cases, hemangiomas are present in extrahepatic sites, including skin, lungs, gastrointestinal tract, and adrenal glands. Interestingly, the endothelial cells in infantile hemangiomas express type 3 iodothyronine deiodinase, an enzyme that inactivates thyroid hormone and often leads to acquired hypothyroidism.[2]

Current management of symptomatic tumors typically involves drug therapy (eg, propranolol) as a first-line option, with resection or arterial embolization in patients who fail to respond to drug therapy.

Histology

The tumors can be unifocal or multifocal or can diffusely involve the liver. Infantile hemangiomas are usually well demarcated and nonencapsulated. They range in size from subcentimeter incidental findings to 15 cm. The neoplasms may derive their blood supply from the hepatic artery and/or extrahepatic arteries, as well as the portal vein.

Infantile hemangiomas are composed of dilated and irregular, capillary-like vessels in a collagenous background (Figure 19.2). Entrapped bile ducts are common at the periphery of the hemangioma. While infantile hemangiomas are well demarcated on gross examination, about one-third of tumors have an infiltrative margin on histologic examination. In these cases, the hepatocytes at the interface can take on a ductular morphology. In some cases, the hepatocytes at the margins can produce large amounts of α-fetoprotein (AFP).[3,4] The center of the tumor can have a cavernous hemangiomalike appearance, with larger caliber vessels and areas of thrombosis, myxoid change, fibrosis, and calcification. The neoplastic endothelial cells are plump to flattened and have no cytologic atypia. Up to 12 mitoses per 10 high-power field (HPF) have been reported, but high mitoses do not impact prognosis; instead, they reflect the transient but rapid postnatal growth.

Although rare, infantile hemangiomas do have a risk of developing malignancy and should be examined for areas of atypia. Architectural atypia can include papillary tufts (Figure 19.3) as well as solid areas (Figure 19.4).

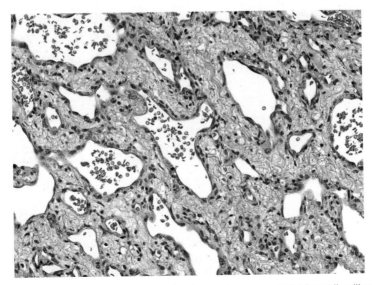

FIGURE 19.2 **Infantile hemangioma.** The tumor is composed of small-caliber vessels embedded in moderate amounts of connective tissue.

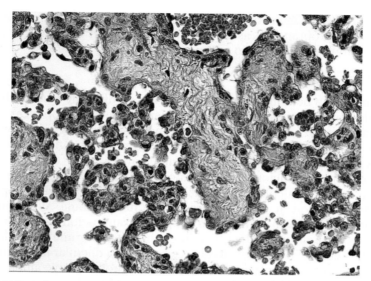

FIGURE 19.3 **Infantile hemangioma with atypia.** The endothelial cells in this area have enlarged nuclei and show tufting.

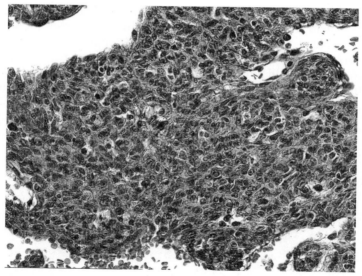

FIGURE 19.4 **Infantile hemangioma with atypia.** A focal area of solid growth is seen.

Other patterns of atypia include spindly, kaposiform-like areas. Currently, cytologic and/or architectural atypia appears to be the best available histologic marker for aggressive potential. While the clinical outcome is similar in most cases regardless of the presence or absence of atypia, almost all tumors with aggressive behavior have histologically atypical areas. Tumor recurrence is more common than metastases.

Immunostains

Infantile hemangiomas stain with vascular markers including ERG, CD31, and CD34. They show strong and diffuse staining for GLUT-1, in contrast to vascular malformations, which are GLUT-1 negative.[1]

Differential Diagnosis

Several studies have suggested that infants can also have congenital hemangiomas. The congenital hemangioma is thought to be analogous to the more common cutaneous *rapidly involuting congenital hemangioma* (RICH). In contrast to infantile hemangiomas, congenital hemangiomas are often diagnosed before birth, are fully formed at birth, and do not have a rapid growth phase after birth (all this is in contrast to most infantile hemangiomas).[5] In addition, congenital hemangiomas are typically unifocal lesions, are less frequently associated with hemangiomas elsewhere in the skin, are GLUT-1 negative, and do not lead to acquired hypothyroidism.[5] The histologic findings are similar and the distinction is made mostly on clinical grounds, although GLUT-1 staining can be helpful. The congenital hemangioma can be followed up without therapy if it is asymptomatic.

MESENCHYMAL HAMARTOMA

Definition

This is a benign tumor composed of loose connective tissue, often with cystic changes, admixed with benign bile ducts and occasional small islands or cords of hepatocytes.

Clinical Findings

Mesenchymal hamartomas usually present with nonspecific clinical findings. Serum AFP levels can be elevated in a subset of cases.[6,7] There is a slight male predominance and 85% of patients present before the age of 3 years.[8] Mesenchymal hamartomas can also be detected by prenatal ultrasound. Rare cases first present in adults.[9] Most mesenchymal hamartomas are single, but rare multifocal cases have been described.[7]

The etiology remains unclear, but chromosome 19q13 alterations are common.[10,11] Recently, cases have been shown to have germline *DICER1* mutations.[12] Multiple case reports have also reported an association between mesenchymal hamartomas and placental mesenchymal dysplasia.[13]

Histology

Mesenchymal hamartomas are mostly composed of loose connective tissue, with scattered benign bile ducts and occasional small hepatocyte islands (Figure 19.5, eFig. 19.1); the latter two findings are best found at the periphery of the tumor. The connective tissue can show varying appearances but is usually edematous with low cellularity and scattered, small, spindled cells without cytologic atypia (Figure 19.6); some areas may be more densely

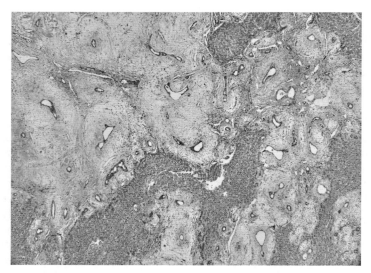

FIGURE 19.5 **Mesenchymal hamartoma**. At low-power magnification, this mesenchymal hamartoma shows disorganized hepatocyte lobules and bile ducts in loose fibrous tissue.

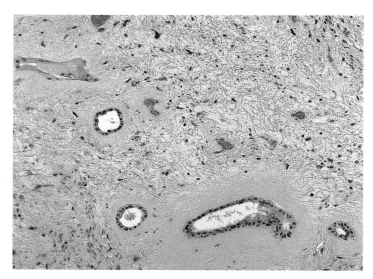

FIGURE 19.6 **Mesenchymal hamartoma**. Occasional bile ducts are seen embedded in loose connective tissue of low cellularity.

collagenized or myxoid. Degenerative, cystic changes are common (Figure 19.7). Osseous metaplasia can rarely occur.[14] The bile duct epithelium is bland with no atypia and low or no mitotic activity. In some cases, the bile ducts will show a ductal plate malformation pattern, while in other cases the ducts may be dilated and form small cysts. The biliary cysts can be microscopic in size or can be up to several centimeters. Also, a small-vessel vascular proliferation

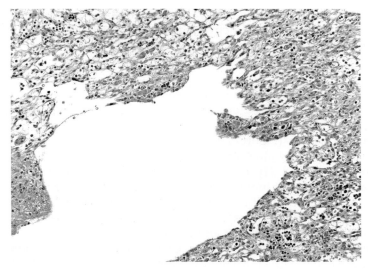

FIGURE 19.7 **Mesenchymal hamartoma, cystic areas.** This cyst has no lining and probably represents cystic degeneration of the tumor's loose connective tissue.

can be seen at the periphery of some cases.[8] The lesions generally show little or no inflammation, but extramedullary hematopoiesis is common. Although mesenchymal hamartomas are benign, some cases can undergo malignant transformation to embryonal sarcoma.

Immunostains

The epithelium lining the biliary cysts and forming the bile duct structures are CK7 and CK19 positive. The loose connective tissue is typically vimentin positive and can also be smooth muscle actin positive.[15] The hepatocytes can be glypican 3 positive[16] but are not malignant. In cases with elevated serum AFP levels, the hepatocyte islands and bile ducts within the hamartoma can be AFP positive by immunostaining, but again are not malignant.[6]

EMBRYONAL SARCOMA

Definition

Embryonal sarcomas are undifferentiated sarcomas most commonly seen in the pediatric population. In the literature, the terms *undifferentiated embryonal sarcoma* or *hepatic undifferentiated sarcoma* are used as synonyms.

Clinical Findings

There is an equal male-to-female ratio, and the median age at presentation is around 10 years.[17] However, patients can also rarely present as adults. The etiology is unknown, although a proportion of embryonal sarcomas arise out of mesenchymal hamartomas.[18] The 5-year overall survival is 86%.[19] Sequencing studies have shown frequent chr19q13 structural changes (also found in mesenchymal hamartomas) as well as mutations or copy loss of *TP53*.[20]

Histologic Findings

Most embryonal sarcomas are composed of undifferentiated spindled cells with significant and diffuse cytologic atypia (Figure 19.8). The tumor cells tend to be medium to large in size and often have scattered areas of giant cell transformation (Figure 19.9). The tumor cellularity can vary, with some areas becoming more fibrotic, whereas in other areas the stroma can be loose and myxoid. Hyaline globules can be seen in the tumor cells and sometimes outside the tumor cells, but they are not necessary for diagnosis and are not present in all tumors. Periodic acid-Schiff (PAS) stain can be used to highlight the globules; the globules will also be resistant to diastase. Cystic degeneration can occur and can dominate the radiologic and gross findings in some cases.[21,22] Remnants of a mesenchymal hamartoma may be seen, in particular with embryonal sarcomas arising in younger individuals.

Immunohistochemistry

In general, immunostains are used to rule out other malignancies, as there are no useful affirmative stains. There are a lot of case reports that describe immunostain findings, but relatively few larger series. Nonetheless, the tumor cells tend to express a variety of cytokeratins, including cytokeratins AE1/AE3 and CAM5.2.[23-25] In most cases, the cytokeratin staining is patchy. Some studies have reported a perinuclear dotlike positivity for cytokeratins AE1/AE3 and CAM5.2.[23] Vimentin and CD68 are routinely positive.[25,26]

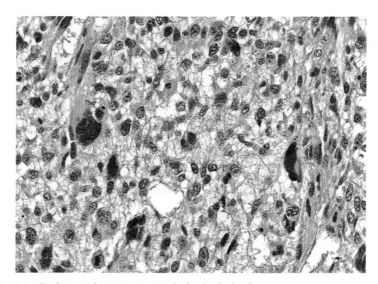

FIGURE 19.8 **Embryonal sarcoma.** Atypical spindled cells are seen.

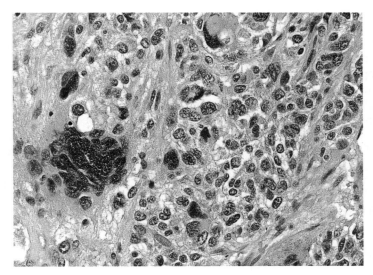

FIGURE 19.9 **Embryonal sarcoma.** Giant cell change is seen within the tumor.

The tumor cells can show membranous CD56 staining and focal membranous CD10 staining.[23] Other stains that have been reported to be positive in a proportion of cases include α1-antitrypsin (positive in most cases, but a rather dirty stain that can be hard to interpret, at least in many laboratories), alpha-1-antichymotrypsin, BCL2, and P53.[24,25] Desmin and alpha-smooth muscle actin show patchy staining in between 30% and 50% of cases.[24,25,27] Tumor cells can be either diffusely or focally positive for glypican 3.[16]

Negative stains include myoglobin (focal positivity in rare cases), smooth muscle myosin, h-caldesmon, CD34 (focal positivity in rare cases), Alk-1, S100 (focal positivity in rare cases), GFAP, HMB45, CD117, and HepPar1.[24,25] Myogenin is also negative.[17,24]

Differential

In children, the primary differential is biliary tract rhabdomyosarcoma. Biliary tract biliary rhabdomyosarcomas tend to lack the diffuse and striking anaplasia seen in embryonal sarcomas. Immunostains are very helpful, as myogenin and the myogenic regulatory protein D1 (MyoD1) are negative in embryonal sarcomas but positive in most biliary tract rhabdomyosarcomas.[17] In adults, metastatic sarcomas should be ruled out, including gastrointestinal stromal tumors.

ANGIOSARCOMAS

Angiosarcomas in the pediatric population are very rare and published data is sparse. They show similar morphologic changes to adult angiosarcomas, including kaposiform morphology, with solid areas of spindle cell growth containing small vascular slits. The tumors are CD31, CD34, and ERG-positive.

RHABDOMYOSARCOMA

Rhabdomyosarcomas are also called *embryonal rhabdomyosarcomas*. This tumor usually affects the extrahepatic bile ducts,[28] but it can present as an intrahepatic mass.[29] There classically is a hypercellular cuff of tumor cells right underneath the bile ducts, a finding referred to as a *cambium layer* (Figure 19.10). The tumor cells can be spindled (Figure 19.11) with eosinophilic inclusions, or they can be more rounded. Intermediate shaped cells that resemble racquets can also be seen. Mitotic activity tends to be high, and there can be areas of necrosis and hemorrhage. As the tumor surrounds the bile duct, it can compress the duct, leading to biliary obstruction. Cross-striations are hard to find in tumor cells, especially on a biopsy, and immunostains are important for establishing the diagnosis; myogenin and myogenic regulatory protein D1 (MyoD1) are positive in most biliary tract rhabdomyosarcomas.[17]

MALIGNANT RHABDOID TUMOR

Definition

Malignant rhabdoid tumors of the liver are defined by the loss of nuclear INI-1 expression or by molecular testing showing mutations/deletions of *SMARCB1*. Most cases will show rhabdoid cytologic features and should not show features of hepatocellular carcinoma or cholangiocarcinoma, as these tumors can rarely show secondary, nonspecific loss of INI-1 staining.[30]

Because of the rarity of this tumor, clinical colleagues can easily confuse the term "rhabdoid tumor" with "rhabdomyosarcoma" and reports can sometimes benefit from a specific statement saying the tumor is not a rhabdomyosarcoma.

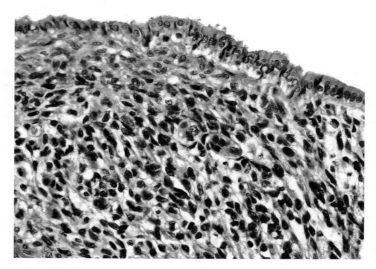

FIGURE 19.10 **Rhabdomyosarcoma.** The tumor grows as a condensed layer cuffing the bile duct.

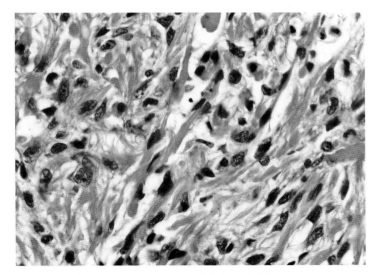

FIGURE 19.11 **Rhabdomyosarcoma.** Spindled, bright pink tumor cells are seen.

Clinical Findings

About 30% of patients have germline mutations in *SMARCB1*,[31] but no other risk factors are known. There is no gender predilection and most patients are children, with an average age at presentation of 2 years[32] and a median of 8 months,[31,33] although occasional patients will present later, in their teenage years.[33] Rare cases have also been reported in adults.[34,35]

Most patients present with nonspecific clinical findings, such as abdominal discomfort, lethargy, and anorexia. Physical examination and/or imaging shows a liver mass. Serum AFP levels are normal or show mild, nonspecific elevations in most cases. Rare cases with very high levels of serum AFP have been reported. The tumors are very aggressive, and two-thirds of patients have metastatic disease at presentation. The prognosis is poor, with a median survival of about 1.5 months.[33]

Histologic Findings

The tumors are composed of moderate-sized, epithelioid cells with abundant cytoplasm, growing in somewhat discohesive sheets (Figure 19.12, eFig. 19.2); there may also be areas of trabecular or nested growth. The tumor cells show vesiculated chromatin, show prominent nucleoli, and can have PAS-positive, perinuclear cytoplasmic inclusion. In some areas, the tumor cells can have a spindled morphology. There often is significant necrosis, which can elicit a marked histiocytic infiltrate; in some cases, the marked histiocytic inflammation can obscure the true diagnosis. The centers of the tumors are often hemorrhagic and necrotic.

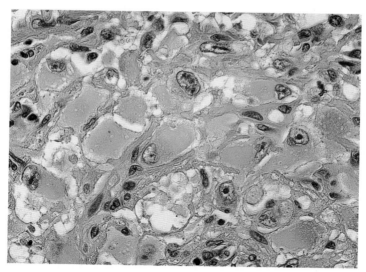

FIGURE 19.12   **Rhabdoid tumor.** The tumor cells have abundant cytoplasm and can have eccentrically located nuclei.

Immunohistochemical Findings

The tumors uniformly show loss of nuclear INI-1 immunostaining (Figure 19.13). Vimentin (eFig. 19.3) is positive in greater than 90% of cases and can highlight perinuclear inclusions. Smooth muscle actin is positive in about 40% of cases. There is at least some cytokeratin staining in most cases, although there is considerable variability in the specific keratin expression pattern, so a broad panel approach is best. Pan-keratin staining is seen in 60% of cases (eFig. 19.4) and Cam5.2 in about 60% of cases (eFig. 19.5). Glypican 3 is positive in about two-thirds of cases and represents an important pitfall, sometimes leading to a misdiagnosis of hepatoblastoma or hepatocellular carcinoma. Rhabdoid tumors are negative for HepPar1 and arginase1.[36,37]

Synaptophysin is positive in about two-thirds of cases, and S100 cytoplasmic staining can be seen in a third of cases (eFig. 19.6). Other positive stains include polyclonal CEA (cytoplasmic, membranous), CD34, and EGFR (eFigs. 19.7-19.9). Tumors have a high Ki-67 proliferative rate. Immunostains are negative for chromogranin, CD34, HMB-45, desmin, myoglobin, and GFAP.

CALCIFYING NESTED STROMAL-EPITHELIAL TUMOR

Definition

Calcifying nested stromal-epithelial tumors are rare primary tumors of the liver that are composed of both epithelial nests and reactive stromal elements.

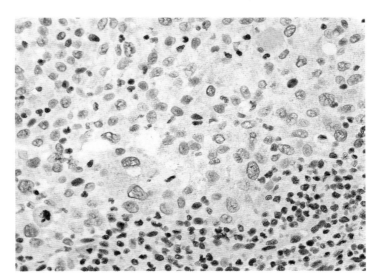

FIGURE 19.13 **Rhabdoid tumor.** An immunostain for INI-1 shows loss of staining in the tumor cells. Infiltrating inflammatory cells are positive.

Clinical Findings

Calcifying nested stromal-epithelial tumors most commonly affect young patients, with an age range of 2 to 33 years.[38] Most patients are teenaged women with the tumors found incidentally,[39] although some patients present with elevated adrenocorticotropic hormone (ACTH) levels, leading to the Cushing syndrome.[38,39] Serum AFP levels are normal or show mild, nonspecific elevations. The prognosis is favorable, but tumors can recur after resection, can metastasize, and can rarely cause death.[40-42]

Histologic Findings

The tumor is composed of epithelial cells forming well-defined nests. The tumor nests are irregularly shaped and surrounded by bands of stroma (Figure 19.14). The stroma can be loose and edematous, more commonly at the periphery of the tumor, or densely collagenized and desmoplastic, a pattern more commonly seen in the center of tumor. In fact, the center of the tumors can become almost completely replaced by fibrous scar tissue (Figure 19.15). The tumor has no capsule and the nests of tumor cells can be seen invading at the tumor front (Figure 19.16); in these areas, stroma is typically absent.

The epithelial nests are solid, with no gland formation and no trabecular formation, but can show areas of cystic degeneration. Small duct-like structures (? reactive) can also be located at the edges of the tumor nests (Figure 19.17). The tumor cells are mostly epithelioid but can be more spindled in some nests. The epithelial nests also frequently show calcification/ossification (à la the tumor's name) (Figure 19.18). Rarely, foci of

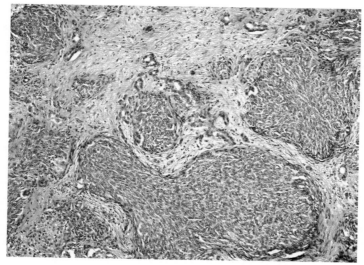

FIGURE 19.14 **Calcifying nested stromal-epithelial tumor.** There are nests of epithelial tumor cells in a background of dense stroma.

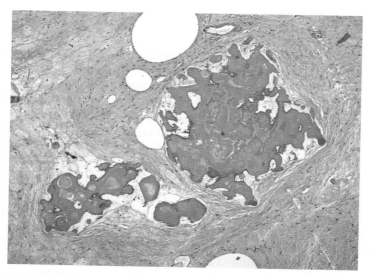

FIGURE 19.15 **Calcifying nested stromal-epithelial tumor.** The center of this tumor is acellular, replaced by fibrous scar and calcifications.

dedifferentiation can be seen, with growth of tumor cells in nonspecific trabeculae (Figure 19.19).

Immunohistochemical Findings

The tumors cells show nuclear accumulation of β-catenin, as well as abnormal cytoplasmic staining (Figure 19.20).[43,44] The tumor cells are positive for

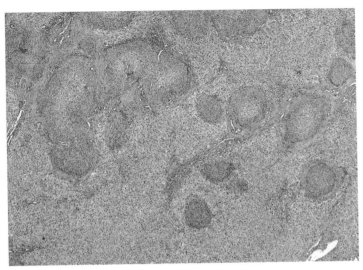

FIGURE 19.16 **Calcifying nested stromal-epithelial tumor.** The interface of the tumor shows nests of infiltrated tumor cells with little stroma.

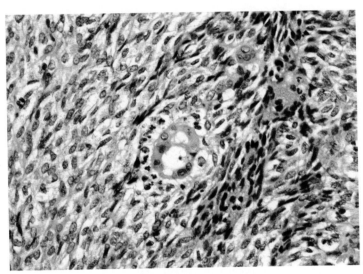

FIGURE 19.17 **Calcifying nested stromal-epithelial tumor.** Small duct-like structures can be seen at the edges of some tumor nests.

cytokeratins AE1/AE3 and CAM5.2, while other keratins such as CK7 and CK19 are positive in a variable number of cases. CK20 is negative. In addition to keratins, tumor cells are positive for NSE, WT-1, and vimentin.[38,39,45] Markers of hepatocellular differentiation are consistently negative, including polyclonal CEA (negative for canalicular staining), arginase, HepPar1,

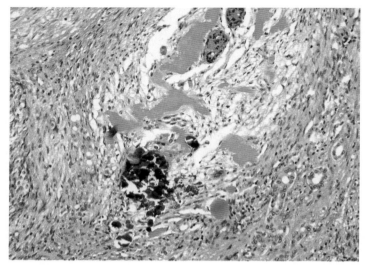

FIGURE 19.18 Calcifying nested stromal-epithelial tumor. This tumor nest shows ossification.

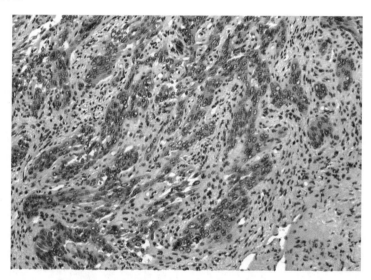

FIGURE 19.19 Calcifying nested stromal-epithelial tumor. An area of tumor dedifferentiation shows tumor cells growing in thin trabeculae.

AFP, and albumin in situ hybridization.[38,39,45,46] CD56 is often positive but this does not indicate neuroendocrine differentiation; chromogranin and synaptophysin stains are negative. The stroma that surrounds the epithelial nests appears to be reactive and can show smooth muscle actin staining, usually weakly and focally, while desmin and myogenin immunostains are negative.

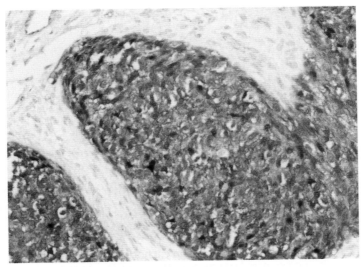

FIGURE 19.20 **Calcifying nested stromal-epithelial tumor.** β-Catenin immunostain shows cytoplasmic and nuclear staining.

BENIGN NODULAR LESIONS IN CHOLESTATIC PEDIATRIC LIVER DISEASE

Approximately 5% of livers with cirrhosis secondary to biliary atresia can develop large nodules that on imaging studies are worrisome for hepatocellular carcinoma.[47] The nodules average 5 cm in size, but some can be larger than 10 cm. Almost all these cases are macroregenerative nodules (Figure 19.21) and not hepatocellular carcinoma. However, hepatocellular carcinomas rarely occur in the setting of cirrhosis from biliary atresia (<1% of cases),[48] so biopsies are often performed. The diagnosis of a macroregenerative nodule or hepatocellular carcinoma should be made using the same criteria as in adults.

FOCAL NODULAR HYPERPLASIA

FNHs develop in up to 8% of children who receive chemotherapy for various malignancies.[49] They can occur many years after therapy, with a median interval of about 10 years.[49] The reported frequencies of pediatric FNH in this setting varies significantly, likely reflecting the length of follow-up as well as the chemotherapeutic agent. Some studies have suggested a link with high-dose alkylating agents or radiotherapy.[50] The diagnosis of an FNH should be made using the same criteria as in adults. In this author's experience, the most common difficulty in making this diagnosis in children is the underappreciation that this lesion occurs in children.

PEDIATRIC HEPATIC ADENOMAS

Hepatic adenomas in children are rare, but occur in several settings. The most common setting is glycogen storage diseases, type I, type III, and

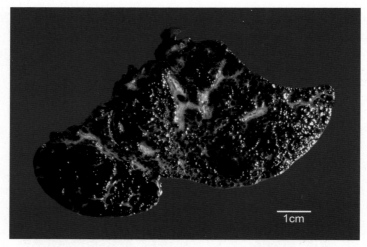

FIGURE 19.21 **Macroregenerative nodule in cirrhosis from biliary atresia.** The nodule stands out as a deep-green nodule on the surface (lower left of image).

less commonly type VI.[51-53] Rare cases of hepatic adenomas have also been reported in Hurler syndrome, severe combined immunodeficiency, Fanconi anemia, and many other rare inherited genetic diseases.[54] Hepatic adenomas in the setting of Fanconi anemia are most commonly associated with androgen therapy and some can show significant cytologic atypia.[54] In cases of glycogen storage disease, most hepatic adenomas are of the inflammatory type or are unclassified.[55]

The histologic diagnosis is made in the same manner as for adult hepatic adenomas. Hepatic adenomas in all these conditions have a risk for malignant transformation, similar to sporadic adenomas in adults.

HEPATOBLASTOMAS

Definition

Hepatoblastomas are malignant epithelial tumors that show varying degrees of hepatic differentiation and may have a malignant sarcomatous component. An epithelial component is required.

Clinical Findings

Epidemiologic studies indicate that 91% of all pediatric liver tumors in patients less than 5 years of age are hepatoblastomas.[56] The median age at presentation is approximately 18 months. Up to 5% of tumors are diagnosed at birth, and approximately 70% are diagnosed before the age of 2 years. Hepatoblastomas can also be first diagnosed after the age of 5 years, but this is very rare and hepatoblastomas are almost never seen past the age of 12 years. There are several dozen case reports of hepatoblastomas occurring in adults,[57] and you can never say never, but many of these appear likely to have better diagnoses. Overall, this group of cases reported as adult hepatoblastomas is likely a mixture of different types of tumors, including many poorly differentiated hepatocellular carcinomas with sarcomatoid features and metastatic carcinosarcomas.

Risk factors for hepatoblastomas are poorly understood, but there is a clear association with prematurity and low birth weight, especially with birth weights less than 1500 g. A modest male predominance of 2:1 has been consistently identified. There is a large list of congenital anomalies that can co-occur with hepatoblastomas, but the frequency of any given finding is low. Overall, an estimated 15% of hepatoblastomas arise in the setting of known genetic syndromes.[58] Of these, the strongest association to date has been with familial adenomatosis polyposis and the Beckwith-Wiedemann syndrome. Regardless of whether or not there is an associated genetic disorder, the background livers show no histologic evidence of chronic liver disease and no fibrosis.

The clinical presentation is nonspecific but typically includes an enlarging abdomen and some degree of weight loss and anorexia. Many paraneoplastic syndromes have been described, but most of them are rare and do not provide unique insight into the diagnosis or the etiology of hepatoblastomas.

Serum AFP levels are markedly elevated in >95% of cases and play an important role in patient workup and in monitoring response to tumor therapy. About 2% to 4% of cases will have normal or mild elevations in serum AFP levels at the time of diagnosis (less than 100 ng/mL).[59] Hepatoblastomas that lack serum AFP level elevations have a worse prognosis and are strongly associated with the small cell undifferentiated morphology.

Histologic Findings

OVERVIEW. Many hepatoblastomas are treated in order to shrink the tumor before resection. Biopsies are often performed before the introduction of therapy. Currently, there are seven generally accepted growth patterns that can be seen within hepatoblastomas (Table 19.1); these patterns are important for prognostication. In order to correctly classify resected hepatoblastomas, at least one section per centimeter of tumor should be submmited.[60] Hepatoblastomas are also classified on biopsy specimens, realizing that the resection specimen may have histologic findings that change the final classification. For clinical care, the most important patterns are (1) the pure fetal pattern with low mitotic activity and (2) the small cell undifferentiated pattern; the first is cured by complete resection, without need for adjuvant chemotherapy, while the small cell undifferentiated pattern is treated with more aggressive chemotherapy.

Examination of resected hepatoblastomas shows that about 40% have both mesenchymal and epithelial components, although the frequency of

	Small Cell		
Feature	Undifferentiated	Embryonal	Fetal
Cell size	Small cells (5-10 µm)	Medium-sized cells (10-15 µm)	Larger cells (10-20 µm)
Cytoplasm	Scant, pale to amphophilic, sometimes more basophilic	Basophilic, high N:C ratio	Moderate amounts of eosino- philic to clear cytoplasm
Nucleus	Fine chromatin	Angulated	Clumpy chromatin
	Inconspicuous nucleoli	Small nucleoli	Variably promi- nent nucleoli
Architecture	• Often discohesive • Solid or nested growth pattern • Negative for well-defined tra- beculae, acini, or pseudoglands	• Solid growth pattern • Pseudoglands	• Solid growth pattern • Trabecular growth pattern • Alternating "light and dark"
Immunostains	• Glypican 3- negative or -positive (focal)	• Glypican 3 posi- tive with coarse, clumpy cytoplas- mic staining	• Glypican 3- negative or -positive with light stippled cytoplasmic staining
	• HepPar1-negative	• HepPar1-positive	• HepPar1- positive
	• Arginase-negative	• Arginase-positive	• Arginase-positive

TABLE 19.1 **Major Epithelial Types in Hepatoblastomas**

mesenchymal tissue is lower in biopsy specimens. The epithelial components will have varying degrees of hepatocellular differentiation evident on
morphology and immunostains, which to some degree recapitulates the normal embryologic development of the liver. The epithelium is classified by the
degree of maturity, going from the least mature to most mature as follows:
small cell undifferentiated, embryonal, fetal, and macrotrabecular. Mixed
patterns are common (about 80% of cases). When a single, pure pattern is
present, most will show a fetal pattern. Overall, the most common patterns
are the embryonal and fetal, with the fetal pattern present at least focally in
about 80% of cases and the embryonal pattern in about 30% of cases.[61,62]
The remaining patterns are less frequent, each found in 5% or fewer cases.

SMALL CELL UNDIFFERENTIATED PATTERN. The small cell undifferentiated morphologic pattern is composed of small, basophilic tumor cells (Figure 19.22).
In some cases, the tumor cells resemble blastemal cells (Figure 19.23).

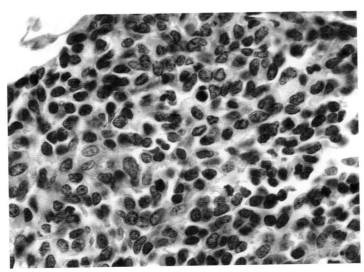

FIGURE 19.22 **Hepatoblastoma, small cell undifferentiated pattern.** The tumor cells are small with scant cytoplasm.

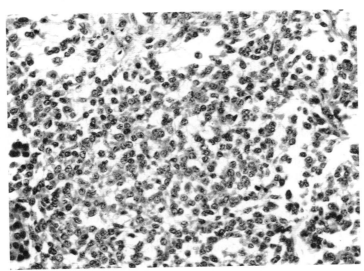

FIGURE 19.23 **Hepatoblastoma, small cell undifferentiated pattern.** The tumor cells in this image resemble blastemal cells.

The tumor cells grow in large sheets that are often poorly cohesive. The also lack pseudoglands and trabeculae. Mitotic activity is high and the cells are small (5-10 μm) with scant cytoplasm. The nuclear chromatin is coarse with small indistinct nucleoli. In most cases, the small cell undifferentiated pattern is admixed with embryonal and fetal patterns (Figure 19.24). For treatment and prognosis, the best cutoff for the minimum percentage of tumor with a small cell undifferentiated pattern has not been

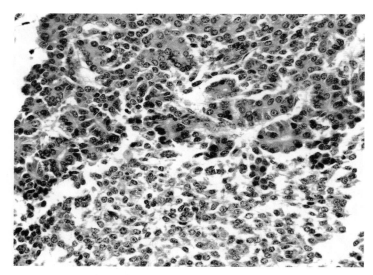

FIGURE 19.24 **Hepatoblastoma, small cell undifferentiated pattern.** Small nests of small cell undifferentiated tumor cells are seen juxtaposed to the embryonal pattern.

fully established, but until that happens, any definite component of small cell undifferentiated pattern should be mentioned in the pathology report.

Markers of hepatic differentiation include immunostains for cytokeratins and (at least historically) electron microscopy for fat, glycogen, bile, and bile canaliculi. Overall, immunostains for cytokeratins are the most sensitive, with CK19 or broad-spectrum cytokeratins performing the best. Tumor cells are often patchy-positive for vimentin. Glypican 3 is generally negative[63] or only focally positive.[64] Immunostains for HepPar1 are negative.[65] β-Catenin shows strong and diffuse nuclear staining.[63] INI-1 immunostaining is used to exclude a rhabdoid tumor (INI-1 shows retained nuclear staining in small cell undifferentiated hepatoblastomas).

EMBRYONAL PATTERN. Embryonal epithelium is almost always seen in conjunction with fetal epithelium. Embryonal epithelium is composed of small basophilic cells with scant cytoplasm and angulated nuclei (Figure 19.25). Cells can be seen growing in sheets and often form small rosettes or pseudoglands. Embryonal epithelium is easiest to find at low power, as the small basophilic cells contrast with the larger, more eosinophilic epithelium of the fetal type growth pattern. Immunostains are positive for HepPar1 and arginase.[64] Glypican 3 shows a strong, granular, cytoplasmic staining pattern (Figure 19.26). Immunostaining for β-catenin shows nuclear accumulation, often accompanied by cytoplasmic staining.

FETAL PATTERN. The fetal pattern is the most common pattern in hepatoblastomas, and most hepatoblastomas have at least a minor component of the fetal pattern. In the fetal pattern, tumor cells show morphologic evidence for hepatic differentiation on hematoxylin-eosin (H&E) (ie, they look like

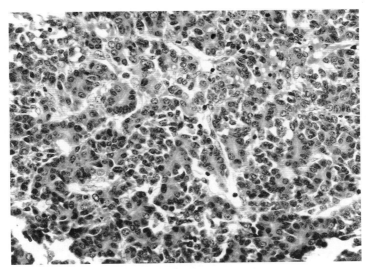

FIGURE 19.25 **Hepatoblastoma, embryonal pattern.** There are small angulated and basophilic tumor cells with rosette formation.

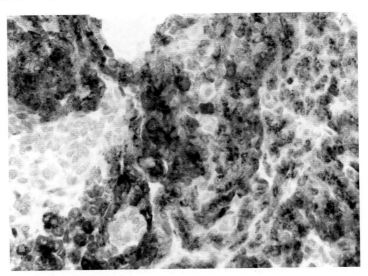

FIGURE 19.26 **Hepatoblastoma, embryonal pattern, glypican 3.** There is strong, granular cytoplasmic staining. A nest of small cell undifferentiated cells are essentially negative.

hepatocytes) and grow in solid sheets or in trabeculae (Figure 19.27). In addition, the tumor cells can produce bile. They can also have varying degrees of glycogen accumulation that causes a "light and dark pattern" at low power (Figure 19.28), which can be further accentuated with a PAS stain. This finding is very distinctive but is not specific for hepatoblastoma and can sometimes be seen in conventional hepatocellular carcinoma. Also, do not mistake alternating areas of embryonal/fetal epithelium as a

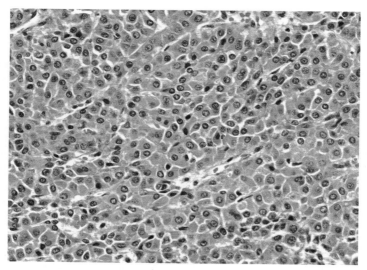

FIGURE 19.27 **Hepatoblastoma, fetal pattern.** The tumor cells show hepatocellular differentiation on hematoxylin-eosin (H&E) staining.

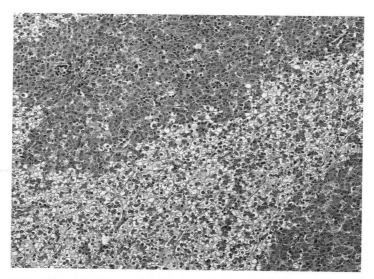

FIGURE 19.28 **Hepatoblastoma, fetal pattern.** A fetal growth pattern is shown, with light and dark areas of the tumor.

"light and dark pattern," as this pattern refers only to variegated glycogen accumulation in fetal epithelium.

It is not uncommon to find cells that are somewhat in between the fetal and embryonal morphology, and the final classification is based on the predominant pattern. In fetal epithelium, immunostains are positive for HepPar1, arginase, and ALB-ISH. In contrast to the embryonal pattern, glypican 3 in the fetal pattern is negative or shows a weak, stippled, cytoplasmic staining pattern (Figure 19.29); this observation can be helpful in

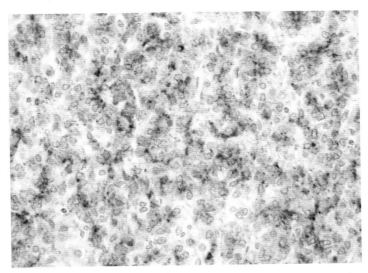

FIGURE 19.29 **Hepatoblastoma, fetal pattern, glypican 3.** There is weaker, stippled cytoplasmic staining.

distinguishing the fetal pattern from the embryonal pattern in difficult cases, but should be used in conjunction with the morphology. β-Catenin is positive for nuclear accumulation, but usually with only scattered positive nuclei; overall less nuclear staining is seen than that in the embryonal pattern.

FETAL HEPATOBLASTOMA SUBTYPES. If the histology shows a pure fetal growth pattern (no small cell undifferentiated or embryonal component, no mesenchymal component), then the next step is to count mitotic figures and assess the degree of cytologic atypia. The pure fetal pattern with low mitotic activity has no more than 1 mitotic figure in 10 high-power fields and no areas of striking cytologic atypia. This pattern has an excellent prognosis and can be cured by resection alone. If the hepatoblastoma has a pure fetal growth pattern but 2 or more mitoses in 10 high-power fields, then it is classified as a mitotically active fetal hepatoblastoma (an alternative term is crowded fetal hepatoblastoma).

PLEOMORPHIC HEPATOBLASTOMA. If the hepatoblastoma has more striking cytologic atypia than is typical for hepatoblastomas (Figure 19.30), with cytologic atypia that is reminiscent of a conventional hepatocellular carcinoma, then the pattern is called *pleomorphic hepatoblastoma*. The tumor cells may show features of either crowded fetal or embryonal patterns. Most cases of pleomorphic hepatoblastoma have greater than 2 mitoses in 10 high-power fields, and atypical mitotic figures can be seen. This pattern may show histologic overlap with conventional hepatocellular carcinoma; a good diagnostic approach is to look for other hepatoblastoma patterns to establish the diagnosis of hepatoblastoma.

MACROTRABECULAR HEPATOBLASTOMA. In this pattern, the tumor cells grow in thickened trabecula that can be 5 to 30 cells in thickness (Figure 19.31). In most cases, the macrotrabecular growth pattern is a minor component

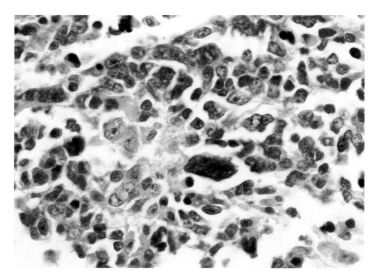

FIGURE 19.30 **Hepatoblastoma, pleomorphic.** There is marked nuclear pleomorphism.

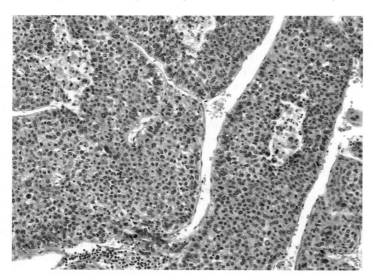

FIGURE 19.31 **Hepatoblastoma, macrotrabecular.** The tumor is growing in thick bulbous plates.

of the tumor but can be seen focally in about 10% of hepatoblastomas.[66,67] The cells have moderate amounts of cytoplasm and thus resemble fetal type epithelium overall, but the cytoplasm can range from basophilic to eosinophilic. The results of tumor stains are similar to those for fetal epithelium, with positive staining for HepPar1, arginase, and often glypican 3.

This pattern shows considerable overlap with similar changes seen in some conventional hepatocellular carcinomas. In both cases, serum AFP levels are usually elevated, so the distinction from a conventional hepatocellular carcinoma is best made by looking for other more typical hepatoblastoma patterns within the same tumor. If no other hepatoblastoma patterns are present, then the most likely diagnosis is conventional hepatocellular carcinoma, as hepatoblastomas with a pure macrotrabecular growth pattern are exceptionally rare, if they exist. In addition, patients older than 5 years at presentation are, in general, more likely to have a conventional hepatocellular carcinoma.

CHOLANGIOBLASTIC PATTERN. The cholangioblastic pattern (sometimes called *cholangiocellular*) shows biliary differentiation, usually with rather poorly formed glands. Overall, this pattern is very rare, is usually focal, and tends to be associated with areas of mesenchymal differentiation, rather than with areas of embryonal or fetal differentiation. There are ductlike structures embedded in a mesenchymal component (Figure 19.32). The cholangioblastic pattern appears to be more common after treatment with chemotherapy. Treated specimens may also have areas of benign bile ductular reaction at the edges of the tumor bed, where the tumor bed interfaces with the background liver. In most cases, this benign, reactive process can be differentiated from the cholangioblastic pattern because of the lack of atypia and mitotic figures. In difficult cases, nuclear accumulation of β-catenin in the glandular cells may be helpful, indicating a diagnosis of malignant cells.

Mesenchymal Components

All hepatoblastomas have an epithelial component by definition, but about 40% will also have a mesenchymal component. For hepatoblastomas with mixed epithelial and mesenchymal features, the epithelium is typically of the fetal type, but should be classified as discussed earlier. The mesenchymal tissue is usually a mixture of mature and immature fibrous tissue and osteoid material (80% of cases) (Figures 19.33 and 19.34). In most cases,

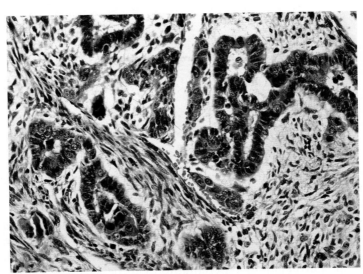

FIGURE 19.32 **Hepatoblastoma, cholangioblastic.** A focus of atypical glandular growth is seen.

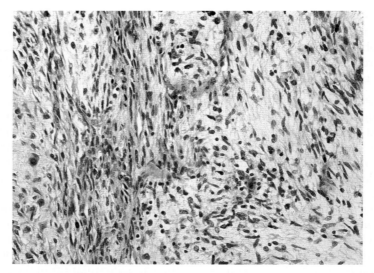

FIGURE 19.33 **Hepatoblastoma, mesenchymal.** Immature and cytologically atypical fibrous tissue is seen within this hepatoblastoma.

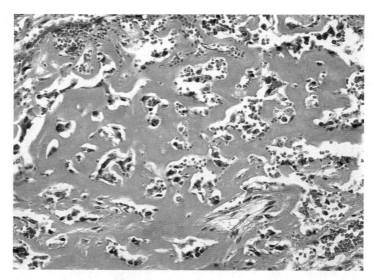

FIGURE 19.34 **Hepatoblastoma, osteoid.** The mesenchymal tissue in this hepatoblastoma shows osteoid material.

the mesenchymal tissue is composed of cytologically bland, plump, and spindled cells that do not show much differentiation. The mesenchymal component can range from being loose and myxoid (most cases) to dense and cellular. Cartilaginous differentiation can be seen, as well as, rarely, skeletal muscle.

Teratoid Hepatoblastoma

To qualify as a teratoid hepatoblastoma, there should be areas of epithelial, mesenchymal, and neuroectodermal differentiation. The epithelial component can show mucinous epithelium or stratified squamous epithelium (Figure 19.35), but be aware that squamous differentiation can also be a nonspecific, posttherapeutic finding. The mesenchymal component can be composed of mature or immature fibrous tissue, which sometimes can show striking myxoid changes, osteoid, or striated muscle. The neuroectodermal component can be melanin-containing cells (Figure 19.36), neural cells, or glial elements. The melanin-containing cells may be seen as small foci scattered in the epithelial components.

Prognosis

The most important prognostic feature is complete resection. Low serum AFP levels indicate a worse prognosis. As noted earlier, this is because low serum AFP levels are strongly associated with a small cell undifferentiated morphology, which has a worse prognosis. Angiolymphatic invasion has also been identified as a bad prognostic sign in some studies.

Diagnostic Challenges

The diagnosis is comfortably made in most cases by paying attention to the typical serum AFP level elevations and the well-described histologic patterns. There are three main areas of potential diagnostic challenges. First, the differential for small cell undifferentiated hepatoblastomas can include metastatic small round blue cell tumors such as Wilms tumor and

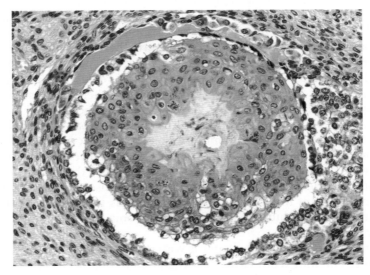

FIGURE 19.35 **Hepatoblastoma, stratified squamous epithelium.** A small nest is present.

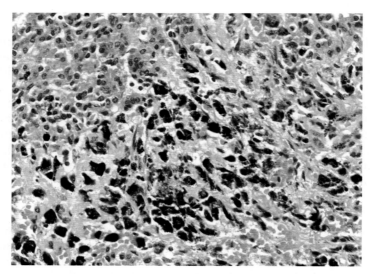

FIGURE 19.36 **Hepatoblastoma, neuroectodermal tissue.** Pigmented cells are seen.

neuroblastoma. In these cases, the immunostain can confirm the diagnosis in most cases. There is a small subset of tumors, however, in which the diagnosis remains unclear based on the histology and immunostain findings, and the best diagnosis on a biopsy specimen may be a prioritized differential.

The second potential diagnostic challenge is primary liver cancers that occur in older children and adolescents. Most of these cancers will be conventional hepatocellular carcinomas. In difficult cases, the presence of underlying liver disease strongly favors hepatocellular carcinoma, so get as much clinical information as you can and carefully examine the background, nonneoplastic liver. When you examine the tumor, do not force a diagnosis of hepatoblastoma if it is not clearly there. The most challenging cases are when your differential is that of pure fetal type of hepatoblastoma, or fetal with minor components of embryonal, versus typical hepatocellular carcinoma. The serum AFP levels can often help differentiate these two possibilities; if the serum AFP level is high, it is not helpful, but a low serum AFP level would argue strongly against a hepatoblastoma. If you have a full resection, then submit more blocks to look for typical hepatoblastoma areas. In terms of the morphology, it can be very helpful to pull a few cases of known hepatoblastomas from your files that have fetal areas and compare the histology to your current case. Also, do no overinterpret the significance of finding "light and dark" areas in a tumor, as they can be seen in typical adult hepatocellular carcinoma too; PAS stains are not terribly helpful either.

The final diagnostic challenge is with rhabdoid tumors of the liver; the main differentiating features are that rhabdoid tumors will show INI-1 loss and are negative for markers of hepatocellular differentiation. There was some data that suggested a subset of small cell undifferentiated carcinomas could show INI-1 loss, but currently those are considered to best classified as rhabdoid tumors of the liver.

Molecular Findings

Mutational analysis currently does not play a role in diagnosis, subtyping, or prognosis. Hepatoblastomas have a high frequency of mutations in genes that code for proteins in the Wnt signaling pathway. Of these, β-catenin mutations (*CTNNB1*) are the most common,[68] with a frequency of about 80%.[68,69] Other mutations in the Wnt signaling pathway include *AXIN1*[70] and *AXIN2*.[71] The *APC* gene can also be mutated, but most commonly in individuals with familial adenomatosis polyposis.[72] Other recurrent molecular changes include *TP53* mutations (25% of cases), microsatellite instability (80%),[73] *NFE2L2* mutations (10%), and *TERT* mutations (6%).[74]

HEPATOCELLULAR MALIGNANT NEOPLASM NOT OTHERWISE SPECIFIED

This terminology has been proposed for tumors in which the pathologist is uncomfortable committing to a diagnosis of either hepatoblastoma or conventional hepatocellular carcinoma.[61] An older (and the original) term for this same entity is *transitional liver cell carcinoma*.[75] The lesions have features that resemble both hepatoblastoma and hepatocellular carcinomas. Serum AFP level is typically elevated. Immunostains have not been shown to be helpful in clarifying the diagnosis. Clinical outcomes are mixed, with some behaving more like conventional hepatocellular carcinomas[75] and others more like hepatoblastomas.[76] Molecular studies to date have not solved the riddle on how to best classify this group of tumors. It can be helpful when reporting out these cases to indicate if the tumor has a predominant pattern, for example, "The tumor morphology is predominantly that of conventional hepatocellular carcinoma, but focal areas of embryonal type growth are seen."

In this author's experience, most of these cases can be reasonably classified as conventional hepatocellular carcinomas, especially those that arise in teenaged patients. The histologic areas that resemble embryonal or fetal type differentiation are typically minor morphologic variations or are foci of tumor cells that are less well-differentiated.

PEDIATRIC HEPATOCELLULAR CARCINOMA

Pediatric hepatocellular carcinomas are rare, but are a well-recognized complication of chronic liver disease. Hepatitis B infection is probably the most common worldwide cause of pediatric hepatocellular carcinoma. Cirrhosis from other causes is also an important risk factor, including biliary atresia, tyrosinemia, bile salt deficiency diseases, and glycogen storage disorders.

As for adults, hepatocellular carcinomas can develop in both cirrhotic and noncirrhotic livers. Some hepatocellular carcinomas that arise in noncirrhotic livers will have background liver disease, such as portal vein loss in the Abernethy syndrome,[77] whereas in other cases, there may be no clear clinical or histologic evidence of chronic liver disease. Fibrolamellar carcinomas can arise in children and teenaged youths, but the median age is in the mid-20s, so these carcinomas are discussed in detail in Chapter 21.

Morphology

The morphologic features of pediatric hepatocellular carcinomas are the same as in adults and the diagnosis is made in the same manner (Figure 19.37). There is relatively little data on the immunohistochemical profile, but pediatric hepatocellular carcinomas appear to have a higher frequency of CK7 staining than adults.[78]

PEDIATRIC BILIARY TUMORS

Bile duct hamartomas and bile duct adenomas are exceptionally rare in children, but they can be seen in cirrhotic livers. Cholangiocarcinomas are rare in the pediatric population, but chronic biliary tract disease from Caroli disease and primary sclerosing cholangitis are recognized risk factors.[79,80] *ABCB11* mutation, leading to bile salt export pump (BSEP) deficiency, is also an important risk factor.[81] The morphologic findings (Figure 19.38) and diagnostic criteria for pediatric cholangiocarcinoma are the same as for adults.

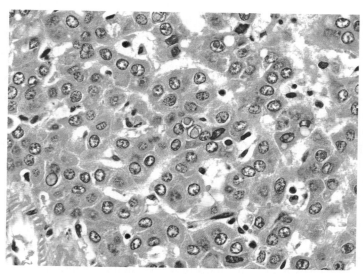

FIGURE 19.37 **Pediatric hepatocellular carcinoma.** This well-differentiated hepatocellular carcinoma was found in a child with cryptogenic cirrhosis.

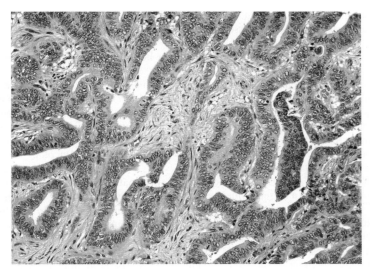

FIGURE 19.38 **Pediatric hepatocellular carcinoma.** The morphologic findings are essentially identical to those seen in adults.

REFERENCES

1. Mo JQ, Dimashkieh HH, Bove KE. GLUT1 endothelial reactivity distinguishes hepatic infantile hemangioma from congenital hepatic vascular malformation with associated capillary proliferation. *Hum Pathol*. 2004;35:200-209.
2. Huang SA, Tu HM, Harney JW, et al. Severe hypothyroidism caused by type 3 iodothyronine deiodinase in infantile hemangiomas. *N Engl J Med*. 2000;343:185-189.
3. Han SJ, Tsai CC, Tsai HM, et al. Infantile hemangioendothelioma with a highly elevated serum alpha-fetoprotein level. *Hepatogastroenterology*. 1998;45:459-461.
4. Sari N, Yalcin B, Akyuz C, et al. Infantile hepatic hemangioendothelioma with elevated serum alpha-fetoprotein. *Pediatr Hematol Oncol*. 2006;23:639-647.
5. Kulungowski AM, Alomari AI, Chawla A, et al. Lessons from a liver hemangioma registry: subtype classification. *J Pediatr Surg*. 2012;47:165-170.
6. Ito H, Kishikawa T, Toda T, et al. Hepatic mensenchymal hamartoma of an infant. *J Pediatr Surg*. 1984;19:315-317.
7. Fretzayas A, Moustaki M, Kitsiou S, et al. Long-term follow-up of a multifocal hepatic mesenchymal hamartoma producing a-fetoprotein. *Pediatr Surg Int*. 2009;25:381-384.
8. Stringer MD, Alizai NK. Mesenchymal hamartoma of the liver: a systematic review. *J Pediatr Surg*. 2005;40:1681-1690.
9. Papastratis G, Margaris H, Zografos GN, et al. Mesenchymal hamartoma of the liver in an adult: a review of the literature. *Int J Clin Pract*. 2000;54:552-554.
10. Speleman F, De Telder V, De Potter KR, et al. Cytogenetic analysis of a mesenchymal hamartoma of the liver. *Canc Genet Cytogenet*. 1989;40:29-32.
11. Rakheja D, Margraf LR, Tomlinson GE, et al. Hepatic mesenchymal hamartoma with translocation involving chromosome band 19q13.4: a recurrent abnormality. *Canc Genet Cytogenet*. 2004;153:60-63.
12. Apellaniz-Ruiz M, Segni M, Kettwig M, et al. Mesenchymal hamartoma of the liver and DICER1 syndrome. *N Engl J Med*. 2019;380:1834-1842.

13. Mack-Detlefsen B, Boemers TM, Groneck P, et al. Multiple hepatic mesenchymal hamartomas in a premature associated with placental mesenchymal dysplasia. *J Pediatr Surg.* 2011;46:e23-e25.

14. Rahadiani N, Stephanie M, Putra J. Recurrent hepatic mesenchymal hamartoma with osseous metaplasia. *Liver Int.* 2018;38:1875.

15. Shintaku M, Watanabe K. Mesenchymal hamartoma of the liver: a proliferative lesion of possible hepatic stellate cell (Ito cell) origin. *Pathol Res Pract.* 2010;206:532-536.

16. Levy M, Trivedi A, Zhang J, et al. Expression of glypican-3 in undifferentiated embryonal sarcoma and mesenchymal hamartoma of the liver. *Hum Pathol.* 2012;43:695-701.

17. Nicol K, Savell V, Moore J, et al. Distinguishing undifferentiated embryonal sarcoma of the liver from biliary tract rhabdomyosarcoma: a Children's Oncology Group study. *Pediatr Dev Pathol.* 2007;10:89-97.

18. Lauwers GY, Grant LD, Donnelly WH, et al. Hepatic undifferentiated (embryonal) sarcoma arising in a mesenchymal hamartoma. *Am J Surg Pathol.* 1997;21:1248-1254.

19. Shi Y, Rojas Y, Zhang W, et al. Characteristics and outcomes in children with undifferentiated embryonal sarcoma of the liver: a report from the National Cancer Database. *Pediatr Blood Canc.* 2017;64.

20. Setty BA, Jinesh GG, Arnold M, et al. The genomic landscape of undifferentiated embryonal sarcoma of the liver is typified by C19MC structural rearrangement and overexpression combined with TP53 mutation or loss. *PLoS Genet.* 2020;16:e1008642.

21. Buetow PC, Buck JL, Pantongrag-Brown L, et al. Undifferentiated (embryonal) sarcoma of the liver: pathologic basis of imaging findings in 28 cases. *Radiology.* 1997;203:779-783.

22. Yoon JY, Lee JM, Kim do Y, et al. A case of embryonal sarcoma of the liver mimicking a hydatid cyst in an adult. *Gut Liver.* 2010;4:245-249.

23. Perez-Gomez RM, Soria-Cespedes D, de Leon-Bojorge B, et al. Diffuse membranous immunoreactivity of CD56 and paranuclear dot-like staining pattern of cytokeratins AE1/3, CAM5.2, and OSCAR in undifferentiated (embryonal) sarcoma of the liver. *Appl Immunohistochem Mol Morphol.* 2010;18:195-198.

24. Kiani B, Ferrell LD, Qualman S, et al. Immunohistochemical analysis of embryonal sarcoma of the liver. *Appl Immunohistochem Mol Morphol.* 2006;14:193-197.

25. Zheng JM, Tao X, Xu AM, et al. Primary and recurrent embryonal sarcoma of the liver: clinicopathological and immunohistochemical analysis. *Histopathology.* 2007;51:195-203.

26. Nishio J, Iwasaki H, Sakashita N, et al. Undifferentiated (embryonal) sarcoma of the liver in middle-aged adults: smooth muscle differentiation determined by immunohistochemistry and electron microscopy. *Hum Pathol.* 2003;34:246-252.

27. Lepreux S, Rebouissou S, Le Bail B, et al. Mutation of TP53 gene is involved in carcinogenesis of hepatic undifferentiated (embryonal) sarcoma of the adult, in contrast with Wnt or telomerase pathways: an immunohistochemical study of three cases with genomic relation in two cases. *J Hepatol.* 2005;42:424-429.

28. Lack EE, Perez-Atayde AR, Schuster SR. Botryoid rhabdomyosarcoma of the biliary tract. *Am J Surg Pathol.* 1981;5:643-652.

29. Kebudi R, Gorgun O, Ayan I, et al. Rhabdomyosarcoma of the biliary tree. *Pediatr Int.* 2003;45:469-471.

30. Wagner BJ, Plum PS, Apel K, et al. Protein-loss of SWI/SNF-complex core subunits influences prognosis dependent on histological subtypes of intra- and extrahepatic cholangiocarcinoma. *Oncol Lett.* 2021;21:349.

31. Trobaugh-Lotrario AD, Finegold MJ, Feusner JH. Rhabdoid tumors of the liver: rare, aggressive, and poorly responsive to standard cytotoxic chemotherapy. *Pediatr Blood Cancer.* 2011;57:423-428.

32. Martelli MG, Liu C. Malignant rhabdoid tumour of the liver in a seven-month-old female infant: a case report and literature review. *Afr J Paediatr Surg.* 2013;10:50-54.

33. Oita S, Terui K, Komatsu S, et al. Malignant rhabdoid tumor of the liver: a case report and literature review. *Pediatr Rep.* 2015;7:5578.

34. Sibileau E, Moroch J, Teyssedou C, et al. Malignant rhabdoid tumors of the liver: an exceptional tumor in adults – a case report and literature review. *Eur J Gastroenterol Hepatol.* 2011;23:104-108.

35. Marzano E, Lermite E, Nobili C, et al. Malignant rhabdoid tumour of the liver in the young adult: report of first two cases. *HPB Surg.* 2009;2009:628206.

36. Kohashi K, Nakatsura T, Kinoshita Y, et al. Glypican 3 expression in tumors with loss of SMARCB1/INI1 protein expression. *Hum Pathol.* 2013;44:526-533.

37. Chan ES, Pawel BR, Corao DA, et al. Immunohistochemical expression of glypican-3 in pediatric tumors: an analysis of 414 cases. *Pediatr Dev Pathol.* 2013;16:272-277.

38. Makhlouf HR, Abdul-Al HM, Wang G, et al. Calcifying nested stromal-epithelial tumors of the liver: a clinicopathologic, immunohistochemical, and molecular genetic study of 9 cases with a long-term follow-up. *Am J Surg Pathol.* 2009;33:976-983.

39. Heerema-McKenney A, Leuschner I, Smith N, et al. Nested stromal epithelial tumor of the liver: six cases of a distinctive pediatric neoplasm with frequent calcifications and association with cushing syndrome. *Am J Surg Pathol.* 2005;29:10-20.

40. Brodsky SV, Sandoval C, Sharma N, et al. Recurrent nested stromal epithelial tumor of the liver with extrahepatic metastasis: case report and review of literature. *Pediatr Dev Pathol.* 2008;11:469-473.

41. Hommann M, Kaemmerer D, Daffner W, et al. Nested stromal epithelial tumor of the liver – liver transplantation and follow-up. *J Gastrointest Cancer.* 2011;42:292-295.

42. Heywood G, Burgart LJ, Nagorney DM. Ossifying malignant mixed epithelial and stromal tumor of the liver: a case report of a previously undescribed tumor. *Cancer.* 2002;94:1018-1022.

43. Malowany JI, Merritt NH, Chan NG, et al. Nested stromal epithelial tumor of the liver in Beckwith-Wiedemann syndrome. *Pediatr Dev Pathol.* 2013;16:312-317.

44. Assmann G, Kappler R, Zeindl-Eberhart E, et al. beta-Catenin mutations in 2 nested stromal epithelial tumors of the liver—a neoplasia with defective mesenchymal-epithelial transition. *Hum Pathol.* 2012;43:1815-1827.

45. Hill DA, Swanson PE, Anderson K, et al. Desmoplastic nested spindle cell tumor of liver: report of four cases of a proposed new entity. *Am J Surg Pathol.* 2005;29:1-9.

46. Grazi GL, Vetrone G, d'Errico A, et al. Nested stromal-epithelial tumor (NSET) of the liver: a case report of an extremely rare tumor. *Pathol Res Pract.* 2010;206:282-286.

47. Liang JL, Cheng YF, Concejero AM, et al. Macro-regenerative nodules in biliary atresia: CT/MRI findings and their pathological relations. *World J Gastroenterol.* 2008;14:4529-4534.

48. Hadzic N, Quaglia A, Portmann B, et al. Hepatocellular carcinoma in biliary atresia: King's College Hospital experience. *J Pediatr.* 2011;159:617-622.e1.

49. Smith EA, Salisbury S, Martin R, et al. Incidence and etiology of new liver lesions in pediatric patients previously treated for malignancy. *AJR Am J Roentgenol.* 2012;199:186-191.

50. Bouyn CI, Leclere J, Raimondo G, et al. Hepatic focal nodular hyperplasia in children previously treated for a solid tumor. Incidence, risk factors, and outcome. *Cancer.* 2003;97:3107-3113.

51. Labrune P, Trioche P, Duvaltier I, et al. Hepatocellular adenomas in glycogen storage disease type I and III: a series of 43 patients and review of the literature. *J Pediatr Gastroenterol Nutr.* 1997;24:276-279.

52. Alshak NS, Cocjin J, Podesta L, et al. Hepatocellular adenoma in glycogen storage disease type IV. *Arch Pathol Lab Med.* 1994;118:88-91.

53. Manzia TM, Angelico R, Toti L, et al. Glycogen storage disease type Ia and VI associated with hepatocellular carcinoma: two case reports. *Transplant Proc.* 2011;43:1181-1183.

54. Resnick MB, Kozakewich HP, Perez-Atayde AR. Hepatic adenoma in the pediatric age group. Clinicopathological observations and assessment of cell proliferative activity. *Am J Surg Pathol*. 1995;19:1181-1190.

55. Sakellariou S, Al-Hussaini H, Scalori A, et al. Hepatocellular adenoma in glycogen storage disorder type I: a clinicopathological and molecular study. *Histopathology*. 2012;60:E58-E65.

56. Darbari A, Sabin KM, Shapiro CN, et al. Epidemiology of primary hepatic malignancies in U.S. children. *Hepatology*. 2003;38:560-566.

57. Rougemont AL, McLin VA, Toso C, et al. Adult hepatoblastoma: learning from children. *J Hepatol*. 2012;56:1392-1403.

58. Tomlinson GE, Kappler R. Genetics and epigenetics of hepatoblastoma. *Pediatr Blood Cancer*. 2012;59:785-792.

59. De Ioris M, Brugieres L, Zimmermann A, et al. Hepatoblastoma with a low serum alpha-fetoprotein level at diagnosis: the SIOPEL group experience. *Eur J Cancer*. 2008;44:545-550.

60. Finegold MJ, Lopez-Terrada DH, Bowen J, et al. Protocol for the examination of specimens from pediatric patients with hepatoblastoma. *Arch Pathol Lab Med*. 2007;131:520-529.

61. Lopez-Terrada D, Alaggio R, de Davila MT, et al. Towards an international pediatric liver tumor consensus classification: proceedings of the Los Angeles COG liver tumors symposium. *Mod Pathol*. 2014;27:472-491.

62. Ishak KG, Goodman ZD, Stocker JT, et al. *Tumors of the Liver and Intrahepatic Bile Ducts*. Armed Forces Institute of Pathology; 2001:356.

63. Cho SJ. Pediatric liver tumors: updates in classification. *Surg Pathol Clin*. 2020;13:601-623.

64. Zynger DL, Gupta A, Luan C, et al. Expression of glypican 3 in hepatoblastoma: an immunohistochemical study of 65 cases. *Hum Pathol*. 2008;39:224-230.

65. Badve S, Logdberg L, Lal A, et al. Small cells in hepatoblastoma lack "oval" cell phenotype. *Mod Pathol*. 2003;16:930-936.

66. Gupta K, Rane S, Das A, et al. Relationship of beta-catenin and postchemotherapy histopathologic changes with overall survival in patients with hepatoblastoma. *J Pediatr Hematol Oncol*. 2012;34:e320-e328.

67. Chen TC, Hsieh LL, Kuo TT. Absence of p53 gene mutation and infrequent overexpression of p53 protein in hepatoblastoma. *J Pathol*. 1995;176:243-247.

68. Lopez-Terrada D, Gunaratne PH, Adesina AM, et al. Histologic subtypes of hepatoblastoma are characterized by differential canonical Wnt and Notch pathway activation in DLK+ precursors. *Hum Pathol*. 2009;40:783-794.

69. Park WS, Oh RR, Park JY, et al. Nuclear localization of beta-catenin is an important prognostic factor in hepatoblastoma. *J Pathol*. 2001;193:483-490.

70. Taniguchi K, Roberts LR, Aderca IN, et al. Mutational spectrum of beta-catenin, AXIN1, and AXIN2 in hepatocellular carcinomas and hepatoblastomas. *Oncogene*. 2002;21:4863-4871.

71. Koch A, Weber N, Waha A, et al. Mutations and elevated transcriptional activity of conductin (AXIN2) in hepatoblastomas. *J Pathol*. 2004;204:546-554.

72. Hirschman BA, Pollock BH, Tomlinson GE. The spectrum of APC mutations in children with hepatoblastoma from familial adenomatous polyposis kindreds. *J Pediatr*. 2005;147:263-266.

73. Curia MC, Zuckermann M, De Lellis L, et al. Sporadic childhood hepatoblastomas show activation of beta-catenin, mismatch repair defects and p53 mutations. *Mod Pathol*. 2008;21:7-14.

74. Eichenmuller M, Trippel F, Kreuder M, et al. The genomic landscape of hepatoblastoma and their progenies with HCC-like features. *J Hepatol*. 2014;61:1312-1320.

75. Prokurat A, Kluge P, Kosciesza A, et al. Transitional liver cell tumors (TLCT) in older children and adolescents: a novel group of aggressive hepatic tumors expressing beta-catenin. *Med Pediatr Oncol.* 2002;39:510-518.

76. Zhou S, Venkatramani R, Gupta S, et al. Hepatocellular malignant neoplasm, NOS: a clinicopathological study of 11 cases from a single institution. *Histopathology.* 2017;71:813-822.

77. Lisovsky M, Konstas AA, Misdraji J. Congenital extrahepatic portosystemic shunts (Abernethy malformation): a histopathologic evaluation. *Am J Surg Pathol.* 2011;35:1381-1390.

78. Klein WM, Molmenti EP, Colombani PM, et al. Primary liver carcinoma arising in people younger than 30 years. *Am J Clin Pathol.* 2005;124:512-518.

79. Deneau M, Adler DG, Schwartz JJ, et al. Cholangiocarcinoma in a 17-year-old boy with primary sclerosing cholangitis and inflammatory bowel disease. *J Pediatr Gastroenterol Nutr.* 2011;52:617-620.

80. Tanaka S, Kubota M, Yagi M, et al. An 11-year-old male patient demonstrating cholangiocarcinoma associated with congenital biliary dilatation. *J Pediatr Surg.* 2006;41:e15-9.

81. Scheimann AO, Strautnieks SS, Knisely AS, et al. Mutations in bile salt export pump (ABCB11) in two children with progressive familial intrahepatic cholestasis and cholangiocarcinoma. *J Pediatr.* 2007;150:556-559.

20

ADULT BENIGN AND MALIGNANT MESENCHYMAL TUMORS

PSEUDOTUMORS OF THE LIVER

Pseudotumors of the liver can be composed of hepatocytes, inflammatory cells, or mesenchymal cells (Table 20.1). The major pseudotumors that are composed of inflammatory cells or mesenchymal cells are considered in this chapter, while epithelial pseudotumors are considered in the respective chapters on biliary and hepatocellular neoplasms.

ECTOPIC SPLEEN

Ectopic spleens result from blunt-force abdominal trauma that leads to implantation of splenic fragments into the liver, or from incomplete surgical resection of spleens. Ectopic spleens may be found both on the liver capsule and within the hepatic parenchyma.[1] Biopsies of an ectopic spleen look like splenic tissue (Figure 20.1), with lymphoid tissue and sometimes prominent sinusoids, but since the lesion is rare, it can be a trickster, and the first impression can be a vascular neoplasm or a lymphoma. The endothelial cells of the splenic sinusoids are strongly CD8 positive (Figure 20.2), and immunostains show a mixed population of lymphocytes, without features of lymphoma.

SEGMENTAL ATROPHY OF THE LIVER AND NODULAR ELASTOSIS

Definition

Segmental atrophy of the liver is a benign pseudotumor of the liver associated with parenchymal loss and replacement by elastosis and fibrosis.

Clinical

These mass lesions are most commonly subcapsular and have a modest female predominance. The most common presentation is nonspecific, right-sided, upper-quadrant abdominal pain. These pseudotumors range in size from 1 to 10 cm.

TABLE 20.1 **Pseudotumors of the Liver**	
Pseudotumor	**Brief Description**
Focal nodular hyperplasia	Nodules of hepatocytes surrounded by bands of fibrosis containing mild ductular proliferation, often with central scars. Eccentrically thick-walled vessels may be seen in the central scars.
Regenerative hepatic pseudotumor	Mass lesion; portal tracts throughout; vascular thrombi; other regenerative changes related to vascular flow abnormalities
Segmental atrophy and nodular elastosis	Collapsed hepatic parenchyma/elastosis
Hypoxic pseudolobular necrosis	Necrotic hepatocytes
Arteriovenous malformation	Mimics vascular neoplasm
Inflammatory pseudotumor	Inflamed fibrous tissue
Reactive lymphoid hyperplasia	Reactive lymphoid follicles
Ectopic spleen	Benign splenic parenchyma
Sarcoidoma	Confluent granulomas and fibrosis
Amyloidoma	Composed of amyloid

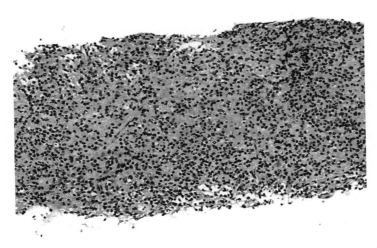

FIGURE 20.1 **Ectopic spleen.** There is a mixture of inflammatory cells and sinusoids.

Histological Findings

The histological findings of this pseudotumor evolve over time, and the findings in a specific case will depend on the relative age of the lesion.[2]

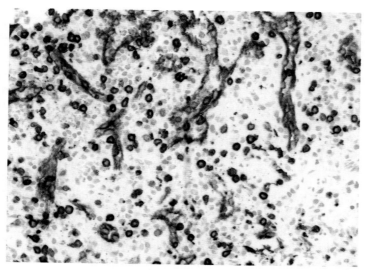

FIGURE 20.2 **Ectopic spleen, CD8.** The sinusoids of the splenic tissue are highlighted.

Early lesions demonstrate parenchymal collapse with marked bile ductular proliferation and mixed inflammation composed of lymphocytes and neutrophils. With time, the inflammation and ductular proliferation abates, and there is increasing amounts of elastosis in the areas of parenchymal loss (Figure 20.3; eFig. 20.1). Biliary cysts are also common at this stage and can rarely dominate the histological findings, especially if they rupture, as this can induce an intense inflammatory response. The biliary cysts are retention-type cysts that result from obstructed, entrapped bile ducts.

In time, the amount of elastosis will increase. At this stage, abundant, amphophilic, extracellular deposits dominate the histological findings, a stage called *nodular elastosis*. Small islands of residual, normal-appearing hepatocytes are common (Figure 20.4), surrounded by extracellular matrix. The distinctive extracellular matrix is composed of admixed reticulin and elastic fibers, which can be highlighted by reticulin and elastic stains. The elastosis often involves the liver capsule (eFig. 20.2). At high power, there will be scattered spindle cells in the matrix without atypia or mitoses (Figure 20.5). These cells will stain with vimentin, which also highlights dendritic-type extensions (Figure 20.6).

Eventually, fibrosis will increase and can ultimately lead to distinctive nodular scars (Figure 20.7). Occasional small calcifications may be present (eFig. 20.3). In all stages, thrombosed and fibrotic vessels are commonly found (Figure 20.8; eFig. 20.4), suggesting a vascular injury as the etiology. In later stages, the histological differential can include a sclerosed hemangioma, and sometimes, the findings may be nonspecific. Findings that support a diagnosis of the end-stage of segmental atrophy

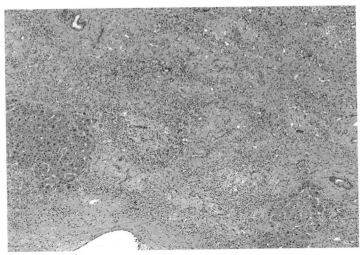

FIGURE 20.3 **Segmental atrophy pseudotumor.** This subcapsular mass lesion shows parenchymal collapse with mild chronic inflammation and patchy bile ductular proliferation. Early elastosis changes can be seen.

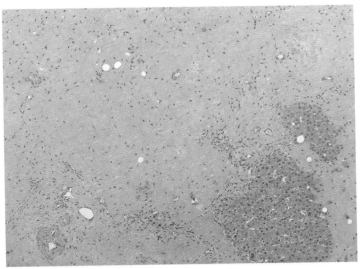

FIGURE 20.4 **Nodular elastosis.** Scattered islands of residual hepatocytes are embedded in a dense extracellular matrix composed of elastic fibers and reticulin fibers.

include islands of residual hepatocytes, floating in a sea of trichrome-blue collagen, and finding thick-walled vessels obliterated by fibrosis.

Rarely, small foci of elastosis can be seen as isolated finding on liver biopsies but are not associated with mass lesions (eFig. 20.5). These small foci are often located in close proximity to the central vein. They are not the same as nodular elastosis and are currently without clinical significance.

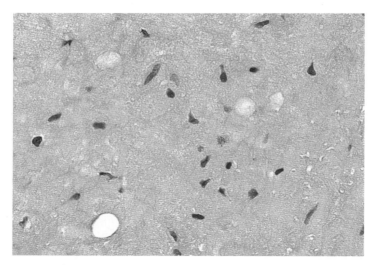

FIGURE 20.5 **Nodular elastosis**. At high power, the spindled cells within the extracellular matrix have no atypia or mitotic activity.

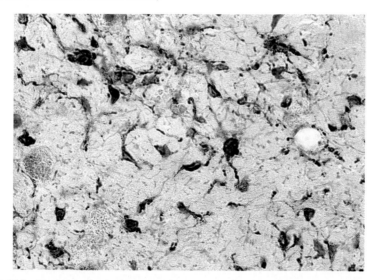

FIGURE 20.6 **Nodular elastosis, vimentin.** The cells have a dendritic morphology.

INFLAMMATORY PSEUDOTUMOR

Definition

Inflammatory pseudotumors are benign, reactive lesions composed of varying degrees of fibrosis and chronic inflammation.

Clinical

Inflammatory pseudotumors of the liver have generated more than their fair share of the literature, with several hundred case reports. There is about a 2:1 male predominance and the average age is 50 years.[3] Most

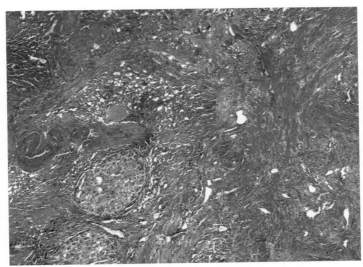

FIGURE 20.7 **Segmental atrophy pseudotumor, fibrotic stage**. End-stage lesions can show a nodule of dense fibrosis with small residual islands of otherwise unremarkable hepatocytes.

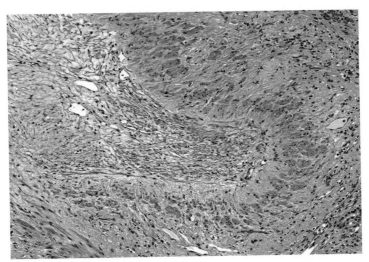

FIGURE 20.8 **Segmental atrophy pseudotumor, thrombosed vessel**. A central vein shows remote thrombosis.

cases represent resolving hepatic bacterial abscesses, which may spontaneously regress or regress after antibiotic therapy. Other recognized causes including IgG4 disease and syphilis infections.

Histology

Inflammatory pseudotumors can be single lesions (approximately 2/3 of cases) or multiple lesions (approximately 1/3 of cases).[3] Single lesions tend to be larger in size than the multifocal lesions. Overall, inflammatory pseudotumors are more common in noncirrhotic livers than in cirrhotic livers.

There are many entities that can mimic an inflammatory pseudotumor, so make this diagnosis with special care. Inflammatory pseudotumors are composed of admixed fibroblasts and inflammatory cells with varying amounts of collagen (Figure 20.9). Early lesions tend to have more inflammation and less fibrosis, while later lesions are the opposite, with less inflammation and more fibrosis. The collagen can be dense and have a whorled appearance in some cases (Figure 20.10). A storiform appearance to the fibrosis is not highly sensitive, nor specific, in biopsy specimens, but is more commonly seen with IgG4 disease; immunostains for IgG4 disease are useful in all cases, even those without storiform fibrosis. Phlebitis can also be seen (Figure 20.11) but is likewise not specific for etiology. Phlebitis tends to involve medium- to larger-sized veins and is more commonly seen in single lesions. There should be no atypia in the spindle cells, and mitoses are absent to rare. The inflammation is lymphocytic (mostly T-cells) and is often rich in plasma cells. B-cells are generally localized to lymphoid aggregates or germinal centers. Multifocal lesions are more commonly seen in the setting of chronic biliary tract disease. The spindled cells in inflammatory pseudotumors are vimentin positive and can be smooth muscle actin positive. They can also show patchy cytokeratin staining.[3]

Differential

Several hematopoietic tumors can closely mimic inflammatory pseudotumors, including Hodgkin lymphoma,[4] dendritic cell sarcomas, and

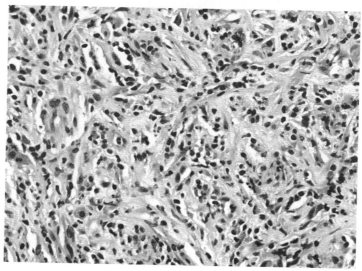

FIGURE 20.9 **Inflammatory pseudotumor.** Inflammatory pseudotumors are composed of chronic inflammation with varying amounts of fibrosis. The inflammation is predominately lymphocytic in this case, with scattered plasma cells and eosinophils.

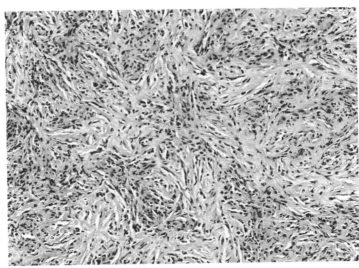

FIGURE 20.10 **Inflammatory pseudotumor.** A storiform pattern of growth is seen on low power.

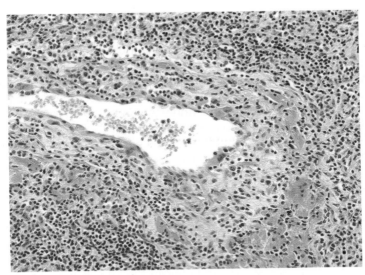

FIGURE 20.11 **Inflammatory pseudotumor, phlebitis.** This large vein shows active inflammation with intimal thickening.

inflammatory myofibroblastic tumors.[5] Anaplastic lymphoma kinase (ALK) staining should be negative; if positive, the lesion is classified as an inflammatory myofibroblastic tumor.

Not surprising given the pathogenesis of most inflammatory pseudotumors, the differential also includes the wall of an abscess; in these cases, the diagnosis is secured by looking for pools of neutrophils representing residual abscess; this is often found at the edge of the biopsy core. IgG4 disease and syphilis should also be ruled out in all cases (please see respective chapters).

Other tumors can have areas that closely resemble inflammatory pseudotumors, including angiomyolipmas[6] and liposarcomas.[7] Also, of note, inflammatory pseudotumors are rarely associated with carcinomas, including cholangiocarcinomas or other tumors that obstruct the common bile duct, with subsequent infectious cholangitis and inflammatory pseudo-tumor formation.[8] Thus, after a diagnosis of an inflammatory pseudotumor is made, the patient should be further worked up for other disease processes, including neoplasms and biliary tract lesions.

CAVERNOUS HEMANGIOMA

Definition

Cavernous hemangiomas are benign vascular tumors composed of dilated, thin-walled vessels. Some authors have suggested that cavernous hemangiomas of the liver are not neoplasms but instead are malformations, but this is not true.

Clinical Findings

Hemangiomas are the most common tumor of the adult liver, affecting approximately 5% of all livers. Hemangiomas are enriched in young adult women and can enlarge during pregnancy or with estrogen therapy, although a direct causative link with estrogen therapy has been disputed. Approximately, 90% of hemangiomas are single tumors. Pain is the most common symptom, but most hemangiomas are incidental findings without symptoms. In general, symptoms are rare unless the tumor is greater than 4 cm.

Hemangiomas are rarely biopsied because the diagnosis is comfortably made by imaging studies in most cases. They are often biopsied, however, when imaging findings are atypical; many of the lesions with atypical imaging findings represent partially sclerosed hemangiomas.

Histology

Most hemangiomas are cavernous hemangiomas. They are composed of a well-circumscribed and unencapsulated aggregate of large-caliber and thin-walled vessels; the stroma in between the vessels can vary from thin to thick and is composed of collagen, sometimes with mild lymphocytic inflammation (Figure 20.12; eFig. 20.6). The vessels are lined by flat endothelial cells without atypia or mitotic figures. The vessels are either empty or filled with red blood cells, and may have fibrin thrombi. The centers of the lesions can be hemorrhagic or infarcted and have abundant hemosiderin-laden macrophages. In these central areas, the vessels may no longer be apparent, replaced by loose myxoid stroma or dense fibrosis (eFig. 20.7). In some cases, the central fibrosis will coalesce into a larger central scar that can be seen grossly and on imaging studies. Calcifications may be

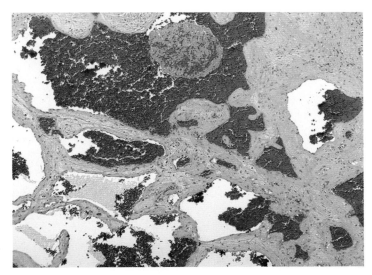

FIGURE 20.12 **Cavernous hemangioma.** This cavernous hemangioma is composed of large dilated vessels. A thrombus is forming in the top vessel.

present in the fibrotic centers. Hemangiomas have no malignant potential and some will entirely regress or undergo fibrosis with time, leading to a sclerosed hemangioma that can often be recognized by residual ghost-like vessel outlines (Figure 20.13).

When cavernous hemangiomas are greater than 8 cm in diameter, they are called *giant cavernous hemangiomas*. Their histological findings are similar to that of smaller hemangiomas, but they are more likely to have an ill-defined border with proliferation of smaller vessels that extends into the adjacent parenchyma (in about 40% of cases) (Figure 20.14).[9,10] Similar findings also can be found focally in smaller hemangiomas.

CAPILLARY HEMANGIOMA

The capillary hemangioma,[11] also called *lobular hemangioma* at times, is morphologically similar to capillary hemangiomas in other organs but is rare in liver. Capillary hemangiomas have a modest female predominance and a wide range of reported ages. A possible predilection for Asian ethnicity has also been suggested.[12] This tumor is composed of small, thin-walled vessels, often growing in a vague lobular arrangement (Figure 20.15). The tumors can be single or rarely multiple. The vascular lumens can be inconspicuous in some areas, leading to a more solid appearance (eFig. 20.8). Occasional larger caliber vessels can be present both at the periphery and center of the tumor. Some of the large-caliber vessels can show myxoid change in their walls. Cytologically, the tumor cells are plump but without atypia or mitotic activity. Extramedullary hematopoiesis may also be present. Immunostains such as CD34 (eFig. 20.9) or ERG can confirm vascular differentiation.

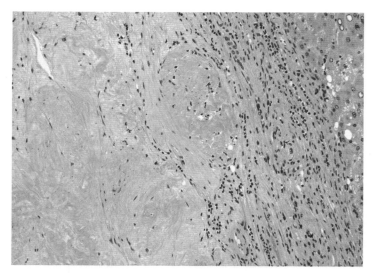

FIGURE 20.13 **Sclerosed hemangioma.** The lesion is composed entirely of fibrous scar, with no residual vascular lumens, but residual "ghost" lumens can be seen, wherein fibrous scars have a circular, whorled morphology representing the old vascular spaces.

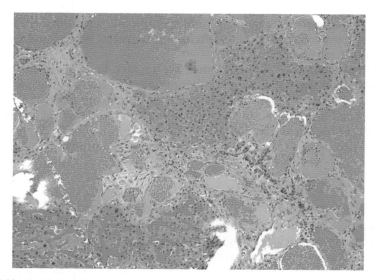

FIGURE 20.14 **Hemangiomatosis at the periphery of a large cavernous hemangioma.** The interface with the liver shows smaller-sized vessels (lower half of the image) that infiltrate the surrounding liver parenchyma.

ANASTOMOSING HEMANGIOMA

The anastomosing hemangioma has only recently been described. Overall, it is most common in the retroperitoneum, kidney, and genital tract.[13,14] The hemangioma is composed of well-formed, small-sized vessels that can show interanastomosing vascular channels (Figure 20.16). One of the distinctive

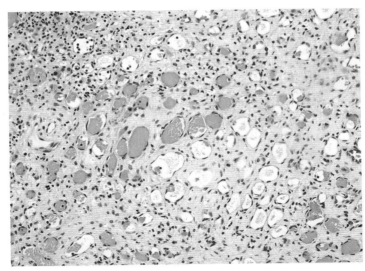

FIGURE 20.15 **Capillary hemangioma.** A capillary hemangioma is composed of small-sized blood vessels.

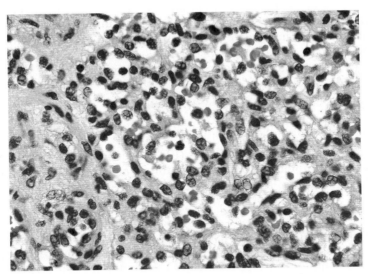

FIGURE 20.16 **Anastomosing hemangioma.** The tumor is composed of small vessels with an interanastomosing growth pattern.

features is the cytology, as the small-sized vessels are lined by endothelial cells that often have hobnail morphology (Figure 20.17).[15] The endothelial cells may show mild cytological atypia, but they lack the severe atypia typical of angiosarcomas. Anastomosing hemangiomas also have no necrosis and no mitotic figures. The stromal between the vessels is usually scant but often contains mild inflammation, including mast cells.[15] The interface

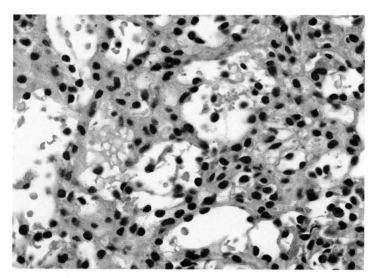

FIGURE 20.17 **Anastomosing hemangioma.** The endothelial cells are not flat but protrude into the lumen (hobnail).

between the anastomosing hemangioma and the background liver typically is poorly circumscribed, showing intermixing of tumor and nontumor liver. These tumors with infiltrative edges have also been reported using the terminology *hepatic small vessel neoplasm*.[16] *GNAQ*, *GNA11*, and *GNA14* mutations are common in anastomosing hemangiomas.[16,17]

EPITHELIOID HEMANGIOENDOTHELIOMA

Definition

Epithelioid hemangioendotheliomas (EHE) are malignant vascular tumors composed of epithelioid and dendritic tumor cells embedded in a myxoid or hyalinized stroma. They have a better prognosis than angiosarcoma.

Clinical Findings

The average age at presentation is 47 years, but the highest tumor incidence is between the ages of 30 and 40.[18] There is a slight female predominance.[18] Presenting symptoms are generally mild and often include vague abdominal pain; patients may have weight loss and jaundice. Approximately, 40% of tumors are incidental findings.

Histological Findings

EHEs are multifocal and involve both lobes of the liver in over 80% of cases. The tumors range in size from subcentimeter to 14 cm. They arise in noncirrhotic livers. However, vascular spread of the tumor can lead to marked secondary atrophy and regeneration of the liver, occasionally mimicking cirrhosis on imaging studies. Microscopically, the tumors are generally of moderate cellularity, but there is variability, and some tumors show low cellularity. and rare cases show marked cellularity. In general, tumor cellularity tends to be denser at the periphery and sparse in the center of the tumor, which can even become densely sclerotic. The sclerotic areas can have calcifications. Some tumors may show areas of necrosis and hemorrhage. In all cases, the neoplastic cells are embedded in abundant extracellular matrix. The extracellular matrix is quite distinctive and is a good first clue to the diagnosis (Figures 20.18 and 20.19). The extracellular matrix is often loose and amphophilic but can have a more hyalinized and eosinophilic appearance, resembling desmoplasia.

Cytologically, the tumor cells have an epithelioid morphology (Figure 20.20). The tumor cells are pale-to-eosinophilic and have moderate amounts of cytoplasm, vacuolated nuclei, and inconspicuous nucleoli. In almost all cases, especially with a large biopsy or full resection, some of the epithelioid cells will have a signet-ring cell–like morphology (Figure 20.21, eFig. 20.10), occasionally with red blood cells in the lumen. The signet-ring–like cells are mucicarmine negative. Cells with a dendritic appearance can also be found, although this feature is best seen on immunostains. Mitotic figures tend to be absent or rare. In some cases, focal areas of better-formed vessels may be present (eFig. 20.11).

EHEs grow as nodular lesions, but, at the microscopic level, tumor cells frequently extend considerable distances from the tumor mass, extending along the sinusoids or portal or central veins, sometimes causing atrophy or drop-out of the hepatocytes. Entrapped portal tracts are common at the edges of nodular areas of tumor growth. The portal veins and the central veins are often involved by tumor, including within and away from the main nodules

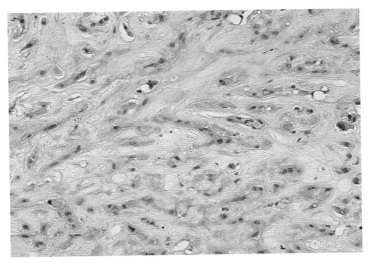

FIGURE 20.18 **Epithelioid hemangioendothelioma.** Epithelioid cells are seen in an epithelioid hemangioendothelioma. Note the characteristic extracellular matrix.

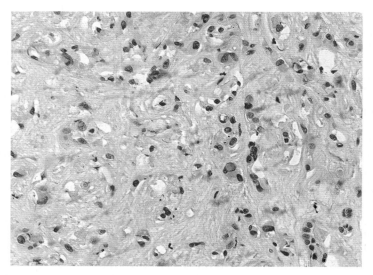

FIGURE 20.19 **Epithelioid hemangioendothelioma.** Another example of the characteristic extracellular matrix.

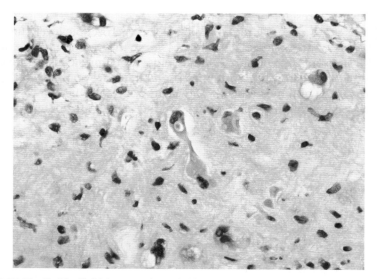

FIGURE 20.20 **Epithelioid hemangioendothelioma.** The tumor cells show moderately abundant eosinophilic cytoplasm.

of tumor growth. The most common pattern of vascular involvement is fibro-obliteration of the veins, with tumor cells within a fibrotic matrix (Figure 20.22). However, the tumor can also grow as small polypoid nodules of tumor cells within a nonobliterated vascular lumen. Uncommonly, hepatic arteries can be involved. The tumor involves the liver capsule in about half of cases. Most tumors have minimal to mild inflammation that is most commonly

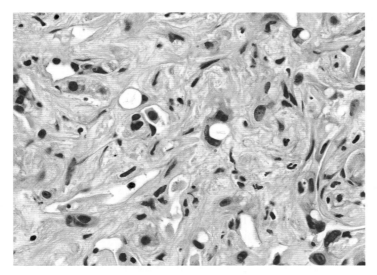

FIGURE 20.21 **Epithelioid hemangioendothelioma, signet ring cells.** Some of the epithelioid cells have a signet ring cell morphology.

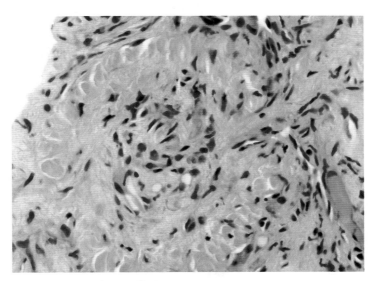

FIGURE 20.22 **Epithelioid hemangioendothelioma, venous involvement.** The central vein has been infiltrated and obliterated by the tumor.

lymphocytic but rarely can be neutrophil-rich. In a few cases, there can be marked inflammation. Of the various histological findings, marked tumor cellularity is the strongest risk factor for aggressive behavior, but all EHE are malignant and have potential for aggressive behavior.

Historically, a high proportion of cases submitted to consult practices were submitted with a preliminary diagnosis of cholangiocarcinoma, because the tumors can have signet-ring–type cells and abundant extracellular matrix.[18] Other common misdiagnoses include angiosarcoma and metastatic carcinomas. Overall, the distinctive extracellular matrix and the distinctive cell types (epithelioid, signet-ring–like, dendritic) will point you to the correct diagnosis in essentially all cases, a diagnosis which can then be confirmed by immunostains.

Immunostains

Immunostains are used to confirm vascular differentiation, with approximate frequencies of positivity as follows[18,19]: ERG (>99%), factor VIII (>99%), CD34 (95%), and CD31 (85%). Smooth muscle actin is positive in 26% of cases and cytokeratin AE1/AE3 in up to 67% of cases.[20] Other keratins, such as OSCAR and CK7, are commonly positive (Figure 20.23).[20] Also, of note, CD10 is positive in most EHE,[21] which can sometimes be confusing if the biopsy is small and the distinctive hematoxylin and eosin (H&E) findings are not well represented. In general, the epithelioid areas stain better with vascular markers than the dendritic areas.

Most cases (~90%) have *WWTR1-CAMTA1* gene fusions.[22] Immunostains for CAMTA-1 can be diagnostically useful (positive in ~90% of cases) and show strong nuclear positivity (Figure 20.24),[23] but are not necessary if the histology and immunostain findings are typical. For the rare EHE that are negative for the *WWTR1-CAMTA1* gene fusion, molecular testing has identified fusions in other genes, including *TFE, FOS*, and *FOSB*.

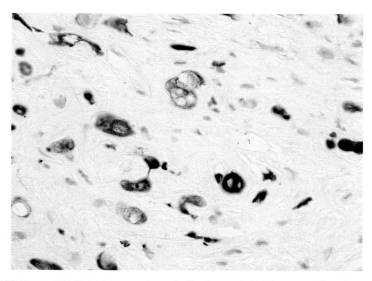

FIGURE 20.23 **Epithelioid hemangioendothelioma, CK7.** The strong keratin expression can lead to a misdiagnosis of carcinoma.

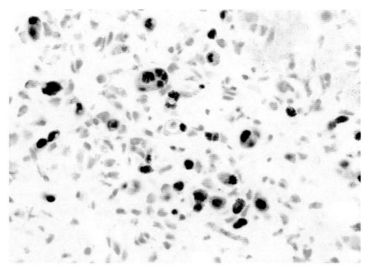

FIGURE 20.24 **Epithelioid hemangioendothelioma, CAMTA1.** There is nuclear staining in the malignant cells.

ANGIOSARCOMA

Definition

Angiosarcomas are high-grade malignant sarcomas with evidence for vascular differentiation by morphology and/or immunostains.

Clinical Findings

Angiosarcomas of the liver can be challenging to recognize on liver biopsy because they are rare and often mimic other tumors. Angiosarcomas can be primary to the liver or metastatic. Recognized risk factors for primary angiosarcomas include arsenic (found in the groundwater in some parts of the world), androgen therapy, Thorotrast (a radiocontrast agent no longer in use), and vinyl chloride exposure. However, no cause is identified in 70% of cases. Most patients are older men. The prognosis is dismal with few individuals surviving greater than 6 months after diagnosis.

Histological Findings

Angiosarcomas can be challenging to diagnose as they can mimic benign processes (eFig. 20.12) or other malignancies (eFig. 20.13). Angiosarcomas can be unifocal or multifocal. In the majority of cases, the diagnosis of malignancy is obvious, as the tumor cells show significant atypia and numerous mitotic figures. Mass-forming tumors can be further classified by their predominant pattern of growth into those that are vasoformative (Figure 20.25), those that are nonvasoformative and are composed of spindled cells (Figure 20.26), and those that are nonvasoformative and

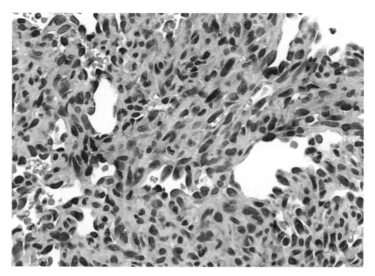

FIGURE 20.25   **Angiosarcoma.** The tumor shows focal poorly formed blood vessels.

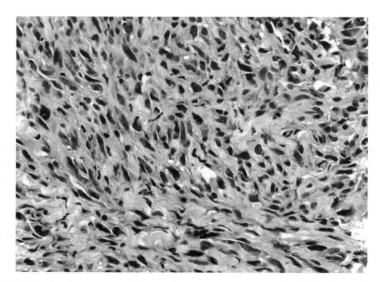

FIGURE 20.26   **Angiosarcoma.** This angiosarcoma is growing in solid sheets of spindled cells.

have a solid, epithelioid growth pattern (Figure 20.27).[24] In all of these patterns, malignant cells can spread along the sinusoids, often inconspicuously, with tumor cells extending considerably beyond the grossly visible tumor. In resection specimens, mixed patterns are frequently seen, but a single morphological pattern is common in biopsy specimens. For all of these three main patterns of growth, larger tumors may undergo central

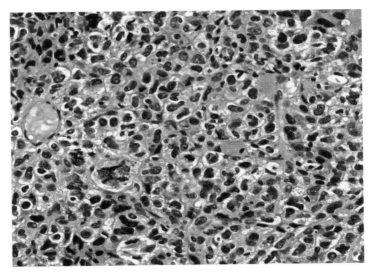

FIGURE 20.27 **Angiosarcoma.** This angiosarcoma shows a growth pattern of epithelioid cells that mimics carcinoma.

cavitating necrosis. In some cases, the necrosis is extensive, leaving behind only a thin rim of malignant cells surrounding a cavity filled with blood, fibrin, and necrotic debris.

In addition to well-defined mass lesions, angiosarcomas can have a subtle growth pattern where malignant cells extend along the sinusoids, but no grossly visible mass lesion is seen. Imaging can show subtle abnormalities that lead to liver biopsy. The diagnosis in this pattern of angiosarcoma can be particularly subtle and challenging.

In these cases, the tumor cells replace the normal, benign sinusoidal endothelial cells, but leave the hepatic plates relatively intact, without forming a distinct mass (Figure 20.28; eFig. 20.14).[24] This growth pattern can lead to sinusoidal dilatation and sometimes to microscopic blood-filled cysts lined by tumor cells. The neoplastic cells show mild to moderate atypia, atypia that is best appreciated when compared to an area of normal liver, as the atypia can be subtle. The cytological atypia does not always reach the level seen in mass-forming angiosarcomas. This pattern is often misdiagnosed initially as vascular outflow disease. A Ki-67 can be helpful by demonstrating a high-proliferate rate in the atypical endothelial cells (Figure 20.29). Immunostains for p53 can also be helpful if they show strong and bright positive staining (about 50% of cases).[25]

Finally, some angiosarcomas with a sinusoidal infiltrative growth pattern can cause complete or near-complete loss of hepatocytes and the biopsy findings may be dominated by parenchymal collapse and proliferating bile ductules. The atypical endothelial cells of the angiosarcoma can be easily overlooked (Figure 20.30) but can be brought out by immunostains for vascular differentiation.

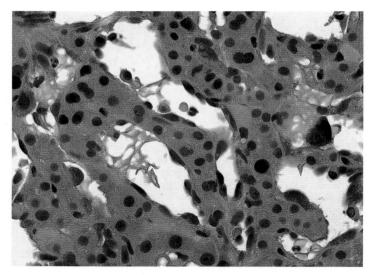

FIGURE 20.28 **Angiosarcoma, sinusoidal pattern.** This angiosarcoma shows atypical cells growing along sinusoids, with intact hepatic plates.

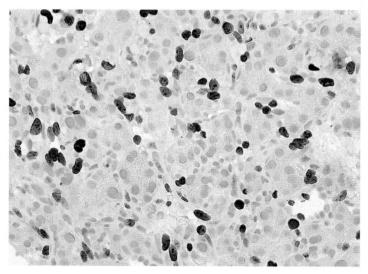

FIGURE 20.29 **Angiosarcoma, sinusoidal pattern.** A Ki-67 on this case shows a very high proliferative rate.

Immunostains

Immunostains are used to confirm vascular differentiation, including ERG (positive in >99%), factor VIII (positive in 80%-90% of cases), CD34 (75%), and CD31 (30%); these are midrange numbers published in the literature, but experiences vary from lab to lab. In general, ERG works very well and is easy to interpret. Some carcinomas, most notably prostate carcinomas, can be ERG positive, so correlation with H&E findings and other immunostain

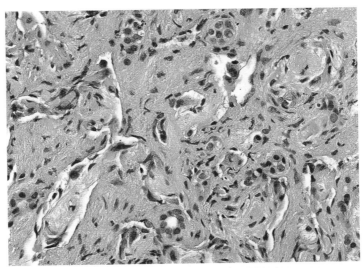

FIGURE 20.30 **Angiosarcoma**. This subtle angiosarcoma has led to substantial collapse of the hepatic parenchyma. Residual bile ducts can be seen.

results is important. Angiosarcomas can also be positive for keratins. For example, aberrant cytokeratin AE1/AE3 positivity is seen in about 45% of angiosarcomas and CAM5.2 in 30% of cases, representing an important diagnostic pitfall.[26] Pankeratins, such as OSCAR, are also frequently positive.[20]

ANGIOMYOLIPOMA

Definition

Angiomyolipomas are benign mesenchymal tumors composed of myoid cells, typically admixed with fat and large irregular vessels.

Clinical

Most angiomyolipomas of the liver (90%) are sporadic and are not part of the tuberous sclerosis complex. In most cases, a single tumor is present (90%), but rare multifocal cases have been reported. The average age at diagnosis is 49 years, and there is a strong female predilection.[27] The background liver is typically nondiseased and not fibrotic. Angiomyolipomas can be challenging to diagnose, with some studies indicating that half of cases are initially misdiagnosed.[27]

Histology

Angiomyolipomas are composed of tumor cells showing up to three lines of differentiation: fatty change, smooth muscle or "myoid" differentiation, and large thick-walled vessels (Figure 20.31). The myoid component can be composed of spindle (Figure 20.32) or epithelioid cells (Figure 20.33). The proportion of each component varies considerably between tumors. A subset of tumors is composed mostly of fat, and some of these can have lipoblast-like

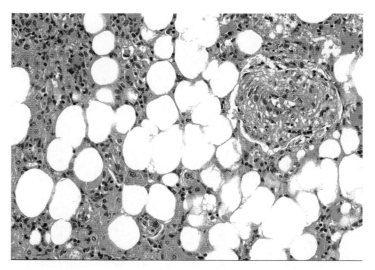

FIGURE 20.31 **Angiomyolipoma.** This image shows the fat, myoid cells, and large irregular vessels. Many biopsies of angiomyolipomas will sample only some of these three elements.

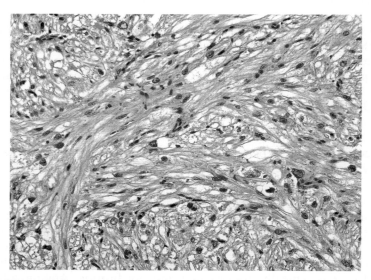

FIGURE 20.32 **Angiomyolipoma, spindle growth pattern.** This growth pattern can mimic metastatic gastrointestinal stromal tumors and other spindle cell tumors.

cells with multivacuolated cytoplasm and indented nuclei, mimicking lipomas or liposarcomas.[27,28] In fat predominant tumors, the best place to find myoid components are around thick-walled vessels. Other angiomyolipomas are composed mostly of spindled myoid cells and can mimic smooth muscle tumors.[29] In yet another subset of angiomyolipomas, the epithelioid myoid cells predominant; this variant can closely mimic hepatocellular carcinoma, with tumor cells showing abundant, eosinophilic cytoplasm and moderate nuclear atypia. They can even have a trabecular growth pattern that further

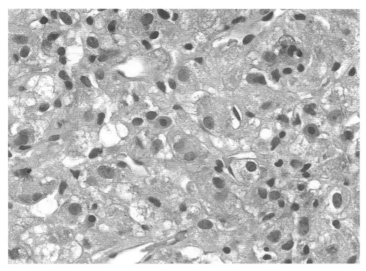

FIGURE 20.33 **Angiomyolipoma, epithelioid.** The myoid cells in this angiomyolipma are epithelioid and can mimic hepatocellular carcinoma.

resembles a hepatocellular carcinoma.[27] In some cases, tumor pigment can provide a clue to the diagnosis of an angiomyolipoma (Figure 20.34). In other epithelioid variants, the cytoplasm will have a clear appearance and engender the differential for clear cell tumors. In fully resected specimens, at least minor components of all elements (fatty, myoid, epithelioid) are commonly seen, but one morphological growth pattern can predominate in biopsy specimens, so a high index of suspicion is helpful.

Other histological findings may include extramedullary hematopoiesis, which can be seen in small amounts in about half of resected specimens and is most evident in cases with lots of fatty differentiation. Hemorrhage, necrosis, and cholesterol clefts are present in a small proportion of cases. Rare angiomyolipomas can show striking peliosis, often associated with hemorrhage,[27] and can mimic an inflammatory hepatic adenoma (Figure 20.35). Also, of note, a subset of cases can have markedly inflamed areas that closely mimic inflammatory pseudotumors of the liver. Finally, about 10% of cases have foci of striking giant cell change, with large, pleomorphic, and sometimes multinucleated epithelioid cells (Figure 20.36). Cases with similar atypia in the spindle-cell component have also been reported.[30] This atypia does not indicate malignancy.

The vast majority of angiomyolipomas are benign, but rare cases behave aggressively. Unfavorable factors include vascular invasion.[31] As noted above, cytological atypia alone does not indicate malignancy. Some studies have suggested that coagulative necrosis,[32] loss of CD117 immunostaining,[32] marked cytological atypia with increased mitoses,[33] or p53 positivity[33] may be markers for more aggressive behavior, but the overall rarity of malignancy makes it difficult to develop well-defined histological factors that predict aggressive behavior. For example, others have subsequently

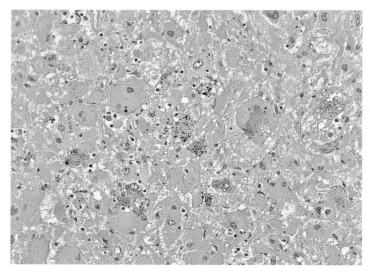

FIGURE 20.34 **Angiomyolipoma, pigment.** Melanin-type pigment is seen in this angiomyolipoma.

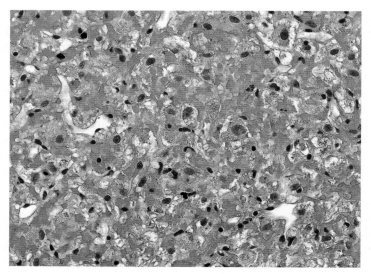

FIGURE 20.35 **Angiomyolipoma, telangiectatic area.** Some angiomyolipomas can have areas of telangiectasia and may raise the differential of an inflammatory hepatic adenoma.

reported p53 positivity in epithelioid angiomyolipomas that were not overtly malignant.[34] On the other hand, late tumor metastasis has also been reported from an angiomyolipoma that was histologically benign.[35]

Immunostains

Angiomyolipomas are negative for cytokeratins[27] and for hepatic markers such as Arginase and HepPar1. HMB45 is the most important positive stain

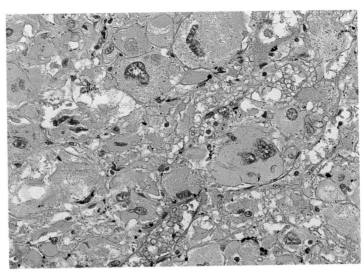

FIGURE 20.36 **Angiomyolipoma with bizarre giant cells.** This angiomyolipoma showed scattered giant cells with bizarre nuclei. This is not evidence for malignancy.

and all cases should be positive (Figure 20.37). Of note, HMB45 staining can be patchy, especially in fatty areas, a finding that must be taken into consideration on biopsy specimens. The myoid component will typically have strong, granular, cytoplasmic staining. Melan A is positive in 90% of cases. Smooth muscle actin is positive in most cases, although the literature indicates a wide range of positivity, from as low as 50% to as high as 100% of cases.[27,36] In general, the spindle cell areas stain best for smooth muscle actin. CKIT (CD117) is also positive in nearly all cases,[36] so make sure to distinguish the angiomyolipoma from a metastatic gastrointestinal stromal tumor (GIST) based on morphology and other immunostains. S100 stains are positive in most of the fatty areas and about half of the myoid areas.[27] Angiomyolipomas are also CD68-positive (Figure 20.38). This can be important to know because epithelioid angiomyolipomas can sometimes mimic fibrolamellar carcinomas on small biopsies, as both can have tumor cells with abundant oncocytic cytoplasm. HMB45 will be positive in angiomyolipomas but not fibrolamellar carcinomas, while HepPar1/Arginase and CK7 will be positive in fibrolamellar carcinomas but not angiomyolipomas.

SOLITARY FIBROUS TUMOR

Definition

Solitary fibrous tumors (SFTs) are rare, benign spindle-cell tumors of uncertain origin.

Clinical

Most SFTs are first diagnosed in women over the age of 40 years,[37] but there is a wide range of ages and both genders can be affected. A rare

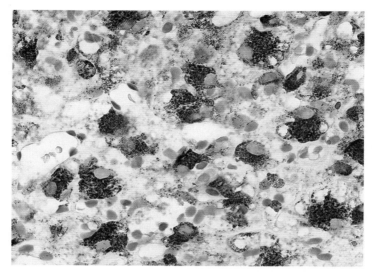

FIGURE 20.37 **Angiomyolipoma, HMB45 immunostain.** The myoid cells in angiomyolipomas show granular cytoplasmic staining with HMB45.

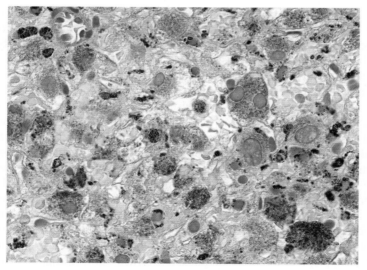

FIGURE 20.38 **Angiomyolipoma, CD68 immunostain.** Angiomyolipomas are CD68-positive.

presentation is hypoglycemia due to production of insulin-like growth factor II by tumor cells.[38,39] Despite the term "solitary" in the name of the entity, rare cases can be multifocal. Most SFTs are intraparenchymal, with only a small subset directly associated with the liver capsule.[37]

Histology

The tumors are generally of low cellularity, with tumor cells embedded in a fibrous stroma (Figures 20.39 and 20.40). The stroma and the tumor cells

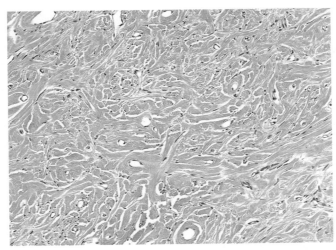

FIGURE 20.39 **Solitary fibrous tumor.** A solitary fibrous tumor shows scattered small spindle cells with dense fibrosis growing in a "patternless pattern."

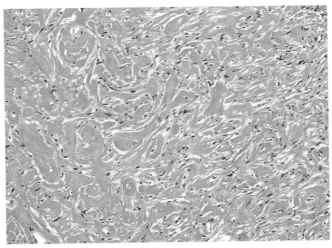

FIGURE 20.40 **Solitary fibrous tumor.** The tumor cells are cytologically bland.

do not have a distinct growth pattern, a finding termed a *patternless pattern*. Of note, some areas of an SFT can become sclerosed while other areas can have myxoid change. Most SFTs are benign, but approximately, 10% of cases have changes that suggest the potential for more aggressive behavior, including increased mitoses, necrosis, and cytological atypia. In some cases, SFT can transform into a frank, high-grade fibrosarcoma.[39]

Rare cases can encase portal tracts, leading to secondary biliary cysts (Figure 20.41). These portal areas may also have small clusters of proliferating bile ducts at their periphery (Figure 20.42), which may demonstrate pancreatic or hepatic metaplasia.

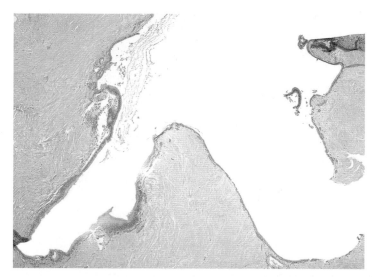

FIGURE 20.41 **Solitary fibrous tumor with bile ductular proliferation.** A secondary biliary cyst is seen.

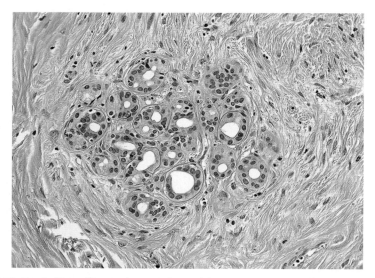

FIGURE 20.42 **Solitary fibrous tumor.** The periphery of these tumors can have entrapped peribiliary-type glands.

Immunostains

The H&E impression of SFT can be confirmed by immunostains for STAT 6 (Figure 20.43). BCL2 (eFig. 20.15) and CD34 (eFig. 20.16) are also frequently positive. The tumor cells are positive for vimentin but are negative for S100, desmin, CKIT (CD117), smooth muscle actin, and cytokeratins.

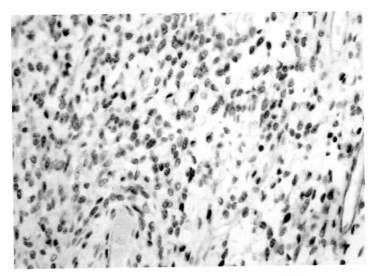

FIGURE 20.43 **Solitary fibrous tumor.** The tumor is strongly STAT6-positive.

OTHER MESENCHYMAL TUMORS

Other rare mesenchymal tumors of the liver include lipomas, liposarcomas, and leiomyomas. In general, their histological and immunostain findings are similar to that of tumors from other sites.

REFERENCES

1. Gandhi D, Sharma P, Garg G, et al. Intrahepatic splenosis demonstrated by diffusion weighted MRI with histologic confirmation. *Radiol Case Rep.* 2020;15:602-606.

2. Singhi AD, Maklouf HR, Mehrotra AK, et al. Segmental atrophy of the liver: a distinctive pseudotumor of the liver with variable histologic appearances. *Am J Surg Pathol.* 2011;35:364-371.

3. Tang L, Lai EC, Cong WM, et al. Inflammatory myofibroblastic tumor of the liver: a cohort study. *World J Surg.* 2010;34:309-313.

4. Anthony PP, Sarsfield P, Clarke T. Primary lymphoma of the liver: clinical and pathological features of 10 patients. *J Clin Pathol.* 1990;43:1007-1013.

5. Granados R, Aramburu JA, Rodriguez JM, et al. Cytopathology of a primary follicular dendritic cell sarcoma of the liver of the inflammatory pseudotumor-like type. *Diagn Cytopathol.* 2008;36:42-46.

6. Kojima M, Nakamura S, Ohno Y, et al. Hepatic angiomyolipoma resembling an inflammatory pseudotumor of the liver. A case report. *Pathol Res Pract.* 2004;200:713-716.

7. Argani P, Facchetti F, Inghirami G, et al. Lymphocyte-rich well-differentiated liposarcoma: report of nine cases. *Am J Surg Pathol.* 1997;21:884-895.

8. Tsou YK, Lin CJ, Liu NJ, et al. Inflammatory pseudotumor of the liver: report of eight cases, including three unusual cases, and a literature review. *J Gastroenterol Hepatol.* 2007;22:2143-2147.

9. Kim GE, Thung SN, Tsui WM, et al. Hepatic cavernous hemangioma: underrecognized associated histologic features. *Liver Int.* 2006;26:334-338.

10. Jhaveri KS, Vlachou PA, Guindi M, et al. Association of hepatic hemangiomatosis with giant cavernous hemangioma in the adult population: prevalence, imaging appearance, and relevance. *AJR Am J Roentgenol.* 2011;196:809-815.

11. Abaalkhail F, Castonguay M, Driman DK, et al. Lobular capillary hemangioma of the liver. *Hepatobiliary Pancreat Dis Int.* 2009;8:323-325.

12. Jhuang JY, Lin LW, Hsieh MS. Adult capillary hemangioma of the liver: case report and literature review. *Kaohsiung J Med Sci.* 2011;27:344-347.

13. Montgomery E, Epstein JI. Anastomosing hemangioma of the genitourinary tract: a lesion mimicking angiosarcoma. *Am J Surg Pathol.* 2009;33:1364-1369.

14. O'Neill AC, Craig JW, Silverman SG, et al. Anastomosing hemangiomas: locations of occurrence, imaging features, and diagnosis with percutaneous biopsy. *Abdom Radiol (NY).* 2016;41:1325-1332.

15. Lin J, Bigge J, Ulbright TM, et al. Anastomosing hemangioma of the liver and gastrointestinal tract: an unusual variant histologically mimicking angiosarcoma. *Am J Surg Pathol.* 2013;37:1761-1765.

16. Joseph NM, Brunt EM, Marginean C, et al. Frequent GNAQ and GNA14 mutations in hepatic small vessel neoplasm. *Am J Surg Pathol.* 2018;42:1201-1207.

17. Liau JY, Tsai JH, Lan J, et al. GNA11 joins GNAQ and GNA14 as a recurrently mutated gene in anastomosing hemangioma. *Virchows Arch.* 2020;476:475-481.

18. Makhlouf HR, Ishak KG, Goodman ZD. Epithelioid hemangioendothelioma of the liver: a clinicopathologic study of 137 cases. *Cancer.* 1999;85:562-582.

19. Miettinen M, Wang ZF, Paetau A, et al. ERG transcription factor as an immunohistochemical marker for vascular endothelial tumors and prostatic carcinoma. *Am J Surg Pathol.* 2011;35:432-441.

20. Lee HE, Torbenson MS, Wu TT, et al. Aberrant keratin expression is common in primary hepatic malignant vascular tumors: a potential diagnostic pitfall. *Ann Diagn Pathol.* 2020;49:151589.

21. Weinreb I, Cunningham KS, Perez-Ordonez B, et al. CD10 is expressed in most epithelioid hemangioendotheliomas: a potential diagnostic pitfall. *Arch Pathol Lab Med.* 2009;133:1965-1968.

22. Errani C, Zhang L, Sung YS, et al. A novel WWTR1-CAMTA1 gene fusion is a consistent abnormality in epithelioid hemangioendothelioma of different anatomic sites. *Genes Chromosomes Cancer.* 2011;50:644-653.

23. Shibuya R, Matsuyama A, Shiba E, et al. CAMTA1 is a useful immunohistochemical marker for diagnosing epithelioid haemangioendothelioma. *Histopathology.* 2015;67:827-835.

24. Yasir S, Torbenson MS. Angiosarcoma of the liver: clinicopathologic features and morphologic patterns. *Am J Surg Pathol.* 2019;43:581-590.

25. Zen Y, Sofue K. Sinusoidal-type Angiosarcoma of the liver: imaging features and potential diagnostic utility of p53 immunostaining. *Am J Surg Pathol.* 2019;43:1728-1731.

26. Meis-Kindblom JM, Kindblom LG. Angiosarcoma of soft tissue: a study of 80 cases. *Am J Surg Pathol.* 1998;22:683-697.

27. Tsui WM, Colombari R, Portmann BC, et al. Hepatic angiomyolipoma: a clinicopathologic study of 30 cases and delineation of unusual morphologic variants. *Am J Surg Pathol.* 1999;23:34-48.

28. Nonomura A, Mizukami Y, Shimizu K, et al. Angiomyolipoma mimicking true lipoma of the liver: report of two cases. *Pathol Int.* 1996;46:221-227.

29. Nonomura A, Minato H, Kurumaya H. Angiomyolipoma predominantly composed of smooth muscle cells: problems in histological diagnosis. *Histopathology.* 1998;33:20-27.

30. Nonomura A, Mizukami Y, Takayanagi N, et al. Immunohistochemical study of hepatic angiomyolipoma. *Pathol Int.* 1996;46:24-32.

31. Dalle I, Sciot R, de Vos R, et al. Malignant angiomyolipoma of the liver: a hitherto unreported variant. *Histopathology*. 2000;36:443-450.

32. Nguyen TT, Gorman B, Shields D, et al. Malignant hepatic angiomyolipoma: report of a case and review of literature. *Am J Surg Pathol*. 2008;32:793-798.

33. Deng YF, Lin Q, Zhang SH, et al. Malignant angiomyolipoma in the liver: a case report with pathological and molecular analysis. *Pathol Res Pract*. 2008;204:911-918.

34. Bing Z, Yao Y, Pasha T, et al. p53 in pure epithelioid PEComa: an immunohistochemistry study and gene mutation analysis. *Int J Surg Pathol*. 2012;20:115-122.

35. Parfitt JR, Bella AJ, Izawa JI, et al. Malignant neoplasm of perivascular epithelioid cells of the liver. *Arch Pathol Lab Med*. 2006;130:1219-1222.

36. Makhlouf HR, Remotti HE, Ishak KG. Expression of KIT (CD117) in angiomyolipoma. *Am J Surg Pathol*. 2002;26:493-497.

37. Moran CA, Ishak KG, Goodman ZD. Solitary fibrous tumor of the liver: a clinicopathologic and immunohistochemical study of nine cases. *Ann Diagn Pathol*. 1998;2:19-24.

38. Fama F, Le Bouc Y, Barrande G, et al. Solitary fibrous tumour of the liver with IGF-II-related hypoglycaemia. A case report. *Langenbeck's Arch Surg*. 2008;393:611-616.

39. Chan G, Horton PJ, Thyssen S, et al. Malignant transformation of a solitary fibrous tumor of the liver and intractable hypoglycemia. *J Hepatobiliary Pancreat Surg*. 2007;14:595-599.

21

HEPATOCELLULAR PSEUDOTUMORS AND TUMORS

REGENERATIVE HEPATIC PSEUDOTUMOR

This pseudotumor of the liver has only recently been described.[1] The regenerative hepatic pseudotumor occurs in equal frequency in men and women, with an average age at presentation of 48 years, with range from 28 to 73 years. Most patients have a hypercoagulable medical condition, such as recently treated malignancies in various nonliver sites. Patients typically do not present with symptomatic liver disease. Instead, the lesions are identified on imaging studies performed for other reasons. The lesions can be single or multiple and occur in both lobes of the liver. The lesions to date have only been reported in noncirrhotic livers.[1] The radiology differential is often broad and may include hepatic adenoma, focal nodular hyperplasia, low-grade hepatocellular carcinoma, and metastatic disease. Over time, the lesions can remain stable or regress, when followed up by imaging.

These pseudotumors have vague borders without capsules and can be subtle and challenging to see on gross examination, but they are often visible as lesions with ill-defined borders, in juxtaposition to the normal liver. They lack nodularity within the lesion, central scars, hemorrhage, and necrosis.

The pseudotumor is associated with vascular thrombi, which can be located in either the portal veins or the central veins (Figure 21.1). The thrombi are usually focal and can be subtle or striking. The remaining pathologic findings, detailed later, are reactive/regenerative changes that result from localized changes in vascular flow. While the diagnosis is best secured in resected specimens, it can be suggested or included in the differential on biopsy specimens when all the features are present, including the vascular thrombi. In all cases, it is important for the radiologist to be confident they sampled the lesion, as peritumoral parenchymal changes can have some of these findings.

Histologically, there are portal tracts throughout the regenerative hepatic pseudotumor (Figure 21.2), but they often have abnormal spacing,

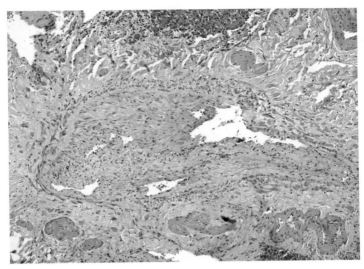

FIGURE 21.1 **Regenerative hepatic pseudotumor.** Several remote portal vein thrombi are seen.

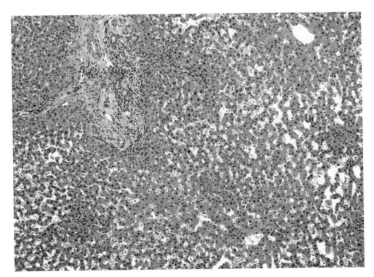

FIGURE 21.2 **Regenerative hepatic pseudotumor.** Sections show patchy but prominent sinusoidal dilation. A portal tract can also be seen.

with some areas with closely approximated portal tracts and other areas with abnormally widely spaced portal tracts. The presence of portal tracts throughout the lesion is a key distinguishing feature from true neoplasms, such as hepatic adenomas and hepatocellular carcinomas. The portal tracts frequently show patchy vascular abnormalities, including hyperplasia and hypertrophy of hepatic arteries (Figure 21.3); some cases may show irregular

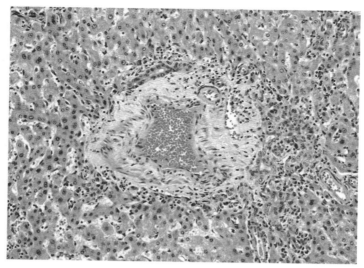

FIGURE 21.3 **Regenerative hepatic pseudotumor.** The portal tract shows an abnormal hepatic artery and an atrophic portal vein.

fibrotic thickening of the hepatic arteries. Portal veins can be dilated or herniated. Focal portal tracts may show mild bile ductular proliferation and there also can be patchy sinusoidal dilatation (Figure 21.2).

The hepatocytes are negative for cytologic atypia, the lobules have no loss of reticulin, and there is no increase in Ki-67 staining. Small, aberrant (or naked) arteries can be present in the lobules. The central veins can be irregularly spaced. Some central veins may have a thicker cuff of glutamine-synthetase-positive hepatocytes than those seen in the normal liver, but a maplike staining pattern is never present. The regenerative hepatic pseudo-tumor also lacks the parenchymal nodularity and bands of fibrosis seen in focal nodular hyperplasia. In keeping with the reactive nature of this pseudotumor, immunostains for C-reactive protein (CRP) and serum amyloid A (SAA) are negative for strong and diffuse staining patterns, while liver fatty acid binding protein (LFABP) shows a retained staining pattern.

FOCAL NODULAR HYPERPLASIA

Definition

Focal nodular hyperplasia is a benign, reactive, nodular pseudotumor composed of hepatocytes and bands of fibrosis that develops in a noncirrhotic liver.

Clinical

Focal nodular hyperplasias are reactive lesions that develop as a result of localized shunting of blood flow. They have no malignant potential. There are rare reports of hepatocellular carcinomas in proximity to focal nodular hyperplasias, often at the edges,[2] but the focal nodular hyperplasias are reactive to the tumor and not the source.

Focal nodular hyperplasias are usually single lesions, but they are multiple in about 20% of cases. Focal nodular hyperplasias occur most commonly in young and middle-aged women. The female-to-male ratio is 10:1, with a median age of 41 years. Overall, 75% of focal nodular hyperplasias occur between the ages of 20 and 50 years. Approximately 7% occur in patients younger than 20 years, with only rare cases seen before the age of 5 years. Focal nodular hyperplasias in children and teenagers are often preceded by chemotherapy for carcinoma in other organs. In this setting, there is often a time lag of many years between the chemotherapy and the development of the focal nodular hyperplasia. Focal nodular hyperplasias rarely occur in liver allografts.[3] In the end, the precise cause is unknown for most focal nodular hyperplasias. Oral contraception does not cause focal nodular hyperplasias, but estrogens can increase the size of focal nodular hyperplasia, at least in some cases.[4]

Histology

Focal nodular hyperplasias are composed of nodules of normal-appearing hepatocytes separated by fibrous bands (Figure 21.4), which may coalesce into a larger central scar. A central scar is seen in most cases of focal nodular hyperplasias larger than 4 cm, but in only about half of smaller cases. In smaller focal nodular hyperplasias, the nodularity may be less developed and the low-power findings may resemble "bridging fibrosis" rather than

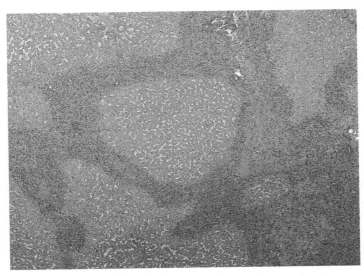

FIGURE 21.4 **Focal nodular hyperplasia.** On low-power examination, the lesion resembles cirrhosis with nodularity and bands of fibrosis.

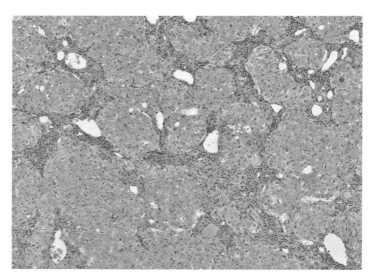

FIGURE 21.5 **Focal nodular hyperplasia.** In smaller focal nodular hyperplasias, and at the periphery of some of the larger focal nodular hyperplasias, the nodularity may be incomplete and the overall pattern can resemble that of bridging fibrosis. Smaller focal nodular hyperplasias with this pattern are often misinterpreted as telangiectatic adenomas.

"focal cirrhosis" (Figure 21.5). The hepatocytes lack cytologic atypia, and a reticulin stain demonstrates a normal reticulin pattern. The fibrous bands typically have proliferating bile ductules, a finding sometimes called bile ductular metaplasia (Figure 21.6; eFig. 21.1). Both the periphery and the center of the lesion often show large vessels with abnormal walls that are eccentrically thickened (Figure 21.7). Focal nodular hyperplasias do not have capsules and do not have true portal tracts. Because focal nodular hyperplasias lack adequate bile drainage, they often show mild cholate stasis at the edges of the fibrous bands. Most cases will also demonstrate mild copper accumulation on copper stain.[5] Of note, mild copper deposition is typical for focal nodular hyperplasia (95% of cases are positive) but is not specific, with copper stains also positive in 40% of inflammatory hepatic adenomas.[6]

A subset of focal nodular hyperplasias can have ballooning and Mallory hyaline (Figure 21.8). When fat is also present, the findings can mimic steatohepatitic hepatocellular carcinoma.[7] The overall architecture and the cytologic features usually allow distinction of these two entities on hematoxylin-eosin (H&E) staining. In challenging cases, glutamine synthetase stains can be helpful. A maplike staining pattern supports a diagnosis of focal nodular hyperplasia. A strong and diffuse staining pattern would be more consistent with a well-differentiated hepatocellular carcinoma. Overall, approximately one-half of hepatocellular carcinomas are diffusely glutamine synthetase positive. Other stains that are helpful to

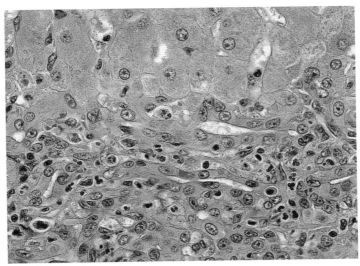

FIGURE 21.6 **Focal nodular hyperplasia.** A bile ductular proliferation (also called metaplasia) is seen at the interface of the hepatic parenchyma and fibrous bands.

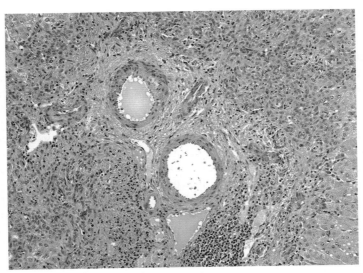

FIGURE 21.7 **Focal nodular hyperplasia.** Abnormal, thick-walled arteries are present in the center of fibrous bands.

exclude a well-differentiated hepatocellular carcinoma include reticulin, Ki-67, and glypican 3.

The background liver in cases of focal nodular hyperplasia should be noncirrhotic. Cirrhotic livers frequently have vascular shunting and sometimes develop nodules that resemble focal nodular hyperplasia. Perhaps unfortunately, this has led to the suggestion to use the term "focal nodular

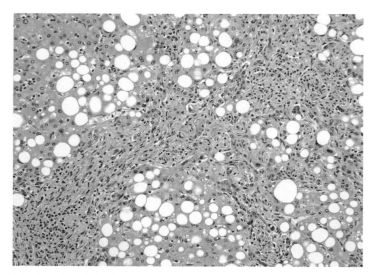

FIGURE 21.8 **Focal nodular hyperplasia.** This case shows fat and balloon cells.

hyperplasia" in the context of cirrhosis. Any upside to expanding the definition of focal nodular hyperplasia to include lesions in cirrhotic livers, however, is offset by the risk of obscuring the biology and clinical correlates of traditional focal nodular hyperplasias.

Papers have been published emphasizing that pathologists confidently diagnose focal nodular hyperplasia on needle biopsy in only approximately 50% of cases on H&E staining. This literature can give the wrong impression, however, as a reliable histologic diagnosis can be readily made in the vast majority of cases. It is true that pathologists cannot do much with suboptimal or inadequate samples, but we are not magicians. Or course, there can be sampling issues and multiple passes will increase the likelihood of a nonequivocating diagnosis. In many cases, however, this "lack of diagnosis" is mostly because a final diagnosis of focal nodular hyperplasia is best made after correlating the histologic findings with the imaging findings. Thus, a pathologist frequently notes that the histologic findings are consistent with focal nodular hyperplasia *after* correlation with imaging studies. Finally, there is an increasing trend to not biopsy lesions that are typical focal nodular hyperplasias on imaging and instead to biopsy lesions that have atypical imaging findings, which in turn can be challenging histologically. Immunostaining for glutamine synthetase can help clarify many of these difficult cases.[8]

Immunohistochemical Stains

Glutamine synthetase normally stains a thin rim of zone 3 hepatocytes, staining a layer of hepatocytes that is a few cells thick, surrounding the central veins. In contrast, staining in focal nodular hyperplasias will show an irregular "map-like" or "geographic" pattern (Figure 21.9). This pattern can

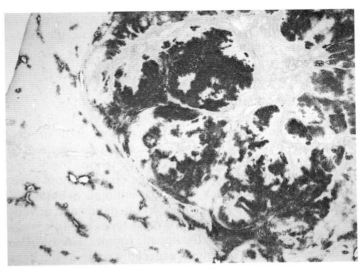

FIGURE 21.9 **Focal nodular hyperplasia, glutamine synthetase stain.** The normal liver shows zone 3 hepatocyte staining (left side of image), while the tumor shows an irregular blotchy staining pattern that is "maplike."

significantly increase the confidence in making a diagnosis of focal nodular hyperplasia over that of H&E findings alone.[8] In the map-like staining pattern, there is irregular, blotchy staining that tends to spare the hepatocytes immediately adjacent to the bands of fibrosis. Of note, about 10% of otherwise ordinary focal nodular hyperplasias may lack the typical map-like staining pattern.[9] Other stains that are occasionally useful include a cytokeratin stain to highlight the proliferating bile ductules, a copper stain to highlight the cholate stasis, and a reticulin stain to help rule out malignancy.

Differential

On H&E staining, the differential for focal nodular hyperplasia primarily includes inflammatory hepatic adenomas. Elements that favor a focal nodular hyperplasia include parenchymal nodularity, bands of fibrosis, abnormal thick-walled vessels, and a bile ductular proliferation located within the fibrous bands. Inflammatory hepatic adenomas may also have bile ductular proliferations, but these are located in faux portal tracts and not fibrous bands. Immunostains for glutamine synthetase, CRP, and SAA are helpful in difficult cases.

The differential also includes focal nodular hyperplasia–like areas that develop around a mass lesion that has caused vascular shunting. Neoplasms that can cause this rim of focal nodular hyperplasia–like changes include hemangiomas, hepatocellular carcinoma, fibrolamellar carcinoma,[10] metastatic neuroendocrine tumors, colon adenocarcinoma, and gastrointestinal stromal tumors (GISTs). This finding is overall very rare and appears to be associated with portal vein involvement by the main tumor mass.[2] In these cases, this reactive rim of hepatocyte changes can be indistinguishable from an otherwise ordinary focal nodular hyperplasia on needle biopsy, including a maplike staining pattern on glutamine synthetase.

HEPATIC ADENOMA

Definition

Hepatic adenomas are benign neoplasms composed of hepatocytes. Synonyms include *hepatocellular adenoma* and *liver adenoma* (the latter one is largely obsolete). They do not occur in cirrhotic livers.

As you read the literature be aware that some authors have used the term "adenoma" to refer to any well-differentiated neoplasm, including those that develop in men with chronic viral hepatitis and advanced fibrosis. The term "adenoma," when used for these types of cases is essentially a synonym for "very well-differentiated hepatic tumor." For this reason, some adenomas described in the literature, especially some of the beta-catenin-activated adenomas and those that arise in cirrhotic livers, would be called well-differentiated hepatocellular carcinomas in many medical centers.

Clinical

Hepatic adenomas occur primarily in young to middle-aged women with a history of oral contraceptive use. However, any population with estrogen use for medical purposes can develop adenomas. Fatty liver disease, which is associated with increased estrogen levels, is also an important risk factor, especially for inflammatory hepatic adenomas.[11] Likewise, exogenous androgen use is a recognized risk factor for hepatic adenomas.[12] In adenomas due to exogenous sex hormone exposure, the background livers are without other liver disease (with the exception of fatty liver disease) and show no fibrosis. Other recognized risk factors for hepatic adenomas include glycogen storage disorders, especially type I and type III.[13] Hepatic adenomas have also been reported with other glycogen storage diseases such as type IV.[14] Interestingly, adenomas in the setting of glycogen storage disease were more common in male patients than female patients in one large study.[13]

Histology

Hepatic adenomas are well-differentiated hepatic neoplasms. Hepatic adenomas should have essentially no cytologic atypia (Figure 21.10) and no mitotic activity. Inflammatory adenomas and androgen-related adenomas can show patchy large cell change, but small cell change, nuclear atypia that is noticeably different from the background liver, or nodule-in-nodule growth, all push strongly towards a diagnosis of hepatocellular carcinoma.

Hepatic adenomas are not encapsulated, but in some areas, they may have a network of thin-walled vessels at the interface of the tumor and non-tumor, which may grossly resemble a capsule. Hepatic adenomas are so well differentiated that it is usually difficult at high power to tell if you are in tumor

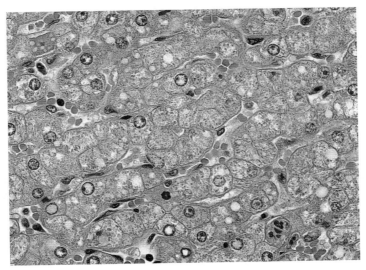

FIGURE 21.10 **Hepatic adenoma.** No cytologic atypia is seen.

or nontumor. On biopsy specimens, the loss of portal tracts is a key feature to recognize neoplastic tissue. Finding aberrant lobular arteries can also be helpful (eFig. 21.2), but this finding is not specific for adenomas, as it is also found in focal nodular hyperplasias, hepatocellular carcinomas, and livers with abnormal vascular flow. Some adenomas can have fatty change, which tends to be just steatosis, without the Mallory hyaline, balloon cells, inflammation, or intratumoral fibrosis that make up the histologic pattern seen with the steatohepatitic variant of hepatocellular carcinoma. When balloon cells or Mallory hyaline is present, it is essentially always in the setting of a patient with the metabolic syndrome,[15] who also has steatohepatitis in the background liver. As an exception, hepatic adenomas that develop in the setting of glycogen storage disease type Ia can have striking steatohepatitis type changes.[16]

HEPATIC ADENOMA VERSUS WELL-DIFFERENTIATED HEPATOCELLULAR CARCINOMA. How do you distinguish a well-differentiated hepatocellular carcinoma from a hepatic adenoma? Hepatic adenomas should have no cytologic atypia (focal large cell change is acceptable in inflammatory hepatic adenomas and androgen adenomas; eFig. 21.3), inconspicuous nucleoli that are the same as those seen in the background liver, no mitotic activity, and a low Ki-67 proliferative rate, usually less than 2%.[17] One exception is that there may be focal, mildly increased proliferation near areas of tumor necrosis (eFig. 21.4). Hepatic adenomas are rarely cholestatic and rarely if ever have a pseudoacinar growth pattern, with the exception of androgen-related adenomas. If bile production or pseudoglands are present, a well-differentiated hepatocellular carcinoma should be carefully excluded. The tumor cells in hepatic adenomas do not have cytoplasmic inclusions (Figures 21.11 and 21.12).

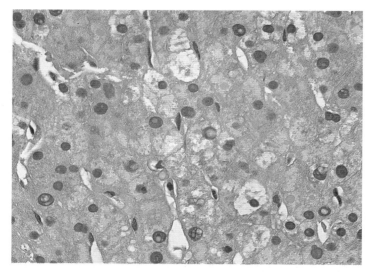

FIGURE 21.11 **Well-differentiated hepatocellular carcinoma.** This well-differentiated hepatocellular carcinoma was originally submitted for consultation as a presumptive hepatic adenoma. However, focal balloon cells and prominent megamitochondria provided a clue that this was not an adenoma.

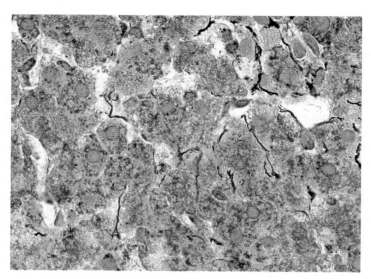

FIGURE 21.12 **Well-differentiated hepatocellular carcinoma.** A reticulin stain showed extensive loss of reticulin (same case as the preceding figure).

Hepatic adenomas should have essentially no reticulin loss. Reticulin staining is a critical tool to exclude malignancy, but there are several caveats. First, definite reticulin loss should push the diagnosis to hepatocellular carcinoma, but the significance of focal equivocal reticulin loss is less clear. Also, the reticulin framework can be artificially disrupted near areas of hemorrhage. In addition, benign hepatic tumors with abundant fatty change can have small foci of reticulin reduction due to the steatosis. Finally, very rare well-differentiated hepatocellular carcinomas do not show reticulin loss on biopsy (Figure 21.13).[18] Thus, as is true for all stains, reticulin interpretation should take place in the context of other histologic findings. These caveats are important but do not diminish the important role of the reticulin stain as a diagnostic tool when evaluating well-differentiated hepatic tumors: essentially all hepatic tumors that behave aggressively have recognizable reticulin loss.

Approach the diagnosis of hepatic adenoma with added care if there are no risk factors if the patient is a man, or if the patient is a woman over the age of 60 years; hepatic adenomas do occur in all these settings, but well-differentiated hepatocellular carcinoma should be carefully excluded. If there are clinical or histologic findings that are not a good fit for a hepatic adenoma on the liver biopsy, then it is best to use a term such as "well-differentiated hepatic neoplasm" and give the differential in a note. Relevant to this, there is a small subset of well-differentiated hepatocellular neoplasms that are difficult to classify, even when fully resected (<1%). They have definite but very mild cytologic or architectural atypia, yet they do not have the full features of hepatocellular carcinoma. Currently there is no definitive way to determine if these types of cases are atypical adenomas or well-differentiated hepatocellular carcinoma. If you send these cases to expert hepatic pathologists, you will get different opinions. The good news is that these cases are cured by resection. Given that rare well-differentiated

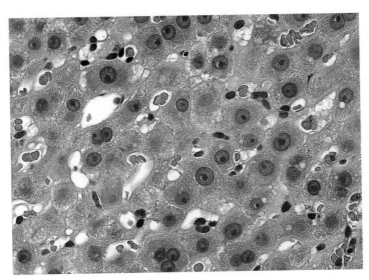

FIGURE 21.13 **Hepatic adenoma mimic.** Well-differentiated hepatocellular carcinoma with no reticulin loss. This hepatocellular carcinoma is very well differentiated and has no reticulin loss, closely mimicking a hepatic adenoma. Note, however, the prominent nucleoli and the occasional bi- and trinucleated cells.

hepatocellular tumors are difficult to classify when fully resected, it should be fully anticipated that occasional biopsy specimens are best approached by a diagnosis of a "well-differentiated hepatic neoplasm" followed by a description and prioritized differential in the comment section of the pathology report.

Hepatic Adenoma Subtypes

Once a diagnosis of hepatic adenoma is made, the adenoma can be subtyped (Table 21.1). If you still are uncertain as to whether a tumor is a hepatic adenoma or a well-differentiated hepatocellular carcinoma, do not try to subtype the tumor as an aid to determine if the neoplasm is benign or malignant: make the diagnosis first, then subtype, as each of the stains

TABLE 21.1 Histologic and Immunostain Findings Used to Subtype Hepatic Adenomas			
H&E Findings	HNF1α Inactivated	Inflammatory	Unclassified
Diffuse steatosis	Often present	Can be present	Infrequent
Faux portal tracts	Negative	Often present	Negative
Sinusoidal dilatation	±	Often present and can be prominent	±
Inflammation	Absent to minimal	Often present	Absent to minimal
Immunostains			
Liver fatty acid binding protein	Lost	Retained	Retained
Serum amyloid A	Negative to patchy nonspecific patterns	Strong and diffuse	Negative to patchy nonspecific patterns
C-reactive protein	Negative to patchy nonspecific patterns	Strong and diffuse	Negative to patchy nonspecific patterns
Risks for malignant transformation			
Frequency of beta-catenin activation	Rare, less than 1%	Highest, about 10%	Intermediate, about 5%
Frequency of heavy pigmentation	Occasional cases, mostly in older patients	Very rare	Very rare
Frequency of myxoid change	Rare, mostly in older patients	Not reported to date	Not reported to date

H&E, hematoxylin-eosin.

used to subtype adenomas can also show similar staining patterns in conventional hepatocellular carcinoma.[19] Subtyping is primarily performed to predict the risk of malignancy in hepatic adenomas, but it also provides information on the risk for hemorrhage. Overall, hepatic adenomas that are inflammatory and/or have beta-catenin activation have a higher risk for malignant transformation, compared with HNF1α-inactivated adenomas. Specific morphologic subtypes (myxoid, pigmented) and androgen-related adenomas also have a higher risk for malignancy.

APPROACH TO MORPHOLOGIC SUBTYPING. One useful way to think about hepatic adenoma subtypes is that there are three major baseline subtypes: HNF1A inactivated, inflammatory, and unclassified.[20] Any of these three subtypes can then have additional, secondary, genetic changes that increase the risk for malignancy. Overall, HNF1A-inactivated adenomas have a higher frequency of becoming pigmented adenomas or myxoid adenomas, while inflammatory and unclassified adenomas are more likely to develop secondary beta-catenin mutations. Thus, classification can include both the underlying type of hepatic adenoma and any additional findings that increase the risk for malignant transformation, for example morphologic findings or beta-catenin activation.

Is full immunostain subtyping of hepatic adenomas necessary for patient care? Currently, management is based primarily on tumor size, clinical findings, atypical radiologic findings, or atypical histologic findings, wherein a well-differentiated hepatocellular carcinoma cannot be completely excluded. Hepatic adenoma subtypes that have an increased risk for malignancy (beta-catenin activated, myxoid, pigmented, androgen related) are also useful for guiding therapy, and this pushes management toward definite therapy, such as complete resection. For these reasons, some medical centers do more focused subclassification of hepatic adenomas by (1) looking for high-risk morphologic features and (2) performing stains to look for beta-catenin activation.

HNF1A-INACTIVATED ADENOMAS make up about 35% of all hepatic adenomas in most case series. Rare cases occur in patients with mature onset diabetes of the young type 3 (MODY3), who have one germline mutation in *HNF1A*, but most HNF1A-inactivated adenomas are sporadic. They are defined by the loss of LFABP expression (a downstream target of HNF1A). They only rarely show beta-catenin activation, and, when they do, it is typically via strong and diffuse glutamine synthetase staining and not by nuclear accumulation of beta-catenin. They have the lowest risk for malignant transformation, although it is not zero and appears to increase in older patients.

HNF1A-inactivated adenomas often have macrovesicular steatosis, ranging from mild to severe, but they typically do not show features of steatohepatitis (Figure 21.14). On the other hand, some HNF1A-inactivated adenomas have no fatty change. In any case, they are defined by having compatible morphology and loss of liver-binding fatty acid protein expression on immunostaining (Figure 21.15). The differential for HNF1A-inactivated hepatic adenomas with fatty change is primarily that of the

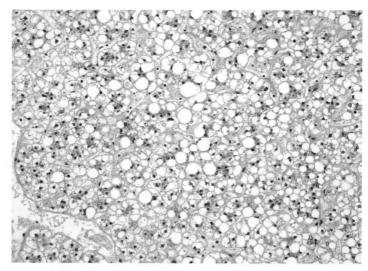

FIGURE 21.14   **Hepatic adenoma, HNF1α inactivated.** This adenoma has moderate fatty change.

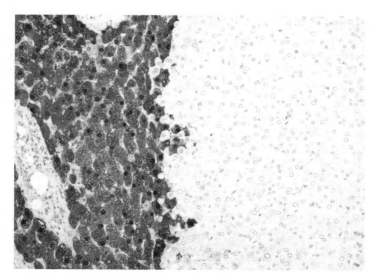

FIGURE 21.15   **Hepatic adenoma, HNF1α-inactivated, liver-binding fatty acid protein.** The background liver is positive, while the tumor is negative.

steatohepatitic variant of hepatocellular carcinoma. In contrast to hepatic adenomas, the steatohepatitic variant of hepatocellular carcinoma typically has more variable-sized fat droplets, balloon cells, often Mallory hyaline, and intratumoral fibrosis. The hepatocellular carcinoma should also have increased mitoses, cytologic atypia, and reticulin loss, as well as can be glypican 3 positive. Both can have mild intratumor inflammation.

INFLAMMATORY HEPATIC ADENOMA. This subtype was first described at the morphologic level as the *telangiectatic variant* of hepatic adenoma but was renamed following refinement of the histological features and molecular studies to the *inflammatory adenoma*. Inflammatory adenomas make up about 50% of all hepatic adenomas in most case series. An important risk factor for this subtype of adenoma is the metabolic syndrome and fatty liver disease. About 10% of all inflammatory adenomas will also show beta-catenin activation, which is much higher than in HNF1A-inactivated adenomas.

Morphologically, many *inflammatory* hepatic adenomas have a classic morphology, a triad of findings composed of dilated (ie, telangiectatic) and congested sinusoids (Figure 21.16), mild to sometimes moderate patchy lymphocytic inflammation in the lobules (Figure 21.17), and distinctive faux portal tracts, with vessels embedded in a fibrous stroma surrounded by a bile ductular proliferation (Figure 21.18; eFigs 21.5-21.7). Not all cases have this morphology, and the diagnosis in the end is based solely on immunostain positivity for CRP and/or SAA (Figure 21.19) in a hepatic adenoma. The staining should be strong and diffuse to be called positive, as moderate to strong, but patchy, staining is commonly seen as a nonspecific staining pattern in focal nodular hyperplasia, other hepatic adenomas, and other reactive lesions. Inflammatory adenomas that arise in the setting of the metabolic syndrome, where the background liver shows steatosis/steatohepatitis, can also show fatty change (eFig. 21.8) and rarely steatohepatitis.

BETA-CATENIN-ACTIVATED ADENOMA. This subtype of hepatic adenoma is defined either by sequencing that identifies *CTNNB1* mutations (which encodes beta-catenin), or by immunostains, which show the presence of

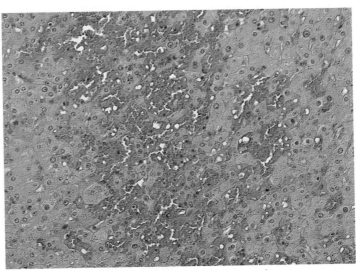

FIGURE 21.16 **Inflammatory hepatic adenoma.** In this area of the adenoma, the parenchyma shows dilated and congested sinusoids or telangiectasia.

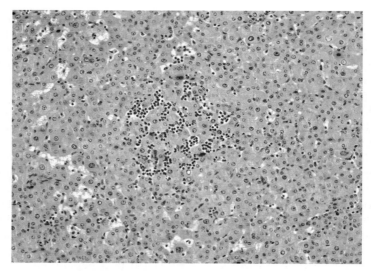

FIGURE 21.17 **Inflammatory hepatic adenoma.** Mild patchy lobular inflammation is seen.

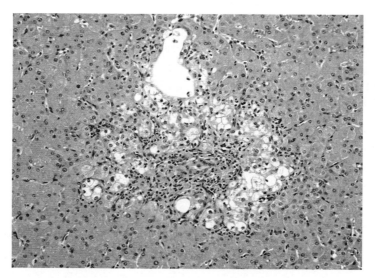

FIGURE 21.18 **Inflammatory hepatic adenoma.** This adenoma has areas that resemble portal tracts, with a circumscribed area of arteries surrounded by a ductular proliferation.

nuclear accumulation of beta-catenin (Figure 21.20) and/or strong and diffuse glutamine synthetase expression (Figure 21.21). The beta-catenin activation, in most cases at least, appears to represent a secondary event in an inflammatory adenoma, unclassified adenoma, or rarely an HNF1α mutated adenoma. Beta-catenin activation in any of these settings is a key

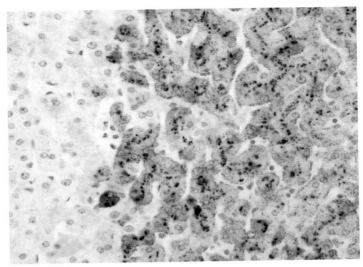

FIGURE 21.19   **Inflammatory hepatic adenoma, serum amyloid A.** The adenoma is positive but the surrounding liver is negative.

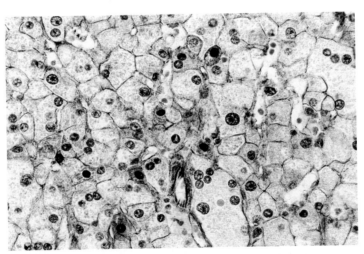

FIGURE 21.20   **Hepatic adenoma, beta-catenin activated.** Nuclear accumulation of beta-catenin is seen.

risk factor for malignant transformation, so some authors lump them all into one basket called *beta-catenin-activated adenomas.*

When evaluating the beta-catenin immunostain, any degree of nuclear staining is considered positive, even a single cell, although the amount of staining does have relevance as discussed later. Glutamine synthetase can show several staining patterns. Because the stain can be "dirty" as a result of background staining, it is important to compare

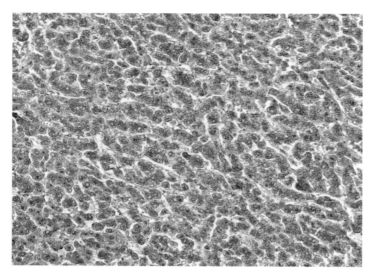

FIGURE 21.21 **Hepatic adenoma, beta-catenin activated.** There is strong and diffuse staining for glutamine synthetase.

the intensity and distribution within the tumor to that seen in the background liver. The background liver should show strong staining of a thin rim of zone 3 hepatocytes. In the adenomas, the most important pattern for identifying an increased risk for malignant transformation is a strong and diffuse staining pattern, with a staining intensity that matches that seen in zone 3 hepatocytes in the background nonneoplastic liver; this pattern indicates beta-catenin activation, even if the beta-catenin immunostain is negative for nuclear staining. A second positive pattern for glutamine synthetase staining shows moderately strong expression that is diffuse (present throughout the tumor) but heterogeneous (not all cells are positive), a pattern sometimes called the "starry sky pattern" (Figure 21.22); this finding is also associated with beta-catenin activation, but with mutations that lead to lower levels of gene activation. Finally, there are a number of nonspecific staining patterns that include weak, patchy staining or perivenular staining.

The type of *CTNNB1* mutation affects the risk for malignant transformation. Large exon 3 deletions and exon 3D32-D37 deletions have the strongest risk, while exon 3 T41 mutations have a moderate risk and exon 3 S45, K335, N387 and other less common mutations all have low risk.[21] These molecular findings show general correlations with beta-catenin and glutamine synthetase staining patterns: tumors with greater than 1% positivity for nuclear accumulation and/or strong and diffuse glutamine synthetase staining correlate with the mutations that have higher risk. The lower risk mutations tend to show rare (less than 1%) or absent nuclear staining and nonspecific glutamine synthetase staining patterns; they are often identified only by sequencing studies. The risk for malignancy is not

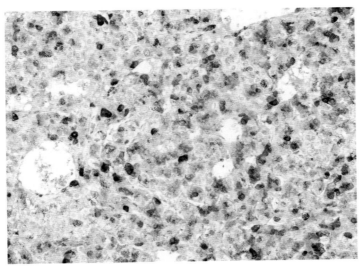

FIGURE 21.22 **Hepatic adenoma, beta-catenin activated.** Staining is heterogeneous but diffuse. This is also referred to as the starry sky pattern.

well defined in hepatic adenomas that have *CTNNB1* mutations identified by sequencing, but lack beta-catenin nuclear accumulation or abnormal glutamine synthetase staining; however, presumably the risk is significantly lower than that of adenomas with immunostain positivity.

PIGMENTED ADENOMA. This finding, like beta-catenin activation, appears to be a secondary event in most cases. Light, subtle lipofuscin is common in many HNF1α-inactivated adenoma, but the pigmented hepatic adenoma is defined by dense, abundant, brown, cytoplasmic pigment made of lipofuscin (Figure 21.23).[22] Many pigmented adenomas appear dark brown or black on gross examination because of the heavy pigmentation. They can demonstrate mild cytologic atypia and in some cases can progress to frank malignancy.[23] In fact, many cases truly straddle the histologic fence between atypical hepatic adenoma and hepatocellular carcinoma, and they can appear as either in the literature. The largest series to date reported that 27% of cases showed early malignant transformation, with male gender being an additional important risk factor. Subtyping shows that about two-thirds of pigmented hepatic adenomas have loss of LFABP expression and one-third are CRP and/or SAA positive.

MYXOID ADENOMAS are defined by the presence of abundant myxoid material that dissects the sinusoids of the hepatic adenoma (Figures 21.24 and 21.25).[24] There is no gland formation and the hepatic adenoma shows histology that is otherwise conventional, with tumor cells composed of mature-appearing hepatocytes with no cytologic atypia. The myxoid material can be weakly alcian blue or mucicarmine positive but does not have the strong staining of true glandular mucin. The percentage of any given

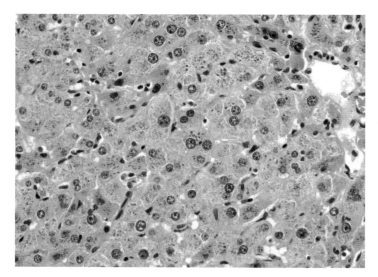

FIGURE 21.23   **Pigmented adenoma.** Abundant cytoplasmic pigment is seen.

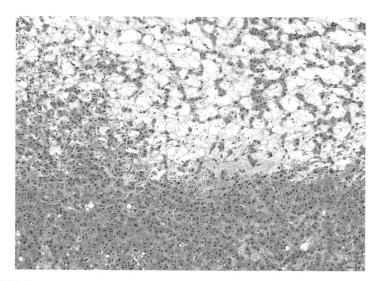

FIGURE 21.24   **Myxoid adenoma.** Abundant myxoid material dissects the sinusoids.

adenoma that shows myxoid change ranges from 30% to 90%. All cases show loss of LAFBP by immunostaining,[24] but these hepatic adenomas have a high risk for malignant transformation, in contrast to the low risk of conventional HNF1α-inactivated adenomas, so they should not be lumped together.

ANDROGEN-ASSOCIATED ADENOMAS by definition arise in persons taking androgens for medical therapy, bodybuilding, or other reasons. About

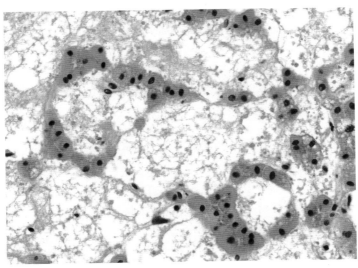

FIGURE 21.25   **Myxoid adenoma.** At higher power, the myxoid material is thin and flocculent. The tumor cells are cytologically bland.

two-thirds occur in men and one-third in women. Subtyping shows that
20% are inflammatory adenomas and 10% are HNF1A-inactivated adenomas, with the rest unclassified.[12] Any of these three subtypes can also show
beta-catenin activation, with about 80% of all androgen-related adenomas
showing beta-catenin activation based on immunostains for beta-catenin
and/or glutamine synthetase.

Morphologically, androgen adenomas frequently show large cell
change (Figure 21.26), pseudoglands (Figure 21.27), and bile production.
A diagnosis of malignant transformation is made in the usual way. Many
reports of malignant transformation can be found in the literature, but the
prognosis is excellent with complete resection.

GNAS-MUTATED ADENOMA. This subtype of hepatic adenoma shows SAA
staining, so early studies classified it with inflammatory adenomas.[25] The
morphology, however, is distinctive and shows intratumoral fibrosis, balloon cells, hyaline bodies, and sometimes Mallory hyaline (Figure 21.28);
the features can be somewhat reminiscent of a fibrolamellar carcinoma.

UNCLASSIFIED ADENOMA. About 10% of hepatic adenomas are unclassified,
as they have none of the morphologic or immunostain findings listed earlier. They may have steatosis (Figure 21.29), and patients often have the
ordinary risk factors of adenomas that can be subclassified.

SONIC HEDGEHOG HEPATIC ADENOMA AND ARGININOSUCCINATE HEPATIC ADENOMA.
This group of proposed adenomas was identified by studying adenomas
that are unclassified using conventional immunostains and morphology:

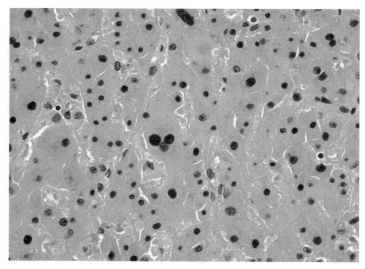

FIGURE 21.26 **Hepatic adenoma, androgen related.** This adenoma arose in a young man using androgens for bodybuilding. Large cell change is evident.

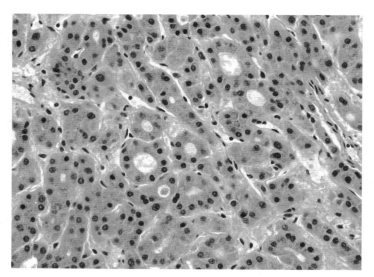

FIGURE 21.27 **Hepatic adenoma, androgen related.** Pseudogland formation is seen.

they look like ordinary adenomas by morphology, show retained LFABP expression, and are negative for SAA and CRP. They are defined by their molecular and immunostain findings. Their clinical relevance is currently under investigation, with early studies suggesting an increased risk for hemorrhage.[26]

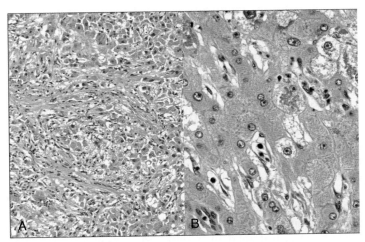

FIGURE 21.28 Hepatic adenoma, GNAS mutated. A, The tumor at low power. The center of the tumor shows fibrosis and ballooning. B, On high power, the tumor cells are cytologically bland, with variably prominent nucleoli. Mallory hyaline is common toward the center of the tumor.

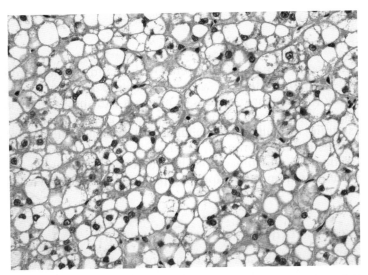

FIGURE 21.29 **Hepatic adenoma, unclassified type**. The adenoma shows fatty change, but immunostains for subtyping were all negative.

Atypical Hepatic Adenomas

In some biopsies of well-differentiated hepatocellular tumors, the histologic features have more atypia than conventional adenomas, but do not reach the level of definite malignancy. Often, these cases are approached by using a diagnosis of *well-differentiated hepatocellular neoplasm, please see note,* and then explaining in the note which features are atypical. In some cases, the atypia is mild but an overall diagnosis of hepatic adenoma is still appropriate. In these cases, the term *atypical hepatic adenoma* can be used. This term is also commonly used when the neoplasm is definitely an adenoma but has risk factors for malignant transformation, such as beta-catenin activation, heavy lipofuscin pigment deposition, or myxoid changes. If the tumor cannot be classified as benign versus malignant, then another proposed term is *hepatocellular neoplasm of uncertain malignant potential* (HUMP).[27]

Cytologic changes may include mild and focal but definite nuclear atypia, cytoplasmic inclusions, or clearly abnormal N:C ratios. Focal or patchy large cell change is acceptable as an expected finding in conventional inflammatory hepatic adenomas or androgen-related adenomas, but small cell change is not seen in hepatic adenomas. Bile production with bile visible on H&E staining is also an atypical finding, one that is absent in most conventional hepatic adenomas, except those that are androgen related. Architectural atypia in atypical adenomas may include pseudogland formation, equivocal nodule-in-nodule growth patterns, and focal equivocal reticulin loss.

Immunostains

Hepatic adenomas should have no reticulin loss and very low proliferation rates on Ki-67 immunostaining, with most being 2% or less.[17] One caveat is that the tumor cells near the areas of necrosis can show mildly increased proliferative rates. Hepatic adenomas should be glypican 3 negative. CD34 immunostaining typically shows patchy sinusoidal staining in hepatic adenomas, versus diffuse staining in hepatocellular carcinoma, but does not reliably distinguish adenomas from hepatocellular carcinoma. Additional information on immunostains for subtyping hepatic adenomas is included in Table 21.1.

Malignant Transformation of Hepatic Adenomas

The overall risk of malignant transformation has not been well defined, but approximately 10% of resected hepatic adenomas reported in the literature have underwent malignant transformation.[28] About 60% of malignancies arise in beta-catenin-activated adenomas. In most cases of malignant transformation, the adenomas are 5 cm or more in greatest dimension. Thus, current management guidelines are based in large part on size and the general recommendation is for adenomas greater than 5 cm to be resected. Histologic subtypes with an increased risk for malignancy can also drive therapy-related decisions.

MACROREGENERATIVE NODULES

Macroregenerative nodules are benign and develop in cirrhotic livers. The basic notion of this lesion is simple: a benign nodule that stands out as being significantly bigger than its peers in a cirrhotic liver (Figure 21.30). Usually the macroregenerative nodule is between 10 and 20 mm.[29] The frequency is approximately 15% in explanted livers. Macroregenerative nodules can also be seen in noncirrhotic livers that have undergone extensive parenchymal loss, with large areas of panacinar collapse, for example, from fulminant hepatitis; in these cases, the macroregenerative nodules can be considerably larger, sometimes up to 5 cm.

Macroregenerative nodules have no significant cytologic or architectural atypia, no loss of reticulin, and no other features to suggest malignancy. The hepatocytes within macroregenerative nodules look essentially the same as hepatocytes located outside the nodule. The nodules show intermingled portal tracts, although the portal tracts may show abnormal spacing. A Ki-67 staining shows a low proliferation rate, one that is the same as the background liver. Because of the size criterion, a diagnosis of a macroregenerative nodule is best made on a resection or wedge biopsy and not a needle biopsy, although the diagnosis can be included in the differential on a needle biopsy specimen when appropriate.

DYSPLATIC NODULE

Dysplastic nodules occur only in cirrhotic livers. They stand out from the background liver on gross examination because of their larger size or the differences in color. Most are less than 2 cm in size. Dysplastic nodules by

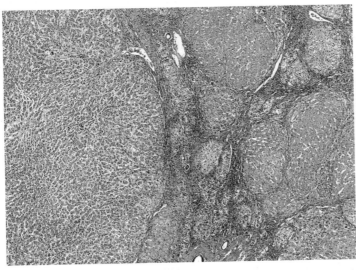

FIGURE 21.30 **Macroregenerative nodule.** The large nodule on the left side of the image is noticeably larger than its peers.

definition show atypia (dysplasia) that is evident in the lesion but not the background liver, yet the atypia does not reach the full criteria of definite hepatocellular carcinoma. Portal tracts are often present within dysplastic nodules, more so in low-grade than high-grade dysplastic nodules.

This essential notion of dysplastic nodules is straightforward, but the minimal criteria needed to distinguish a macroregenerative nodule from a low-grade dysplastic nodule have been difficult to standardize. Likewise, distinguishing a high-grade dysplastic nodule from a well-differentiated hepatocellular carcinoma can be challenging. In general, biopsy specimens are best approached by deciding if the lesion can be definitely classified as benign or malignant. If there is definitive atypia, but the atypia does not reach the level diagnostic of hepatocellular carcinoma, then the best diagnosis is often descriptive, with a note indicating that the differential includes a dysplastic nodule versus a well-differentiated hepatocellular carcinoma.

The histologic atypia in dysplastic nodules is further divided into low-grade and high-grade dysplasia. This distinction is routine in research studies and is reasonably applied to nodules in resected liver specimens, but it can be challenging to use in clinical practice with biopsy specimens because of sampling concerns; the core elements are shown in Table 21.2. In addition, the distinction between a low-grade dysplastic nodule and a macroregenerative nodule can be fairly arbitrary using currently available methods, but the basic notion is that the low-grade dysplastic nodule has mild but noticeable cytological atypia that is not present in the background liver.

Atypical histologic features may include areas of pseudogland formation (less helpful in cholestatic livers), mild nuclear atypia, intraparenchymal arterioles, and complex architecture with a "nodule within a nodule" appearance. Large cell change or small cell change may also be seen (Figures 21.31 and 21.32) (Table 21.2). Often, large cell change is also present in the background cirrhotic liver; in these cases, the large cell change should be more striking or more diffuse in comparison to the background liver in order to be helpful in suggesting the lesion is a dysplastic nodule.

To exclude hepatocellular carcinoma, there should be no loss of reticulin, no mitotic figures, and a Ki-67 proliferation rate that is similar to the background liver. α-Fetoprotein (AFP) immunohistochemistry is negative. Beta-catenin immunostaining is negative for nuclear accumulation. Glutamine synthetase is negative for strong and diffuse staining.

HEPATOCELLULAR CARCINOMA: GENERAL PRINCIPLES

Definition

Hepatocellular carcinomas are malignant liver tumors that show hepatocellular differentiation.

TABLE 21.2   Differentiating Features in Macroregenerative Nodules, Dysplastic Nodules, and Low-Grade Hepatocellular Carcinoma

Histologic Features	Macroregenerative Nodule	Dysplastic Nodule, Low Grade	Dysplastic Nodule, High Grade	Hepatocellular Carcinoma
Cytology				
Small cell change	–	–	±	±
Large cell change	–	±	±	±
Subclone-like areas of growth	–	–	±	±
Architectural changes				
Portal tracts	Present	Present	Present, focal	Absent
Pseudogland/ acinar changes	–	–	±	±
Lobular arterialization	–	±	±	+
Stromal invasion[a]	–	–	–	±
Nodule in Nodule Growth	–	–	–	±
Immunohistochemical stains				
Reticulin framework	Intact	Intact	Intact	Usually at least focal loss
Ki-67	No increase compared to background liver	No increase compared to background liver	No or minimal increase compared to background liver	Increased compared to background liver
Glypican 3	–	–	–	±
Strong, diffuse glutamine synthetase staining	–	–	–	±

(Continued)

TABLE 21.2 Differentiating Features in Macroregenerative Nodules, Dysplastic Nodules, and Low-Grade Hepatocellular Carcinoma (Continued)

Histologic Features	Macroregenerative Nodule	Dysplastic Nodule, Low Grade	Dysplastic Nodule, High Grade	Hepatocellular Carcinoma
Beta-catenin nuclear staining	–	–	–	±

[a]This finding is most useful in cirrhotic livers and in resection specimens; it is rarely if ever helpful in biopsy specimens. Stromal invasion is defined as malignant cells extending into the portal tracts or fibrous stroma as small clusters of cells or as single cells. Stromal invasion is also associated with a loss of the normal ductular reaction that is present around cirrhotic nodules; stains for CK7 or CK19 can help evaluate for the presence or absence of a ductular reaction.

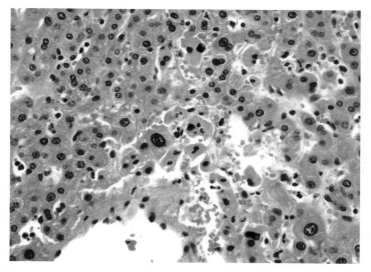

FIGURE 21.31 **Large cell change.** Several hepatocytes have large, hyperchromatic nuclei, but they also have abundant cytoplasm, with near normal N:C ratios.

Clinical

Older men with chronic liver disease are at the highest risk for hepatocellular carcinoma. The incidence increases dramatically after the age of 40 years, and the average age at diagnosis is approximately 65 years. Overall, the most important risk factor is cirrhosis from any cause. Worldwide, chronic hepatitis B is the most common risk factor, but in the United States, much of Europe, and Japan, chronic hepatitis C is also a common risk factor. The metabolic syndrome is both a contributing factor for carcinoma in patients with chronic viral hepatitis[30] and an independent risk

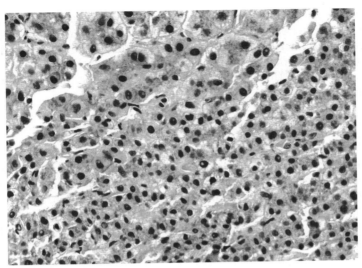

FIGURE 21.32 **Small cell change.** The hepatocytes in the upper left corner of the image are normal in size, in contrast to the hepatocytes with small cell change.

factor for hepatocellular carcinoma.[31] With the advent of highly effective antiviral therapy, modeling suggests that in time, hepatocellular carcinomas in cirrhotic livers from fatty liver disease will become more common than viral-hepatitis-associated hepatocellular carcinoma. Other important causes include alcohol-related liver disease and hemochromatosis. Cirrhosis from chronic biliary tract disease is also a risk factor.

Of note, 15% to 20% of hepatocellular carcinomas arise in noncirrhotic livers.[32] Of these cases, approximately 50% will have chronic liver disease that is thought to have caused the cancer, despite the lack of cirrhosis. Chronic hepatitis B,[33] chronic hepatitis C,[34] HFE-related hemochromatosis,[35] fatty liver disease,[36,37] and malignant transformation of hepatic adenomas[28] have all been linked to hepatocellular carcinoma in noncirrhotic livers. No cause is identified in the remaining subset of cases, despite full clinical and pathologic evaluation.

SERUM FINDINGS. Serologic findings are helpful when there is a liver mass on imaging. The most commonly used serum markers are AFP, lens culinaris agglutinin-reactive AFP (AFP-L3), and des-gamma-carboxyprothrombin (DCP). All of these markers have both diagnostic value and prognostic value, as higher levels indicate a worse prognosis.[38] For serum AFP, normal levels are less than 20 ng/mL in healthy adults. Overall, about one-third of hepatocellular carcinomas have significantly elevated serum AFP levels at the time of diagnosis. AFP levels greater than 400 ng/mL are generally considered to be diagnostic for hepatocellular carcinoma in a person with a liver mass, chronic viral hepatitis, and cirrhosis. AFP-L3 measures a glycosylated form of AFP that is more specific for hepatocellular carcinoma and typically uses a cutoff of 10%, but when levels reach 35%, the specificity increases to nearly 100%.[39] DCP has a sensitivity of about 75% and a specificity of about 70% for hepatocellular carcinoma.[40] DCP is an abnormal form of prothrombin and is also known as prothrombin induced by vitamin K absence II (PIVKA II). In many centers, combinations of all three markers are used.

How to Make the Histologic Diagnosis of Hepatocellular Carcinoma

Many hepatocellular carcinomas are recognizable on H&E stains, whereas others require confirmation with special stains. In the process of choosing which special stains to perform, a useful first step is to ask yourself this question: is the tissue clearly liver parenchyma, but I am not sure if it is benign or malignant? Or, alternatively, the relevant question could be this: I am sure there is cancer on the biopsy, but is the cancer a hepatocellular carcinoma or metastatic disease? The stains you should perform will depend substantially on the answer to this question (Tables 21.3 and 21.4). If the tissue in question is clearly well-differentiated hepatocytes and the background liver is noncirrhotic, then the differential is typically that of a focal nodular hyperplasia, hepatic adenoma, or well-differentiated hepatocellular carcinoma; however, the differential for a well differentiated hepatocellular lesion in a cirrhotic liver is a regenerative nodule, dysplastic nodule, and well-differentiated hepatocellular carcinoma. Stains that will help with this differential are shown in Table 21.3. In contrast, if the tumor is clearly malignant, but you are not sure if it is metastatic disease or hepatocellular carcinoma, then stains for hepatocellular differentiation will help you make the diagnosis (Table 21.4). A common misstep is not making this distinction up front, which can lead to unnecessary stains and sometimes to exhaustion of the block before a full diagnosis can be made.

Hepatocellular Grading

Hepatocellular grading is an important part of the pathology report. Research studies commonly use the modified Edmondson-Steiner grading system, which is focused on nuclear changes, as summarized in Table 21.5.[42] Grading for clinical purposes tends to be more holistic, assessing nuclear changes as well as cytoplasmic changes. The WHO approach is shown in Table 21.6[43] and can be summarized as **well differentiated**—the tissue is clearly liver, but stains are needed to make sure it is cancer (Figure 21.33; eFig. 21.9); **moderately differentiated**—on H&E stain the tissue is clearly cancer *and* hepatocellular differentiation is morphologically evident (Figure 21.34); and **poorly differentiated**—on H&E stain the tissue is clearly cancer, but immunostains are needed to be sure it has hepatocellular differentiation (Figures 21.35 and 21.36; eFig. 21.10). Regardless of the system used, two or more nuclear grades can be present, in which case the tumor is classified according to the worse nuclear grade.

TABLE 21.3 Stains to Distinguish Benign From Malignant Liver Lesions

Stains	Comment
Reticulin	A very small proportion of hepatocellular carcinomas will not have reticulin loss.
Ki-67	Only helpful if significantly higher than background liver.
Glypican 3	Positive in about 50% of well-differentiated hepato-cellular carcinomas. Can be very focally positive in both benign livers with significant inflammation and in high dysplastic nodules.
AFP	Negative in benign lesions; positive in about one-third of all hepatocellular carcinomas.
EZH2	Overexpression favors hepatocellular carcinoma.[41]
Beta-catenin	In a cirrhotic liver only, positive staining supports hepatocellular carcinoma; not very sensitive, so negative staining is not informative.
Glutamine synthetase	In a cirrhotic liver only, positive staining supports hepatocellular carcinoma; not very sensitive, so negative staining is not informative.
CD34	Strong diffuse staining is commonly seen in hepatocel-lular carcinoma, but it is not specific and should not be the sole or primary feature supporting a diagnosis of hepatocellular carcinoma.

AFP, α-fetoprotein; EZH2, enhancer of zeste homolog 2.

UNDIFFERENTIATED CARCINOMA OF THE LIVER. With the wise use of immu-nostain panels, nearly all carcinomas primary to the liver can be classi-fied as hepatocellular carcinoma versus cholangiocarcinoma. The few that remain (<1%) are sufficiently undifferentiated that a final diagnosis of a carcinoma primary to the liver can be ascertained only by the imaging and clinical findings; in these cases, the histology and immunostain results do not provide sufficient evidence to confidentially distinguish hepatocellu-lar carcinoma from cholangiocarcinoma. Some of these cases will show at least patchy albumin in situ hybridization staining, but this finding does not differentiate a poorly differentiated hepatocellular carcinoma from a poorly differentiated cholangiocarcinoma.

Background Liver

Do not forget the importance of examining the background liver for active injury and for fibrosis stage. To do this, a section(s) should be taken as far away from the tumor as possible, ideally at least 1 cm. With biopsy specimens, this is of course problematic unless a separate biopsy was intentionally taken away from the mass lesion. If the only back-ground liver tissue available for assessment is adjacent to the tumor, the

TABLE 21.4 Stains to Identify Hepatocellular Differentiation in a Definite Carcinoma	
Stains	**Comment**
In situ hybridization for albumin	• Positive in >95% of all HCCs
	• Also positive in most intrahepatic cholangiocarcinomas
HepPar-1	• Positive in 90% of all HCCs
	• Poorly differentiated HCCs are most likely to be negative.
Arginase-1	• Positive in 90% of all HCCs
	• HCC can be negative at either end of the differentiation spectrum: well-differentiated or poorly differentiated HCCs
Glypican 3	• Positive in 70%-90% of moderately to poorly differentiated carcinomas
	• Positive in 50% of well-differentiated carcinomas
	• Can be positive in other types of cancer
Polyclonal CEA (canalicular pattern)	• Positive in 60%-80% of all HCCs
	• Poorly differentiated HCCs are frequently negative
CD10 (canalicular pattern)	• Positive in 60%-80% of all HCCs
	• Only a canalicular pattern of staining provides evidence for hepatocellular differentiation; other patterns of staining, such as membranous, are fine for HCC, but are not specific
	• Poorly differentiated HCCs are frequently negative
AFP	• Positive in about one-third of all HCCs

AFP, α-fetoprotein; CEA, carcinoembryonic antigen; HCC, hepatocellular carcinoma.

findings can be inaccurate, as estimates of fat, inflammation, cholestasis, and fibrosis can be strongly influenced by the nearby tumor mass and may not reflect the background liver. Also, with resection specimens avoid the cauterized resection edges as much as possible when evaluating the background liver.

Prognosis

The single most important prognostic factor is tumor resectability. Other prognostic findings include age (the younger, the better), gender (women, better), and the presence or absence of cirrhosis (absence, better). Comorbid conditions such as heart disease also strongly influence survival.

Histology findings that influence survival include tumor grade, tumor size, tumor number, and the presence of angiolymphatic invasion (eFigs. 21.11

TABLE 21.5 Modified Edmondson-Steiner Grading System for Hepatocellular Carcinoma

Grade	Criteria
1	Abundant cytoplasm; minimal nuclear atypia
2	Mild nuclear atypia with prominent nucleoli, hyperchromasia, and nuclear irregularity
3	Moderate nuclear atypia with greater hyperchromasia and nuclear irregularity
4	Marked nuclear pleomorphism, marked hyperchromasia, and anaplastic giant cells

TABLE 21.6 WHO[43] Grading Schema for Hepatocellular Carcinomas

Grade	Criteria
Well differentiated	• **Overview:** on H&E, tumor could be benign or malignant and hepatocellular differentiation is clearly evident on H&E • **Nuclear atypia:** minimal to mild • **Cytoplasm:** typically eosinophilic, abundant to moderately abundant • **N:C ratio:** normal or very slightly increased
Moderately differentiated	• **Overview:** tumor is clearly malignant on H&E, yet the morphology strongly suggests hepatocellular origin. Stains are useful to confirm hepatocellular differentiation • **Nuclear atypia:** mild to moderate • **Cytoplasm:** ranges from eosinophilic to basophilic; moderately abundant in most cases • **N:C ratio:** clearly increased by light microscopy when compared to neighboring nonneoplastic hepatocytes
Poorly differentiated	• **Overview:** tumor is clearly malignant on H&E. The differential would include a range of poorly differentiated carcinomas; immunostains are used to confirm hepatocellular differentiation • **Nuclear atypia:** moderate[a] to marked • **Cytoplasm:** usually basophilic, moderately abundant[b] to scant • **N:C ratio:** clearly increased by light microscopy when compared to neighboring nonneoplastic hepatocytes

H&E, hematoxylin-eosin.
[a]Tumor cells with moderate nuclear atypia but scant cytoplasm, leading to very high N:C ratios, are classified as poorly differentiated.
[b]Tumor cells with moderately abundant cytoplasm but severe nuclear atypia are classified as poorly differentiated.

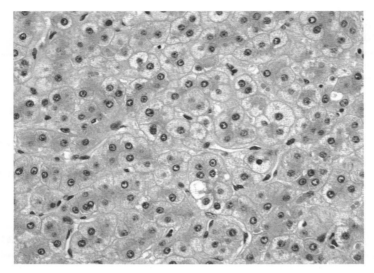

FIGURE 21.33 **Hepatocellular carcinoma, well differentiated.**

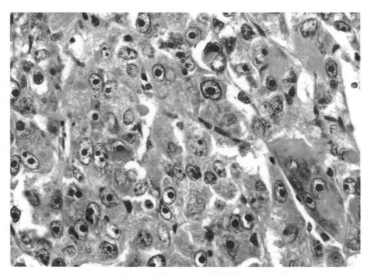

FIGURE 21.34 **Hepatocellular carcinoma, moderately differentiated.**

and 21.12). The last three factors are key elements in most tumor staging systems. For angiolymphatic invasion, large vessel invasion is defined as vessels that are large enough to identify on imaging or gross examination. Large vessel invasion has a worse prognosis than small vessel invasion, the latter being identified only on microscopy. The portal veins are the most common

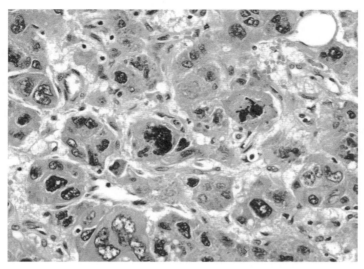

FIGURE 21.35 **Hepatocellular carcinoma, poorly differentiated.** There is moderately abundant cytoplasm but striking nuclear atypia.

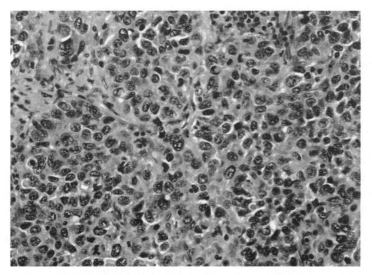

FIGURE 21.36 **Hepatocellular carcinoma, poorly differentiated.** In this example the tumor cells have scant cytoplasm and less nuclear atypia.

site of tumor invasion and the best place to search for vascular invasion is at the tumor-nontumor interface. Tumor grade also influences prognosis, as do morphologic variants discussed later, but neither have the prognostic power of tumor stage.

Histology

- Two-thirds of hepatocellular carcinomas show conventional morphology.
- One-third of hepatocellular carcinomas can be further subtyped into about 12 recognized histologic variants/subtypes.
- The morphologic findings below can be seen with conventional morphology and any subtypes.

  - **Findings within tumor cells**
    - Bile production
    - Hyaline bodies
    - Mallory hyaline
    - Pale bodies
    - Fat accumulation in tumor cells
    - Glycogen accumulation in tumor cells
    - Ballooning

  - **Architectural findings in hepatocellular carcinoma**
    - Nodule within nodule growth
    - Peliosis
    - Four histologic growth patterns: trabecular (70%), solid (20%), pseudoglandular (10%), and macrotrabecular (1%). Most cases have mixed growth patterns.

  - **Stromal changes in hepatocellular carcinoma**
    - Intratumoral inflammation
    - Intratumoral fibrosis
    - Clusters of foamy macrophages in tumor sinusoids (rare)
    - Myxoid changes, usually focal (rare)

Cytologic findings and architectural growth patterns show considerable variation in hepatocellular carcinomas (eFigs. 21.13-21.16). Well-differentiated hepatocellular carcinomas have abundant pink cytoplasm and round nuclei with dispersed chromatin and variably prominent nucleoli. Aberrant arteries (because they are located in the lobules and not the portal tracts) are not specific for hepatocellular carcinoma, but they can be a useful finding in distinguishing well-differentiated tumors from the background liver (eFigs. 21.17 and 21.18). The cytoplasm of tumor cells can have fatty change, clear cell change, or eosinophilic inclusions. As tumors become poorly differentiated, they tend to have less cytoplasm and increasingly basophilic cytoplasm, along with increasing degrees of nuclear atypia.

Hepatocellular carcinomas have four histologic growth patterns (Figures 21.37-21.40; eFigs. 21.19 and 21.20), which are defined by the H&E findings: trabecular (70%), solid (also known as compact, 20%), pseudoglandular (also known as pseudoacinar, 10%), and macrotrabecular (1%). These growth patterns are important to know mostly so you recognize the patterns of growth that are consistent with hepatocellular carcinoma.

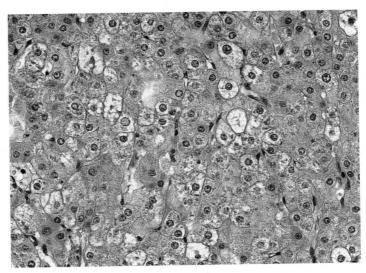

FIGURE 21.37 Hepatocellular carcinoma, solid growth pattern.

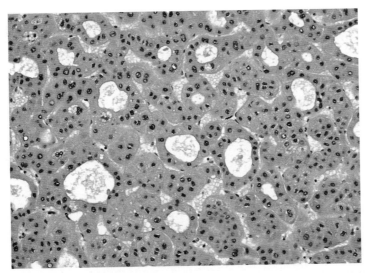

FIGURE 21.38 Hepatocellular carcinoma, pseudoglandular growth pattern.

Overall, the pseudoglandular growth pattern has an association with beta-catenin mutations,[44] while the macrotrabecular growth pattern tends to have a worse prognosis.[45] For research purposes, a minimum cutoff of 5% is used to say that a growth pattern is present. Most hepatocellular carcinomas have a mixture of these growth patterns, and any of these patterns can be found in the various hepatocellular carcinoma subtypes.

The trabecular growth pattern has clearly evident trabeculae on H&E staining, while the solid growth pattern grows in solid sheets. The solid growth pattern can also result from a compressed trabecular pattern, and

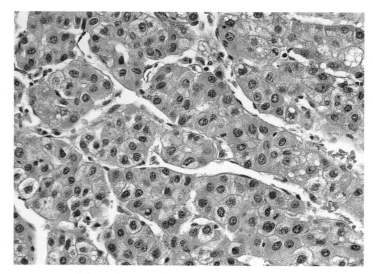

FIGURE 21.39 Hepatocellular carcinoma, trabecular growth pattern.

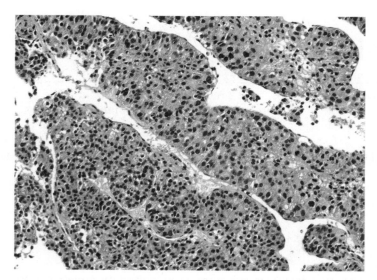

FIGURE 21.40 Hepatocellular carcinoma, macrotrabecular growth pattern.

they often coexist and blend imperceptibly into each other. The macrotrabecular growth pattern is defined as trabeculae that are at least 10 cells thick (some authors prefer 6; there is no data to really say which is better). The pseudoglandular pattern has tumor cells lining circular gland-like structures that represent dilated bile canalicular structures (at least in many cases) and can have actual bile or thin, flocculent eosinophilic material. The pseudoglands can range in size from very small to very large, with the larger ones resembling the size of thyroid follicles. A synonym for the pseudogland growth pattern is pseudoacinar growth pattern.

Histochemical Stains and Immunostains

Four Immutable Laws of Immunohistochemistry

Law 1. Special stains (or molecular tests) should be interpreted in conjunction with the H&E findings. A good example, and one that is frequently encountered, is the use of stains for hepatocellular differentiation (HepPar1, Arginase, glypican 3, and albumin in situ hybridization). To date, none of these stains are entirely specific, all being positive in a small proportion of metastatic carcinomas. Nonetheless, this potential problem is substantially mitigated when the morphologic findings are taken into account when looking at the stains. In fact, diagnostic specificity approaches its maximum when (1) using a panel of stains, (2) fully integrating their interpretation with the morphologic features, and (3) performing correlation of tissue diagnosis with clinical/imaging findings.

Law 2. The sensitivity and specificity of any immunostain is best in the first reports, gets worse in subsequent reports, and reaches its true test characteristics only after many years. So true! The literature bears witness to this time and again. The first set of papers reports the best specificity and sensitivity. More robust understanding of a stain's performance, however, develops only after many years, during which time the stains are used at many different medical centers in many different situations.

Law 3. Discrepancies between the morphology and immunohistochemical findings are resolved by more investigation. This seems obvious but continues to be a recurrent diagnostic pitfall. The most common example is to diagnose hepatocellular carcinoma based on a positive HepPar-1 or arginase-1 stain, when the H&E findings are not typical for hepatocellular carcinoma, or to exclude hepatocellular carcinoma, when the H&E findings are typical for that diagnosis, only because a single marker of hepatocellular differentiation was negative, such as HepPar-1 or arginase-1. In these cases, the diagnosis is resolved with additional immunostains or sometimes with additional sections (on resection specimens).

Law 4. A difficult case is the worst time to first use an unfamiliar stain. This also seems a bit obvious but continues to be a recurrent diagnostic pitfall, leading to a fair number of consults where new stains that were applied to a difficult case turn out to be positive and then the pathologist is unsure what the staining means. To wisely use a new stain, it takes time and experience with the stain to fully understand its strengths and weaknesses. Much of this is best performed when first validating the new stain for use in your laboratory; it is good practice to stain many cases expected to be positive and many that are in the same H&E differential but are expected to be negative.

Most cases of liver tumors benefit from additional stains to confirm or establish the diagnosis. As discussed previously, there are two distinct situations in which most stains are used. The first situation is making a diagnosis on well-differentiated hepatocellular lesions; the second situation is to confirm hepatic differentiation in moderately to poorly differentiated carcinomas. It is best to make this distinction before you order your stains.

There are four fundamental laws that govern the application of immunostains to diagnostic histopathology (see box). Some additional observations are also helpful for understanding the literature on immunostains and hepatocellular carcinoma. There is a large body of literature that pits one stain against another and has them duke it out to see who is the number 1 champ for diagnosing hepatocellular carcinoma. Keep these issues in mind as you read this type of literature, or hear talks, or read books that summarize this literature. First, a stain's performance characteristics will depend on the grade of the tumor. For example, a general trend in the literature is that HepPar-1 beats glypican 3 in well-differentiated tumors, while glypican 3 beats HepPar-1 in poorly differentiated tumors. A second important observation is that other factors, such as the presence or absence of cirrhosis and the underlying liver disease, can also influence the overall performance of a stain. For example, glypican 3 is more likely to be positive in hepatocellular carcinomas that arise in the setting of cirrhosis and have chronic hepatitis B as the underlying cause of liver disease. Thus, the published results from a given center can be strongly influenced by the overall mix of tumor grades in their study population, as well as other histologic findings such as background fibrosis. A third important observation, which naturally follows the first two, is that the first reports in the literature generally have the highest sensitivities and specificities for any given marker. The sensitivities and specificities invariably drop off with additional experiences at other institutions. Finally, sometimes a group or an author can become overly committed to the superiority of a single marker. In the end, however, essentially all expert pathologists prefer to use a panel of stains in their daily practice, and many published articles have drawn the same conclusion.

A last note regarding staining specificity—many immunostains that detect hepatocellular differentiation are also positive at low frequencies in a wide range of non-hepatocellular carcinomas. Although this is important to know, it is less of a problem than the literature sometimes makes it out to be because you also have a powerful ally—the H&E findings. As one example, a small proportion of adenocarcinomas from many different sites can be HepPar-1 positive, but generally this is only a small concern, as adenocarcinomas typically do not look like hepatocellular carcinomas on H&E staining. Thus, as a practical matter, in most cases, this is not really a practical matter after all. For those cases that are truly problematic, for example, a biopsy with only a very small amount of poorly differentiated tumor, the best approach lies in doing a panel of stains.

RETICULIN STAIN. The reticulin stain has been a true workhorse for the diagnosis of hepatocellular carcinoma. In the normal liver, the reticulin stain will highlight the hepatocyte trabecular architecture, with trabecula composed of single or double layers of hepatocytes. Sometimes the trabeculae are even a bit thicker in rapidly regenerating livers (three to four cells, focally). In hepatocellular carcinomas, the hepatic trabeculae are even thicker and the reticulin stain brings this out. However, as many hepatocellular carcinomas do not grow in trabecular growth pattern and so may not show "thickened trabecula," another useful diagnostic approach is that hepatocellular carcinomas demonstrate "loss of reticulin". In benign livers, all hepatocytes touch reticulin on at least one of their borders (Figure 21.41). With hepatocellular carcinoma, there is reduction in the amount of reticulin, and there will be aggregates of hepatocytes that do not touch a reticulin fiber on any of their surfaces (Figures 21.42 and 21.43). Regardless of which approach you prefer remember that the reticulin findings should be more than focal and minimal to have diagnostic significance. Also of note, a small proportion of well-differentiated hepatocellular carcinomas (less than 1%) will have a normal reticulin staining pattern on liver biopsy.[46] The diagnosis in these cases has to be made by other features, primarily cytologic atypia, increased proliferation rates, and/or abnormal staining for markers such as glypican 3. Fatty tumors can represent an additional diagnostic pitfall, as benign livers with macrovesicular steatosis can have focal and patchy reticulin loss that mimics hepatocellular carcinoma.[47]

CD34 STAIN. Immunostains for CD34 highlight the zone 1 sinusoids of the normal liver (eFig. 21.21), but there tends to be strong, diffuse sinusoidal staining in hepatocellular carcinomas (Figure 21.44). However, some hepatocellular carcinomas will lack this staining pattern, and some

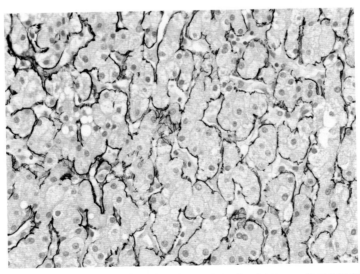

FIGURE 21.41 **Reticulin stain, normal liver.** The hepatic plates are all one to two cells in thickness, and each hepatocyte is touching the reticulin on one of its surfaces.

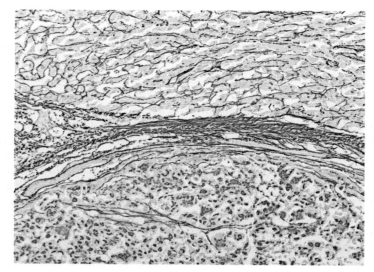

FIGURE 21.42 **Reticulin loss in hepatocellular carcinoma.** The reticulin framework is preserved in the nonneoplastic liver (upper part of image) but the tumor shows substantial loss of reticulin (lower part of image).

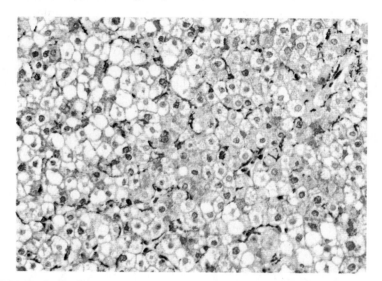

FIGURE 21.43 **Reticulin loss in hepatocellular carcinoma.** A hepatic plate architecture is not evident in this tumor, which has a solid growth pattern, but there is extensive reticulin loss as evidenced by the numerous tumor cells that are not touching reticulin on any surface.

adenomas can show strong and diffuse sinusoidal staining, especially on biopsy specimens, so CD34 is not as useful as many of the other available stains. Hepatocellular carcinomas with a macrotrabecular growth have a distinctive staining pattern, where CD34 highlights the very thick trabeculae (eFig. 21.22).

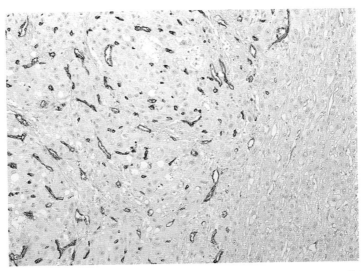

FIGURE 21.44 **Hepatocellular carcinoma, CD34 immunostain in hepatocellular carcinoma**. A CD34 stain shows diffuse sinusoidal positivity in this hepatocellular carcinoma. The nonneoplastic liver seen in the right side of the image is negative.

STAINS FOR HEPATOCELLULAR DIFFERENTIATION

Stains for hepatocellular differentiation include makers of canaliculi such as CD10,[48] polyclonal carcinoembryonic antigen (pCEA), and bile salt export pump (BSEP).[49] These stains are positive in approximately 70% to 90% of hepatocellular carcinomas, and all require a canalicular pattern of staining to be diagnostically useful (Figure 21.45). As with all stains for hepatocellular differentiation, they perform best on well-differentiated and moderately differentiated hepatocellular carcinomas and less well, and often not at all, in poorly differentiated hepatocellular carcinomas. Of note, about 10% to 15% of hepatocellular carcinomas will have membranous and/or cytoplasmic CD10 staining alone, instead of the canalicular pattern. Although this finding is not diagnostically useful, in that it does not distinguish hepatocellular carcinoma from non-hepatocellular carcinoma, this pattern is still consistent with hepatocellular carcinoma. Noncanalicular staining patterns for pCEA and CD10 often coexist with canalicular staining patterns (about a third of cases), and this combination still provides specific support for a diagnosis of hepatocellular carcinoma, as long as a canalicular component is present.[50] Overall, a lack of canalicular staining is more common with poorly differentiated hepatocellular carcinomas, and this can be taken into account when working up a case. Put another way, the lack of a canalicular staining for pCEA, CD10, or BSEP in a well-differentiated or moderately differentiated tumor provides stronger evidence against a diagnosis of hepatocellular carcinoma than it does in a poorly differentiated tumor. Overall, these stains have been

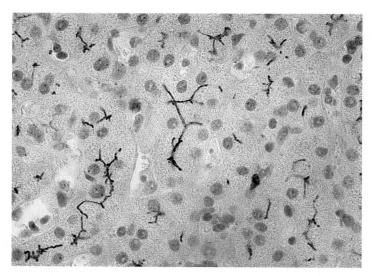

FIGURE 21.45 **Hepatocellular carcinoma, CD10 with canalicular staining pattern.** To demonstrate hepatic differentiation, CD10 stains show a canalicular staining pattern. A similar pattern should be seen with immunostains for polyclonal carcinoembryonic antigen (pCEA).

largely supplanted by HepPar-1, glypican 3, arginase-1, and albumin in situ hybridization.

The HepPar-1 stain was one of the first widely used stains specifically designed to identify hepatocellular differentiation[51]; this stain revolutionized the approach of diagnosing hepatocellular carcinomas. HepPar-1 recognizes a mitochondrial antigen[52] and demonstrates granular cytoplasmic staining (Figure 21.46) in approximately 85% to 95% of hepatocellular carcinomas.[53] HepPar-1 performs very well in tumors that are well and moderately differentiated, with some loss of sensitivity and specificity in poorly differentiated tumors. Even when positive, HepPar-1 staining can be patchy, especially in moderately and poorly differentiated tumors, so do not insist on diffuse staining when making a diagnosis in this setting. Other carcinomas that can be HepPar-1 positive include those with morphologic hepatoid differentiation (eg, from the stomach, pancreas) as well as gastric adenocarcinomas, esophageal adenocarcinoma arising in the setting of Barrett mucosa, colon adenocarcinoma, adrenal cortical carcinoma, lung adenocarcinoma, bladder carcinoma, pancreas carcinoma, neuroendocrine carcinoma, ovarian carcinoma, and cervical carcinoma.[54-56] Although this list appears discouragingly long, it is a bit deceptive, as almost none of these entities have H&E findings that resemble hepatocellular carcinoma. Thus, HepPar-1 tends to perform very well in cases in which hepatocellular carcinoma *is actually in the differential based on the H&E findings* (Figures 21.47 and 21.48). The most relevant diagnostic pitfall is that of oncocytic tumors, as oncocytic carcinomas can mimic hepatocellular carcinoma on H&E stain with their large

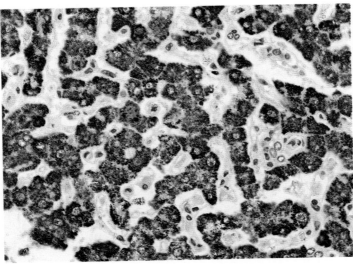

FIGURE 21.46 **Hepatocellular carcinoma, HepPar-1 with cytoplasmic staining.** This moderately differentiated hepatocellular carcinoma shows strong granular cytoplasmic staining.

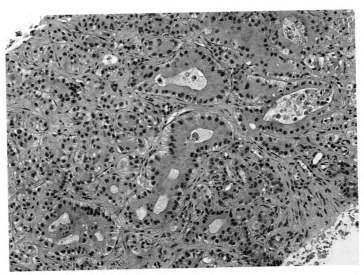

FIGURE 21.47 **Metastatic adenocarcinoma.** This adenocarcinoma is metastatic from the pancreas to the liver. HepPar-1 stain is strongly positive (see next figure), but the morphology is inconsistent with a hepatocellular carcinoma.

pink cells and can also be strongly HepPar-1 positive, although commonly the staining in this setting is patchy. Another important diagnostic pitfall is that some tumors can have entrapped benign hepatocytes that will stain strongly with HepPar-1—always go back and check the H&E when staining is patchy or limited to scattered single cells or small clusters of cells.

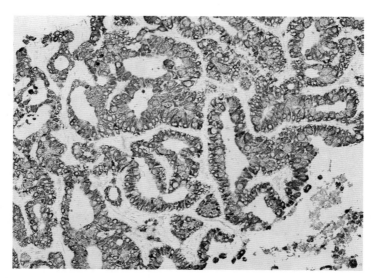

FIGURE 21.48 **Metastatic adenocarcinoma, HepPar-1 positive.** Same case as preceding figure; a HepPar-1 stain is strongly positive.

Glypican 3 shows cytoplasmic staining (Figure 21.49; eFig. 21.23) and is positive in approximately 80% to 85% of hepatocellular carcinomas. In contrast to stains for true hepatocellular differentiation, glypican 3 does not stain the background liver. However, if the background liver is significantly inflamed, then even nonneoplastic hepatocytes may show very focal glypican 3 positivity.[57] For workup of tumors, glypican 3 performs poorly in well-differentiated hepatocellular carcinomas, with only 50% being positive.[58] Glypican 3, however, is very useful in diagnosing well-differentiated tumors as hepatocellular carcinoma when the stain is positive, because glypican 3 is negative in hepatic adenomas and in focal nodular hyperplasia.[58-60] Also of note, glypican 3 positivity in hepatocellular carcinoma is influenced by other clinical and histologic factors. For example, glypican 3 is more likely to be positive in tumors that arise in cirrhotic livers[58] and in tumors that arise in the setting of chronic hepatitis B.[61] Glypican 3 positivity is also influenced by the hepatocellular carcinoma subtype. For example, only about 50% of fibrolamellar carcinomas are glypican 3 positive.

Other carcinomas that can be positive for glypican 3 include squamous cell carcinoma of the lung, ovarian carcinoma, and melanoma. As noted for HepPar-1, this is generally a manageable problem, as the H&E findings, along with other stains used in a panel approach, will indicate the non- hepatocellular carcinoma nature of these tumors.

Arginase-1 is a very useful addition to the diagnostic armamentarium that was first reported in 2010.[62] Arginase-1 is positive in both benign and malignant hepatocytes (Figure 21.50) and appears to have performance characteristics that are slightly better than both glypican 3 and HepPar-1, at least for poorly differentiated hepatocellular carcinomas. On the other

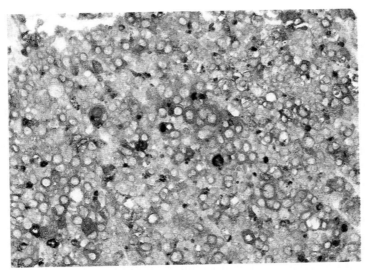

FIGURE 21.49 **Glypican 3 in hepatocellular carcinoma.** Strong diffuse cytoplasmic staining is seen.

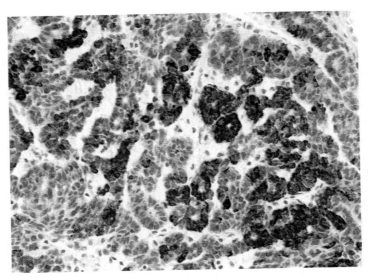

FIGURE 21.50 **Arginase-1 in hepatocellular carcinoma.** Strong but patchy cytoplasmic staining is seen.

hand, about 10% of well-differentiated hepatocellular carcinomas are arginase negative.[63] For poorly differentiated carcinomas, a panel of immunostains that includes arginase-1, HepPar-1, and glypican 3 is the best approach to diagnose hepatocellular carcinoma. AFP staining can also be helpful in poorly differentiated tumors, but it is positive in only approximately 35%

of overall cases (eFig. 21.24). Thus, a negative staining result is generally not very useful.

In situ hybridization for albumin is positive in 95% or more of hepatocellular carcinomas, being positive in essentially all well-differentiated tumors, but it can become patchy or even negative in some poorly differentiated hepatocellular carcinomas. Intrahepatic cholangiocarcinomas are positive for albumin in situ hybridization, so correlation with morphology and other immunostains is important. Metastatic carcinomas can also sometimes be positive for albumin in situ hybridization, including about one-third of acinar cell carcinomas of the pancreas[64] and a few percentage of adenocarcinomas from a wide variety of locations, including the lung and upper gastrointestinal (GI) tract.

CYTOKERATIN STAINS. Normal hepatocytes express cytokeratin (CK)8 and CK18, and these keratins are positive in almost all hepatocellular carcinomas. The CAM5.2 stain is not synonymous with CK8 and CK18, but instead labels primarily CK8 and to some degree CK7.[65] Nonetheless, CAM5.2 is positive in essentially all hepatocellular carcinomas. CK7 staining can be seen in 20% to 40% of hepatocellular carcinomas.[66,67] Hepatocellular carcinomas that are cholestatic or that arise in younger patients (aged less than 40 years) are more likely to be CK7 positive.[68] Also, CK7 is positive in fibrolamellar carcinomas.[69]

CK20 positivity is seen in approximately 5% of hepatocellular carcinomas. CK7 positivity can be seen alone or in combination with CK20. In contrast, CK20 staining alone is rare for hepatocellular carcinomas. CK19 positivity is seen in approximately 10% to 15% of cases and is associated with a worse prognosis.[66,67] Similar to the observations on CK20, CK19 expression without accompanying CK7 expression is uncommon.[66,67]

OTHER IMMUNOSTAINS. Hepatocellular carcinomas can also be positive for a number of immunostains not traditionally associated with hepatocellular differentiation (Table 21.7), such as villin, CDX2,[70] and SATB2.[71] This information is helpful when working up tumors, as positivity for these markers can sometimes confound the diagnosis if you are unaware that hepatocellular carcinomas can be positive for these markers.

OTHER FINDINGS. Hepatocellular carcinomas are often embolized before surgery. The embolic beads are not typically seen on liver biopsy, but when present, they are round to oval structures. Their appearances vary depending on their composition (eFig. 21.25) and they can be found in necrotic tumor, in viable tumor, and in the liver parenchyma substantially away from the tumor. Necrotic tumors often have "ghost cells." In many cases, the ghost cells allow some degree of interpretation as to whether the dead tissue is benign or malignant, but in other cases the necrosis leads to the loss of all features and the tissue cannot be further assessed.

TABLE 21.7 Frequency of Positive Staining for Nonhepatocyte Markers in Hepatocellular Carcinoma

Immunostain	Approximate Frequency in HCC	Comments
Cam5.2	>99%	
Cytokeratin AE1/3	15%	
CK19	15%	Positive tumors have a worse prognosis
		Positive cases typically co-express CK7
CK7	30%	HCCs that are cholestatic or occur in younger individuals (<40 y) are positive in the majority of cases
CK20	10%	Positive cases typically co-express CK7
CDX2	5%	More common in poorly differentiated HCCs; 30% of cholangiocarcinomas are also CDX2 positive
SATB2	40%	
Villin	10%–30% (noncanalicular)	A canalicular staining pattern can be seen in 20%–30% of well-differentiated and moderately differentiated HCCs, supporting the diagnosis of HCC; membranous or cytoplasmic staining can also be seen and is not specific
EMA	5%	
Glutamine synthetase	30–50%	Strong and diffuse staining
MOC31 (anti-EpCam)	35%	Usually focal or patchy
SALL4	45%	Usually patchy, may be a marker of "stemness"
Vimentin	10%	About 10% of typical HCCs are positive. Sarcomatoid HCCs are positive in most cases. Vimentin expression is associated with more aggressive behavior and with epithelial to mesenchymal transition
CD117 (CKIT)	70%	

(Continued)

TABLE 21.7 **Frequency of Positive Staining for Nonhepatocyte Markers in HCC (Continued)**		
Immunostain	Approximate Frequency in HCC	Comments
CD138	65%	Nonneoplastic hepatocytes will also be positive. Membranous staining is seen in both tumors and nontumors.
WT1	>80%	

HCC, hepatocellular carcinoma.

Differential Diagnoses

HEPATOCELLULAR CARCINOMA VERSUS CHOLANGIOCARCINOMA

A common differential for hepatocellular carcinoma includes intrahepatic cholangiocarcinoma. This occurs in three primary settings: (1) cholangiocarcinomas that have solid or trabecular growth patterns, (2) scirrhous hepatocellular carcinoma or fibrolamellar carcinoma, or (3) poorly differentiated carcinomas without definite morphologic differentiation on H&E staining. Albumin in situ hybridization is positive in both intrahepatic cholangiocarcinoma and hepatocellular carcinoma, while positive staining for arginase, HepPar-1, and glypican 3 favors hepatocellular carcinoma. Most cholangiocarcinomas will show strong and diffuse staining for CK7, CK19, and MOC31. Of note, patchy staining for any of these markers is not uncommon in hepatocellular carcinomas, so these stains are informative primarily when they are negative (making cholangiocarcinoma less likely) or when they show strong and diffuse staining (favoring cholangiocarcinoma). Mucicarmine positivity is also helpful when positive, indicating the tumor is an adenocarcinoma, but is noninformative when negative, as intrahepatic small duct cholangiocarcinomas are typically mucicarmine negative. In most cases, especially if the tumor is not well differentiated, a panel of stains is important; a panel is most useful when it contains several markers for hepatocellular differentiation and several markers that would favor cholangiocarcinoma.

HEPATOCELLULAR CARCINOMA VERSUS METASTATIC DISEASE

For poorly differentiated carcinomas, the best approach in most cases is to use a panel of stains to exclude hepatocellular carcinoma, choosing several (and often all) of the four big markers: HepPar-1, glypican 3, arginase, and albumin in situ hybridization. Mucicarmine and strong and diffuse staining for MOC31 or CEA can help evaluate for adenocarcinoma, while p40 and CK5/6 are helpful for excluding squamous cell carcinomas.

Several well-differentiated metastatic neoplasms can have large eosinophilic cells and prominent nuclei, can grow in solid or trabecular growth patterns, and can closely mimic several features of well-differentiated hepatocellular carcinoma; the most common of these are well-differentiated neuroendocrine tumors and renal oncocytic tumors, but others that closely mimic hepatocellular carcinoma include acinar cell carcinoma of the pancreas, paragangliomas, adrenal cortical carcinoma, nonkeratinizing squamous cell carcinomas, and epithelioid angiomyolipomas. The best stains for hepatocellular differentiation in well-differentiated tumors are HepPar-1 and albumin in situ hybridization, as glypican 3 is negative in up to 50% of cases and arginase in up to 10% of well-differentiated hepatocellular carcinomas. These stains for hepatocellular differentiation are used in conjunction with other relevant markers, such as synaptophysin and chromogranin.

HEPATOCELLULAR CARCINOMA VERSUS METASTATIC HEPATOID CARCINOMA

Most hepatoid carcinomas that metastasize to the liver are adenocarcinomas or neuroendocrine tumors. The most common sites for the primary tumor are the upper GI tract, pancreas, and lungs. By definition, a hepatoid carcinoma should have morphology and growth patterns that suggest hepatocellular differentiation, plus some evidence for hepatocellular differentiation by immunostains/in situ hybridization.

Hepatoid carcinomas can be positive for all of the markers of hepatocellular differentiation, including HepPar-1, arginase, glypican 3, and albumin in situ hybridization.[72-74] These tumors can closely mimic hepatocellular carcinomas and are easily misdiagnosed. Well-differentiated to moderately differentiated metastatic hepatoid carcinomas are more likely to be mistaken for hepatocellular carcinomas than poorly differentiated metastatic hepatoid carcinomas, probably because poorly differentiated tumors tend to receive a more extensive workup by immunohistochemistry.

Clinical and imaging findings are important clues, as many patients will have imaging that shows both liver tumor(s) and tumors in other organs. At the morphologic level, the best clues are findings that do not fit the usual, expected patterns for hepatocellular carcinoma. Some examples include nuclear chromatin that is finely dispersed and without at least somewhat prominent nucleoli (raising the possibility of a neuroendocrine tumor); tumors that have an epithelioid morphology, but lack distinct cell membranes and have irregular nuclear spacing (consider an epithelioid angiomyolipoma, epithelioid GIST, melanoma); or focal areas of gland formation. As hepatocellular carcinomas can have pseudoglands, mucicarmine stains are helpful.

Other clues to the correct diagnosis are derived from immunostain patterns that would be atypical for hepatocellular carcinomas. The most common are strong and diffuse staining for MOC31, CK19, CK20, and other markers of organ differentiation such as CDX2 or synaptophysin/chromogranin; discordant staining patterns for hepatocellular markers, such as only focal staining for HepPar-1 or albumin in situ hybridization in a well-differentiated to moderately differentiated tumor; or well-differentiated tumors that show strong diffuse HepPar-1 staining but are negative for albumin in situ hybridization.

HEPATOCELLULAR CARCINOMA SUBTYPES

> ### Hepatocellular Carcinoma Subtypes Have Four Critical Elements
>
> 1. **Consistent H&E histologic findings.** There will be some variation around a central core pattern.
> 2. **Test results that confirm the H&E morphologic findings.** Most tests will be immunostains or molecular assays.
> 3. **Clinical correlates.** These may include risk factors, average age at diagnosis, gender, and prognosis.
> 4. **Molecular findings.** These often form the basis for improvements in the methods of diagnosis (see step 2) and can serve as the basis for treatment decisions.

Hepatocellular carcinomas have a large range of cytologic features and histologic growth patterns. Some of these findings cluster into distinctive patterns and have been designated as unique subtypes of hepatocellular carcinoma. The standard approach for defining morphologic hepatocellular carcinoma subtypes is shown in the box[75]; these four elements are not equally well developed when a subtype is first described, often taking many years to fully mature. The terms *hepatocellular carcinoma subtype* and *hepatocellular carcinoma variant* can be used interchangeably. There are about 12 fairly well-established subtypes (Table 21.8).

These subtypes are important for several reasons. First, many of them have specific diagnostic pitfalls that are important to know for routine surgical pathology practice. Second, a few subtypes have specific surgical or chemotherapy treatment differences, compared to conventional hepatocellular carcinoma (primarily, fibrolamellar carcinoma, combined hepatocellular carcinoma-cholangiocarcinoma, combined hepatocellular carcinoma-neuroendocrine carcinoma, carcinosarcoma). Finally, several of the subtypes have prognostic differences compared to conventional hepatocellular carcinoma. The subtypes are discussed in the following sections in their approximate order of frequency. They do not need to be specifically mentioned in the pathology report, except for fibrolamellar carcinoma and the combined tumors (combined hepatocellular carcinoma-cholangiocarcinoma, combined hepatocellular carcinoma-neuroendocrine carcinoma, and carcinosarcoma). Given the emerging evidence that the steatohepatitic variant of hepatocellular carcinoma may be less likely to respond to checkpoint inhibitor therapy, clinical teams may want this variant specified in the future.

TABLE 21.8 Hepatocellular Carcinoma Subtypes

Subtype	Frequency[a]	Prognosis[b]	Major Tumor Findings
Steatohepatitic	20%	Similar	Fat, inflammation, and fibrosis
Clear cell	7%	Better	Glycogen accumulation
Scirrhous	4%	Similar to better	Dense diffuse intratumoral fibrosis
Chromophobe	5%	Similar	Chromophobic cytoplasm, sudden anaplasia, microscopic pseudocysts
Macrotrabecular massive	5%–20%	Worse	Very thick trabeculae
Fibrolamellar carcinoma	1%	Similar to better	Abundant eosinophilic cytoplasm, vesiculated nuclear chromatin, prominent nucleoli, and intratumoral fibrosis
Combined hepatocellular carcinoma-cholangiocarcinoma	1%	Worse	Two distinct morphologies: hepatocellular carcinoma and cholangiocarcinoma
Lymphocyte rich	<1%	Better	Marked intratumoral lymphocytes
Granulocyte colony-stimulating-factor producing	<1%	Worse	Poorly differentiated with moderate to marked intratumoral neutrophils
Carcinosarcoma	<1%	Worse	Two distinct morphologies: hepatocellular carcinoma and sarcoma
Combined hepatocellular carcinoma and neuroendocrine carcinoma	<1%	Worse	Two distinct morphologies: hepatocellular carcinoma and neuroendocrine carcinoma

(Continued)

TABLE 21.8 **Hepatocellular Carcinoma Subtypes** **(Continued)**

Subtype	Frequency[a]	Prognosis[b]	Major Tumor Findings
Distinctive growth patterns	**Comment**		
Fibronodular	Unclear if there are overlaps/associations with other subtypes		
Macrotrabecular	Best way to distinguish the growth pattern from the subtype has not been clearly determined by data; see text for more detail		
Sarcomatoid	Focus of poorly differentiated carcinoma with spindle cell growth		
Beta-catenin mutated	Well-differentiated tumor cells, small thin trabeculae, pseudoglands, often bile; pattern has a strong statistical association with *CTNNB1* mutations but is neither sensitive nor specific		
Diffuse	Defined by the gross growth pattern; often regarded as a subtype, but still not clear if it is a subtype or a growth pattern. The observation that some diffuse growth patterns can have clear cell morphology or steatohepatitic morphology tends to favor this is not a true or pure subtype.		

[a]The frequencies of the more aggressive subtypes are typically higher in autopsy studies.
[b]Compared to conventional hepatocellular carcinoma.

Steatohepatitic Hepatocellular Carcinoma

- Key morphologic features: at least 5% fat, plus tumor cell ballooning, intratumoral inflammation, and intratumoral fibrosis.
- Frequency: 20%.
- Clinical correlates: steatosis/steatohepatitis in the background liver from either the metabolic syndrome or alcohol.
- Stains for hepatocellular differentiation: tumor cells stain in the usual fashion.
- Prognosis: similar to conventional hepatocellular carcinoma; may be less likely to respond to checkpoint inhibitor therapy.
- Molecular correlates: less likely to have beta-catenin mutations.
- Potential pitfall: well-differentiated cases may mimic benign steatohepatitis.

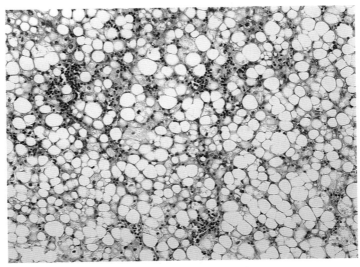

FIGURE 21.51 **Steatohepatitic hepatocellular carcinoma.** This growth pattern of hepatocellular carcinoma is associated with the metabolic syndrome and can be seen in individuals with fatty liver disease alone or with fatty liver disease plus other chronic liver diseases such as chronic hepatitis C. The tumor shows fat, balloon cells, inflammation, and intratumoral fibrosis. These tumors can mimic benign fatty liver disease on biopsy specimens.

This variant of hepatocellular carcinoma has all the features of steatohepatitis within the tumor itself, including fat, inflammation, balloon cells, Mallory hyaline, and pericellular fibrosis (Figure 21.51; eFigs. 21.26 and 21.27).[76-80] The minimum amount of fat needed to make the diagnosis of steatohepatitic hepatocellular carcinoma has not been rigorously defined, and studies have used minimal criteria as low as 5%, all the way up to 50%. Likewise, intratumoral fibrosis has not been a requirement for many studies. Current recommendations are that the diagnosis requires at least 5% fat, plus other features of steatohepatitis.[78]

This pattern occurs in two distinct settings: first, a typical hepatocellular carcinoma can accumulate fat and features of steatohepatitis, much as the background liver, in the setting of the metabolic syndrome or alcoholic hepatitis (>95% of cases of the steatohepatitic variant); second, rare hepatocellular carcinomas have tumor-specific molecular changes that lead to this distinctive morphology (<5% of cases). In the latter setting, the metabolic syndrome is absent and there is no significant fat in the background liver.[81]

Many hepatocellular carcinomas with the steatohepatitic morphology will be well-differentiated tumors and an important diagnostic pitfall is to recognize them as hepatocellular carcinomas and not miss the tumor diagnosis by focusing on the changes of steatohepatitis. The usual findings of hepatocellular carcinoma will be present in these cases and will help make the diagnoses, including lack of portal tracts, cytologic atypia, increased proliferation, and loss of reticulin. However, reticulin loss should be more than focal, as benign fatty liver can have focal areas of reticulin loss that mimic hepatocellular carcinoma.[47]

Clear Cell Carcinoma

- Key morphologic features: tumor cells have clear cytoplasm. A cutoff of 50% has been used in some papers; a better cutoff is 90%, providing purer group of tumors.
- Frequency: 5% to 10%.
- Clinical correlates: none to date.
- Prognosis: better, at least when using higher threshold definitions.
- Stains for hepatocellular differentiation: tumor cells stain in the usual fashion.
- Molecular correlates: possible link to IDH1 mutations.[82]
- Potential pitfall: tumors may mimic other clear cell carcinomas. About 35% of clear cell carcinomas of the ovary were HepPar-1 positive in one study, although the total number of studied cases was small.[56] Clear cell carcinomas of the kidney are HepPar-1 negative.[83]

Clear cell hepatocellular carcinomas have been recognized as a histologic variant for many years, but this has not led to a uniform definition for this entity, which has likely obscured some important aspects of this tumor. Clear cell hepatocellular carcinomas should have at least 50% of tumor cells with clear cell change (Figure 21.52; eFig. 21.28). The purest group of tumors, however, and probably the best definition, is that all the tumor cells, or nearly all (90% or greater), should show clear cell change.

In general, clear cell carcinomas are well-differentiated to moderately differentiated hepatocellular carcinomas with moderate to abundant cytoplasm that appears "clear" on H&E stains. Hepatocellular

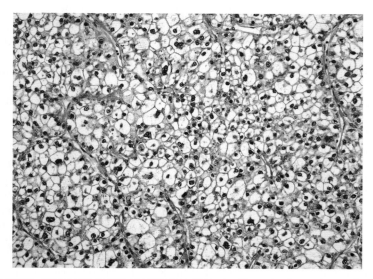

FIGURE 21.52 **Clear cell hepatocellular carcinoma.** The cytoplasm shows clearing due to glycogen accumulation.

carcinomas with focal clear cell change are not classified as clear cell hepatocellular carcinoma. Fatty change (macrovesicular steatosis) is present in some clear cell carcinomas. Clear cell hepatocellular carcinomas stain like conventional hepatocellular carcinomas. Many possible clinical correlates have been identified, but few have been consistently identified. An overall better prognosis has been found by several, but not all, studies.[84,85]

It seems likely that "clear cell hepatocellular carcinoma," as currently defined, actually represents several biologically different types of tumors. For example, those tumors with 100% clear cell change are likely different than those tumors with 50% clear cell change (thus the recommendation to use a higher cutoff). In addition, hepatocellular carcinomas that have clear cell change from glycogen are probably different from the smaller subset that has clear cell change from lipid accumulation.[86] Likewise, some clear cell hepatocellular carcinomas have patchy but focally abundant macrovesicular steatosis, perhaps representing clear cell carcinomas in the setting of the metabolic syndrome, but potentially representing different genetic pathways than those of conventional clear cell carcinoma. Finally, even within those tumors that diffusely have the classic clear cell morphology, there is a subset that consistently has high-grade nuclear changes, including significant nuclear irregularity and prominently vacuolated nuclei; these may be biologically different than those clear cell carcinomas that have low-grade nuclei.

Scirrhous Hepatocellular Carcinoma

- Key morphologic features: abundant intratumoral fibrosis that is a dominant histologic finding.
- Frequency: 5%.
- Prognosis: similar to better.
- Stains for hepatocellular differentiation: HepPar-1 is negative in about 50% of biopsy specimens.[87] Arginase and glypican 3 are typically positive.
- Molecular correlates: higher frequency of TSC1/TSC2 mutations.[88]
- Potential pitfalls: fibrolamellar carcinoma, cholangiocarcinoma, and metastatic disease.

While many definitions have been proposed for scirrhous hepatocellular carcinoma, the best definition at this point is that the fibrosis component should make up 50% or more of the tumor area.[89] The frequency is less than 1%. They occur in both cirrhotic and noncirrhotic livers[90] but are more likely to arise in noncirrhotic livers than typical hepatocellular carcinomas (about two-thirds of cases). The overall prognosis appears to be similar to conventional hepatocellular carcinoma,[90,91] although some studies have suggested this subtype is less likely to respond to chemotherapy.[92]

The neoplastic cells (Figure 21.53; eFig. 21.29) grow in trabecula or cords that are often somewhat atrophic. The fibrosis can have varying

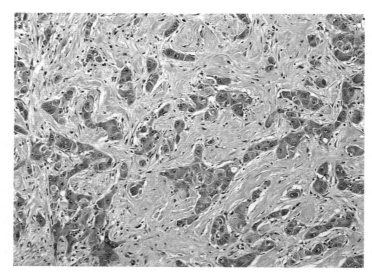

FIGURE 21.53 **Scirrhous hepatocellular carcinoma.** The carcinoma grows in atrophic cords and irregular aggregates and is embedded in a dense fibrous background.

patterns. In some cases, the fibrosis appears to be tracking along and filling in the sinusoids, in other cases the fibrosis is distinctly lamellar (thus, make sure to exclude fibrolamellar carcinoma), and in some other cases the fibrosis is present in irregular but interconnected clumps, leaving the tumor cells to grow as irregular nodules and misshapen trabecula. Imaging studies are often not typical for hepatocellular carcinoma, and one group reported that 36% of scirrhous hepatocellular carcinomas were originally diagnosed by contrast computed tomography (CT) as cholangiocarcinomas, metastatic carcinomas, or biphenotypic hepatocellular carcinoma.[93]

Scirrhous hepatocellular carcinomas are often subcapsular in location.[93] They typically have no capsule[91,93] and grow as an aggregate of adjacent tumor nodules. Entrapped intratumoral portal tracts are common, in particular near the tumor-nontumor interface. Some cases may have fatty change or clear cell change. Hepatocyte inclusions can also be present, including both pale bodies and hyaline bodies.[91] A subset of cases show the steatohepatitic morphology.[89] The fibrous areas can sometimes show moderate, or rarely marked, lymphocyte-rich inflammation.

As noted earlier, the differential may include cholangiocarcinoma or metastatic carcinoma. On H&E alone, it can be difficult to distinguish hepatocellular carcinomas with abundant fibrosis stroma from cholangiocarcinomas, even for experienced hepatopathologists,[94] but the diagnosis can be established when using the morphology in conjunction with immunostains. Scirrhous hepatocellular carcinomas should have no gland formation, no mucin, and have definite evidence of hepatocellular differentiation by immunohistochemistry. Of note, scirrhous hepatocellular carcinomas are less likely to be HepPar-1 positive than conventional hepatocellular carcinomas (about 40% are positive),[91] while glypican 3 and arginase-1 both perform better than HepPar-1 (about 80% positive each).[87] CK7 staining is seen in about 50% of cases and CK19 in about 25% of cases.[87]

Macrotrabecular Massive

- Key morphologic features: macrotrabecular growth pattern.
- Frequency: 5% to 20%.
- Prognosis: worse.
- Clinical correlates: elevated serum AFP levels, enriched for chronic hepatitis B.
- Stains for hepatocellular differentiation: tumor cells stain in the usual fashion.
- Molecular correlates: TP53 mutations and FGF19 amplification.

This tumor variant is incompletely defined and there remain several key points of uncertainty. As originally defined, this tumor subtype had a macrotrabecular growth pattern plus tumor cells that were small and basophilic (Figure 21.54), and cases were strongly associated with elevated serum AFP levels and chronic hepatitis B as an underlying disease.[95] Subsequent studies have used the sole criterion of a macrotrabecular growth pattern,[96,97] which likely leads to a more heterogeneous group of tumors, as areas of macrotrabecular growth are not uncommon when many different subtypes

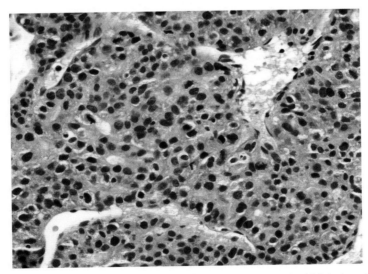

FIGURE 21.54 **Macrotrabecular massive.** The tumor cells grow in thick trabeculae.

become less well differentiated. Likewise, the best criterion for how thick the trabeculae need to be has not been fully evaluated, with different approaches using >6 or 10 or greater tumor cells in thickness.

Chromophobe Hepatocellular Carcinoma

- Key morphologic features: chromophobic cytoplasm, sudden nuclear anaplasia, and microscopic pseudocysts.
- Frequency: 5%.
- Clinical correlates: none to date.
- Prognosis: unclear.
- Stains for hepatocellular differentiation: tumor cells stain in the usual fashion.
- Molecular correlates: positive for alternative lengthening of telomeres (ALT).

This subtype of hepatocellular carcinoma shows tumor cells that have a background morphology of chromophobic to eosinophilic cytoplasm (Figure 21.55) with low-grade tumor nuclei.[75] Within this background morphology, there are small, scattered foci of tumor cells with distinctly higher grade nuclear cytology (Figure 21.56), a finding referred to as *sudden anaplasia*. In addition, the tumor typically has scattered, irregular, pseudocyst-like structures that lack the well-defined outlines of true pseudoglands and are filled with pink flocculent material (Figure 21.57).

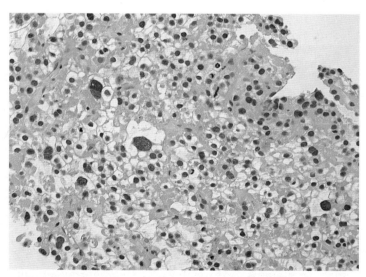

FIGURE 21.55 **Hepatocellular carcinoma, chromophobe subtype.** This tumor has a chromophobe type cytoplasmic change and shows patchy but striking nuclear atypia. This tumor morphology is strongly correlated with the alternative lengthening of telomeres (ALT) phenotype by telomere fluorescence in situ hybridization (FISH).

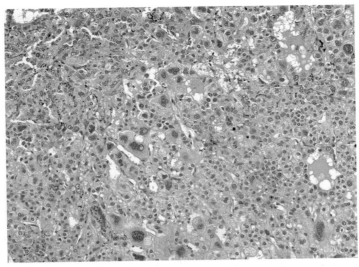

FIGURE 21.56 **Hepatocellular carcinoma, chromophobe subtype.** This tumor has a more eosinophilic cytoplasmic change but also shows patchy and striking nuclear atypia. This tumor showed the alternative lengthening of telomeres (ALT) phenotype by telomere fluorescence in situ hybridization (FISH).

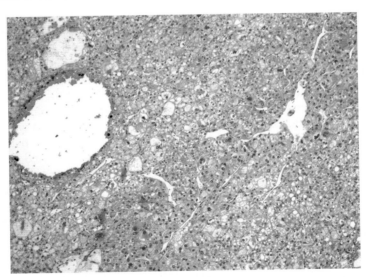

FIGURE 21.57 **Hepatocellular carcinoma, chromophobe subtype.** Pseudocysts are also seen in the tumor parenchyma.

Most hepatocellular carcinomas maintain their telomeres through *TERT* promoter mutations or through *TERT* gene rearrangements, but this subtype of hepatocellular carcinoma uses an alternative mechanism[75] that involves homologous recombination and is called *alternative lengthening of telomeres*.

Fibrolamellar Carcinoma

- Key morphologic features: large eosinophilic tumor cells, prominent nucleoli, and prominent intratumoral fibrosis.
- Frequency: 1%.
- Clinical correlates: younger individuals (median age, 22 years).[69] No underlying liver disease.[98,99]
- Prognosis: similar to conventional hepatocellular carcinomas arising in noncirrhotic livers.[69]
- Stains for hepatocellular differentiation: tumor cells stain in the usual fashion; most cases also show co-expression of CD68 (KP1 clone, lysosomal marker) and CK7.
- Molecular correlates: microdeletion on chromosome 19 leads to *DNAJB1-PRKACA* fusion.
- Potential pitfall: can be mistaken for scirrhous hepatocellular carcinoma or for cholangiocarcinoma. Conventional hepatocellular carcinomas can be misdiagnosed as fibrolamellar carcinoma if they occur in young individuals with noncirrhotic livers.

Fibrolamellar carcinoma arise in noncirrhotic livers with no underlying liver disease, typically in older children and young adults. The tumor cells have abundant cytoplasm, large vesiculated nuclei, and prominent nucleoli. Intratumoral fibrosis is prominent, and often lamellar, but the fibrosis can show regional variability within tumors, which may have areas of more solid growth.

Fibrolamellar carcinomas generally present with vague, nonspecific clinical signs and symptoms, including abdominal pain, weight loss, malaise,[100] and occasionally gynecomastia.[100] AFP levels are normal or show mild nonspecific elevations[69]; nonetheless, patients with mild elevations may have a worse prognosis.[101] Serum fibrinogen levels can also be elevated, as can serum neurotensin levels. Finally, PIVKA-II, also known as DCP, levels are elevated in 70% to 90% of fibrolamellar carcinoma cases. Of note, none of these serum markers are specific for fibrolamellar carcinoma, but they can be useful in monitoring for tumor recurrence.

Fibrolamellar carcinomas have no strong gender predilection.[69] Fibrolamellar carcinomas strongly cluster in the young, with 80% of all cases occurring between the ages 10 and 35 years.[69] Cancer registry studies have suggested a possible second peak of tumor incidence in the elderly,[102] but this remains unverified by histologic or molecular studies. Also of note, conventional hepatocellular carcinomas remain the most common form of liver cancer in children and young adults, where they account for between 60% and 80% of liver cancers.[69] Hilar lymph node metastatic disease is more common in fibrolamellar carcinoma than in conventional hepatocellular carcinoma, so surgeons often do a hilar lymph node dissection. Complete resectability is the single most important prognostic feature for fibrolamellar carcinoma.[103-106]

Fibrolamellar carcinomas are driven by activation of protein kinase A. Protein kinase A is composed of both activating and inhibiting subunits. In most cases (>99%), fibrolamellar carcinoma results from a microdeletion on chromosome 19 that leads to a *DNAJB1-PRKACA* fusion. This fusion leads to unregulated expression of one of the activation subunits (PRKACA) and overactivation of protein kinase A. In rare cases, fibrolamellar carcinomas can also arise through biallelic mutations that inactivate one of the protein kinase A inhibitory subunits, *PRKAR1A*. *PRKAR1A* mutations in fibrolamellar carcinoma are usually found in the setting of the Carney complex, but also in rare sporadic cases, usually in older persons.[107]

HISTOLOGIC FINDINGS

The background livers are noncirrhotic and without chronic liver disease, although mild, nonspecific portal inflammation can be present, as well as occasional epithelioid granulomas.

The tumor cells are large and polygonal, with abundant eosinophilic cytoplasm, vesiculated nuclear chromatin, and large nucleoli (Figure 21.58). Those three cytologic findings, in conjunction with the lamellar fibrosis, are the characteristic features of fibrolamellar carcinoma. The abundant eosinophilic cytoplasm is rich in mitochondria and lysosomes. In approximately half of cases, the tumor cells can have round, amphophilic, cytoplasmic inclusions called "pale bodies" (Figure 21.59). Hyaline bodies (cytoplasmic inclusions that are eosinophilic and tend to be smaller than pale bodies) are also present in nearly half of fibrolamellar carcinomas (Figure 21.60). A diagnosis of fibrolamellar carcinoma, however, should not be based on the presence of these inclusions alone, as similar

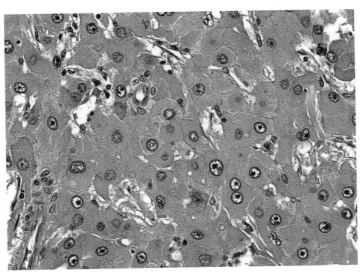

FIGURE 21.58 **Fibrolamellar carcinoma.** Fibrolamellar carcinomas have eosinophilic tumor cells with abundant cytoplasm and prominent nucleoli.

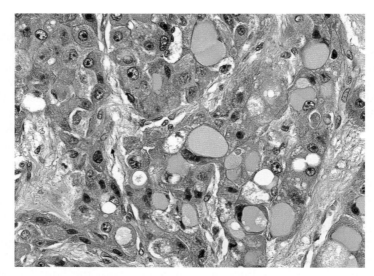

FIGURE 21.59 **Fibrolamellar carcinoma with pale bodies.** Pale bodies are prominent in this fibrolamellar carcinoma.

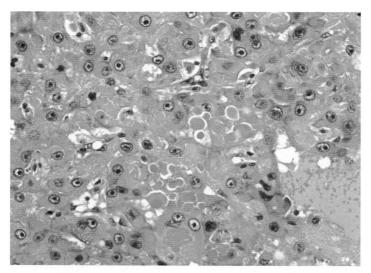

FIGURE 21.60 **Fibrolamellar carcinoma with hyaline bodies.** Numerous hyaline globules are seen.

inclusions can occasionally be found in conventional hepatocellular carcinomas. Intratumoral cholestasis is seen in many fibrolamellar carcinomas, with canalicular bile plugs being the most common pattern. Because of the cholestasis, fibrolamellar carcinomas frequently have copper deposition. On the other hand, copper accumulation is also common in conventional hepatocellular carcinomas that are cholestatic, so it is not a diagnostic feature of fibrolamellar carcinoma.

One of the most characteristic low-power features of fibrolamellar carcinoma is the presence of intratumoral fibrosis (Figure 21.61; eFigs. 21.30 and 21.31), which is present in all primary tumors and in most metastatic deposits. In many fibrolamellar carcinomas, the fibrosis will be deposited in parallel, or "lamellar," bands. However, a lamellar pattern of fibrosis is not a requirement for the diagnosis and many cases will have more irregular patterns of intratumoral fibrosis. In addition, the amount of fibrosis within fibrolamellar carcinomas can vary, leading to some areas that have a solid appearance with little or no fibrosis; sometimes this has been mistaken for a mixed fibrolamellar carcinoma-hepatocellular carcinoma. In about two-thirds of fibrolamellar carcinomas, particularly larger tumors, the fibrosis will coalesce into central scars with radiating fibrous bands. Calcifications are seen in two-thirds of fibrolamellar carcinomas by CT studies,[108] and small calcifications are often seen histologically, located in the central scar, fibrous bands, or tumor cells (Figure 21.62). Some cases show perineural invasion, especially those involving the hilum of the liver (eFig. 21.32).

Some fibrolamellar carcinomas have prominent pseudoglands, which are circular to ovoid, cystic structures lined by neoplastic cells (Figure 21.63; eFig. 21.33).[100] The lining cells may be somewhat smaller than the cells in the more typical areas of fibrolamellar carcinoma, but are otherwise morphologically similar. The secretions within the pseudoglands can be mucicarmine positive (albeit usually weakly) in just over half the cases and are alcian blue positive in most cases.[69] The presence of mucin positivity sometimes elicits a debate as to whether these areas should be called true glands or pseudoglands, but in either case, certainly do not call these cases

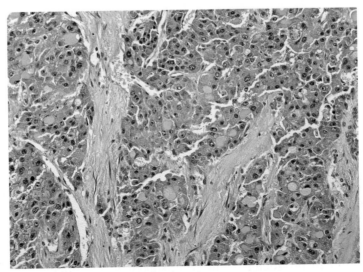

FIGURE 21.61 **Fibrolamellar carcinoma and fibrosis.** Fibrolamellar carcinomas have variable but often striking intratumoral fibrosis. The fibrosis can be organized into parallel or lamellar bands, but this is not necessary for the diagnosis.

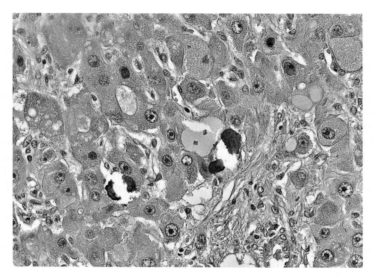

FIGURE 21.62 **Fibrolamellar carcinoma.** Calcifications are seen within the tumor cells.

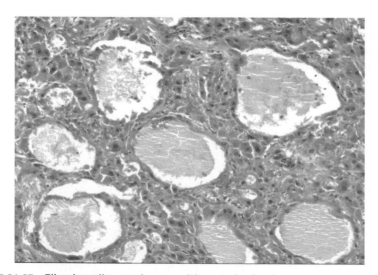

FIGURE 21.63 **Fibrolamellar carcinoma with pseudoglands.**

combined hepatocellular carcinoma-cholangiocarcinoma or combined fibrolamellar carcinoma-cholangiocarcinoma.

Metastases to lymph nodes and other organs mostly retain the typical cytologic features (eFig. 21.34), including the intratumoral fibrosis (eFig. 21.35). In some cases, the metastatic disease can appear more glandular, have mucin production, and be mistaken for a cholangiocarcinoma. However, immunostains for HepPar-1, CK7, and CD68 show the typical staining pattern of fibrolamellar carcinoma.

Immunohistochemistry

The tumor cells in fibrolamellar carcinoma are strongly HepPar-1 positive in all cases, even in areas with pseudoglandular differentiation and mucin production.[69] In contrast, glypican 3 is positive in only a subset of cases from 20% to 60%.[69] Immunostains for AFP are negative. The neoplastic cells not only show expression of the expected hepatocellular CK8 and CK18 but also are strongly positive for CK7 (Figure 21.64)[109] and occasionally for CK19 (between 5% and 25%). Immunostains for CD68 (KP-1 clone) are also positive because of abundant tumor lysosomes (Figure 21.65).[109] CD68 staining varies in intensity from weak to strong and can be patchy, but at least focal staining is seen in most specimens, even biopsy specimens. Co-expression of CK7 and CD68 is characteristic of fibrolamellar carcinoma.

Fibrolamellar Carcinoma Versus Conventional Hepatocellular Carcinoma

In general, the H&E stain findings are sensitive for suggesting a diagnosis of fibrolamellar carcinoma, but a small proportion of conventional hepatocellular carcinomas can have some areas that focally and strongly resemble fibrolamellar carcinoma; many of these cases have BAP1 mutations.[110] On the other hand, some fibrolamellar carcinomas can have areas that resemble conventional or scirrhous hepatocellular carcinoma (eFig. 21.36). To aid in correctly diagnosing these tumors, molecular testing can be used to detect the *PRKACA-DNAJB1* fusion, including polymerase chain reaction (PCR) and fluorescence in situ hybridization (FISH).[111,112] The presence of this fusion gene is highly sensitive and specific for fibrolamellar carcinoma, in the context of a primary liver tumor in which fibrolamellar carcinoma

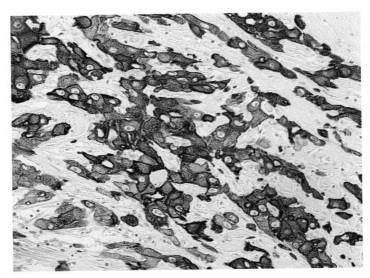

FIGURE 21.64 **Fibrolamellar carcinoma, immunostain for CK7.** The CK7 immunostain shows strong cytoplasmic staining.

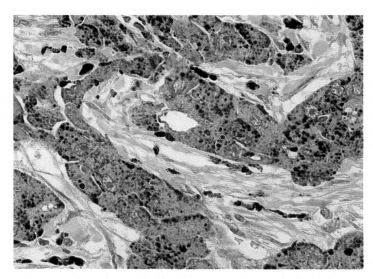

FIGURE 21.65 **Fibrolamellar carcinoma, immunostain for CD68.** The CD68 immunostain shows strong granular cytoplasmic staining.

is in the histologic differential. Identical fusions can occur in intraductal oncocytic papillary neoplasms of the pancreas and bile duct,[113] but this poses no diagnostic barrier, as the morphology and other basic immunostain findings are distinct. Thus, molecular testing for the fusion is a very useful and highly recommended diagnostic tool.[114]

If molecular testing is not available, CK7 and CD68 immunostains can be useful, as fibrolamellar carcinomas should be positive for both markers. This assumes, of course, that the stains worked well. For CD68, the KP1 clone should be used, as it cross reacts with lysosomes; a good internal control is the Kupffer cells in the sinusoids of the background liver. Of note, a subset of conventional hepatocellular carcinomas is positive for either CK7 or CD68 (for CD68, especially those hepatocellular carcinomas with a steatohepatitic morphology), so correlation with H&E findings is important.

Additional findings that suggest a diagnosis of fibrolamellar carcinoma is probably wrong include the following: the presence of significant fibrosis in the background liver, serum AFP level elevations greater than 200 ng/mL or AFP positivity in the tumor cells by immunostaining, and areas of tumor that lack the key histologic features of fibrolamellar carcinoma (remembering that the intratumoral fibrosis will vary in density throughout the tumor).

The differential diagnosis for fibrolamellar carcinoma may include scirrhous hepatocellular carcinoma. The presence of chronic liver disease can be helpful, as this finding would make fibrolamellar carcinoma unlikely. Immunostains are helpful, as fibrolamellar carcinoma will be CK7, CD68,[115] and HepPar-1 positive, while scirrhous carcinomas are CD68 negative and HepPar-1 negative in about half the cases. CK7 is positive in all fibrolamellar carcinomas and many scirrhous hepatocellular carcinomas. The diagnosis can also be established by using molecular tests for the PRKACA-DNAJB1 fusion found in fibrolamellar carcinoma, including FISH. The differential for fibrolamellar carcinoma may also include cholangiocarcinoma or other adenocarcinomas because of the intratumoral fibrosis and the pseudoglands.[116] The distinctive H&E findings of large oncocytic cells and prominent nuclei will indicate the proper diagnosis of fibrolamellar carcinoma in most cases, which can be confirmed by immunostains for hepatocellular differentiation.

Combined Hepatocellular Carcinoma-Cholangiocarcinoma

- Key morphologic features: biphenotypic tumor; there is an H&E component of hepatocellular carcinoma and an H&E component of cholangiocarcinoma.
- Frequency: 1%.
- Clinical correlates: both serum CA19-9 and AFP levels are elevated in 50% of cases.[117]
- Prognosis: worse.
- Stains for hepatocellular differentiation: the hepatocellular carcinoma component as well as the cholangiocarcinoma component stain in the usual fashion.
- Molecular correlates: no consistent findings to date.
- Potential pitfall: if the tumor is morphologically homogenous, then it is not a combined hepatocellular carcinoma-cholangiocarcinoma, even if there is aberrant staining. Examples include a tumor with a hepatocellular carcinoma morphology but patchy CK19 or MOC31 staining or a tumor with a cholangiocarcinoma morphology but patchy glypican 3 or HepPar-1 staining.

Combined hepatocellular carcinoma-cholangiocarcinoma are grossly single tumors that have two physically separate and histologically distinct morphologies within the same tumor—one that looks and stains like hepatocellular carcinoma and one that looks and stains like cholangiocarcinoma (Figure 21.66). The two morphologies are in direct contact and may have a small transition zone. Their frequency is approximately 1% to 3%.[118] Synonyms include *mixed hepatocellular carcinoma-cholangiocarcinoma* and *biphenotypic hepatocellular carcinoma-cholangiocarcinoma*. Prior publications of "collision tumors" appear in many cases to describe this same tumor, but the term "collision tumor" is no longer used. A true collision tumor is very rare, showing two grossly separate nodules of tumor—one that is hepatocellular carcinoma and one that is cholangiocarcinoma—that happen to touch at one of their borders, often only focally, but are actually separate primaries.

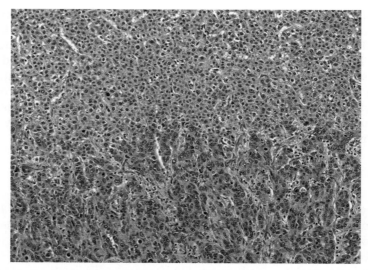

FIGURE 21.66 **Combined hepatocellular carcinoma.** The carcinoma shows areas of conventional hepatocellular carcinoma (top) and cholangiocarcinoma (bottom).

The morphology in combined hepatocellular carcinoma-cholangiocarcinoma is confirmed by immunostains. The hepatocellular carcinoma component demonstrates a typical immunostain pattern for hepatocellular differentiation (for example, positive for HepPar-1, arginase, etc.), while the cholangiocarcinoma should be negative for hepatocellular markers and be strongly and diffusely positive for keratins, such as CK7, CK19, or CKAE1/AE3 (Figures 21.67 and 21.68). Aberrant expression of biliary-type keratins, often patchy, in an otherwise ordinary hepatocellular carcinoma should not be called a biphenotypic hepatocellular carcinoma. Not all cholangiocarcinomas produce mucin, so mucin production is not a requirement for the cholangiocarcinoma component.

Potential diagnostic pitfalls include pseudoglands in conventional hepatocellular carcinomas, which might mimic the glands of cholangiocarcinoma. Pseudoglands, however, are scattered throughout an otherwise typical hepatocellular carcinoma. Immunostains for hepatic differentiation can be used in difficult cases, as the tumor cells that make up pseudoglands stain with markers of hepatocellular differentiation. Also, hepatocellular carcinomas can sometimes elicit a robust ductular reaction at the tumor-nontumor liver interface; do not overinterpret this process as cholangiocarcinoma. Immunostains will not help you much here, but the bland cytology of the ductular reaction, versus the atypia of cholangiocarcinomas, will clarify the diagnosis.

The overall risk factors and demographics for combined hepatocellular carcinoma-cholangiocarcinoma appear similar to those of conventional hepatocellular carcinoma. They arise in both cirrhotic and noncirrhotic

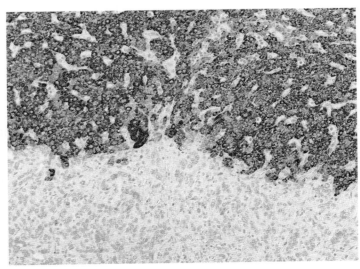

FIGURE 21.67 **Combined hepatocellular carcinoma, HepPar-1.** This image is from the same tumor and same field that is shown in the preceding figure. The HepPar-1 stain is strongly positive in the hepatic component.

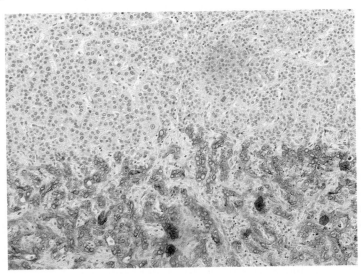

FIGURE 21.68 **Combined hepatocellular carcinoma, cytokeratin AE1/AE3.** This image is from the same tumor and same field that is shown in the two preceding figures. Cytokeratin AE1/AE3 is positive in the cholangiocarcinoma component.

livers. The prognosis is in between cholangiocarcinoma and hepatocellular carcinoma, befitting its mixed growth patterns: better than cholangiocarcinoma and worse than hepatocellular carcinoma.[118] Patients are more likely to have hilar lymph node metastatic disease. Thus, if the diagnosis is known before surgery, lymph node dissections are commonly performed.

Lymphocyte-Rich Hepatocellular Carcinoma

- Key morphologic features: lymphocytes within the tumor are striking, typically outnumbering tumor cells.
- Frequency: <1%.
- Clinical correlates: none to date.
- Prognosis: better.
- Stains for hepatocellular differentiation: tumor cells stain in the usual fashion.
- Molecular correlates: no consistent findings to date.
- Potential pitfalls: histology can mimic a lymphoma. Rarely, metastatic lymphoepithelioma-like carcinomas can metastasize from other organs; lymphoepithelioma-like cholangiocarcinomas should also be excluded.

The cause for lymphocyte-rich hepatocellular carcinoma is unknown. The average age at presentation is in the late 60s, and there is a possible female predominance.[119] While data is limited because of the tumor's rarity, the overall prognosis appears to be better than conventional hepatocellular carcinoma.[120] Lymphocyte-rich hepatocellular carcinomas occur in both cirrhotic and noncirrhotic livers.

Lymphocyte-rich hepatocellular carcinomas are distinguished by marked intratumoral lymphocytosis (Figure 21.69; eFigs. 21.37 and 21.38), often with scattered germinal centers. There are varying definitions on how many lymphocytes are needed, but probably the best approach is that tumors should have as many or more lymphocytes than they do tumor cells in most high-power fields; in other words, there should be both diffuse and striking lymphocytosis within the tumor. The lymphocytes are reactive T cells, with B cells largely restricted to occasional germinal centers. Of note, there are many conventional hepatocellular carcinomas with mild to moderate but patchy lymphocytic inflammation; these cases should not be diagnosed as lymphocyte-rich hepatocellular carcinoma. In addition, inflammation primarily located in fibrous bands within the tumor does not count.

Focal pale bodies are not uncommon (Figure 21.70). The neoplastic tumor cells stain like a typical hepatocellular carcinoma. Epstein-Barr virus (EBV) stains are routinely negative.

Lymphoepithelioma-like hepatocellular carcinoma is often used as a synonym for lymphocyte-rich hepatocellular carcinoma, based on the notion that the lymphoepithelioma-like hepatocellular carcinoma is the poorly differentiated version of lymphocyte-rich hepatocellular carcinoma. Lymphoepithelioma-like hepatocellular carcinomas have irregular, poorly differentiated, syncytial sheets of epithelial cells with numerous admixed lymphocytes. It is not entirely clear, however, if these are actually the same

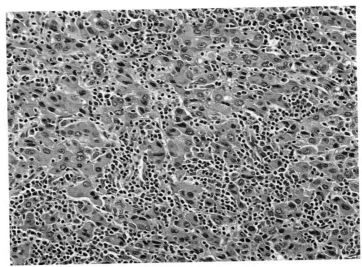

FIGURE 21.69 **Lymphocyte-rich hepatocellular carcinoma.** The hepatocellular carcinoma shows diffuse, intense lymphocytosis.

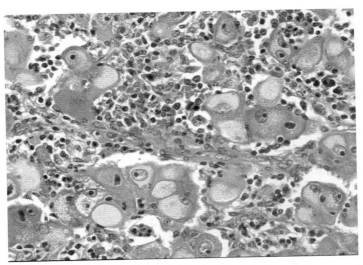

FIGURE 21.70 **Lymphocyte-rich hepatocellular carcinoma.** The tumor cells in this lymphocyte-rich hepatocellular carcinoma focally show pale bodies.

tumors, but just different grades. In some cases of lymphoepithelioma-like hepatocellular carcinoma, more typical areas of lymphocyte-rich hepatocellular carcinoma can be found.

In terms of diagnostic pitfalls, lymphomas can sometimes mimic lymphocyte-rich hepatocellular carcinomas, but the overall clinical, histologic, and immunostain findings sort out most cases pretty quickly. The other tumor in the differential is lymphoepithelioma-like cholangiocarcinoma. To separate these two, lymphocyte-rich hepatocellular carcinomas should show definite evidence of hepatocellular differentiation by morphology and/or immunostains. In addition, lymphoepithelioma-like cholangiocarcinomas are almost always EBV positive (the tumor cells, not the lymphocytes), while lymphocyte-rich hepatocellular carcinomas are not EBV positive. Molecular findings are sparse, but the distinctive lymphocytic inflammation in lymphocyte-rich hepatocellular carcinoma is not associated with higher tumor mutation burden.[121]

Granulocyte Colony-Stimulating Factor–Producing Hepatocellular Carcinoma

- Key morphologic features: striking neutrophil infiltrates.
- Frequency: <1%.
- Clinical correlates: elevated peripheral white blood cell counts, elevated serum interleukin (IL)-6 levels, and elevated serum CRP levels.
- Prognosis: worse.
- Stains for hepatocellular differentiation: tumor cells stain in the usual fashion.
- Potential pitfalls: rare cholangiocarcinomas and metastatic carcinomas can produce granulocyte colony-stimulating factor and have striking neutrophilic tumor infiltrates.

Granulocyte colony-stimulating factor–producing (GCSFP) hepatocellular carcinoma is very rare, much less than 1% of hepatocellular carcinomas. It is defined histologically by striking neutrophilic infiltrates. This variant suffers from a very long name but is an interesting and histologically striking tumor. These tumors tend to occur in older individuals, are often poorly differentiated, and have a poor prognosis.[122] Clinically, a very high white blood cell count is typical. Fevers and elevated CRP[122-126] and IL-6[122,124-126] levels are common.

Histologically, the tumors tend to be moderately to poorly differentiated and there may be sarcomatoid areas.[122] The most striking histologic feature is enormous numbers of neutrophils within the tumor stroma (Figure 21.71; eFig. 21.39). When poorly differentiated, these tumors will have only weak or patchy staining for hepatocellular markers (arginase, HepPar, glypican 3, albumin in situ hybridization), but evidence for hepatocellular differentiation is needed in order to make the diagnosis (eFig. 21.40), as carcinomas from other organ systems can also produce granulocyte colony-stimulating factor and have striking neutrophilia within the tumor. Some cholangiocarcinomas can also have neutrophil-rich infiltrates (eFig. 21.41). An otherwise typical hepatocellular carcinoma that has been embolized, or treated with chemotherapy, can have focal areas of

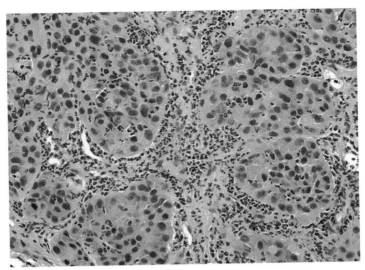

FIGURE 21.71 **Granulocyte colony-stimulating factor–producing hepatocellular carcinoma.** The hepatocellular carcinoma is poorly differentiated and shows numerous tumor-infiltrating neutrophils.

neutrophilic inflammation, but such cases should not be classified as the GCSFP variant of hepatocellular carcinoma.

Other Morphologic Rare Subtypes

CARCINOSARCOMA

Carcinosarcoma is one of the three types of biphenotypic differentiation seen in adult hepatocellular carcinomas, the others being combined hepatocellular carcinoma-cholangiocarcinoma and combined hepatocellular carcinoma-neuroendocrine carcinoma. The frequency is less than 1%. The prognosis is worse than conventional hepatocellular carcinoma. Molecular studies have not unlocked specific findings to date. By morphology, the tumors show a hepatocellular carcinoma component plus a distinctly different component of sarcoma (Figure 21.72). In some cases, the malignant epithelial component is not hepatocellular carcinoma, but instead is either cholangiocarcinoma or undifferentiated carcinoma, and the final diagnosis is then modified appropriately. In general, the diagnosis for both the epithelial component and the sarcoma component are made in the usual way. Overall, the most common types of sarcomas are leiomyosarcoma, rhabdomyosarcoma, chondrosarcoma, fibrosarcoma, or osteosarcoma.[126-128]

The differential diagnosis is primarily that of a sarcomatoid hepatocellular carcinoma. The distinction is not always easily made, especially on a biopsy or small sample, but as a general rule, the sarcoma component in carcinosarcoma is keratin negative or only focally positive and often shows specific mesenchymal differentiation by morphology and immunostains.

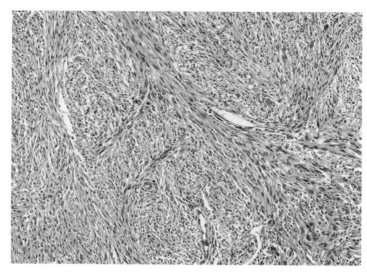

FIGURE 21.72 **Carcinosarcoma.** The sarcoma component is shown.

In sarcomatoid hepatocellular carcinoma, however, the spindle cell component shows stronger and more abundant keratin staining and is negative for specific mesenchymal differentiation on morphology and immunostains.

COMBINED HEPATOCELLULAR CARCINOMA-NEUROENDOCRINE CARCINOMA

This subtype is very rare, much less than 1%, and relatively few details are known about this variant, other than that it occurs. The prognosis appears to be worse. By definition, there must be two distinct morphologies, one of hepatocellular carcinoma and one of neuroendocrine carcinoma. The hepatocellular carcinoma is usually well to moderately differentiated, while the neuroendocrine component is usually a small cell carcinoma, with the small cell carcinoma growing as focal nests in the sinusoids of the hepatocellular carcinoma component (Figure 21.73). Immunostains can be used to confirm both the components. Occasional hepatocellular carcinomas can show aberrant staining for synaptophysin or CD56, but this would not qualify as the combined hepatocellular carcinoma-neuroendocrine carcinoma.

Other Growth Patterns

DIFFUSE HEPATOCELLULAR CARCINOMA

Diffuse hepatocellular carcinoma is also called *cirrhotomimetic hepatocellular carcinoma* and is defined by the growth pattern seen on gross examination. Currently, data is not sufficiently clear to determine if the distinctive findings should be classified as subtype or a growth pattern.

Diffuse hepatocellular carcinoma grows in small nodules that closely mimic cirrhosis (Figure 21.74; eFig. 21.42). The cancer burden can be enormous, yet imaging studies and gross examination may fail to show a tumor

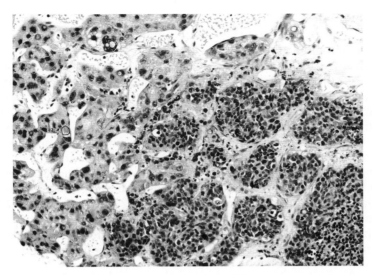

FIGURE 21.73 **Combined hepatocellular carcinoma-small cell carcinoma.** The small cell carcinoma is located within the sinusoids of the well-differentiated hepatocellular carcinoma.

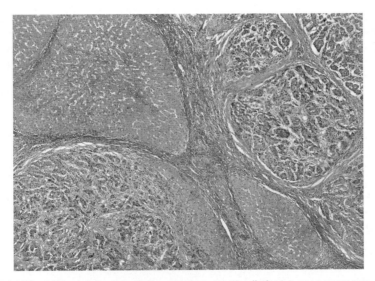

FIGURE 21.74 **Diffuse hepatocellular carcinoma.** No distinct tumor mass was seen by imaging studies or on gross examination in this case. The carcinoma grows as small nodules that closely resemble cirrhotic nodules.

or show a much smaller tumor burden than what is actually present. These nodules of hepatocellular carcinoma are evident primarily on microscopic examination, as the nodules blend into the background cirrhotic liver on gross examination. Although most cases have been reported in cirrhotic livers, an identical growth pattern (innumerable small nodules of tumor through the liver) can rarely be seen in noncirrhotic livers.

The carcinoma tends to be composed of small, basophilic tumor cells that grow in small nodules that are spread throughout the liver. In many cases, original cirrhotic nodules appear to have been "transformed" into cancer, leaving adjacent cirrhotic nodules untouched. Tiny tumorlets, smaller than a cirrhotic nodule, can also be seen (Figure 21.75). In some cases, the tumor nodules in the center will coalesce into a larger dominant nodule that can be seen grossly. Diffuse hepatocellular carcinomas are typically moderately to poorly differentiated and their staining patterns are similar to those of conventional hepatocellular carcinoma. The prognosis is not clear because of the rarity of this tumor, but in some cases the liver can enlarge rapidly and the prognosis is poor.[129] In other cases, successful liver transplant has been reported.[130]

The biological explanation for the unusual growth pattern has not been entirely resolved. Microscopic vascular invasion of the portal veins or hepatic veins is not always apparent in the specimen,[131] but the widely dispersed tumor foci suggest hematogenous spread. In fact, autopsy studies suggest that the tumor is often present in the large hilar portal veins, seeding the rest of the liver.[129] Imaging studies also support this explanation for the unusual growth pattern.[132]

One potential pitfall is that conventional hepatocellular carcinomas often have satellite nodules. In contrast to diffuse hepatocellular carcinoma, which almost always has more than 30 small tumor nodules, the number of satellite nodules for conventional hepatocellular carcinoma is typically less

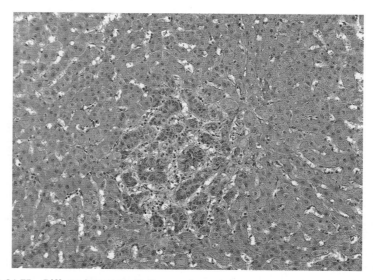

FIGURE 21.75 **Diffuse hepatocellular carcinoma.** In some areas, very small tumorlets can be seen inside benign cirrhotic nodules; these are presumably precursors to the larger cirrhotomimetic nodules of hepatocellular carcinoma.

than 5 (90% of cases) and virtually always than 10 nodules. In addition, satellite nodules associated with conventional hepatocellular carcinomas are located fairly close to the main tumor mass, usually within a centimeter or two, while the nodules in diffuse hepatocellular carcinoma are much more widely dispersed, even in cases where a coalesced aggregate of tumor nodules has formed a mass visible by imaging or on gross examination. Finally, in nearly all cases of satellite nodules, the tumors do not blend into the background cirrhotic liver as they do with the cirrhotomimetic growth pattern, but instead they are often larger or have other distinguishing gross characteristics such as differences in color or texture.

SARCOMATOID HEPATOCELLULAR CARCINOMA

Sarcomatoid hepatocellular carcinoma is defined as a hepatocellular carcinoma with a spindle cell carcinoma component (Figure 21.76). The frequency is less than 1% and the prognosis is worse than conventional hepatocellular carcinoma. The basic notion is the same as that for sarcomatoid carcinomas that arise in other organs: a subclone of the tumor underwent dedifferentiation into a high-grade, spindled, undifferentiated carcinoma.

Sarcomatoid hepatocellular carcinoma is only rarely composed entirely of spindle cells, without a background component of recognizable hepatocellular carcinoma[133]; if they are, it is not possible in most cases to distinguish a sarcomatoid hepatocellular carcinoma from a sarcomatoid cholangiocarcinoma or metastatic sarcomatoid carcinoma. The spindle cells are routinely vimentin positive and show convincing positivity for broad-spectrum cytokeratins. Some spindle cells may also be positive for albumin in situ hybridization or other markers of hepatocellular differentiation.[133,134]

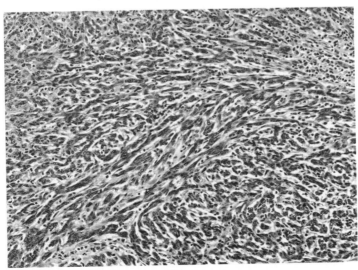

FIGURE 21.76 **Sarcomatoid hepatocellular carcinoma.** Sarcomatoid hepatocellular carcinomas grow as sheets of spindle cells and require staining with markers of hepatic differentiation to confirm the diagnosis.

Nonetheless, in the areas of spindle cell growth, immunostains for hepatocellular differentiation are often negative or only focally positive, so a wide panel of markers for hepatocellular differentiation may be required if that is the only component visible on a specimen. Metastatic spindle cell tumors should be carefully excluded. The main findings used to differentiate a carcinosarcoma from a sarcomatoid hepatocellular carcinoma are (1) the spindle cells in sarcomatoid carcinoma are keratin positive (typically there is stronger and more abundant staining in sarcomatoid carcinomas vs carcinosarcoma, which are usually negative to focally positive) and (2) the spindled areas in sarcomatoid carcinoma do not show specific mesenchymal differentiation by morphology or by immunostains. This diagnostic algorithm works well in most cases, but some cases remain challenging to definitely classify as a sarcomatoid hepatocellular carcinoma or a carcinosarcoma.

FIBRONODULAR GROWTH PATTERN

This distinctive tumor growth pattern can be seen in cirrhotic and noncirrhotic livers. The main tumor mass is composed of an aggregate of smaller tumor nodules, all surrounded by bands of fibrosis (Figure 21.77).[135] These tumors also have distinctive imaging findings.[135] The correlation between this growth pattern and other subtype information has not been fully explored.

BETA-CATENIN GROWTH PATTERN

Hepatocellular carcinomas with beta-catenin mutations tend to be well differentiated, with a thin trabecular growth pattern, along with scattered and sometimes prominent pseudoglands (Figure 21.78).[44,136] Bile plugs are also common, especially in tumors in men. This pattern, however, is neither sensitive nor specific for beta-catenin mutations.

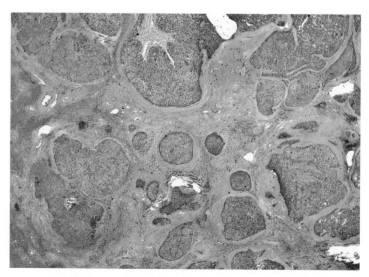

FIGURE 21.77 **Fibronodular growth pattern.** At low power, the tumor is composed of smaller nodules surrounded by bands of fibrosis.

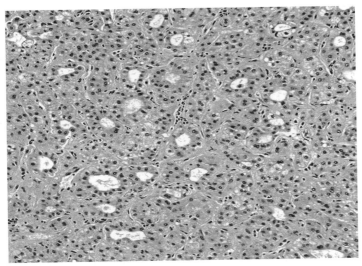

FIGURE 21.78 **Beta-catenin growth pattern.** The tumor is well differentiated with numerous pseudoglands.

RERFERENCES

1. Torbenson M, Yasir S, Anders R, et al. Regenerative hepatic pseudotumor: a new pseudotumor of the liver. *Hum Pathol.* 2020;99:43-52.

2. Arnason T, Fleming KE, Wanless IR. Peritumoral hyperplasia of the liver: a response to portal vein invasion by hypervascular neoplasms. *Histopathology.* 2013;62:458-464.

3. Ra SH, Kaplan JB, Lassman CR. Focal nodular hyperplasia after orthotopic liver transplantation. *Liver Transpl.* 2010;16:98-103.

4. Fukahori S, Kawano T, Obase Y, et al. Fluctuation of hepatic focal nodular hyperplasia size with oral contraceptives use. *Am J Case Rep.* 2019;20:1124-1127.

5. Makhlouf HR, Abdul-Al HM, Goodman ZD. Diagnosis of focal nodular hyperplasia of the liver by needle biopsy. *Hum Pathol.* 2005;36:1210-1216.

6. Chandan VS, Shah SS, Mounajjed T, et al. Copper deposition in focal nodular hyperplasia and inflammatory hepatocellular adenoma. *J Clin Pathol.* 2018;71:504-507.

7. Deniz K, Moreira RK, Yeh MM, et al. Steatohepatitis-like changes in focal nodular hyperplasia, A finding to distinguish from steatohepatitic variant of hepatocellular carcinoma. *Am J Surg Pathol.* 2017;41:277-281.

8. Bioulac-Sage P, Cubel G, Taouji S, et al. Immunohistochemical markers on needle biopsies are helpful for the diagnosis of focal nodular hyperplasia and hepatocellular adenoma subtypes. *Am J Surg Pathol.* 2012;36:1691-1699.

9. Joseph NM, Ferrell LD, Jain D, et al. Diagnostic utility and limitations of glutamine synthetase and serum amyloid-associated protein immunohistochemistry in the distinction of focal nodular hyperplasia and inflammatory hepatocellular adenoma. *Mod Pathol.* 2014;27:62-72.

10. Saxena R, Humphreys S, Williams R, et al. Nodular hyperplasia surrounding fibrolamellar carcinoma: a zone of arterialized liver parenchyma. *Histopathology.* 1994;25:275-278.

11. Paradis V, Champault A, Ronot M, et al. Telangiectatic adenoma: an entity associated with increased body mass index and inflammation. *Hepatology.* 2007;46:140-146.

12. Gupta S, Naini BV, Munoz R, et al. Hepatocellular neoplasms arising in association with androgen use. *Am J Surg Pathol.* 2016;40:454-461.

13. Labrune P, Trioche P, Duvaltier I, et al. Hepatocellular adenomas in glycogen storage disease type I and III: a series of 43 patients and review of the literature. *J Pediatr Gastroenterol Nutr*. 1997;24:276-279.

14. Alshak NS, Cocjin J, Podesta L, et al. Hepatocellular adenoma in glycogen storage disease type IV. *Arch Pathol Lab Med*. 1994;118:88-91.

15. Liu Y, Zen Y, Yeh MM. Steatohepatitis-like changes in hepatocellular adenoma. *Am J Clin Pathol*. 2020;154:525-532.

16. Volmar KE, Burchette JL, Creager AJ. Hepatic adenomatosis in glycogen storage disease type Ia: report of a case with unusual histology. *Arch Pathol Lab Med*. 2003;127:e402-e405.

17. Jones A, Kroneman TN, Blahnik AJ, et al. Ki-67 "hot spot" digital analysis is useful in the distinction of hepatic adenomas and well-differentiated hepatocellular carcinomas. *Virchows Arch*. 2021;478:201-207.

18. Yasir S, Chen ZE, Said S, et al. Biopsies of hepatocellular carcinoma with no reticulin loss: an important diagnostic pitfall. *Hum Pathol*. 2021;107:20-28.

19. Liu L, Shah SS, Naini BV, et al. Immunostains used to subtype hepatic adenomas do not distinguish hepatic adenomas from hepatocellular carcinomas. *Am J Surg Pathol*. 2016;40:1062-1069.

20. Torbenson M. Hepatic adenomas: classification, controversies, and consensus. *Surg Pathol Clin*. 2018;11:351-366.

21. Rebouissou S, Franconi A, Calderaro J, et al. Genotype-phenotype correlation of CTNNB1 mutations reveals different ss-catenin activity associated with liver tumor progression. *Hepatology*. 2016;64:2047-2061.

22. Mounajjed T, Yasir S, Aleff PA, et al. Pigmented hepatocellular adenomas have a high risk of atypia and malignancy. *Mod Pathol*. 2015;28:1265-1274.

23. Masuda T, Beppu T, Ikeda K, et al. Pigmented hepatocellular adenoma: report of a case. *Surg Today*. 2011;41:881-883.

24. Salaria SN, Graham RP, Aishima S, et al. Primary hepatic tumors with myxoid change: morphologically unique hepatic adenomas and hepatocellular carcinomas. *Am J Surg Pathol*. 2015;39:318-324.

25. Nault JC, Fabre M, Couchy G, et al. GNAS-activating mutations define a rare subgroup of inflammatory liver tumors characterized by STAT3 activation. *J Hepatol*. 2012;56:184-191.

26. Henriet E, Abou Hammoud A, Dupuy JW, et al. Argininosuccinate synthase 1 (ASS1): a marker of unclassified hepatocellular adenoma and high bleeding risk. *Hepatology*. 2017;66:2016-2028.

27. Bedossa P, Burt AD, Brunt EM, et al. Well-differentiated hepatocellular neoplasm of uncertain malignant potential: proposal for a new diagnostic category. *Hum Pathol*. 2014;45:658-660.

28. Micchelli ST, Vivekanandan P, Boitnott JK, et al. Malignant transformation of hepatic adenomas. *Mod Pathol*. 2008;21:491-497.

29. Torbenson MS, Zen Y, Yeh MM, et al. *Tumors of the Liver*. American Registry of Pathology; 2018. xv:449.

30. Wang CS, Yao WJ, Chang TT, et al. The impact of type 2 diabetes on the development of hepatocellular carcinoma in different viral hepatitis statuses. *Cancer Epidemiol Biomarkers Prev*. 2009;18:2054-2060.

31. Paradis V, Zalinski S, Chelbi E, et al. Hepatocellular carcinomas in patients with metabolic syndrome often develop without significant liver fibrosis: a pathological analysis. *Hepatology*. 2009;49:851-859.

32. Borie F, Bouvier AM, Herrero A, et al. Treatment and prognosis of hepatocellular carcinoma: a population based study in France. *J Surg Oncol*. 2008;98:505-509.

33. Wang Q, Luan W, Villanueva GA, et al. Clinical prognostic variables in young patients (under 40 years) with hepatitis B virus-associated hepatocellular carcinoma. *J Dig Dis.* 2012;13:214-218.

34. Yeh MM, Daniel HD, Torbenson M. Hepatitis C-associated hepatocellular carcinomas in non-cirrhotic livers. *Mod Pathol.* 2010;23:276-283.

35. von Delius S, Lersch C, Schulte-Frohlinde E, et al. Hepatocellular carcinoma associated with hereditary hemochromatosis occurring in non-cirrhotic liver. *Z Gastroenterol.* 2006;44:39-42.

36. Baffy G, Brunt EM, Caldwell SH. Hepatocellular carcinoma in non-alcoholic fatty liver disease: an emerging menace. *J Hepatol.* 2012;56:1384-1391.

37. Alexander J, Torbenson M, Wu TT, et al. Non-alcoholic fatty liver disease contributes to hepatocellular carcinoma in non-cirrhotic liver: a clinical and pathological study. *J Gastroenterol Hepatol.* 2013;28:848-854.

38. Toyoda H, Kumada T, Tada T, et al. Tumor markers for hepatocellular carcinoma: simple and significant predictors of outcome in patients with HCC. *Liver Cancer.* 2015;4:126-136.

39. Leerapun A, Suravarapu SV, Bida JP, et al. The utility of Lens culinaris agglutinin-reactive alpha-fetoprotein in the diagnosis of hepatocellular carcinoma: evaluation in a United States referral population. *Clin Gastroenterol Hepatol.* 2007;5:394-402; quiz 267.

40. Marrero JA, Feng Z, Wang Y, et al. Alpha-fetoprotein, des-gamma carboxyprothrombin, and lectin-bound alpha-fetoprotein in early hepatocellular carcinoma. *Gastroenterology.* 2009;137:110-118.

41. Hajosi-Kalcakosz S, Dezso K, Bugyik E, et al. Enhancer of zeste homologue 2 (EZH2) is a reliable immunohistochemical marker to differentiate malignant and benign hepatic tumors. *Diagn Pathol.* 2012;7:86.

42. Nzeako UC, Goodman ZD, Ishak KG. Comparison of tumor pathology with duration of survival of North American patients with hepatocellular carcinoma. *Cancer.* 1995;76:579-588.

43. *Digestive Systems Tumors.* 5th ed. International Agency fo Research on Cancer; 2019.

44. Kitao A, Matsui O, Yoneda N, et al. Hepatocellular carcinoma with beta-catenin mutation: imaging and pathologic characteristics. *Radiology.* 2015;275:708-717.

45. Lauwers GY, Terris B, Balis UJ, et al. Prognostic histologic indicators of curatively resected hepatocellular carcinomas: a multi-institutional analysis of 425 patients with definition of a histologic prognostic index. *Am J Surg Pathol.* 2002;26:25-34.

46. Hong H, Patonay B, Finley J. Unusual reticulin staining pattern in well-differentiated hepatocellular carcinoma. *Diagn Pathol.* 2011;6:15.

47. Singhi AD, Jain D, Kakar S, et al. Reticulin loss in benign fatty liver: an important diagnostic pitfall when considering a diagnosis of hepatocellular carcinoma. *Am J Surg Pathol.* 2012;36:710-715.

48. Xiao SY, Wang HL, Hart J, et al. cDNA arrays and immunohistochemistry identification of CD10/CALLA expression in hepatocellular carcinoma. *Am J Pathol.* 2001;159:1415-1421.

49. Lagana SM, Salomao M, Remotti HE, et al. Bile salt export pump: a sensitive and specific immunohistochemical marker of hepatocellular carcinoma. *Histopathology.* 2015;66:598-602.

50. Borscheri N, Roessner A, Rocken C. Canalicular immunostaining of neprilysin (CD10) as a diagnostic marker for hepatocellular carcinomas. *Am J Surg Pathol.* 2001;25:1297-1303.

51. Wennerberg AE, Nalesnik MA, Coleman WB. Hepatocyte paraffin 1: a monoclonal antibody that reacts with hepatocytes and can be used for differential diagnosis of hepatic tumors. *Am J Pathol.* 1993;143:1050-1054.

52. Butler SL, Dong H, Cardona D, et al. The antigen for Hep Par 1 antibody is the urea cycle enzyme carbamoyl phosphate synthetase 1. *Lab Invest.* 2008;88:78-88.

53. Chan ES, Yeh MM. The use of immunohistochemistry in liver tumors. *Clin Liver Dis.* 2010;14:687-703.

54. Chu PG, Ishizawa S, Wu E, et al. Hepatocyte antigen as a marker of hepatocellular carcinoma: an immunohistochemical comparison to carcinoembryonic antigen, CD10, and alpha-fetoprotein. *Am J Surg Pathol.* 2002;26:978-988.

55. Kakar S, Muir T, Murphy LM, et al. Immunoreactivity of Hep Par 1 in hepatic and extrahepatic tumors and its correlation with albumin in situ hybridization in hepatocellular carcinoma. *Am J Clin Pathol.* 2003;119:361-366.

56. Fan Z, van de Rijn M, Montgomery K, et al. Hep par 1 antibody stain for the differential diagnosis of hepatocellular carcinoma: 676 tumors tested using tissue microarrays and conventional tissue sections. *Mod Pathol.* 2003;16:137-144.

57. Abdul-Al HM, Makhlouf HR, Wang G, et al. Glypican-3 expression in benign liver tissue with active hepatitis C: implications for the diagnosis of hepatocellular carcinoma. *Hum Pathol.* 2008;39:209-212.

58. Shafizadeh N, Ferrell LD, Kakar S. Utility and limitations of glypican-3 expression for the diagnosis of hepatocellular carcinoma at both ends of the differentiation spectrum. *Mod Pathol.* 2008;21:1011-1018.

59. Libbrecht L, Severi T, Cassiman D, et al. Glypican-3 expression distinguishes small hepatocellular carcinomas from cirrhosis, dysplastic nodules, and focal nodular hyperplasia-like nodules. *Am J Surg Pathol.* 2006;30:1405-1411.

60. Coston WM, Loera S, Lau SK, et al. Distinction of hepatocellular carcinoma from benign hepatic mimickers using Glypican-3 and CD34 immunohistochemistry. *Am J Surg Pathol.* 2008;32:433-444.

61. Yan B, Wei JJ, Qian YM, et al. Expression and clinicopathologic significance of glypican 3 in hepatocellular carcinoma. *Ann Diagn Pathol.* 2011;15:162-169.

62. Yan BC, Gong C, Song J, et al. Arginase-1: a new immunohistochemical marker of hepatocytes and hepatocellular neoplasms. *Am J Surg Pathol.* 2010;34:1147-1154.

63. Clark I, Shah SS, Moreira R, et al. A subset of well-differentiated hepatocellular carcinomas are Arginase-1 negative. *Hum Pathol.* 2017;69:90-95.

64. Askan G, Deshpande V, Klimstra DS, et al. Expression of markers of hepatocellular differentiation in pancreatic acinar cell neoplasms: a potential diagnostic pitfall. *Am J Clin Pathol.* 2016;146:163-169.

65. Han CP, Hsu JD, Koo CL, et al. Antibody to cytokeratin (CK8/CK18) is not derived from CAM5.2 clone, and anticytokeratin CAM5.2 (Becton Dickinson) is not synonymous with the antibody (CK8/CK18). *Hum Pathol.* 2010;41:616-617; author reply 7.

66. Durnez A, Verslype C, Nevens F, et al. The clinicopathological and prognostic relevance of cytokeratin 7 and 19 expression in hepatocellular carcinoma. A possible progenitor cell origin. *Histopathology.* 2006;49:138-151.

67. Uenishi T, Kubo S, Yamamoto T, et al. Cytokeratin 19 expression in hepatocellular carcinoma predicts early postoperative recurrence. *Cancer Sci.* 2003;94:851-857.

68. Klein WM, Molmenti EP, Colombani PM, et al. Primary liver carcinoma arising in people younger than 30 years. *Am J Clin Pathol.* 2005;124:512-518.

69. Torbenson M. Fibrolamellar carcinoma: 2012 update. *Scientifica.* 2012;2012:15.

70. Shah SS, Wu TT, Torbenson MS, et al. Aberrant CDX2 expression in hepatocellular carcinomas: an important diagnostic pitfall. *Hum Pathol.* 2017;64:13-18.

71. Lee W, Li X, Chandan VS. Hepatocellular carcinomas can be Special AT-rich sequence-binding protein 2 positive: an important diagnostic pitfall. *Hum Pathol.* 2020;105:47-52.

72. Chandan VS, Shah SS, Torbenson MS, et al. Arginase-1 is frequently positive in hepatoid adenocarcinomas. *Hum Pathol.* 2016;55:11-16.

73. Terracciano LM, Glatz K, Mhawech P, et al. Hepatoid adenocarcinoma with liver metastasis mimicking hepatocellular carcinoma: an immunohistochemical and molecular study of eight cases. *Am J Surg Pathol.* 2003;27:1302-1312.

74. Yang C, Sun L, Lai JZ, et al. Primary hepatoid carcinoma of the pancreas: a clinicopathological study of 3 cases with review of additional 31 cases in the literature. *Int J Surg Pathol.* 2019;27:28-42.

75. Wood LD, Heaphy CM, Daniel HD, et al. Chromophobe hepatocellular carcinoma with abrupt anaplasia: a proposal for a new subtype of hepatocellular carcinoma with unique morphological and molecular features. *Mod Pathol.* 2013;26:1586-1593.

76. Salomao M, Remotti H, Vaughan R, et al. The steatohepatitic variant of hepatocellular carcinoma and its association with underlying steatohepatitis. *Hum Pathol.* 2012;43:737-746.

77. Salomao M, Yu WM, Brown RS Jr, et al. Steatohepatitic hepatocellular carcinoma (SH-HCC): a distinctive histological variant of HCC in hepatitis C virus-related cirrhosis with associated NAFLD/NASH. *Am J Surg Pathol.* 2010;34:1630-1636.

78. Torbenson MS. Hepatocellular carcinoma: making sense of morphological heterogeneity, growth patterns, and subtypes. *Hum Pathol.* 2021;112:86-101.

79. Qin J, Higashi T, Nakagawa S, et al. Steatohepatitic variant of hepatocellular carcinoma is associated with both alcoholic steatohepatitis and nonalcoholic steatohepatitis: a study of 2 cohorts with molecular insights. *Am J Surg Pathol.* 2020;44:1406-1412.

80. Jain D, Nayak NC, Kumaran V, et al. Steatohepatitic hepatocellular carcinoma, a morphologic indicator of associated metabolic risk factors: a study from India. *Arch Pathol Lab Med.* 2013;137:961-966.

81. Yeh MM, Liu Y, Torbenson M. Steatohepatitic variant of hepatocellular carcinoma in the absence of metabolic syndrome or background steatosis: a clinical, pathological, and genetic study. *Hum Pathol.* 2015;46:1769-1775.

82. Lee JH, Shin DH, Park WY, et al. IDH1 R132C mutation is detected in clear cell hepatocellular carcinoma by pyrosequencing. *World J Surg Oncol.* 2017;15:82.

83. Murakata LA, Ishak KG, Nzeako UC. Clear cell carcinoma of the liver: a comparative immunohistochemical study with renal clear cell carcinoma. *Mod Pathol.* 2000;13:874-881.

84. Liu Z, Ma W, Li H, et al. Clinicopathological and prognostic features of primary clear cell carcinoma of the liver. *Hepatol Res.* 2008;38:291-299.

85. Li T, Fan J, Qin LX, et al. Risk factors, prognosis, and management of early and late intrahepatic recurrence after resection of primary clear cell carcinoma of the liver. *Ann Surg Oncol.* 2011;18:1955-1963.

86. Clayton EF, Furth EE, Ziober A, et al. A case of primary clear cell hepatocellular carcinoma in a non-cirrhotic liver: an immunohistochemical and ultrastructural study. *Rare Tumors.* 2012;4:e29.

87. Krings G, Ramachandran R, Jain D, et al. Immunohistochemical pitfalls and the importance of glypican 3 and arginase in the diagnosis of scirrhous hepatocellular carcinoma. *Mod Pathol.* 2013;26:782-791.

88. Calderaro J, Couchy G, Imbeaud S, et al. Histological subtypes of hepatocellular carcinoma are related to gene mutations and molecular tumour classification. *J Hepatol.* 2017;67:727-738.

89. Hatano M, Ojima H, Masugi Y, et al. Steatotic and nonsteatotic scirrhous hepatocellular carcinomas reveal distinct clinicopathological features. *Hum Pathol.* 2019;86:222-232.

90. Lee JH, Choi MS, Gwak GY, et al. Clinicopathologic characteristics and long-term prognosis of scirrhous hepatocellular carcinoma. *Dig Dis Sci.* 2012;57:1698-1707.

91. Matsuura S, Aishima S, Taguchi K, et al. 'Scirrhous' type hepatocellular carcinomas: a special reference to expression of cytokeratin 7 and hepatocyte paraffin 1. *Histopathology.* 2005;47:382-390.

92. Zakka K, Jiang R, Alese OB, et al. Clinical outcomes of rare hepatocellular carcinoma variants compared to pure hepatocellular carcinoma. *J Hepatocell Carcinoma*. 2019;6:119-129.

93. Kurogi M, Nakashima O, Miyaaki H, et al. Clinicopathological study of scirrhous hepatocellular carcinoma. *J Gastroenterol Hepatol*. 2006;21:1470-1477.

94. Malouf G, Falissard B, Azoulay D, et al. Is histological diagnosis of primary liver carcinomas with fibrous stroma reproducible among experts? *J Clin Pathol*. 2009;62:519-524.

95. Torbenson M. Hepatocellular Carcinoma Variants. *Annual Meeting of the Laennec Liver Pathology Society*; Heidelberg, Germany 2012 (oral presentation).

96. Ziol M, Pote N, Amaddeo G, et al. Macrotrabecular-massive hepatocellular carcinoma: a distinctive histological subtype with clinical relevance. *Hepatology*. 2018;68:103-112.

97. Jeon Y, Benedict M, Taddei T, et al. Macrotrabecular hepatocellular carcinoma: an aggressive subtype of hepatocellular carcinoma. *Am J Surg Pathol*. 2019;43:943-948.

98. Kakar S, Burgart LJ, Batts KP, et al. Clinicopathologic features and survival in fibrolamellar carcinoma: comparison with conventional hepatocellular carcinoma with and without cirrhosis. *Mod Pathol*. 2005;18:1417-1423.

99. Njei B, Konjeti VR, Ditah I. Prognosis of patients with fibrolamellar hepatocellular carcinoma versus conventional hepatocellular carcinoma: a systematic review and meta-analysis. *Gastrointest Cancer Res*. 2014;7:49-54.

100. Torbenson M. Review of the clinicopathologic features of fibrolamellar carcinoma. *Adv Anat Pathol*. 2007;14:217-223.

101. McDonald JD, Gupta S, Shindorf ML, et al. Elevated serum alpha-fetoprotein is associated with abbreviated survival for patients with fibrolamellar hepatocellular carcinoma who undergo a curative resection. *Ann Surg Oncol*. 2020;27:1900-1905.

102. Ramai D, Ofosu A, Lai JK, et al. Fibrolamellar hepatocellular carcinoma: a population-based observational study. *Dig Dis Sci*. 2021;66:308-314.

103. El-Serag HB, Davila JA. Is fibrolamellar carcinoma different from hepatocellular carcinoma? A US population-based study. *Hepatology*. 2004;39:798-803.

104. Katzenstein HM, Krailo MD, Malogolowkin MH, et al. Fibrolamellar hepatocellular carcinoma in children and adolescents. *Cancer*. 2003;97:2006-2012.

105. Stipa F, Yoon SS, Liau KH, et al. Outcome of patients with fibrolamellar hepatocellular carcinoma. *Cancer*. 2006;106:1331-1338.

106. Moreno-Luna LEM, Arrieta OM, Garcia-Leyva JM, et al. Clinical and pathologic factors associated with survival in young adult patients with fibrolamellar hepatocarcinoma. *BMC Cancer*. 2005;5:142.

107. Rondell PG, Lackner K, Terracciano L, et al. Fibrolamellar carcinoma in the Carney complex: PRKAR1A loss instead of the classic DNAJB1-PRKACA fusion. *Hepatology*. 2018;68:1441-1447.

108. Ichikawa T, Federle MP, Grazioli L, et al. Fibrolamellar hepatocellular carcinoma: imaging and pathologic findings in 31 recent cases. *Radiology*. 1999;213:352-361.

109. Ross HM, Daniel HD, Vivekanandan P, et al. Fibrolamellar carcinomas are positive for CD68. *Mod Pathol*. 2011;24:390-395.

110. Hirsch TZ, Negulescu A, Gupta B, et al. BAP1 mutations define a homogeneous subgroup of hepatocellular carcinoma with fibrolamellar-like features and activated PKA. *J Hepatol*. 2020;72:924-936.

111. Graham RP, Yeh MM, Lam-Himlin D, et al. Molecular testing for the clinical diagnosis of fibrolamellar carcinoma. *Mod Pathol*. 2018;31:141-149.

112. Graham RP, Jin L, Knutson DL, et al. DNAJB1-PRKACA is specific for fibrolamellar carcinoma. *Mod Pathol*. 2015;28:822-829.

113. Singhi AD, Wood LD, Parks E, et al. Recurrent rearrangements in PRKACA and PRKACB in intraductal oncocytic papillary neoplasms of the pancreas and bile duct. *Gastroenterology*. 2020;158:573-582.e2.

114. Torbenson MS. Morphologic subtypes of hepatocellular carcinoma. *Gastroenterol Clin North Am*. 2017;46:365-391.

115. Limaiem F, Bouraoui S, Sboui M, et al. Fibrolamellar carcinoma versus scirrhous hepatocellular carcinoma: diagnostic usefulness of CD68. *Acta Gastroenterol Belg*. 2015;78:393-398.

116. du Toit M, Aldera AP. Fibrolamellar carcinoma with predominantly pseudoglandular architecture: a potential diagnostic pitfall. *Int J Surg Pathol*. 2021;29:69-72.

117. Li R, Yang D, Tang CL, et al. Combined hepatocellular carcinoma and cholangiocarcinoma (biphenotypic) tumors: clinical characteristics, imaging features of contrast-enhanced ultrasound and computed tomography. *BMC Cancer*. 2016;16:158.

118. Yeh MM. Pathology of combined hepatocellular-cholangiocarcinoma. *J Gastroenterol Hepatol*. 2010;25:1485-1492.

119. Patel KR, Liu TC, Vaccharajani N, et al. Characterization of inflammatory (lymphoepithelioma-like) hepatocellular carcinoma: a study of 8 cases. *Arch Pathol Lab Med*. 2014;138:1193-1202.

120. Chan AW, Tong JH, Pan Y, et al. Lymphoepithelioma-like hepatocellular carcinoma: an uncommon variant of hepatocellular carcinoma with favorable outcome. *Am J Surg Pathol*. 2015;39:304-312.

121. Chan AW, Zhang Z, Chong CC, et al. Genomic landscape of lymphoepithelioma-like hepatocellular carcinoma. *J Pathol*. 2019;249:166-172.

122. Kohno M, Shirabe K, Mano Y, et al. Granulocyte colony-stimulating-factor-producing hepatocellular carcinoma with extensive sarcomatous changes: report of a case. *Surg Today*. 2013;43:439-445.

123. Joshita S, Nakazawa K, Koike S, et al. A case of granulocyte-colony stimulating factor-producing hepatocellular carcinoma confirmed by immunohistochemistry. *J Korean Med Sci*. 2010;25:476-480.

124. Amano H, Itamoto T, Emoto K, et al. Granulocyte colony-stimulating factor-producing combined hepatocellular/cholangiocellular carcinoma with sarcomatous change. *J Gastroenterol*. 2005;40:1158-1159.

125. Araki K, Kishihara F, Takahashi K, et al. Hepatocellular carcinoma producing a granulocyte colony-stimulating factor: report of a resected case with a literature review. *Liver Int*. 2007;27:716-721.

126. Aita K, Seki K. Carcinosarcoma of the liver producing granulocyte-colony stimulating factor. *Pathol Int*. 2006;56:413-419.

127. Lao XM, Chen DY, Zhang YQ, et al. Primary carcinosarcoma of the liver: clinicopathologic features of 5 cases and a review of the literature. *Am J Surg Pathol*. 2007;31:817-826.

128. Xiang S, Chen YF, Guan Y, et al. Primary combined hepatocellular-cholangiocellular sarcoma: an unusual case. *World J Gastroenterol*. 2015;21:7335-7342.

129. Okuda K, Noguchi T, Kubo Y, et al. A clinical and pathological study of diffuse type hepatocellular carcinoma. *Liver*. 1981;1:280-289.

130. Han YS, Choi DL, Park JB. Cirrhotomimetic type hepatocellular carcinoma diagnosed after liver transplantation – eighteen months of follow-up: a case report. *Transplant Proc*. 2008;40:2835-2836.

131. Jakate S, Yabes A, Giusto D, et al. Diffuse cirrhosis-like hepatocellular carcinoma: a clinically and radiographically undetected variant mimicking cirrhosis. *Am J Surg Pathol*. 2010;34:935-941.

132. Kanematsu M, Semelka RC, Leonardou P, et al. Hepatocellular carcinoma of diffuse type: MR imaging findings and clinical manifestations. *J Magn Reson Imaging*. 2003;18:189-195.

133. Haratake J, Horie A. An immunohistochemical study of sarcomatoid liver carcinomas. *Cancer.* 1991;68:93-97.

134. Oda Y, Katsuda S, Nakanishi I. An autopsy case of hepatic sarcomatoid tumor: immunohistochemical comparison with a sarcomatous component of hepatocellular carcinoma. *Pathol Int.* 1994;44:230-236.

135. Tefera J, Revzin M, Chapiro J, et al. Fibronodular hepatocellular carcinoma—a new variant of liver cancer: clinical, pathological and radiological correlation. *J Clin Pathol.* 2021;74:31-35.

136. Dal Bello B, Rosa L, Campanini N, et al. Glutamine synthetase immunostaining correlates with pathologic features of hepatocellular carcinoma and better survival after radiofrequency thermal ablation. *Clin Cancer Res.* 2010;16:2157-2166.

22

BENIGN AND MALIGNANT BILIARY TUMORS

BILE DUCT HAMARTOMA

Definition

Bile duct hamartomas are benign, generally small lesions composed of interanastomosing bile duct-like structures. Bile duct hamartomas are also called *biliary hamartomas* or *von Meyenburg complexes*. The term bile duct plate malformation is also used, mostly in the context of lesions occurring in the setting of polycystic kidney and liver disease.

Overview of Demographics and Risk Factors

Sporadic lesions are not hamartomas per se but are acquired, clonal lesions. Overall, they are more common in cirrhotic livers than in noncirrhotic livers and have an increased frequency in chronic hepatitis C and alcohol-related liver cirrhosis. Their malignant potential is very low but not zero. Bile duct hamartomas are most commonly encountered at frozen section, when a surgeon sees a small, white, subcapsular lesion while doing abdominal surgery for cancers of other organs, and then biopsies the liver lesion for frozen section in order to rule out metastatic disease.

Histological Findings

Bile duct hamartomas can be single or multiple. Most are small (less than 10 mm). They are composed of small aggregates of bile duct-like structures that have open lumens, often contain bile, and grow in an irregular, interanastomosing fashion (Figure 22.1; eFig. 22.1). They can have abundant stroma, which can be either myxoid or fibrotic. Bile duct hamartomas differ from bile duct adenomas in several key aspects: bile duct adenomas lack an interanastomosing growth pattern and lack bile. Bile duct adenomas on average tend to be somewhat bigger than bile duct hamartomas, but there is significant size overlap.

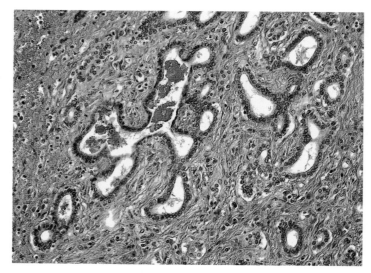

FIGURE 22.1 **Von Meyenburg complex, also called bile duct hamartoma.** The von Meyenburg complex is composed of interanastomosing tubular structures with open lumens containing bile.

Immunostains

Immunostains are not needed to make the diagnosis, but the tumor cells stain similarly to normal bile ducts. They have very low to absent Ki-67 labeling, which can be very helpful if you are worried about malignancy.

BILE DUCT ADENOMA

Definition

Bile duct adenomas are benign aggregates of small, tubular, bile duct-like structures without lumens or bile, growing in variably fibrous stroma.

Demographics and Risk Factors

Like von Meyenburg complexes, bile duct adenomas appear to be acquired lesions and are more common in cirrhotic livers than in non-cirrhotic livers.

Histological Findings

Bile duct adenomas are usually small, single, and subcapsular.[1] Most are less than 2 cm in diameter (average is about 6 mm[1]) but occasional cases can be a bit larger. In about 15% of cases, there can be multiple adenomas.[1] At low power, bile duct adenomas range in appearance from that of plump, small, round glands embedded in scant and loose fibrous stroma, to that of atrophic-appearing glands and tubular structures embedded in dense fibrosis. Bile duct adenomas tend to be well circumscribed, but some irregularity at their edges can be seen, with occasional entrapped hepatocytes.

On higher magnification, the adenomas are composed of small, tubular structures that, in contrast to von Meyenburg complexes, lack lumens, are not interanastomosing, and do not contain bile (Figures 22.2 and 22.3, eFigs. 22.2-22.5). Cytologically, the cells should have consistent nuclear size, smooth round nuclei, and inconspicuous nucleoli. Rarely, the epithelial cells may be oncocytic.[2,3] In patients with alpha-1-antitrypsin deficiency, bile duct adenomas can show periodic acid-Schiff (PAS) with diastase (PASD) positive inclusions composed of alpha-1-antitrypsin protein.[4] Glandular complexity, luminal necrotic debris, or destructive growth is not found. Bile duct adenomas are embedded in a fibrous stroma, often containing mild lymphocytic inflammation.

The epithelial cells have a cytokeratin profile that is typical for biliary-type cells. They also stain positive for *BRAF* V600E mutations in about 50% of cases.[4,5] The Ki-67 rate should be low or absent, and mitotic figures are generally absent and never atypical. Rare cases of malignant degeneration have been reported, but their overall malignant potential is close to none.

Sometimes, bile duct adenomas can be difficult to separate from a well-differentiated cholangiocarcinoma, especially on needle biopsy. These features all favor cholangiocarcinoma: prominent nucleoli, significant variation in nuclear size, glandular complexity, mitotic figures, and luminal

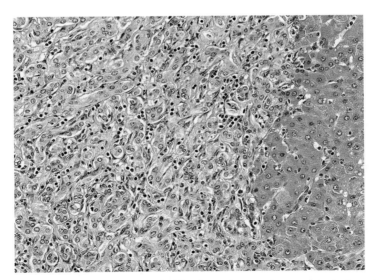

FIGURE 22.2 **Bile duct adenoma.** This bile duct adenoma is composed of small round glands that lack bile and do not interconnect with each other. This Bile duct adenoma has little stroma, but others may have fibrotic stroma.

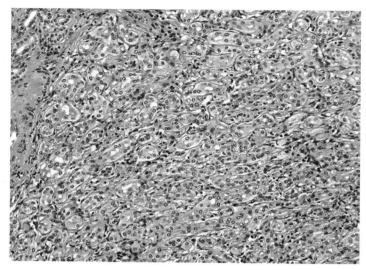

FIGURE 22.3 **Bile duct adenoma.** At high power, the glands are small and well formed, with no cytological atypia. This example has very little intervening stroma.

necrosis. In borderline cases, a firm diagnosis is sometimes impossible on needle biopsy, and the best diagnosis can be that of an atypical bile duct lesion, followed with the differential in a note. Bile duct adenomas stain like normal bile duct cells, and there are no routinely available immunostains that are specific for bile duct adenomas.

CLEAR-CELL BILE DUCT ADENOMA

The clear-cell bile duct adenoma is a rare but distinct type of bile duct adenoma.[6] The neoplastic cells have moderate amounts of cytoplasm with diffuse clear-cell change (Figure 22.4). The cells grow in small nests and cords with round to ovoid nuclei that have no or minimal pleomorphism. The distinctive cytoplasm can result from diffuse, homogeneous clear cell change and/or from numerous tiny vacuoles filling the cytoplasm. They have a low proliferative rate by Ki-67 and otherwise stain like typical bile duct adenomas. The borders of the tumor can be less well-defined than a typical bile adenoma, with patchy, irregular extensions into the adjacent hepatic parenchyma. The stroma often has chronic inflammation (Figure 22.5). The differential includes clear-cell cholangiocarcinoma and metastatic clear-cell carcinomas. Use the cytological features (lack of significant atypia), lack of necrosis, and low proliferative rates to separate the clear-cell bile duct adenoma from malignant clear-cell tumors. If the tumor is malignant, metastatic clear cell carcinomas have to be excluded by clinical and immunostain findings, as the histological findings can show overlap with that of clear-cell cholangiocarcinoma.

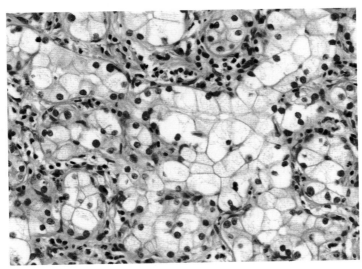

FIGURE 22.4 **Bile duct adenoma, clear cell type.** At high power, the distinctive clear cytoplasm stands out. The cytoplasm can be homogenous clear or have many tiny vacuoles barely at the light microscopy resolution.

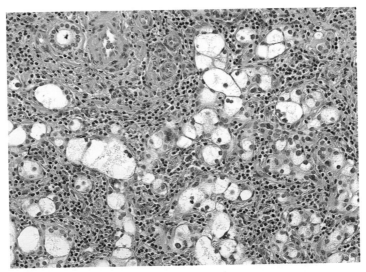

FIGURE 22.5 **Bile duct adenoma, clear cell type.** Lymphocytic inflammation is often present and can be prominent.

CHALLENGING BILE DUCT LESIONS

At times, biopsies for a mass lesion will show an aggregate of bile duct-type structures and the differential is between a benign lesion and a well-differentiated cholangiocarcinoma. Benign lesions in the differential may include bile ductular proliferation in response to a nearby, unsampled mass lesion, as well as a bile duct hamartoma or a bile duct adenoma. Findings that can help sort out these cases include architectural features, cytological changes, and proliferative rates. None is absolutely perfect in isolation and the features work best when considered together. A ductular-like proliferation that remains located at the periphery of fibrous bands would favor a benign reactive process. Luminal necrotic debris is a worrisome finding that favors malignancy (Figure 22.6). Another architectural finding that favors malignancy is incomplete glands, where a gland does not appear to be lined by epithelial cells around its entire circumference (Figure 22.7). Cytological atypia can be very helpful when present (Figure 22.8), but remember that some cholangiocarcinomas are very well differentiated. A Ki-67 immunostain typically shows increased proliferation in cholangiocarcinomas but minimal or absent staining in bile duct adenomas and hamartomas. Studies have fairly consistently found that most cholangiocarcinomas have a proliferative rate of greater than 10%, while benign lesions tend to be 2% or less.[7-9] A ductular reaction can have a high proliferative rate also, but typically in cases of recent, substantial parenchymal injury/collapse. In this situation, the ductular reaction can be more diffuse but still tends to retain a lobular pattern at low power. In addition, residual portal tracts and small islands of hepatocytes are common in areas of benign parenchymal collapse. Strong and diffuse staining for p53 is found in about one-third of intrahepatic cholangiocarcinomas.[7] Of note, weak-to-moderate, but patchy, staining is common in benign biliary lesions.

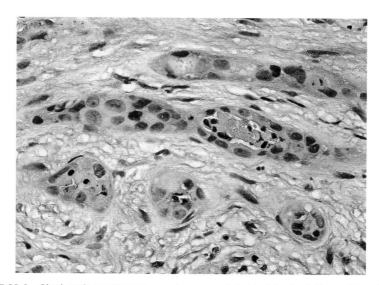

FIGURE 22.6 **Cholangiocarcinoma.** Lumina necrosis in the bile duct-like proliferation and cytological atypia were used to make the diagnosis.

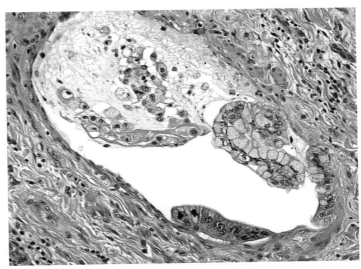

FIGURE 22.7 **Cholangiocarcinoma, "incomplete gland."** This malignant gland appears to lack epithelium in some areas.

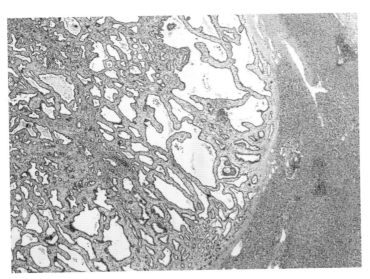

FIGURE 22.8 **Adenofibroma.** Note the areas of cystic change.

Metastatic adenocarcinoma can sometimes enter the differential, but in most cases, the metastatic deposits are overtly malignant, excluding a benign biliary lesion by the morphological changes. In difficult cases, ancillary studies are useful to distinguish a bile duct proliferation from metastatic disease. Biliary lesions are typically CK7 and CK19 positive, while CK20 and CDX2 negative.[10] Benign biliary lesions are also positive for albumin in situ hybridization.[11]

BILIARY ADENOFIBROMA

Biliary adenofibromas are composed of tubulocystic structures that are dilated and embedded in a fibrotic stroma. This tumor is rare and was described relatively recently.[12] Prior to its recognition, these tumors were classified as giant von Meyenburg complexes or as giant bile duct adenomas. They range in size from 5 to 20 cm.[13] Most patients are adults.

The individual glands in adenofibromas tend to be larger than in adenomas or von Meyenburg complexes and can be filled with blood or proteinaceous material and sometimes bile. The glandular structures can be serpentine and interanastomosing in some areas, focally resembling classic von Meyenburg complexes. The glands can also be more circular and form cysts, which can range from small to large in size (Figure 22.9). In some cases, cystic change can dominate the histology. The cells lining the glands are cuboidal and biliary in morphology (Figure 22.9); rarely, the cells can be more columnar. While data is limited, mucin production has not been reported.[14] The tumor glands are embedded in a dense, fibrous stroma and can have entrapped benign hepatocytes at the edges of the tumor. The epithelial cells stain for CK7 and CK19. High-grade dysplasia and/or malignant transformation is seen in about 40% of resected cases.[15]

SIMPLE CYSTS: BILIARY, MESOTHELIAL, AND FOREGUT

Simple Biliary Cyst

A simple biliary cyst is lined by simple, cuboidal epithelium, does not connect to the biliary tree, and lacks ovarian stroma. A simple biliary cyst is only rarely biopsied but can sometimes be removed by a wedge biopsy (Figure 22.10). Simple cysts have a strong female predominance (8:1), and

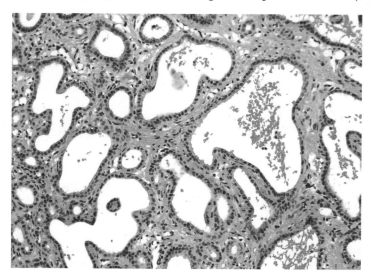

FIGURE 22.9 **Adenofibroma.** This tumor is composed of serpentine and interanastomosing duct structures that somewhat resemble a von Meyenburg complex.

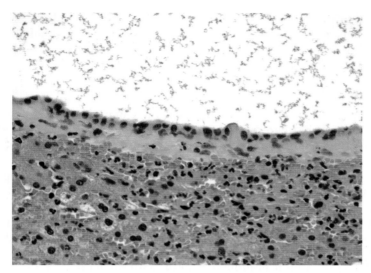

FIGURE 22.10 **Simple biliary cyst.** The epithelium is cuboidal and without atypia.

the average age at identification is in the sixth decade. They are asymptomatic in half of the cases. Grossly, they are usually a single cyst, but occasionally, there can be an aggregate of several smaller cysts. The cysts are lined by simple biliary-type epithelium that lies on a layer of fibrous tissue that can be thin or thick; thicker-walled cysts often show chronic inflammation. In many cases, the epithelium is extensively sloughed off during the processing and you will have to hunt to find the small remaining bits of epithelium. If the cyst has epithelial erosions, the cyst wall can show a marked histiocyte-rich inflammatory response with pigment-laden macrophages. The epithelium may also undergo metaplasia (intestinal, pyloric, squamous) and occasionally shows dysplasia.

Peribiliary Gland Cyst

Small cysts can arise from peribiliary glands located in the hilum of the liver,[16] or near large intrahepatic portal tracts; these are called *peribiliary gland cysts*. They are common in explanted livers, with one study find a frequency of 23% in alcoholic-related cirrhosis.[17] The cysts are small, typically less than 1 cm. The wall may contain small aggregates of bile ducts, peribiliary-type glands, or pancreatic acinar metaplasia/heterotopia. A small percentage of cysts can also show low-grade intraductal papillary neoplasia.[17]

Mesothelial Cyst

In some cases, the differential for a simple biliary cyst may include a mesothelial cyst.[18] Mesothelial cysts are generally small and always subcapsular. They can be seen by the surgeon while doing other abdominal surgeries, leading to intraoperative biopsies. They are lined by mesothelial cells, instead of biliary-type cells, a distinction that is often difficult without the use of immunostains. The surrounding fibrous stroma can have entrapped portal tracts and small aggregates of hepatocytes. The mesothelial cells are positive for calretinin and WT1.

Ciliated Hepatic Foregut Cyst

If the epithelium lining the cyst is columnar and has cilia, then the diagnosis is that of a ciliated hepatic foregut cyst. Ciliated hepatic foregut cysts are uncommon but can be encountered by surgeons doing other abdominal surgeries, leading to intraoperative biopsies. Another common presentation is as an incidental finding on imaging studies. Ciliated hepatic foregut cysts are equal in frequency in men and women and average 4 cm in diameter at the time of surgery—although they can occasionally reach greater than 10 cm. They are unilocular in 90% of cases.[19] Most ciliated hepatic foregut cysts are found in adults, but rarely they are diagnosed in children.[20] Most, but not all, ciliated hepatic foregut cysts are found in segment 4 of the liver (medial section of the left lobe).

The epithelium is columnar overall, with nuclei that appear jumbled and multilayered, with moderate-to-scant apically oriented cytoplasm. Some, but not all, of these lining cells will have cilia (Figure 22.11). In some areas, the lining cells can be more cuboidal or flattened.

The classic description for a ciliated hepatic foregut cyst includes additional layers underneath the distinctive epithelium, in this order: loose subepithelial connective tissue, then irregular bundles of smooth muscle, and finally an outer fibrous layer. These layers are often not evident in biopsy specimens (and not always well seen in resection specimens), so the

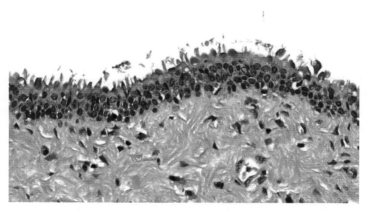

FIGURE 22.11 **Ciliated hepatic foregut cyst**. The epithelium is columnar with scattered ciliated cells.

diagnosis is best made by identifying the distinctive, ciliated epithelium. Rare cases undergo malignant transformation, usually to squamous cell carcinoma[21,22]; most often in cysts that are greater than 10 cm.

MUCINOUS CYSTIC NEOPLASM

Mucinous cystic neoplasms are lined by mucinous or biliary-type epithelium with ovarian-type stroma in the cyst wall. They are the liver analogue of mucinous cystic neoplasms of the pancreas. Ovarian stroma is needed, by definition, to classify a tumor as a mucinous cystic neoplasm. Mucinous cystic neoplasms used to be called *biliary cystadenomas, hepatobiliary cystadenomas,* or *cystadenocarcinomas* (when malignant). They are currently classified as having low-grade dysplasia or high-grade dysplasia. Invasive carcinoma can also arise in mucinous cystic neoplasms.

There is a strong female predominance (essentially all cases) and most occur in the fourth and fifth decade of life. Mucinous cystic neoplasms are solitary and multilocular, with about 70% occurring in the left lobe of the liver.[23] The fluid content is generally thin and clear but can be more mucinous, bloody, or purulent if the cyst has become infected. The cyst typically does not communicate with the bile ducts, although a number of case reports have shown communication can rarely be found, likely resulting from the mucinous cystic neoplasm eroding into a bile duct. Nonetheless, using the combined features of ovarian stroma and lack of communication with bile ducts will separate mucinous cystic neoplasms from intraductal papillary neoplasms in almost all cases.[24]

Histological Findings

The cysts are lined by epithelial cells that are classically columnar, with basally oriented nuclei and apically oriented mucin (mucinous epithelium similar to that seen in the pancreas). In areas, however, the lining cells can show a cuboidal or biliary morphology, or even show flattened epithelium. In fact, one study found that biliary-type epithelium predominated in 50% of cases.[23] Intestinal metaplasia is common and pyloric gland metaplasia and squamous metaplasia can also be seen. Special stains, such as mucicarmine, PAS, or Alcian Blue, will highlight the mucinous areas of the epithelium but are not necessary for diagnosis. The epithelium expresses a range of cytokeratins including CK7, CK19, CK8, and CK18. CK20 will be negative, except in areas of dysplasia.[24] Synaptophysin or chromogranin stains will highlight scattered endocrine cells in the epithelial lining.

Not all mucinous cystic neoplasms of the liver will have demonstrable mucin, especially if your section or biopsy has mostly cuboidal or flattened epithelium. This does not really matter, as the diagnosis is based on finding an epithelial-lined cyst with ovarian-type stroma within the wall (Figure 22.12). Ovarian-type stroma is composed of spindle-shaped cells that are positive for estrogen, progesterone, and alpha-inhibin by immunostaining.[25] Vimentin, actin, and desmin stains also are positive.

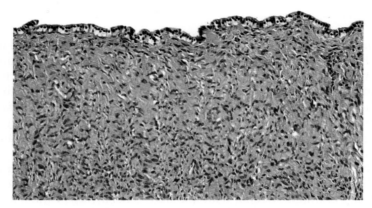

FIGURE 22.12 **Mucinous cystic neoplasm.** The cyst is lined by simple biliary epithelium and has ovarian-type stroma within the cyst wall.

The epithelium is subclassified as low- or high-grade dysplasia. Dysplastic areas may include architectural changes such as crypt-like invaginations of the epithelium into the cyst wall, micropapillary projections into the cyst lumen, or areas of epithelial multilayering. Cytological changes include hyperchromasia and nuclear variability. High-grade dysplasia (formerly called *carcinoma* in situ) has marked papillary projections, often with a complex tubulopapillary architecture, along with increased cellularity, easily found mitotic figures, and more striking nuclear pleomorphism.

In resection specimens, the tumor should be extensively sampled for invasive adenocarcinoma, in particular any areas with mural nodules or other wall thickenings. Adenocarcinoma is found in less than 5% of cases. The adenocarcinoma component typically has a tubular morphology. In general, invasive adenocarcinoma is more common in intraductal papillary neoplasms than in mucinous cystic neoplasms.[24,26]

Differential Diagnoses

ENDOMETRIOTIC CYSTS. Endometriotic cysts can involve the liver and sometimes enter the differential for a mucinous cystic neoplasm. In terms of the stroma morphology, the stroma in mucinous cystic neoplasms tends to be dense and cellular (ovarian-type stroma), while the stroma in endometriotic cysts is less cellular and often contains pigment-laden macrophages (endometrial stroma). These differences in stromal morphology are best seen in resection specimens with classic morphology. In biopsy specimens, the amount of sampled stroma may be small and in some resection specimens, the stromal may be attenuated or hyalinized, leading to nonspecific morphological features. In these difficult cases, immunostains are very helpful. Immunostains for estrogen and progesterone are positive in the stroma of both tumors. In contrast, the cyst epithelium is negative for estrogen and progesterone in mucinous cystic neoplasms, while positive in endometriotic cysts. Other stains can be helpful, especially if the epithelium is largely or completely denuded: the stroma in mucinous cystic neoplasms is inhibin positive, while the stroma in endometriotic cysts is inhibin negative.[27]

MUCINOUS CYSTIC NEOPLASM WITHOUT OVARIAN STROMA. There continues to be occasional cystic biliary tumors that defy the current classification system—ie, they do not connect to the biliary tree (thus, are unlikely to be intraductal papillary neoplasm with marked cystic change) and otherwise appear to be mucinous cystic neoplasms with mixtures of mucinous and biliary-type epithelium, yet lack the ovarian stroma.[28] These cases typically occur in men or postmenopausal women. What to do here? Take more sections and/or perform immunostains. If that fails to identify stromal epithelium, and the findings do not fit for any other cystic neoplasm, then consider using the term *mucinous cystic neoplasm without ovarian stroma* and provide a note of explanation.

SIMPLE BILIARY CYSTS. Simple biliary cysts lack mucinous epithelium (PAS and Alcian Blue stains can be helpful, as needed) and lack ovarian stroma.

INTRADUCTAL PAPILLARY NEOPLASMS OF THE BILE DUCTS (IPNBs). IPNBs lack ovarian stroma, typically have a papillary growth pattern within a dilated bile duct lumen, and are always connected to the biliary tree. In contrast, mucinous cystic neoplasms have ovarian stroma, papillary growth is uncommon unless there is high-grade dysplasia, and they are not connected to the biliary tree.

INTRADUCTAL PAPILLARY NEOPLASMS OF THE BILE DUCT

IPNBs are noninvasive tumors that grow within the biliary tree and can lead to marked cystic changes of the bile duct.[29] A commonly used synonym is *intraductal papillary neoplasm*. This category includes the lesions previously called *biliary papillomatosis* and *biliary papilloma*. IPNBs are analogues of intraductal papillary neoplasms seen within the pancreas.

Intraductal papillary biliary neoplasms have a nearly equal male-to-female ratio, although a modest male predominance has been found in some studies. In any case, they lack the striking female predominance of mucinous cystic neoplasms. The average age at presentation is in the late 60s.[30] A history of intrahepatic biliary stones is present in about 50% of cases.

Gross and Histological Findings

In most cases, the tumors form a single large cyst with multiple subdivisions created by thin, fibrous walls. They connect to the bile duct but sometimes have to be carefully grossed in order to document that finding. Correlation with imaging findings is also very helpful.

Histologically, they are composed of epithelial cells growing within the duct lumen in a micropapillary or complex tubulovillous architecture (Figure 22.13). Some cases are associated with marked dilatation of the bile duct upstream of the papillary neoplasm, which can mimic mucinous cystic neoplasms. The main features used to differentiate these two entities are ovarian-type stroma and connection to the biliary tree (Table 22.1). The epithelium can show a range of morphological findings.[30] Overall, *biliary-type* epithelium is the most common (also called *pancreatobiliary*), where the cells resemble dysplastic biliary epithelium (Figure 22.14). Other epithelial morphologies include intestinal *type*, where the epithelium is composed of tall, thin, columnar cells with basally located nuclei that resemble intestinal epithelium; *gastric type*, where the epithelium is composed of tall, rounded cells with abundant mucin giving them a foveolar appearance (Figure 22.15); and *oncocytic type*, where the epithelium has abundant pink cytoplasm. Oncocytic lesions have *PRKACA* and *PRKACB* fusions leading to activation of the protein kinase A pathway.[31] Fibrolamellar carcinoma also are protein kinase A driven tumors, through *PRKACA-DNJB1* fusions.[32]

There is a high risk of invasive carcinoma, so they should be sectioned well. For example, one large study found stromal invasion in 38% of intraductal papillary neoplasms of the bile ducts.[30] Overall, invasion is most commonly seen with the biliary-type epithelium but can be seen with any of the epithelial types. When cancers develop, tubular adenocarcinoma is the most common morphology. Colloid carcinoma is less common and, when seen, tends to be associated with intestinal-type epithelium.

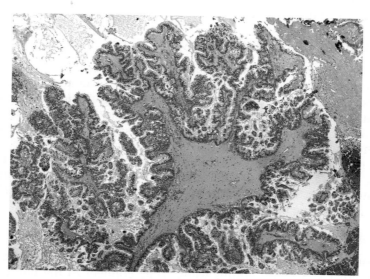

FIGURE 22.13 **Intraductal papillary biliary neoplasm.** There is papillary growth of the tumor.

TABLE 22.1 Comparison of Findings in Mucinous Cystic Neoplasms to That of Intraductal Papillary Neoplasms of the Bile Ducts

Finding	Mucinous Cystic Neoplasm	Intraductal Papillary Biliary Neoplasm
Gender	Strong female predominance	Male: female ratio more equal
Hepatolithiasis	Absent	½ of cases
Gross morphology[a]	80% multicystic	80% multilocular
Ovarian stroma	Present	Absent
Connection to bile duct	Absent	Present
Risk of invasive carcinoma	Low	High

[a]Multicystic appears "grape-like," while multilocular is a large single cyst with subdivisions.

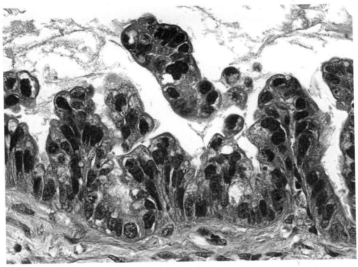

FIGURE 22.14 **Intraductal papillary biliary neoplasm.** The epithelium shows a biliary morphology.

Differential Diagnoses

INTRADUCTAL TUBULOPAPILLARY NEOPLASM. Intraductal tubulopapillary neoplasms were first described in the pancreas but rarely occur within intrahepatic bile ducts. They are generally classified as high-grade dysplastic lesions. They have complex, cribriform growth patterns, with back-to-back glands, in contrast to the papillary growth seen with intraductal papillary biliary neoplasms. They also have a relatively homogenous appearance on low-power examination (Figure 22.16). Foci of comedo-type necrosis are common.

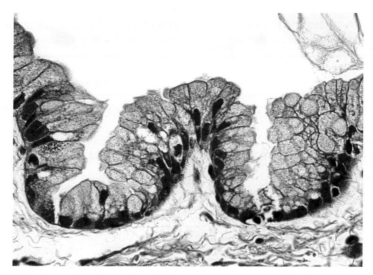

FIGURE 22.15 **Intraductal papillary biliary neoplasm.** The epithelium shows a gastric-type morphology.

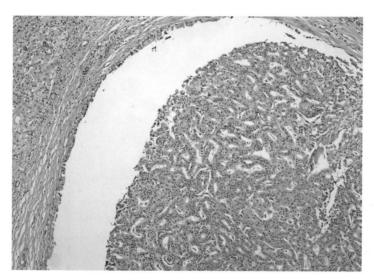

FIGURE 22.16 **Intraductal tubulopapillary neoplasm.** The bile duct is distended by relatively homogenous but complex growth pattern with back-to-back glands.

Intracellular mucin is focal or absent and they are CK7 and CK19 positive. Epithelial membrane antigen (EMA) (also known as MUC1) and MUC6 are commonly positive. MUC5AC is typically negative in intrahepatic tumors but can be positive in tumors arising in the hilum or extrahepatic bile ducts.[33]

BILIARY INTRAEPITHELIAL NEOPLASIA (BilIN). BilIN lesions are microscopic findings that do not lead to grossly visible tumors and are analogues to pancreatic intraepithelial neoplasia (PanIN). They are further classified into low grade and high grade dysplasia based on cytological atypia and architectural complexity. In cirrhotic livers, mostly from chronic hepatitis B or C or alcoholic hepatitis, they are found most commonly in the peripheral, smaller-sized bile ducts. In cases of primary sclerosing cholangitis or other causes of chronic extrahepatic biliary inflammation, they tend to be more commonly found in sections of the liver hilum.

UNDIFFERENTIATED CARCINOMA WITH OSTEOCLAST-LIKE GIANT CELLS

UNDIFFERENTIATED CARCINOMA WITH OSTEOCLAST-LIKE GIANT CELLS was previously called *giant cell tumor of the liver* and is an analogue of the same tumor found in the pancreas. This rare malignancy is characterized by these three elements: (1) undifferentiated tumor cells that are (2) admixed with numerous benign histiocytes as well as (3) benign osteoclast-like giant cells (Figures 22.17 and 22.18). Hemorrhage and abundant hemosiderin can be prominent.

The malignant component of the tumor is composed of undifferentiated, noncohesive tumor cells that can be spindled or epithelioid. Cytokeratin stains can be focally positive or negative and the true line of differentiation for this tumor remains obscure. In the liver, this tumor can be associated with BilIN (Figure 22.19), suggesting they are related to biliary tract dysplasia/neoplasia. *KRAS* and *TP53* mutations are common in tumors of pancreatic origin but liver tumors have not been well studied.

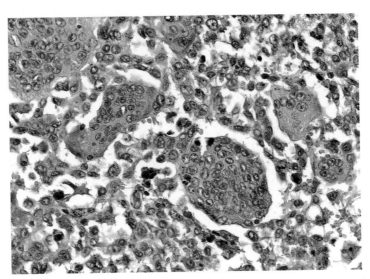

FIGURE 22.17 **Undifferentiated carcinoma with osteoclast-like giant cells.** This tumor is composed of benign histiocytes that form giant cells admixed with small undifferentiated, keratin-negative tumor cells. The giant cells are strongly CD68 positive.

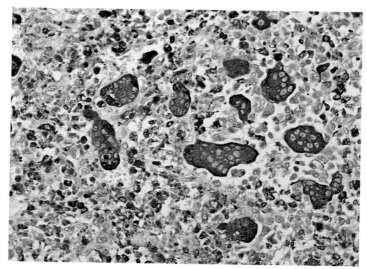

FIGURE 22.18 **Undifferentiated carcinoma with osteoclast-like giant cells.** A CD68 immunostain highlights the numerous benign giant cells.

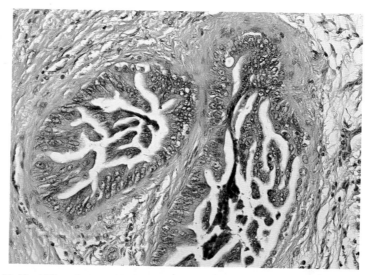

FIGURE 22.19 **Biliary intraepithelial neoplasia (BilIN)-3 associated with undifferentiated carcinoma with osteoclast-like giant cells.** This BilIN-3 lesion was immediately adjacent to the giant cell tumor shown in Figure 22.17.

OTHER RARE PANCREATIC ANALOGUE CARCINOMAS

Rare cases have been reported of acinar cell carcinoma[34,35] and of solid pseudopapillary tumors that appeared to be primary to the liver.[36,37] Of course, metastatic disease has to be carefully excluded.

CHOLANGIOCARCINOMA

Definition

Cholangiocarcinomas are malignant epithelial tumors with biliary differentiation.

Demographics and Risk Factors

Cholangiocarcinomas are clinically divided into those that are intrahepatic, those that are perihilar, and those that are extrahepatic. Perihilar cholangiocarcinomas, also called *Klatskin tumors*, arise from the right or left hepatic duct, or at the junction of the right and left hepatic ducts. The precise location where larger tumors originate is often not clear but is generally assessed based on where the center of the mass lesion is located.

Cholangiocarcinomas arise in both cirrhotic and noncirrhotic livers. Risk factors for intrahepatic cholangiocarcinoma include cirrhosis from any cause including chronic hepatitis C, chronic hepatitis B, alcohol use, and obesity.[38] Of note, in many cases, no etiology is apparent, especially for cholangiocarcinomas arising in noncirrhotic livers. Primary sclerosing cholangitis, liver fluke infections, and hepatolithiasis are important risk factors for perihilar cholangiocarcinomas.

Precursor lesions include BilIN, which is further subdivided according to the degree of dysplasia into types 1, 2, and 3. BilIN-1 is considered low-grade dysplasia, while BilIN-2 and BilIN-3 are high-grade dysplastic lesions. BilIN-1 lesions can be difficult to reliably separate from reactive changes and their frequency in the literature varies accordingly. BilIN-2 and BilIN-3 lesions are most commonly identified in cirrhotic livers, involving medium-sized intrahepatic branches of the biliary tree (Figure 22.20; eFig. 22.6). Peripheral BilIN are most frequent in the setting of chronic hepatitis C and alcohol-related liver disease.[39]

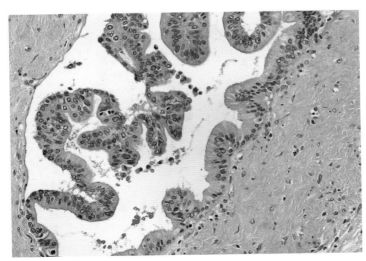

FIGURE 22.20 **Biliary intraepithelial neoplasia (BilIN)-3, hepatitis C related.** This section from a liver transplant for chronic hepatitis C had no cancer but showed BilIN-3 involving larger intrahepatic bile ducts. BilIN involves the upper half of the bile duct in this image.

Histological Findings

Cholangiocarcinomas have a variety of growth patterns. They can be composed of irregular, branching, tubular structures, or be composed of irregular aggregates of infiltrating glands (Figure 22.21; eFigs. 22.7 and 22.8). Cholangiocarcinomas do not always have lumens and can grow in solid trabeculae (Figure 22.22) and solid nests that may mimic hepatocellular carcinoma. Furthermore, any given cholangiocarcinoma often has multiple different growth patterns. There is a rough correlation with anatomic location, however, as centrally located or perihilar cholangiocarcinomas are more likely to have columnar-type epithelial cells, have well-formed glands, and produce mucin; this pattern is called the *large duct pattern of cholangiocarcinoma*. In contrast, cholangiocarcinomas located in the middle of the liver, or in the liver periphery, are more likely to grow as irregular, small, tubular structures lined by low-cuboidal cells that do not produce mucin and in some tumors can somewhat resemble proliferating bile ductules, a morphology called the *small duct pattern of cholangiocarcinoma*.

Rare cholangiocarcinoma can have clear-cell morphology (Figure 22.23; eFig. 22.9), signet-ring morphology (Figure 22.24), colloid morphology (defined as greater than 50% extracellular mucin that contains floating neoplastic cells) (Figure 22.25), sarcomatoid growth (Figure 22.26; eFig. 22.10), or produce granulocyte colony-stimulating factor (GCSF) and have abundant neutrophil-rich stroma. Other cases can show areas of squamous differentiation. Lymphoepithelioma-like cholangiocarcinomas are considered

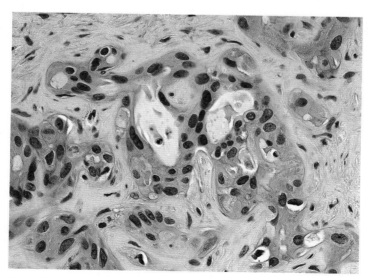

FIGURE 22.21 **Cholangiocarcinoma, gland forming.** This cholangiocarcinoma has a glandular morphology.

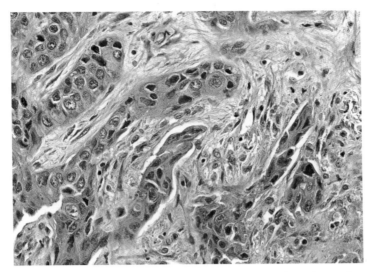

FIGURE 22.22 **Cholangiocarcinoma, trabecular.** This cholangiocarcinoma has a trabecular growth pattern.

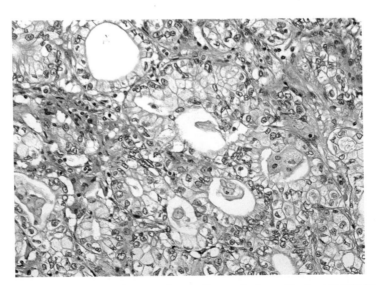

FIGURE 22.23 **Cholangiocarcinoma, clear cell morphology.** The tumor cells have clear cytoplasm.

separately, below. Combined hepatocellular carcinoma-cholangiocarcinoma is considered in more detail in the hepatocellular carcinoma chapter.

Cholangiocarcinomas often elicit a dense, desmoplastic fibrotic response. In some cases, the stroma can also show elastosis (eFig. 22.11). Cholangiocarcinoma rarely colonize and grow along the bile duct epithelium

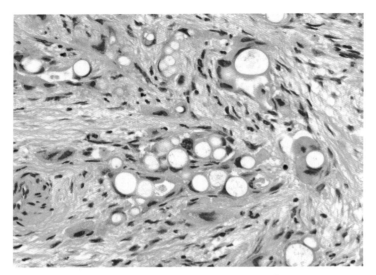

FIGURE 22.24 **Cholangiocarcinoma, signet ring cell morphology.** Signet ring cells are seen.

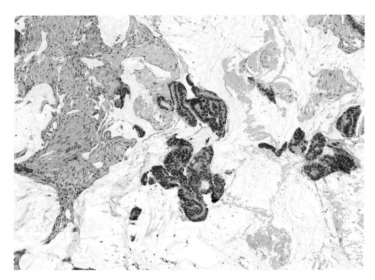

FIGURE 22.25 **Cholangiocarcinoma, colloid morphology.** Small islands of malignant epithelium float in pools of mucin.

(eFig. 22.12). This growth pattern is not specific for cholangiocarcinoma; other tumors can have a similar growth pattern, including metastatic colon adenocarcinoma. Cholangiocarcinomas can also extend along the portal tract stroma, growing within the portal tract connective tissue without direct involvement of the bile duct (eFig. 22.13). This pattern has been called the *periductal infiltrating growth pattern* and is seen more commonly with the

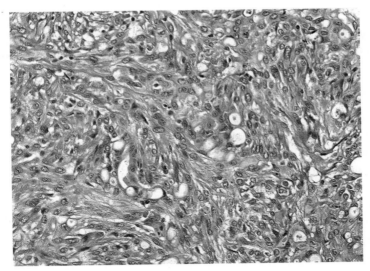

FIGURE 22.26 **Cholangiocarcinoma, spindle morphology.** This tumor has a sarcoma-toid growth pattern. Rare poorly formed glands can be seen. More typical cholangiocarcinoma was seen elsewhere in the tumor.

large duct growth pattern. Cholangiocarcinomas can also show perineural invasion, most commonly the large duct growth pattern.

SMALL DUCT AND LARGE DUCT PATTERNS. These growth patterns help capture the morphological changes seen in most cholangiocarcinomas. They also have strong genetic associations (Table 22.2). These patterns have become the standard nomenclature for research studies, but they do not affect patient care at this time, so do not need to be reported in the clinical pathology reports, unless the clinical team finds them helpful. The key histological findings that distinguish the small and large duct growth patterns can be supplemented with immunostains if desired (Table 22.2).[40] When using this classification schema, the predominant growth pattern drives classification in those tumors that have mixed large duct and small duct patterns of growth. For tumors that have mixed solid and glandular growth patterns, tumors are classified by the glandular component.

The large duct pattern is composed of large-sized malignant glands lined by cells that are usually columnar and have intracellular or luminal mucin (Figure 22.27), which can be highlighted by mucicarmine or PAS stains. In terms of key clinical correlates, large duct cholangiocarcinomas mostly arise in the perihilum and may have a periductal infiltrating growth pattern. In general, the risk factors associated with the large duct pattern of cholangiocarcinoma are similar to those seen for extrahepatic cholangiocarcinomas, including primary sclerosing cholangitis, liver flukes, and other causes of chronic inflammation of the extrahepatic and or large perihilar

TABLE 22.2 Key Morphological and Genetic Differences in Small Duct Versus Large Duct Growth Patterns

Finding	Small Duct Growth Pattern	Large Duct Growth Pattern Frequency of Mutation
Location	Peripheral	Hilar/central
Gland size	Small to absent	Large
Cell morphology	Cuboidal to flattened	Columnar
Mucin production	No	Yes
CRP	95%	5%
CD56	90%	15%
S100P	30%	95%
Genetic changes		
KRAS mutation	2%	20%
PRKACA/PRKACB gene fusions	0%	10%
MDM2 amplification	0%	10%
BAP1 mutation	15%	5%
ARID 1 mutation	25%	10%
IDH1 mutation	15%	0%
FGFR2 amplifications	10%	0%

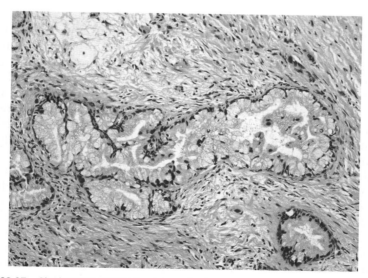

FIGURE 22.27 **Cholangiocarcinoma, large duct morphology.** The large glands are lined by columnar, mucin-producing epithelium.

ducts of the biliary tree. In comparison to the small duct pattern, the large duct pattern is more likely to have lymph node metastases. Overall, they have a worse prognosis in comparison to small duct cholangiocarcinoma.

The small duct pattern is composed of small glands/tubules or can grow as irregular trabeculae with no gland formation (Figure 22.28). The tumor cells in the small duct pattern do not produce mucin and glands, when present, are lined by low-cuboidal to flattened tumor cells. In addition to these definitional findings, the interface between the tumor and nontumor often shows tumor cells directly adjacent to hepatocytes, appearing to be growing along the same trabeculae as the benign hepatocytes; this finding is called *a replacement growth pattern*. The small duct pattern is seen most often in cholangiocarcinomas that arise in the center or the periphery of the liver. While they can occur in noncirrhotic livers, an important risk factor is cirrhosis. Even in noncirrhotic livers, many cases have chronic parenchymal disease, such as chronic hepatitis C, chronic hepatitis B, or alcoholic hepatitis.

In addition to the ordinary small duct growth pattern described above, there are two subtypes of small duct cholangiocarcinoma: *cholangiolocellular* and *ductal plate malformation like*. The cholangiolocellular pattern was first described in 1959 as a tumor that can be deceptively bland, mimicking a bile ductular proliferation.[41] This pattern shows anastomosing duct-like growth with bland cytology and essentially no gland formation (Figure 22.29).

The second subtype, the ductal plate malformation-like pattern, was first suggested as an entity in 2012,[42] it shows a growth pattern that resembles

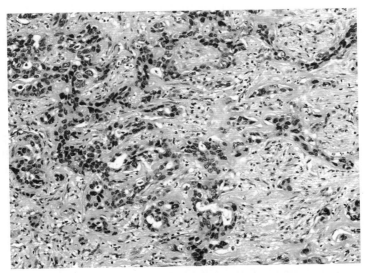

FIGURE 22.28 **Cholangiocarcinoma, small duct morphology.** Small tumor glands are lined by cuboidal to flattened epithelium. The image is at the same magnification as Figure 22.27.

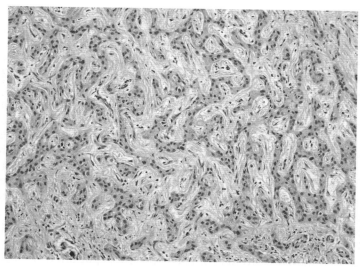

FIGURE 22.29 **Cholangiocarcinoma, cholangiolocellular pattern.** This tumor grows in interanastomosing trabeculae with no gland formation.

a von Meyenburg complex (Figure 22.30). It often has a more fibrotic center, with the morphology best seen at the periphery of the tumor. In contrast to most cholangiocarcinomas, this pattern can have focal, inspissated bile. The tumor cells often have very-low-grade cytology. In many cases, this pattern is admixed with the cholangiolocellular pattern. Regardless of whether these two patterns represent distinct biological entities (still being studied), they represent important diagnostic pitfalls and help extend and clarify the growth patterns that can be seen with cholangiocarcinoma.

Immunostain Findings

There are no positive, affirmative stains specific for identifying biliary differentiation. Instead, the diagnosis is one of exclusion, with other tumors excluded using morphology, immunostains, imaging studies, and clinical findings. Once that is done, a tumor with the appropriate morphology and immunostain findings can be diagnosed as cholangiocarcinoma. The pathologist's role is to make sure the morphological and immunostain findings do not have a better diagnosis.

Cholangiocarcinomas are positive for CK7 in more than 90% of cases, while CK19 is positive in 80% to 90% of cases (Table 22.3). MOC31 is positive in approximately 90% of cases and shows a strong and generally diffuse staining pattern.[43] Of note, the immunostain profile depends on the location and the large duct versus small duct pattern of growth. This has been best documented for CK7 and CK20, where peripheral cholangiocarcinomas are CK7 positive but CK20 negative, while perihilar tumors tend to be both CK7 positive and CK20 positive.[44] CD56 is also more likely to be

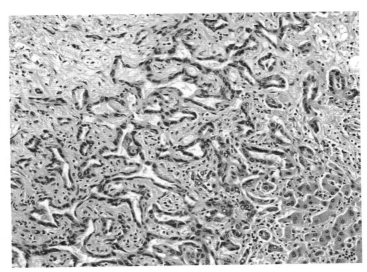

FIGURE 22.30 **Cholangiocarcinoma, bile duct plate malformation-like pattern.** This tumor's growth pattern shows interanastomosing duct-like structures with open lumens. The center of the lesion (upper left corner of image) shows dense fibrosis.

TABLE 22.3	Immunostains and Cholangiocarcinoma
Stains	**Comment**
CK7	90%
CK19	80%-90%
MOC31	80%-90%
Albumin in situ hybridization	50%-90%. 90% small duct; 50% large duct
CK20	Patchy; about 50% of large duct; less common in small duct
CDX2	30%; more common in large duct
SATB2	5%
GATA3	10%. Usually in poorly differentiated tumors or in large duct pattern
ER	Rare
TTF1	30%, mostly extrahepatic and some large duct
Napsin	10%, mostly extrahepatic and some large duct
PAX8	Rare
Arginase 1	1%-5%, focal; usually in small duct
HepPar1	10%, focal; usually in small duct
Glypican 3	1%-5%, focal

These numbers are mid-range of the numbers reported in the literature, but there is a lot of variability between studies.

positive in small duct cholangiocarcinomas, especially if they have a cholangiolocellular pattern.[45] Likewise, focal HepPar1 staining is more commonly seen in peripherally located cholangiocarcinomas, and should not be called combined hepatocellular carcinoma-cholangiocarcinoma. Albumin in situ hybridization is positive in about 90% of cases with a small duct growth pattern (Figure 22.31),[46] although there is considerably lower frequencies of about 50% in the large duct pattern.[47] This stain does not separate a cholangiocarcinoma from a hepatocellular carcinoma, but can be diagnostically useful when the tumor is definitely an adenocarcinoma and staining is reasonably strong and more than minimal; this pattern is cholangiocarcinoma in the vast majority of cases. In addition, tumors with a cholangiolocarcinoma growth pattern or a ductal plate-like malformation pattern can be confirmed as cholangiocarcinomas by their strong and diffuse albumin in situ hybridization staining pattern. Focal staining is less specific and can be seen occasionally with metastatic tumors, especially adenocarcinomas from the lung and upper gastrointestinal (GI) tract. Strong and more diffuse staining can also be seen in about one-third of acinar cell carcinomas of the pancreas.[48]

Differentiating Benign Biliary Lesions From Cholangiocarcinoma

In some cases, sections show a low-grade biliary tumor and the differential is between a benign tumor (von Meyenburg complex, bile duct adenoma) and a well-differentiated cholangiocarcinoma. In these cases, a good approach is to evaluate at low power for architecture, high power for cytology and then to supplement the hematoxylin and eosin (H&E) findings

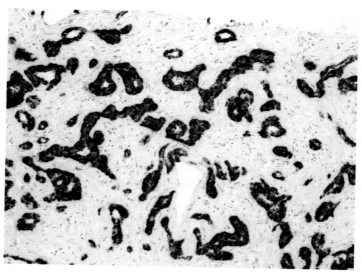

FIGURE 22.31 **Cholangiocarcinoma, albumin** in situ **hybridization.** The tumor cells are strongly positive.

with immunostains. At low power, benign lesions have well-circumscribed growth patterns without tissue destruction and generally without any peritumoral mass effect. The edges of many benign lesions can be a bit irregular, so "tissue invasion" is often a hard feature to assess. In fact, if there is obvious invasion into the adjacent liver parenchyma, then the lesion is typically not low grade. Nonetheless, evaluation of the edges of the lesion is important, looking for irregularly invading tumor cells, either as small nests or less often as single cells. The cytology of the tissue-invasive foci is often subtly but noticeably different than the rest of the tumor; for example, there may be more prominent nucleoli or greater degrees of nuclear hyperchromasia. General cytology findings that help differentiate a benign from a malignant tumor include significant cytological atypia, often manifesting as noticeable nuclear size variability within a single gland and/or between glands. Striking gland-to-gland size variability is not always present in low-grade cholangiocarcinomas but is essentially never seen in bile duct adenomas. Tumor necrosis or dirty luminal necrosis also favors malignancy. Mitotic figures in benign lesions are very rare and never atypical. Immunostains are also helpful, as cholangiocarcinomas typically show an increased Ki-67 proliferative rate of >10%, while most benign lesions are typically closer to 1%.[7-9] Positive staining for S100P (eFig. 22.14) or p53 is also helpful; p53 can show either a strong and diffuse staining pattern or a null phenotype in cholangiocarcinomas. Repeating the p53 for confirmation is useful for the null phenotype. In these difficult low-grade tumors, the best diagnosis requires assessment of all of these features, as an excellent diagnosis rarely rests comfortably on a single, isolated finding.

Differentiating Cholangiocarcinoma From Hepatocellular Carcinoma

The scirrhous pattern of hepatocellular carcinoma can mimic a cholangiocarcinoma, while solid growth patterns of cholangiocarcinoma can mimic hepatocellular carcinoma. At the morphological level, finding fat or Mallory hyaline in a scirrhous-type tumor strongly favors a hepatocellular carcinoma (many scirrhous hepatocellular carcinomas appear to result from progression of steatohepatitic hepatocellular carcinomas and can show residual focal fat or Mallory hyaline). Strong and diffuse staining for MOC31, with absence of staining for hepatocellular markers, favors a cholangiocarcinoma. In terms of markers of hepatocellular differentiation, most cholangiocarcinomas lack expression for HepPar1, arginase, and glypican 3. Of note, HepPar1 is positive in only about 50% of scirrhous hepatocellular carcinomas,[49] so a panel of stains for hepatocellular differentiation is the best approach.

Many cholangiocarcinomas with a solid pattern of growth will still have some gland formation or mucin production, albeit often focal and usually best found at the tumor periphery. Mucicarmine is useful for identifying focal or subtle mucin production. Strong and diffuse staining for MOC31 and CK19 favors a cholangiocarcinoma while strong staining, even if patchy, for HepPar1, arginase, or glypican 3 will favor a hepatocellular carcinoma. Strong and diffuse CK7 positivity is also more common in cholangiocarcinomas, but there is significant overlap in staining in biopsy specimens. In these difficult cases, the use of common sense and a panel approach is recommended, as aberrant staining for any single stain is not uncommon.

Differentiating Cholangiocarcinoma From Metastatic Carcinoma

The gland size and gland morphology are generally not diagnostically useful for separating cholangiocarcinomas from metastatic adenocarcinomas. Areas of trabecular growth are more common in cholangiocarcinoma but are not specific. Likewise, the presence of dense fibrosis is more typical of cholangiocarcinomas than metastatic disease but is not specific.

Immunostain findings are very helpful. The classic immunostain pattern for cholangiocarcinoma is as follows: CK7 positive, CK20 negative or patchy positive, CDX2 negative or positive patchy, MOC31 strong and diffusely positive, and albumin in situ hybridization positive (for small duct pattern in particular). For cases where albumin in situ hybridization is negative or not available, the differential for this CK7/CK20/CDX2 immunostain prolife expands to include adenocarcinomas of the upper GI tract, pancreatic ductal adenocarcinomas, and extrahepatic bile duct adenocarcinomas. Based on the morphology and clinical history, other stains are useful and important for excluding common origins of metastatic disease, including TTF1, NKX3.1, ER, etc. One important diagnostic pitfall is that hilar cholangiocarcinomas and gallbladder adenocarcinomas can be TTF1/napsin positive.[50] After a full histological work-up that shows findings compatible with cholangiocarcinoma, the "final" diagnosis is finally secured when imaging does not identify another primary.

LYMPHOEPITHELIOMA-LIKE CHOLANGIOCARCINOMA

Definition

Lymphoepithelioma-like cholangiocarcinomas are tumors with irregular sheets of poorly defined epithelial cells embedded in an intense lymphocytic infiltrate. A partial synonym is *lymphoepithelioma-like carcinoma*, but note that some of the literature includes both hepatocellular carcinomas and cholangiocarcinomas under this same entity, a practice that does not seem to be very useful for understanding the biology of these tumors, or for patient care.

Clinical Findings

These tumors are very rare (less than 1%) but appear to be more common in Asia compared to the other parts of the world. The prognosis is not completely settled because they are so rare, but they seem to have a better prognosis.

Histological Findings

The tumors show attenuated glandular structures and poorly defined sheets of epithelial cells embedded in a background of intense lymphocytosis (Figure 22.32). In parts of the tumor, especially in resection specimens, there can be areas of more typical cholangiocarcinoma away from the lymphoepithelioma-like morphology. On biopsies you may not see the more typical areas of cholangiocarcinoma, but you can still recognize this tumor by its striking lymphocytosis and poorly formed epithelial and glandular structures. In other cases, a cholangiocarcinoma may be well-to-moderately differentiated, but have striking lymphocytosis (Figure 22.33). The tumors in both settings are cytokeratin positive (CK7 and CK19) and HepPar1 and arginase negative. In situ hybridization for Epstein-Barr virus is strongly positive in the tumor epithelial cells (Figure 22.34).

CHOLANGIOBLASTIC VARIANT OF CHOLANGIOCARCINOMA

The *cholangioblastic variant of cholangiocarcinoma* is a recently described variant of cholangiocarcinoma that tends to affect younger-aged persons (average age about 40) who lack underlying chronic liver disease,[51] with a caveat that very few cases have been reported to date.

Histologically, the tumor shows a wide range of morphology, including areas that are solid, microcystic, trabecular, and blastemal like (Figure 22.35).

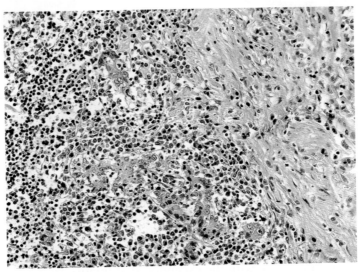

FIGURE 22.32 **Lymphoepithelioma-like cholangiocarcinoma.** The tumor is composed of scant irregular epithelial structures in the background of intense chronic inflammation.

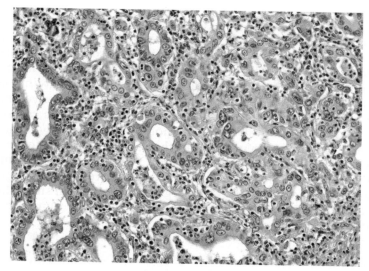

FIGURE 22.33 **Lymphocyte-rich cholangiocarcinoma.** This image shows a gland-forming cholangiocarcinoma that is accompanied by intense lymphocytosis.

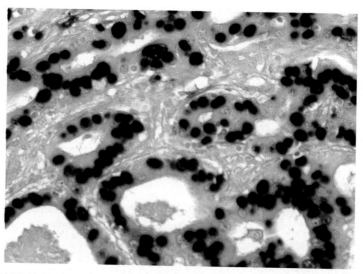

FIGURE 22.34 **Lymphocyte-rich cholangiocarcinoma.** In situ hybridization for Epstein-Barr virus (EBV) is strongly positive in the tumor cells (same case as preceding image).

The cholangioblastic variant of cholangiocarcinoma stains like a typical cholangiocarcinoma, with the exception that tumors are synaptophysin and chromogranin positive, and all cases to date are inhibin positive. Recently, a *NIPBL-NACC1* fusion has been identified and appears to be characteristic of the cholangioblastic variant of cholangiocarcinoma.

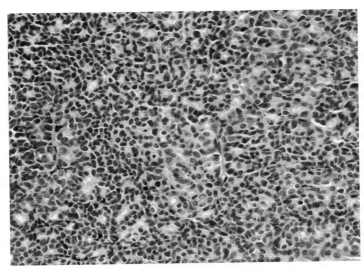

FIGURE 22.35 **Cholangioblastic variant of cholangiocarcinoma.** An area of blastemal-type growth is seen, with small primitive-looking cells that form gland-like structures.

REFERENCES

1. Allaire GS, Rabin L, Ishak KG, et al. Bile duct adenoma. A study of 152 cases. *Am J Surg Pathol.* 1988;12:708-715.
2. Arena V, Arena E, Stigliano E, et al. Bile duct adenoma with oncocytic features. *Histopathology.* 2006;49:318-320.
3. Johannesen EJ, Wu Z, Holly JS. Bile duct adenoma with oncocytic features. *Case Rep Pathol.* 2014;2014:282010.
4. Angkathunyakul N, Rosini F, Heaton N, et al. BRAF V600E mutation in biliary proliferations associated with alpha1 -antitrypsin deficiency. *Histopathology.* 2017;70:485-491.
5. Pujals A, Bioulac-Sage P, Castain C, et al. BRAF V600E mutational status in bile duct adenomas and hamartomas. *Histopathology.* 2015;67:562-567.
6. Albores-Saavedra J, Hoang MP, Murakata LA, et al. Atypical bile duct adenoma, clear cell type: a previously undescribed tumor of the liver. *Am J Surg Pathol.* 2001;25:956-960.
7. Tsokos CG, Krings G, Yilmaz F, et al. Proliferative index facilitates distinction between benign biliary lesions and intrahepatic cholangiocarcinoma. *Hum Pathol.* 2016;57:61-67.
8. Tan G, Yilmaz A, De Young BR, et al. Immunohistochemical analysis of biliary tract lesions. *Appl Immunohistochem Mol Morphol.* 2004;12:193-197.
9. Bertram S, Padden J, Kalsch J, et al. Novel immunohistochemical markers differentiate intrahepatic cholangiocarcinoma from benign bile duct lesions. *J Clin Pathol.* 2016;69:619-626.
10. Hughes NR, Goodman ZD, Bhathal PS. An immunohistochemical profile of the so-called bile duct adenoma: clues to pathogenesis. *Am J Surg Pathol.* 2010;34:1312-1318.
11. Moy AP, Arora K, Deshpande V. Albumin expression distinguishes bile duct adenomas from metastatic adenocarcinoma. *Histopathology.* 2016;69:423-430.
12. Tsui WM, Loo KT, Chow LT, et al. Biliary adenofibroma. A heretofore unrecognized benign biliary tumor of the liver. *Am J Surg Pathol.* 1993;17:186-192.
13. Gurrera A, Alaggio R, Leone G, et al. Biliary adenofibroma of the liver: report of a case and review of the literature. *Patholog Res Int.* 2010;2010:504584.

14. Varnholt H, Vauthey JN, Dal Cin P, et al. Biliary adenofibroma: a rare neoplasm of bile duct origin with an indolent behavior. *Am J Surg Pathol.* 2003;27:693-698.

15. Sturm AK, Welsch T, Meissner C, et al. A case of biliary adenofibroma of the liver with malignant transformation: a morphomolecular case report and review of the literature. *Surg Case Rep.* 2019;5:104.

16. Nakanuma Y, Kurumaya H, Ohta G. Multiple cysts in the hepatic hilum and their pathogenesis. A suggestion of periductal gland origin. *Virchows Arch A Pathol Anat Histopathol.* 1984;404:341-350.

17. Pedica F, Heaton N, Quaglia A. Peribiliary glands pathology in a large series of end-stage alcohol-related liver disease. *Virchows Arch.* 2020;477(6):817-823.

18. Torbenson MS. Hamartomas and malformations of the liver. *Semin Diagn Pathol.* 2019;36:39-47.

19. Sharma S, Dean AG, Corn A, et al. Ciliated hepatic foregut cyst: an increasingly diagnosed condition. *Hepatobiliary Pancreat Dis Int.* 2008;7:581-589.

20. Khoddami M, Kazemi Aghdam M, Alvandimanesh A. Ciliated hepatic foregut cyst: two case reports in children and review of the literature. *Case Rep Med.* 2013;2013:372017.

21. de Lajarte-Thirouard AS, Rioux-Leclercq N, Boudjema K, et al. Squamous cell carcinoma arising in a hepatic forgut cyst. *Pathol Res Pract.* 2002;198:697-700.

22. Vick DJ, Goodman ZD, Ishak KG. Squamous cell carcinoma arising in a ciliated hepatic foregut cyst. *Arch Pathol Lab Med.* 1999;123:1115-1117.

23. Quigley B, Reid MD, Pehlivanoglu B, et al. Hepatobiliary mucinous cystic neoplasms with ovarian type stroma (so-called "hepatobiliary cystadenoma/cystadenocarcinoma"): clinicopathologic analysis of 36 cases illustrates rarity of carcinomatous change. *Am J Surg Pathol.* 2018;42:95-102.

24. Zen Y, Pedica F, Patcha VR, et al. Mucinous cystic neoplasms of the liver: a clinicopathological study and comparison with intraductal papillary neoplasms of the bile duct. *Mod Pathol.* 2011;24:1079-1089.

25. Lam MM, Swanson PE, Upton MP, et al. Ovarian-type stroma in hepatobiliary cystadenomas and pancreatic mucinous cystic neoplasms: an immunohistochemical study. *Am J Clin Pathol.* 2008;129:211-218.

26. Li T, Ji Y, Zhi XT, et al. A comparison of hepatic mucinous cystic neoplasms with biliary intraductal papillary neoplasms. *Clin Gastroenterol Hepatol.* 2009;7:586-593.

27. Hsu M, Terris B, Wu TT, et al. Endometrial cysts within the liver: a rare entity and its differential diagnosis with mucinous cystic neoplasms of the liver. *Hum Pathol.* 2014;45:761-767.

28. Mano Y, Aishima S, Fujita N, et al. Cystic tumors of the liver: on the problems of diagnostic criteria. *Pathol Res Pract.* 2011;207:659-663.

29. Shyu S, Singhi AD. Cystic biliary tumors of the liver: diagnostic criteria and common pitfalls. *Hum Pathol.* 2021;112:70-83.

30. Nakanuma Y, Uesaka K, Okamura Y, et al. Reappraisal of pathological features of intraductal papillary neoplasm of bile duct with respect to the type 1 and 2 subclassifications. *Hum Pathol.* 2021;111:21-35.

31. Singhi AD, Wood LD, Parks E, et al. Recurrent rearrangements in PRKACA and PRKACB in intraductal oncocytic papillary neoplasms of the pancreas and bile duct. *Gastroenterology.* 2020;158:573.e2-582.e2.

32. Honeyman JN, Simon EP, Robine N, et al. Detection of a recurrent DNAJB1-PRKACA chimeric transcript in fibrolamellar hepatocellular carcinoma. *Science.* 2014;343:1010-1014.

33. Akita M, Hong SM, Sung YN, et al. Biliary intraductal tubule-forming neoplasm: a whole exome sequencing study of MUC5AC-positive and -negative cases. *Histopathology.* 2020;76:1005-1012.

34. Wildgruber M, Rummeny EJ, Gaa J. Primary acinar cell carcinoma of the liver. *Rofo*. 2013;185:572-573.

35. Agaimy A, Kaiser A, Becker K, et al. Pancreatic-type acinar cell carcinoma of the liver: a clinicopathologic study of four patients. *Mod Pathol*. 2011;24:1620-1626.

36. Thai E, Dalla Valle R, Silini EM. Primary solid papillary tumor of the liver. *Pathol Res Pract*. 2012;208:250-253.

37. Kim YI, Kim ST, Lee GK, et al. Papillary cystic tumor of the liver. A case report with ultrastructural observation. *Cancer*. 1990;65:2740-2746.

38. Palmer WC, Patel T. Are common factors involved in the pathogenesis of primary liver cancers? A meta-analysis of risk factors for intrahepatic cholangiocarcinoma. *J Hepatol*. 2012;57:69-76.

39. Torbenson M, Yeh MM, Abraham SC. Bile duct dysplasia in the setting of chronic hepatitis C and alcohol cirrhosis. *Am J Surg Pathol*. 2007;31:1410-1413.

40. Akita M, Sawada R, Komatsu M, et al. An immunostaining panel of C-reactive protein, N-cadherin, and S100 calcium binding protein P is useful for intrahepatic cholangiocarcinoma subtyping. *Hum Pathol*. 2021;109:45-52.

41. Steiner PE, Higginson J. Cholangiolocellular carcinoma of the liver. *Cancer*. 1959;12:753-759.

42. Nakanuma Y, Sato Y, Ikeda H, et al. Intrahepatic cholangiocarcinoma with predominant "ductal plate malformation" pattern: a new subtype. *Am J Surg Pathol*. 2012;36:1629-1635.

43. Chan ES, Yeh MM. The use of immunohistochemistry in liver tumors. *Clin Liver Dis*. 2010;14:687-703.

44. Rullier A, Le Bail B, Fawaz R, et al. Cytokeratin 7 and 20 expression in cholangiocarcinomas varies along the biliary tract but still differs from that in colorectal carcinoma metastasis. *Am J Surg Pathol*. 2000;24:870-876.

45. Kozaka K, Sasaki M, Fujii T, et al. A subgroup of intrahepatic cholangiocarcinoma with an infiltrating replacement growth pattern and a resemblance to reactive proliferating bile ductules: 'bile ductular carcinoma'. *Histopathology*. 2007;51:390-400.

46. Ferrone CR, Ting DT, Shahid M, et al. The ability to diagnose intrahepatic cholangiocarcinoma definitively using novel branched DNA-enhanced albumin RNA in situ hybridization technology. *Ann Surg Oncol*. 2016;23:290-296.

47. Avadhani V, Cohen C, Siddiqui MT, et al. A subset of intrahepatic cholangiocarcinomas express albumin RNA as detected by in situ hybridization. *Appl Immunohistochem Mol Morphol*. 2021;29:175-179.

48. Shahid M, Mubeen A, Tse J, et al. Branched chain in situ hybridization for albumin as a marker of hepatocellular differentiation: evaluation of manual and automated in situ hybridization platforms. *Am J Surg Pathol*. 2015;39:25-34.

49. Krings G, Ramachandran R, Jain D, et al. Immunohistochemical pitfalls and the importance of glypican 3 and arginase in the diagnosis of scirrhous hepatocellular carcinoma. *Mod Pathol*. 2013;26:782-791.

50. Surrey LF, Frank R, Zhang PJ, et al. TTF-1 and Napsin-A are expressed in a subset of cholangiocarcinomas arising from the gallbladder and hepatic ducts: continued caveats for utilization of immunohistochemistry panels. *Am J Surg Pathol*. 2014;38:224-227.

51. Braxton DR, Saxe D, Damjanov N, et al. Molecular and cytogenomic profiling of hepatic adenocarcinoma expressing inhibinA, a mimicker of neuroendocrine tumors: proposal to reclassify as "cholangioblastic variant of intrahepatic cholangiocarcinoma." *Hum Pathol*. 2017;62:232-241.

52. Argani P, Palsgrove DN, Anders RA, et al. A novel NIPBL-NACC1 gene fusion is characteristic of the cholangioblastic variant of intrahepatic cholangiocarcinoma. *Am J Surg Pathol*. 2021. doi:10.1097/PAS.0000000000001729.

23

LYMPHOMA AND METASTATIC DISEASE

REACTIVE LYMPHOID HYPERPLASIA

Reactive lymphoid hyperplasia is a mass-forming lesion composed of a well-circumscribed nodule of reactive lymphoid follicles. Other terms in the literature include *pseudolymphoma* and *nodular lymphoid lesion*, but *reactive lymphoid hyperplasia* is preferred.

Reactive lymphoid hyperplasia results from a localized immunological response to various types of antigens, such as infections, neoplasms, or autoimmune antigens. Many patients have immune dysfunction, such as common variable immune deficiency (CVID), or autoimmune diseases, such as autoimmune hepatitis or primary biliary cirrhosis/cholangitis.

Overall, reactive lymphoid hyperplasia is very rare. The average age at presentation is approximately 55 years, but the range is wide and can include teenaged patients. There is an 8 to 1 female predominance.[1] Patients usually present with an incidentally discovered mass lesion. The lesion(s) can be single (80%) or multiple (20%). Most are 1 to 2 cm in greatest dimension, but some reported cases have reached 10 cm.[2]

Reactive lymphoid hyperplasia is composed of a well-circumscribed cluster of lymphoid follicles (Figure 23.1). The follicles are reactive and retain normal organization, with polarized germinal centers surrounded by reactive mantles. The germinal centers show a mixture of centroblasts, centrocytes, and tingible-body macrophages. The follicles do not have the back-to-back arrangement seen in follicular lymphoma and are nondestructive to the adjacent liver, although there can be reactive bile ductules and compressed fibrous tissue at the interface. The follicles are nonclonal by polymerase chain reaction (PCR) studies.

LYMPHOMA AND LEUKEMIA

Lymphoma Overview

Most lymphomas involving the liver represent spread from other sites of origin, and essentially any lymphoma can involve the liver at some point.

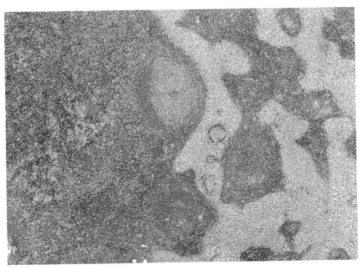

FIGURE 23.1   **Reactive lymphoid hyperplasia.** A wedge biopsy shows a well-circumscribed cluster of reactive lymphoid follicles.

Primary lymphomas of the liver are rare and are most commonly seen in men (approximately gender ratio 2:1), with an average age of 61 years at first diagnosis.[3] The etiology is unknown in most cases, although a link with chronic hepatitis C and B infection has been identified; other risk factors include human immunodeficiency infection (HIV) or other forms of chronic immunosuppression.[4,5] Primary liver lymphomas are typically non-Hodgkin, B-cell lymphomas. The most common type is diffuse large B-cell lymphoma (about 75% of cases), followed by marginal zone lymphoma (20%),[4-7] and Burkett lymphoma (5%)[4,6]; the remaining types of B-cell lymphomas each contribute 1% or less. Hepatosplenic T-cell lymphomas are the most common T-cell lymphoma.

While there is a lot of overlap, different types of B-cell lymphomas have some general histological patterns when they involve the liver (Table 23.1).[8,9] Lymphomas that are mass-forming are most commonly diffuse large B-cell lymphomas. Most non–mass-forming lymphomas are portal based. Important histological clues to a possible lymphoma include lymphoid aggregates that diffusely involve portal tracts (in reactive conditions, lymphoid aggregates tend to be focal or sparse), unusually large lymphoid aggregates in any portal tract (Figure 23.2), or portal lymphocytes with cytological monotony or cytological atypia. For cases with a sinusoidal predominant pattern of growth, diagnostic clues include lymphocytes that have too much cytoplasm or that show definite cytological atypia (Figure 23.3). Unusually, dense sinusoidal lymphocytic infiltrates can also suggest lymphoma, as can atypical patterns of lobular necrosis.

The diagnosis of lymphoma is made following usual criteria, which for space constraints are not reviewed here. For most lymphomas that present with a mass lesion, the atypical lymphoid infiltrates will suggest the

TABLE 23.1	Patterns of Lymphoma in the Liver
Predominant Growth Pattern	Lymphoma
Mass lesion	Diffuse large B-cell lymphoma
	Burkitt lymphoma
	Anaplastic large cell lymphoma
Portal Tract	Marginal zone lymphoma
	Follicular lymphoma
	Mantle cell lymphoma
	Hodgkin
	T-cell–rich B-cell lymphoma
	CLL/SLL
Sinusoidal	Hepatosplenic T-cell lymphoma
	Hairy cell and other leukemia
	Peripheral T-cell lymphoma

CLL, chronic lymphocytic leukemia; SLL, small lymphocytic lymphoma.

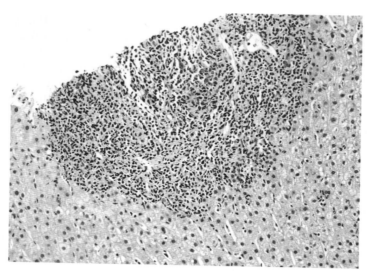

FIGURE 23.2 **Enlarged portal tract, follicular lymphoma.** The portal tract is greatly enlarged by the lymphocytic infiltrate.

correct diagnosis. In some cases, however, especially on biopsies, the cells may appear epithelioid and mimic a carcinoma. Mass-forming B-cell lymphomas often have entrapped hepatocytes, so HepPar1 and keratin stains should be carefully interpreted in association with the hematoxylin and eosin (H&E) findings to lead to the correct diagnosis.

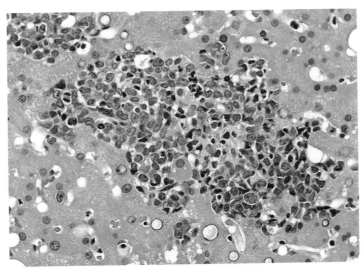

FIGURE 23.3 **Cytological atypia.** The malignant lymphocytes show significant cytological atypia in this case of diffuse large B-cell lymphoma.

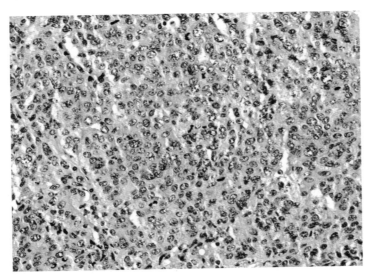

FIGURE 23.4 **Diffuse large B-cell of liver.** In this case, the lymphoma presented as a mass in the liver.

DIFFUSE LARGE B-CELL LYMPHOMAS. Diffuse large B-cell lymphoma is usually a mass-forming tumor and shows sheets of large, loosely cohesive, atypical lymphocytes (Figure 23.4).[10] The lymphocytes may have moderate amounts of eosinophilic-to-amphophilic cytoplasm and mimic a carcinoma on H&E. The lymphoma can also be p63 positive, another diagnostic pitfall (eFig. 23.1).

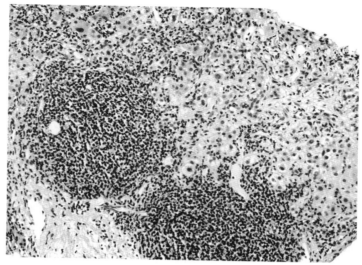

FIGURE 23.5 **Mucosa-associated lymphoid tissue (MALT) lymphoma**. This extranodal marginal zone lymphoma (MALT lymphoma) was primary to the breast but spread to the liver. The portal tracts show a monotonous B-cell nodular infiltrate.

MUCOSA-ASSOCIATED LYMPHOID TISSUE (MALT) LYMPHOMAS. MALT lymphomas can be mass-forming or non–mass-forming lesions. When they do form a mass, they are typically solitary and can be large. In cases that are not mass-forming, or at the edges of mass-forming lesions, the lymphoma shows a distinctly portal-based pattern, where the portal tracts show nodular infiltrates of small-sized lymphocytes (Figure 23.5; eFigs. 23.2-23.5), with occasional germinal centers. MALT lymphoma involves the lobules to a lesser degree. Lymphoma cells can also involve the bile duct, leading to lymphoepithelial lesions similar to those seen in MALT lymphomas of the stomach.

HODGKIN DISEASE. Hodgkin disease typically shows a nodular infiltrate in the liver, involving both the portal tracts and the lobules (Figure 23.6). The nodules are often fibrotic and show mixed inflammation, including lymphocytes, plasma cells, and eosinophils. The nodules can vary in size from small portal-based nodules to large aggregates that fill several low-power microscope fields. Plasma cells can be prominent and the findings can mimic an inflammatory pseudotumor. Other cases can mimic hepatic parenchymal collapse. Reed-Sternberg cells and variants are helpful when present (Figure 23.7).

HEPATOSPLENIC T-CELL LYMPHOMAS. This lymphoma shows a male predominance and affects younger-aged persons, with a median age of 35 years at diagnosis. About 20% of patients have chronic immunosuppression from various causes.[11] Most patients present with hepatosplenomegaly but lack lymphadenopathy or systemic symptoms. Abnormalities in the peripheral

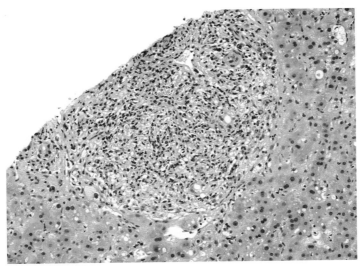

FIGURE 23.6 **Hodgkin disease involving the liver.** A nodular portal infiltrate is seen with mixed cells, including mildly prominent plasma cells.

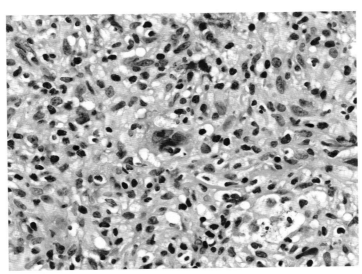

FIGURE 23.7 **Hodgkin disease involving the liver.** Reed-Sternberg cells and variants are helpful clues to the diagnosis when present.

blood, however, are common, including anemia, leukopenia, and thrombocytopenia. These lymphomas show differentiation toward cytotoxic T-cells, usually with γδ T-cell receptor clonality,[12] but a minority of them are of the αβ T-cell receptor (TCR) type.[13]

Histologically, hepatosplenic T-cell lymphomas manifest as atypical lymphoid cells infiltrating the sinusoids, with absent or mild portal tract involvement. Depending on the case, the histological findings can be very subtle and mistaken for a lobular hepatitis. One clue can be the relatively small amount of lobular injury for the degree of sinusoidal infiltrates. The sinusoidal infiltrates are moderate in cellularity and can be somewhat patchy, sometimes mistaken for Kupffer cell hyperplasia. The individual cells tend to have abundant, eosinophilic-to-pale cytoplasm (Figure 23.8). They also have larger and more irregular nuclei than typical lymphocytes, although overall atypia tends to be mild. On immunostain, the lymphoma cells are positive for T-cell markers CD2, CD3, and CD7 but not for CD4, CD5, or CD8. The tumor cells are also positive for TIA-1 but negative for granzyme B.[14,15]

Leukemia Overview

When leukemias involve the liver, they typically lead to diffuse hepato-megaly without causing significant hepatic dysfunction. In most cases, the patient's diagnosis of leukemia is known beforehand and the biopsy is per-formed for some other reason. The biopsy will show infiltrates of imma-ture cells or blasts. In general, myeloid leukemia preferentially involves the sinusoids, while lymphoid leukemia preferentially involves the portal tracts, but a lot of cases do not follow these patterns very well (Figure 23.9).[16] The B-lymphoblasts will be positive for CD34, terminal deoxynu-cleotidyl transferase (TdT), and HLA-DR. T-lymphoblasts are positive for TdT, CD2 and CD3 positive. Myeloblasts are positive for CD34, HLA-DR, myeloperoxidase, CKIT, and TdT (often focal, weak).

In those rare cases where the type of leukemia is not already known, immunostains can be performed to subclassify the leukemia. In general,

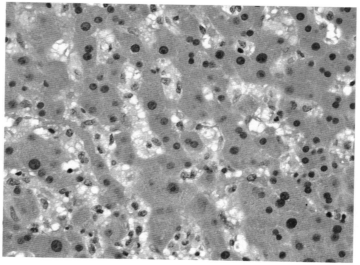

FIGURE 23.8 **Hepatosplenic T-cell lymphoma.** The sinusoids show increased cellularity. The tumor cells have abundant lightly eosinophilic cytoplasm.

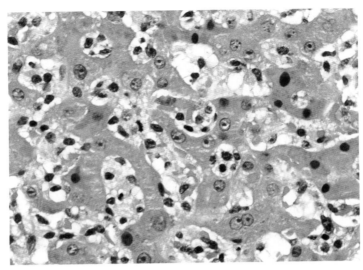

FIGURE 23.9 **Acute lymphoid leukemia, NK-cell type.** The sinusoids are filled with atypical cells.

immunostains should be used as a panel, since aberrant expression, or lack of expression, is common.

HAIRY CELL LEUKEMIA. This leukemia is indolent and mostly affects middle-aged and older men. Hairy cell leukemia is composed of mature B-cells that are small-to-medium sized and have pale cytoplasm, with oval nuclei and inconspicuous nucleoli (Figure 23.10). The tumor cells show predominately a sinusoidal growth pattern but involve the portal tracts to a lesser degree. The classic "fried egg" appearance of tumor cells that is seen in other organs is generally hard to see in liver specimens, although it can be present in the portal infiltrates. In addition to the typical sinusoidal growth pattern, hairy cell leukemia can lead to peliotic-like changes, where pools of red blood cells are lined by neoplastic cells.[17-19]

The leukemia cells are positive for pan-B-cell markers (eg, CD19, CD20, CD79a, PAX-5) and for CD103 (Figure 23.11), CD25, CD11c, and tartrate-resistant acid phosphatase. The tumor cells also have *BRAF* V600E mutations, which can be detected using immunostains or by molecular methods.[20]

FOLLICULAR DENDRITIC CELL SARCOMA

Follicular dendritic cell sarcomas have a strong female predominance and most of the reported cases in the liver come from Asia. They form mass lesions composed of spindled-to-ovoid cells with admixed lymphoplasmacytic inflammation (Figure 23.12). In most cases, they are within the differential diagnosis of an inflammatory pseudotumor. Rare cases can be more

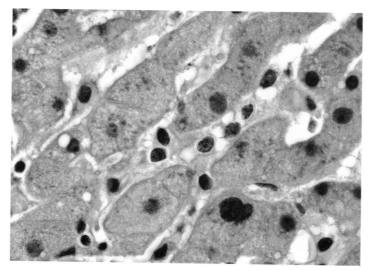

FIGURE 23.10 **Hairy cell leukemia.** The sinusoids contain a subtle infiltrate of atypical cells.

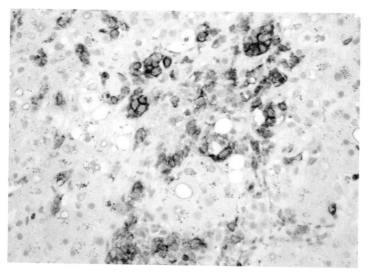

FIGURE 23.11 **Hairy cell leukemia, CD103.** The tumor cells are highlighted.

cellular and lack the distinct inflammatory component. The spindled cells grow in sheets, whorls, or less commonly have a storiform pattern. Foci of multinucleated spindle cells may be seen. The tumor cells are positive for markers of follicular differentiation: CD21, CD23, and CD35. They are also positive for Epstein-Barr encoding region (EBER) and/or Epstein-Barr virus latent membrane protein (EBV LMP).

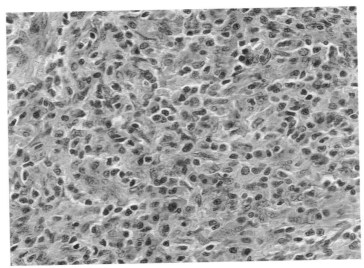

FIGURE 23.12 **Follicular dendritic cell sarcoma.** The tumor cells are ovoid and with admixed lymphoplasmacytic inflammation.

METASTATIC NEOPLASMS

Metastatic disease can involve both cirrhotic and noncirrhotic livers. In cases of liver cirrhosis, metastases are enriched for tumors arising within the gastrointestinal (GI) tract and pancreas. Metastatic neoplasms to the liver are commonly biopsied to identify the site of origin or to obtain tissue for molecular testing. If the tumor is biopsied for the latter purpose, your job is to make sure the morphology is consistent with the clinical diagnosis and then to preserve the tissue for molecular studies; immunostains are only needed for diagnostic purposes if the morphology suggests a different diagnosis.

Most metastatic tumors are mass-forming lesions. Rarely, tumors show an infiltrative pattern and grow largely in the sinusoids (Figure 23.13); this latter pattern is most commonly seen with breast carcinoma, pancreas carcinoma, and melanoma.

There are many different ways to approach the work-up for tumors of unknown site of origin. Regardless of the approach used, it should be systematic and the immunostains should be used in tandem with the H&E findings, that is, do not ignore the H&E findings and rely on a battery or algorithm of immunostains alone. As an illustration, there have been many cases over the years, both submitted as consults as well as internal cases, where either a positive or negative stain was at odds with the H&E findings. Many times, in particular with negative stains, repeat staining demonstrated that the first stain result was a technical error. In addition, remember that a panel of stains that works best in one hospital may be different than the one that work best in another hospital, based on what

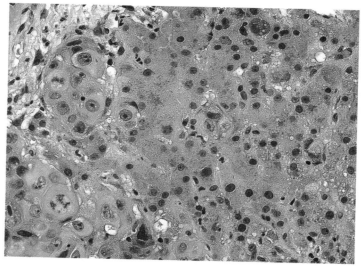

FIGURE 23.13 **Metastatic pancreas adenocarcinoma.** The carcinoma is growing in the sinusoids.

immunostains are available, their quality, and a pathologist's overall familiarity with a particular stain.

Diagnostic Approach

One reasonable systematic approach to establishing a diagnosis is illustrated below and can easily be modified to fit the needs of specific cases.

FIRST, are there any clinical or imaging clues to the primary site? For example, is there diffuse thickening of the stomach wall on imaging studies, or a history of breast carcinoma? If so, the clinical/imaging findings can be combined with the H&E morphological findings to choose the first round of stains.

SECOND, is the tumor a carcinoma? Here, the morphology can usually answer this question, but in difficult cases, immunostains are important. A useful panel includes multiple keratins as well as a broad panel of other stains to determine cell lineage (Table 23.2). Importantly, when a tumor is poorly differentiated, a broad screen for epithelial differentiation is often necessary. A single pankeratin stain is insufficient for this purpose. Vascular stains are also important, as both angiosarcomas and epithelioid hemangioendotheliomas can show aberrant expression of keratins (Figure 23.14). Another recurrent diagnostic pitfall for noncarcinomas is this: a subset of melanomas is strongly CKIT positive.

THIRD, if the tumor is a carcinoma, does it show features to suggest hepatocellular carcinoma? Immunostains can be used to confirm or exclude

TABLE 23.2	**Examples of Useful Panels of Stains**
Situation	Stains
Establish lineage[a]	Keratins: pankeratins such as Oscar; CKAE1/AE3, CAM 5.2, CK5/6
	Lymphoma: CD3, CD20
	Melanoma: S100, SOX10
	Sarcoma: CKIT, DOG1, desmin, myogenin, others based on morphology
Hepatocellular carcinoma vs benign hepatic tumors	Reticulin
	Ki-67 (compare to background liver)
	Glypican 3
Hepatocellular carcinoma vs metastatic disease	HePar1
	Arginase 1
	Glypican 3
	ALB-ISH
Definite adenocarcinoma on morphology	Mucicarmine can confirm glandular mucin
	ALB-ISH staining favors cholangiocarcinoma
	CK7/CK20 can help suggest broad differential
	Organ markers such as CDX2, Napsin, etc
	Adenocarcinomas that are CK7 +/CK20 focal or negative/CDX2 positive or negative; also negative for all other organ markers have this differential: upper GI tract, pancreas, biliary
Carcinoma, but not hepatocellular carcinoma and not adenocarcinoma	CK7/CK20 can help suggest broad differential
	Synaptophysin/chromogranin
	SF1 for adrenal cortical
	p40 for squamous differentiation
	Trypsin for acinar cell carcinoma

ALB-ISH, albumin in situ hybridization; GI, gastrointestinal.
[a]A broad panel is important because aberrant staining of keratins in sarcoma is not uncommon.

hepatocellular differentiation (Table 23.2). In many poorly differentiated hepatocellular carcinomas, the positive staining for any given marker can be focal or patchy, and some stains for hepatocellular differentiation may be negative, so a broad panel is important. Both polyclonal carcinoembryonic

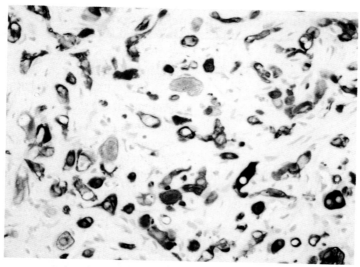

FIGURE 23.14 **Epithelioid hemangioendothelioma, CK7.** The tumor cells are strongly positive; case originally submitted as possible cholangiocarcinoma.

antigen (CEA) and CD10 are less useful markers in poorly differentiated hepatocellular carcinoma. Also, of note, do not make a diagnosis of hepatocellular carcinoma if the H&E findings are not consistent, even if the tumor is positive for alpha-fetoprotein (AFP), or HepPar1, or glypican 3, or arginase1. Each of these stains can occasionally be positive in nonhepatocellular carcinomas (Figure 23.15), but they are very powerful for confirming the diagnosis when they are combined with the H&E findings and a thoughtfully chosen panel of immunostains.

Also, be aware that some well-differentiated tumors can closely mimic hepatocellular carcinoma, showing big pink tumor cells and sometimes a trabecular growth pattern. Thus, an immunostain for hepatocellular differentiation can be helpful even in well-differentiated tumors. Of note, arginase is negative in about 10% of well-differentiated hepatocellular carcinomas, so HepPar1 is preferred in this setting. Examples of tumors that mimic well-differentiated hepatocellular carcinomas on H&E include neuroendocrine tumors (most common) (Figure 23.16), squamous cell carcinoma (Figure 23.17), paragangliomas, renal oncocytic tumors, acinar cell carcinoma, adrenal cortical carcinomas, and epithelioid angiomyolipoma.

FOURTH, after excluding hepatocellular carcinoma based on morphology and/or immunostains, carcinomas can be divided into adenocarcinomas and nonadenocarcinomas. If there is no gland formation and mucicarmine stains are negative, the diagnostic workup can next focus on common nonadenocarcinomas metastatic to the liver, such as neuroendocrine tumors/carcinoma. Immunostains will be positive for synaptophysin and or chromogranin. INSM1 is a newer stain and can occasionally be helpful, rarely positive when synaptophysin or chromogranin stains are equivocal or negative. Neuroendocrine

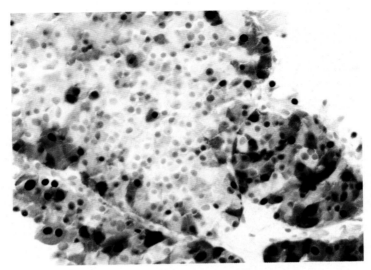

FIGURE 23.15 **Neuroendocrine tumor, arginase positive.** There was focal but strong arginase 1 staining in this neuroendocrine tumor.

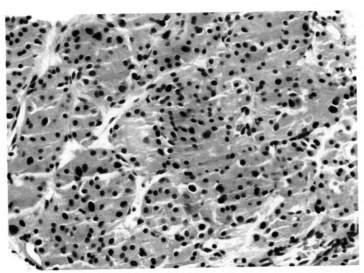

FIGURE 23.16 **Neuroendocrine tumor.** The morphological features at first suggested a hepatocellular carcinoma.

neoplasms are classified as per the current World Health Organization (WHO) criteria into well-differentiated neuroendocrine tumors, neuroendocrine carcinomas, and small cell carcinomas. If the tumor is well differentiated, WHO grading is then applied. Neuroendocrine carcinomas show more cytological and architectural atypia than neuroendocrine tumors and are routinely RB1 positive. In most cases, imaging and clinical findings are sufficient to identify the site of origin for a neuroendocrine tumor involving the liver. If clinically

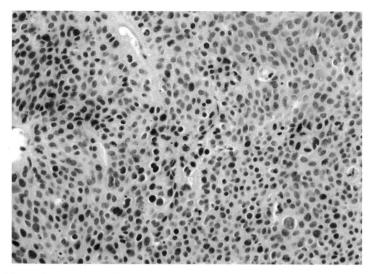

FIGURE 23.17 **Squamous cell carcinoma.** This case was submitted in consultation with a provisional diagnosis of moderately differentiated hepatocellular carcinoma.

requested, immunostains can provide some useful information about possible sites of origin (Table 23.3).

One important diagnostic pitfall is that about 10% of neuroendocrine tumors are HepPar1 positive. Glypican 3 and arginase case also be occasionally positive (less than 5% of cases).

The diagnosis of small cell carcinoma is made in the usual fashion. One pitfall is that the fragile tumor cells can be inapparent on H&E in some biopsies due to crush or other processing artifacts, so immunostains are important if there is clinical concern for small cell carcinoma.

Neuroendocrine tumors should be keratin positive; if not, then the diagnosis is most likely a metastatic paraganglioma. S100 stains are not helpful for identifying sustentacular cells in metastatic paragangliomas (they are usually absent), so the diagnosis of a paraganglioma is established by compatible morphology, immunostains (synaptophysin and or chromogranin positive, keratins negative) and imaging findings.

Other useful diagnostic pearls include the following. Adrenal cortical carcinomas and acinar cell carcinomas can show patchy synaptophysin staining, representing important diagnostic pitfalls. The possibility of a squamous cell carcinomas is often overlooked because they frequently do not show readily apparent keratinization; a p40 stain is very helpful for making the diagnosis. Some intrahepatic cholangiocarcinomas can show solid or trabecular growth patterns, without gland formation; these are typically positive for albumin in situ hybridization.

FIFTH, a diagnosis of adenocarcinoma can be established by morphology and/or mucicarmine positivity. The differential for adenocarcinomas

TABLE 23.3 Immunohistochemical Stains for Nonsmall Cell Neuroendocrine Tumors and Carcinomas

Tumor Primary	CK7	CK20	TTF1[b]	CDX2	Islet-1	SATB2	PAX6
Pancreas	50	30	<5	<5	90	<5	60
Stomach	10	20	<5	<5	10	<5	<5
Duodenum/ jejunum	10	20	<5	<5	90	5	90
Ileum	10	20	<5	90	10	5	<5
Appendix[a]	10	20	<5	100	10	90	20
Colon	10	20	<5	70	10	<5	Insufficient data
Rectum	10	20	<5	10	90	90	80
Lung	60	<5	40	<5	10	10	<5

Note that there is a lot of variability in the result of different studies, so these are only representative numbers.

[a]Goblet cell carcinomas are usually CK20 and CK7 positive.

[b]OTP may be a better marker of lung origin but is not widely available.

includes intrahepatic cholangiocarcinomas as well as metastatic disease from various organs. Most intrahepatic cholangiocarcinomas are positive for CK7, CK19 (90%), and albumin in situ hybridization (90%). In the specific differential of cholangiocarcinoma versus hepatocellular carcinoma, strong and diffuse staining for MOC31 favors cholangiocarcinoma. MOC31, however, is not specific for adenocarcinoma per se, also being seen in many other carcinomas. Also, patchy staining is common in hepatocellular carcinoma.

Once cholangiocarcinoma is excluded, standard stains can be used in conjunction with the CK7/CK20 profile to suggest a site of origin. There are several recurrent pitfalls to be aware of when using the most common stains for site of origin. First, adenocarcinomas from the right side of the colon can be CK20 negative. Second, gallbladder and some hilar cholangiocarcinomas can be TTF1 and napsin positive.[21] Third, there are no stains currently available that reliably separate a metastatic pancreatic adenocarcinoma from an intrahepatic cholangiocarcinoma. This includes DPC4. Fourth, GATA3 is positive in not only breast and urothelial carcinomas but also in many pancreatic ductal adenocarcinomas (about 1/3) and mesotheliomas (1/2).

Representative metastatic carcinomas are shown in eFigures, including colon carcinoma (eFigs. 23.6-23.8), pancreas acinar cell carcinoma (eFig. 23.9), pancreas ductal carcinoma (eFigs. 23.10 and 23.11), neuroendocrine tumor (eFigs. 23.12-23.20), breast adenocarcinoma (eFig. 21), lung adenocarcinoma (eFigs. 23.22-23.27), lung small cell carcinoma (eFigs.

23.28 and 23.29), renal chromophobe carcinoma (eFigs. 23.30-23.34), renal clear cell carcinoma (eFigs. 23.35-23.38), prostate carcinoma (eFigs. 23.39-23.41), melanoma (eFig. 23.42), gastrointestinal stromal tumor (eFig. 23.43), leiomyosarcoma (eFig. 23.44), and nonseminomatous germ cell tumor (eFigs. 23.45-23.47).

Cancer of Unknown Primary

Despite full workup, a site of origin is not identified in about 2% of carcinomas involving the liver; about 45% of these are adenocarcinomas, 35% are undifferentiated carcinomas, and 10% are squamous cell carcinomas. In 40% of these cases, only the liver is involved on full body imaging, suggesting the tumor represents an undifferentiated carcinoma primary to the liver. In addition, when these cases go to autopsy, a primary site is confidently identified in only about one-third of cases; of these, the most common sites of origin are lungs, pancreas, and GI tract.

REFERENCES

1. Yang CT, Liu KL, Lin MC, et al. Pseudolymphoma of the liver: report of a case and review of the literature. *Asian J Surg.* 2017;40(1):74-80.
2. Seitter S, Goodman ZD, Friedman TM, et al. Intrahepatic reactive lymphoid hyperplasia: a case report and review of the literature. *Case Rep Surg.* 2018;2018:9264251.
3. El-Fattah MA. Non-hodgkin lymphoma of the liver: a US population-based analysis. *J Clin Transl Hepatol.* 2017;5:83-91.
4. Bronowicki JP, Bineau C, Feugier P, et al. Primary lymphoma of the liver: clinical-pathological features and relationship with HCV infection in French patients. *Hepatology.* 2003;37:781-787.
5. Kikuma K, Watanabe J, Oshiro Y, et al. Etiological factors in primary hepatic B-cell lymphoma. *Virchows Arch.* 2012;460:379-387.
6. Swadley MJ, Deliu M, Mosunjac MB, et al. Primary and secondary hepatic lymphomas diagnosed by image-guided fine-needle aspiration: a retrospective study of clinical and cytomorphologic findings. *Am J Clin Pathol.* 2014;141:119-127.
7. Eom DW, Huh JR, Kang YK, et al. Clinicopathological features of eight Korean cases of primary hepatic lymphoma. *Pathol Int.* 2004;54:830-836.
8. Loddenkemper C, Longerich T, Hummel M, et al. Frequency and diagnostic patterns of lymphomas in liver biopsies with respect to the WHO classification. *Virchows Arch.* 2007;450:493-502.
9. Baumhoer D, Tzankov A, Dirnhofer S, et al. Patterns of liver infiltration in lymphoproliferative disease. *Histopathology.* 2008;53:81-90.
10. Ugurluer G, Miller RC, Li Y, et al. Primary hepatic lymphoma: a retrospective, multicenter rare cancer network study. *Rare Tumors.* 2016;8:6502.
11. Torbenson MS, Zhang L, Moreira RK. *Surgical Pathology of the Liver.* Wolters Kluwer Health; 2018, xi:740.
12. Swerdlow SH; International Agency for Research on Cancer; World Health Organization. *WHO Classification of Tumours of Haematopoietic and Lymphoid Tissues.* 4th ed. International Agency for Research on Cancer; 2008:439.
13. Macon WR, Levy NB, Kurtin PJ, et al. Hepatosplenic alphabeta T-cell lymphomas: a report of 14 cases and comparison with hepatosplenic gammadelta T-cell lymphomas. *Am J Surg Pathol.* 2001;25:285-296.

14. Krenacs L, Smyth MJ, Bagdi E, et al. The serine protease granzyme M is preferentially expressed in NK-cell, gamma delta T-cell, and intestinal T-cell lymphomas: evidence of origin from lymphocytes involved in innate immunity. *Blood.* 2003;101:3590-3593.

15. Felgar RE, Macon WR, Kinney MC, et al. TIA-1 expression in lymphoid neoplasms. Identification of subsets with cytotoxic T lymphocyte or natural killer cell differentiation. *Am J Pathol.* 1997;150:1893-1900.

16. Sternberg SS, Mills SE, Carter D. *Sternberg's Diagnostic Surgical Pathology.* 5th ed. Wolters Kluwer Lippincott Williams & Wilkins; 2010.

17. Roquet ML, Zafrani ES, Farcet JP, et al. Histopathological lesions of the liver in hairy cell leukemia: a report of 14 cases. *Hepatology.* 1985;5:496-500.

18. Bethel KJ, Sharpe RW. Pathology of hairy-cell leukaemia. *Best Pract Res Clin Haematol.* 2003;16:15-31.

19. Sharpe RW, Bethel KJ. Hairy cell leukemia: diagnostic pathology. *Hematol Oncol Clin North Am.* 2006;20:1023-1049.

20. Turakhia S, Lanigan C, Hamadeh F, et al. Immunohistochemistry for BRAF V600E in the differential diagnosis of hairy cell leukemia vs other splenic B-cell lymphomas. *Am J Clin Pathol.* 2015;144:87-93.

21. Roy M, Jain D, Yadav R, et al. TTF-1 and napsin-A are not markers for biliary phenotype: an immunohistochemical study of gallbladder adenocarcinomas. *Am J Surg Pathol.* 2015;39:1742-1744.

THE LANGUAGE OF LIVER PATHOLOGY: DEFINITIONS OF KEY TERMS

Liver pathology has its own unique vocabulary for describing important histological changes. Locating reasonable definitions for liver pathology terms in the literature can be a challenge, one compounded further by inconsistent usage between different authors. Definitions from internet sources are convenient, but are often incomplete and sometimes wrong. Thus, this section provides a quick reference for important terms that are relatively unique to the field of liver pathology, but will not cover more general pathology terms. As appropriate, the different usages for these terms are also noted. These terms provide the building blocks from which pathology entities are described and diagnosed. Having a firm understanding of these terms will substantially increase your enjoyment and understanding of the liver pathology literature.

The goal of this chapter is not to be a vocabulary scold, but instead to provide a foundation to help understand the pathology literature. Not everyone will completely agree with the definitions provided here, which should be no surprise given the varying usages in the literature, but it is hoped that this section will still have value, providing a reasonable foundation on which to build your understanding of the liver pathology literature. Also, uniform definitions are much more important, for the purposes of this book, for those words used to make a pathology diagnosis. For example, if you prefer "acidophil bodies" or "spotty necrosis" or "hepatocyte apoptosis" to describe scattered dead hepatocytes, it is all fine and your choice of terms matters relatively little. On the other hand, terms that undermine clarity of communication in a surgical pathology report should be avoided. Examples include terms that are easily misinterpreted by clinical colleagues, such as "microgranulomas," and terms that are largely obsolete such as "pericholangitis."

USEFUL DEFINITIONS IN LIVER PATHOLOGY

Aberrant artery/arteriole; *synonym: naked artery.* This term is used for small arteries found in the hepatic lobules, instead of their normal location in the portal tracts (Figure A.1.1). Aberrant arteries can result from

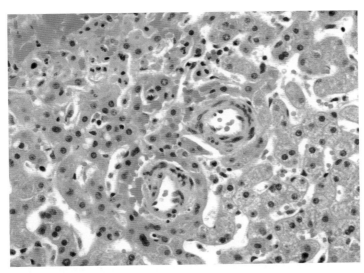

FIGURE A.1.1 **Aberrant artery.** This hepatocellular carcinoma shows several arteries located outside of portal tracts.

chronic lobular ischemia or from tumor factors that lead to arterialization of the lobules. As such, they can be found in both reactive conditions associated with vascular flow changes, such as focal nodular hyperplasia (FNH),[1] regenerative hepatic pseudotumors (RHP),[2] central vein sclerosis in the setting of alcoholic cirrhosis,[3] or hepatic neoplasms such as hepatic adenomas and hepatocellular carcinomas.

Acidophil body; *synonyms: apoptotic body, spotty necrosis (councilman body; historical interest, rarely used today but was used to describe hepatocyte apoptosis in the setting of yellow fever).* Acidophil bodies are single, scattered, dead hepatocytes. They are typically smaller than a normal hepatocyte, with densely eosinophilic cytoplasm and generally lack a nucleus; or it may have a small and shriveled nuclear remnant (Figure A.1.2). Acidophil bodies can be seen in a wide variety of hepatic injuries and are not specific for etiology. Rarely, however, lobular apoptosis is the predominant pattern of injury, where it is unaccompanied by inflammation or cholestasis, or other changes, and in this setting, the differential is primarily that of drug effect, acute viral infection, and low-grade/transient hepatic ischemia.

Acinus; *synonym: lobule (in practical use).* The hepatic acinus is the smallest vascular-hepatocellular functional unit of the liver, a conceptual entity that captures the blood flow moving from the terminal portal tracts through the lobules and out the central veins. It is usually defined as an elliptical or diamond-shaped structure with top and bottom borders formed by the portal tracts and a bulging middle with edges defined by central veins (Figure A.1.3). Perfectly shaped acini are hardly ever seen in human

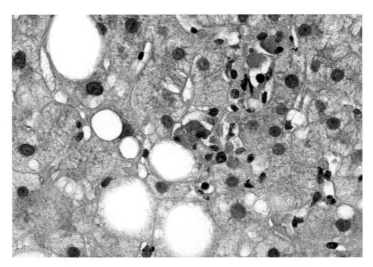

FIGURE A.1.2 **Acidophil body.** Several acidophil bodies are present in the hepatic lobules in this case of steatohepatitis.

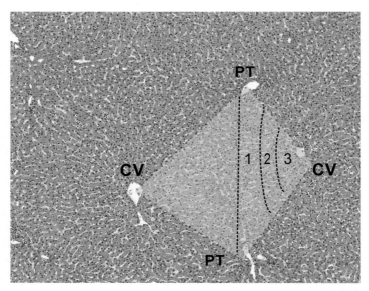

FIGURE A.1.3 **Rappaport hepatic acinus model.** The diamond-shaped acinus outlined by black lines is composed of two triangles with the axis between two portal tracts (PTs) and the acinus divided into zone 1, 2, and 3.

tissue specimens, except in conceptual cartoons. The concept is important, however, as the acinus forms the basis for three approximately equal-sized microscopic liver zones, which can be seen histologically and are useful diagnostically, with zone 1 defined as those hepatocytes near the portal tracts, zone 3 defined as hepatocytes near the central vein, and zone 2 defined as the remaining hepatocytes located in between zones 1 and 3.

In contrast to the hepatic acinus, the hepatic lobule is formally defined as a hexagon-shaped structure with portal tracts at each corner, all draining into a single central vein (Figure A.1.4). In ordinary usage, however, the terms *acini* and *lobule* simply refer to where the hepatocytes are located. The Mall model has the lobule defined by the biliary drainage, creating a triangular lobule with central veins at the vertices, all centered on a portal tract (Figures A.1.5 and A.1.6).[4]

Accessory lobe. Accessory lobes are not uncommon, with a frequency of about 10% based on imaging studies, with the most common type called a *Riedel lobe*. Overall, accessory lobes are more relevant to radiologists, so that they do not mistake the accessory lobes for tumors, and are only rarely encountered in surgical pathology specimens. Accessory lobes can rarely come to surgical attention when they can develop tumors[5-7] or undergo torsion.[8]

Histologically, accessory lobes show benign liver parenchyma that is essentially normal in most cases, but can show loss of bile ducts or portal veins, in which case, they may also show features of nodular regenerative hyperplasia.

Accessory lobes by definition are clearly connected to the liver, in contrast to ectopic hepatic tissue, which has no connection to the liver. Accessory lobes are usually connected by a thick pedicle of essentially normal liver tissue, or less often by a thin fibrovascular core composed of

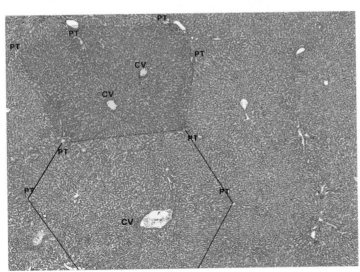

FIGURE A.1.4 **Liver structural units (microanatomy). Kiernan model.** The classical hexagonal lobule outlined by black lines with the central vein (CV) at the center and the portal tracts (PTs) at the corners of the hexagon. Two are shown in this image. Note that that in practice a perfectly shaped hexagon is almost never seen. Also, note that sometimes multiple profiles of the central vein can be seen.

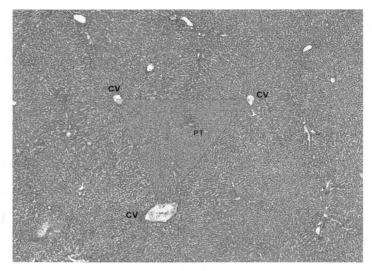

FIGURE A.1.5 **Mall model**: This model tracks the bile drainage, with a triangular lobule centered around a portal tract.

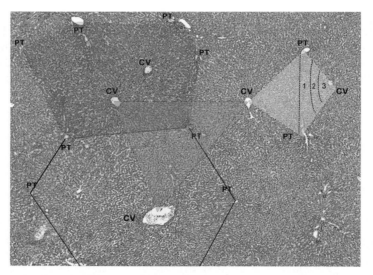

FIGURE A.1.6 **Liver models.** Here, all three models are shown together.

connective tissue containing blood vessels and often bile ducts running through it, along with occasional, scattered small islands of hepatocytes.

Acute hepatitis. In common medical usage, the term "acute hepatitis" refers to any abrupt presentation of liver disease. Formal clinical definitions vary depending on the study, but a common definition is any abrupt-onset hepatitis of less than 6 months in duration. The histological findings will vary considerably, depending on the type of injury, but can be predominately hepatitic, cholestatic, biliary, congested, fatty, or bland necrosis.

Most biopsies show no histological findings that specifically indicate an acute hepatitis (versus a chronic hepatitis), so the term is typically avoided as a pathology diagnosis. As exceptions, moderate diffuse lobular hepatitis, marked lobular hepatitis, or significant necrosis are too damaging to the liver to be a chronic process, indicating either an acute hepatitis or an acute-on-chronic hepatitis. In this regard, the presence of significant fibrosis on a biopsy suggests a flare of chronic liver disease, despite the abrupt onset of the clinical disease. On the other hand, the absence of fibrosis is compatible with both acute and chronic causes of hepatitis.

Acute yellow atrophy of the liver. This term is obsolete, but is still occasionally encountered. Acute yellow atrophy of the liver describes the atrophy associated with acute liver failure from extensive necrosis, often with fatty change in the surviving hepatocytes. Acute yellow atrophy is really a gross pathology term and over the years has been used to describe acute liver failure from a variety of causes, including everything from fatty liver of pregnancy, to massive viral infection, to drug-induced liver injury.

Alcoholic foamy degeneration; *synonym: acute foamy degeneration.* This term refers to diffuse microvesicular steatosis of the hepatocytes, specifically in the context of alcohol use.[9] Alcoholic foamy degeneration represents a rare pattern of injury, with a prevalence of less than 1% in most centers. The precise cause is not clear.

Apoptosis/apoptotic body; *synonyms (for dead hepatocytes): acidophil body, spotty necrosis, councilman body.* An apoptotic body is a single dead cell that has undergone programmed cell death. This is the sciency definition. At a practical, diagnostic pathology level, it can be a single dead hepatocyte, a dead cholangiocyte, or any other single dead cell, with or without accompanying inflammation. In hepatitic patterns of injury, hepatocellular apoptosis is often associated with foci of lobular inflammation and or pigmented macrophages.

Ascending cholangitis. Ascending cholangitis refers to an infection of the extrahepatic biliary tree that has "ascended" up the biliary tree into the liver, typically manifesting as bile ducts that are dilated, lined by attenuated epithelium, and filled with neutrophils (Figure A.1.7). There can also be neutrophils in the portal tract stroma.

Balloon cell; *synonyms: ballooned hepatocyte, balloon cell change, ballooning degeneration (partial synonym).* Balloon cells are hepatocytes that have more cytoplasm than adjacent hepatocytes, a rarified appearance to their cytoplasm, and may contain Mallory bodies. Balloon cells are best diagnosed at lower power magnification, such as 4× or 10× objectives; they should truly stand out from the adjacent hepatocytes (Figure A.1.8). They should not have big droplets of fat in them. Balloon cells can be seen in a wide variety of diseases, but are most commonly encountered in fatty liver

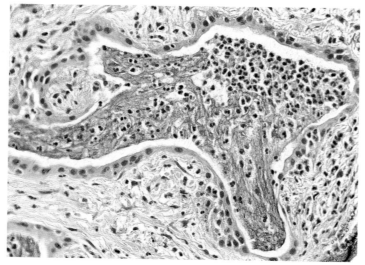

FIGURE A.1.7 **Ascending cholangitis.** A bile duct is distended with numerous neutrophils in this case of ascending cholangitis.

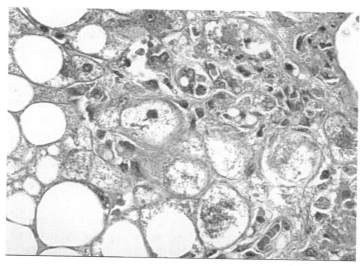

FIGURE A.1.8 **Balloon cell.** Ballooned hepatocytes with Mallory hyaline are shown. The ballooned hepatocytes can be contrasted to hepatocytes with macrovesicular steatosis on the left side of this image.

disease, where they are useful in making the diagnosis of steatohepatitis. In some liver biopsy specimens with fatty change, scattered hepatocytes may have changes that are equivocal for balloon cells, especially if you spend too much time at 40× or 60× objectives. These types of cells generally lack the diagnostic value of classic balloon cells. Both classic ballooned hepatocytes and some equivocal balloon cells will lose their normal expression of CK8/18,[10,11] and this finding may find use diagnostically in the future.

Balloon cells are also commonly seen with chronic cholestasis, as part of a process called cholate stasis, and can also be seen with a variety of different causes of acute hepatitis, usually as scattered injured cells.

Ballooning degeneration. Hepatocytes with ballooning degeneration have lost their usual polygonal shape and are rounded, often with increased cytoplasm that is less eosinophilic than the neighboring cells. At the individual cell level, this finding is essentially the same as balloon cells in fatty liver disease and is often used in that context. The term *ballooning degeneration*, however, is also used to describe groups of cells or rarely the entire lobule, where contiguous swaths of ballooned cells are seen, usually in the setting of marked hepatitis or cholestasis.

Bile duct. The bile duct is the tubular structure that is formed by cholangiocytes and located in the central region of the portal tract (Figure A.1.9). It is usually accompanied by the hepatic artery, which will be located near the bile duct, typically within a distance that is about equal to the bile duct's diameter. The bile duct and the hepatic artery typically are about the same size in diameter. Do not confuse the bile duct with bile ductules (Figure A.1.10), or the medical literature and this book will make no sense.

Bile duct duplication. A portal tract with bile duct duplication will have a small cluster of bile ducts in the center of the portal tract, instead of the normal finding of a single bile duct (Figure A.1.11). This finding is different from that of bile ductular proliferation, where increased ductules are located at the periphery of the portal tract. Bile duct duplication is rare, but is most commonly associated with chronic biliary tract diseases affecting the large intrahepatic bile ducts or the extrahepatic bile ducts, such as primary sclerosing cholangitis.

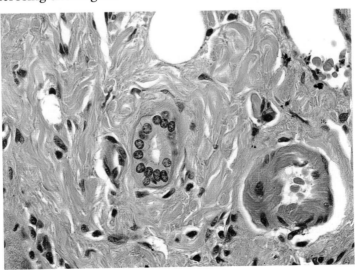

FIGURE A.1.9 **Bile duct.** A normal bile duct is present in the center region of a portal tract.

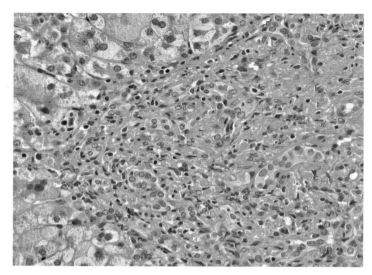

FIGURE A.1.10 **Bile ductules.** Proliferating bile ductules are seen at the edge of the portal tract in this case of extrahepatic biliary atresia.

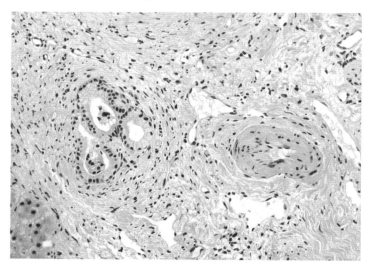

FIGURE A.1.11 **Bile duct duplication.** In this case of primary biliary cholangitis (PBC), there are three bile duct profiles instead of one.

Bile duct lymphocytosis; *synonym: lymphocytic cholangitis.* This term means exactly what it says: the bile ducts have lymphocytes within the epithelium. In some diseases, like acute cellular rejection and some cases of drug induced liver injury, the bile duct lymphocytosis is part of the main pattern of injury, a dominant part of the histology. In these cases, the lymphocytosis can range from mild to severe and from focal to diffuse; it is commonly accompanied by cholangiocyte injury, such as apoptosis.

By way of contrast, focal and mild lymphocytosis is common and nonspecific whenever there is moderate or marked chronic inflammation of the portal tract.

Bile duct hamartoma; *synonyms: ductal plate malformation, von Meyenburg complex.* Bile duct hamartomas are benign duct-like structures embedded in fibrous background, with angulated, inter-anastomosing growth patterns, open lumens, and bile deposits. They are usually incidental findings, with most examples less than 5 mm in size and almost all are less than 15 mm in size. Most cases encountered in surgical pathology are sporadic and appear to be acquired lesions, being more common in cirrhotic than noncirrhotic livers,[12] where they can be single or multifocal. There is one more setting where they are routinely seen: numerous bile duct hamartomas are found in livers with autosomal dominant polycystic kidney and liver disease. They are histologically identical in both settings.

Bile duct metaplasia. Rarely, bile ducts undergo metaplasia. The most common type is intestinal metaplasia, but sometimes there can be pyloric metaplasia or squamous metaplasia or two very rare forms of metaplasia: hepatic metaplasia and clear cell metaplasia.[13] Intestinal, pyloric, and squamous metaplasia are more common in large bile ducts, hepatic metaplasia in small bile ducts, while clear cell change can be found in either small or large bile ducts. When there is intestinal metaplasia, Paneth cells may also be present. Bile duct metaplasia results from chronic injury due to inflammation or ischemia. One last type of change is not a true metaplasia but is sometimes called *oncocytic metaplasia*; in this setting, the small bile duct cells have a densely eosinophilic cytoplasmic appearance that results from increased mitochondrial mass.[14] This finding is rare, but when observed, seems to be mostly in the setting of PBC or alcoholic liver disease.[15]

Bile ductule. Bile ductules are small, epithelial, tubular structures located at the periphery of the portal tracts (see Figure A.1.10). You will not see them in normal portal tracts, but they are observed in a wide variety of disease conditions and, when abundant, can give a clue to the etiology of the disease process. Bile ductules appear to arise from stem-like cells located at the portal tract-lobule interface and can differentiate toward hepatocytes or biliary cells in response to injury. They often do not have a lumen, though they may have bile plugs in badly cholestatic diseases. Bile ductules connect the canals of Hering to the bile duct proper.[16]

Bile ductular proliferation represents part of the normal response to liver injury from many different causes, but is usually mild and best seen with keratin stains. On the other hand, bile ductular proliferation can be particularly prominent with obstruction of the biliary tree.

Bile ductular cholestasis; *synonym: cholangitis lenta.* This term is used when bile plugs are found in the proliferating bile ductules (Figure A.1.12; eFig. A.1.1). In most cases, this is a nonspecific finding in patients with long-standing cholestasis from any cause, including debilitating illnesses, and in this setting, the lobules are also deeply cholestatic.

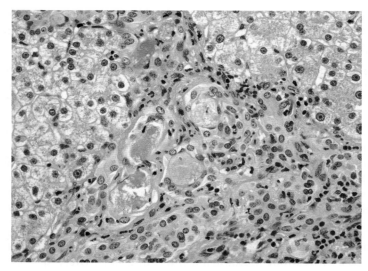

FIGURE A.1.12 **Bile ductular cholestasis.** The bile ductules show plugs of cholestasis.

In some specimens, however, the bile ductular cholestasis pattern is the dominant finding, with little or no lobular cholestasis. In most of these cases, bile ductular cholestasis is an idiopathic finding, but it has been associated with sepsis,[17-19] congestive heart failure, and various chronic debilitating illnesses, including severe alcoholic hepatitis.[17,20]

Of note, the association with sepsis appears to be indirect, as patients with chronic debilitating illnesses are prone to sepsis. Thus, the bile ductular cholestasis is a general reflection of the underlying debilitating illnesses; it is not necessarily caused by sepsis, and it certainly is not the cause of the sepsis. It is possible that sepsis accentuates this pattern of cholestasis, but cholangitis lenta is not evidence of sepsis per se.[17]

Bile ductular proliferation. This term refers to the proliferation of small bile ductules at the periphery of portal tracts (see Figure A.1.10). The bile ductular proliferation can be focal and mild in a wide variety of liver injuries, as the ductules are a source of liver progenitor cells and they proliferate in response to injury. If the ductular reaction is a major pattern in the biopsy, however, then it suggests large duct biliary obstruction. If neutrophils accompany the proliferating ductules, then the pattern is called a ductular reaction. A striking ductular proliferation can sometimes be associated with edema of the portal tracts, especially with acute biliary obstructive disease.

Bile ductular reaction; *synonym: pericholangitis (obsolete).* A bile ductular reaction is defined as a proliferation of bile ductules that is accompanied by neutrophils (Figure A.1.13). The neutrophils should be in the stroma next to the proliferating ductules. In contrast, if neutrophils are present

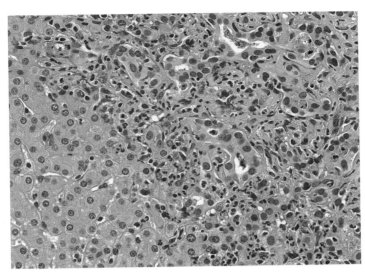

FIGURE A.1.13 **Bile ductular reaction.** The edge of this portal tract shows a brisk bile ductular reaction with numerous admixed neutrophils; image is from a case of large duct biliary obstructive.

in the bile duct proper (the main duct seen within the portal tract), then the pattern has a separate differential and suggests ascending cholangitis, especially if the bile duct is dilated (see Figure A.1.7). An older and obsolete term for a ductular reaction that has neutrophilia is "pericholangitis."

The term *ductular reaction* was used early on by Popper and colleagues[21] where it was further divided into three types[22]: type I, associated with biliary obstruction; type II, associated with significantly active hepatitis; and type III, associated with massive liver necrosis. This terminology is not used anymore, but serves as a useful reminder of the major settings in which a ductular reaction can be observed.

Bile infarct. A bile infarct is a small circumscribed collection of dead and bile stained hepatocytes, usually located right next to a portal tract. This finding often indicates acute high-grade biliary obstruction when found in a biopsy specimen (Figure A.1.14), but can also be a nonspecific finding in livers with long-standing, profound cholestasis.

Bridging fibrosis; *synonym: septal fibrosis, fibrous septa (inconsistently used).* Bridging fibrosis is defined as fibrosis that extends from portal tract to portal tract or from portal tract to central vein. While the terms *septal fibrosis* or *fibrous septa* are generally considered to be synonyms, some authors use *fibrous septa* when portal tracts have short fibrous extensions that do not fully connect two portal tracts, and thus would not be the same as bridging fibrosis. The term *bridging fibrosis* has the advantage of unambiguous meaning.

Bridging necrosis. This term describes necrosis that extends from portal tract to portal tract or from portal tract to central veins. Bridging necrosis is most commonly seen in the setting of markedly active hepatitis or toxin

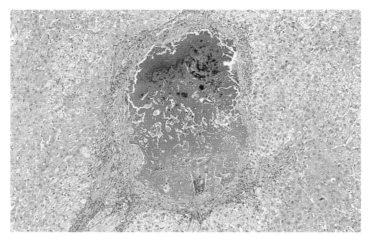

FIGURE A.1.14   **Bile infarct.** A bile infarct is seen in a case of acute high-grade obstruction.

exposure. The areas of necrosis often stain blue on trichrome and can thus mimic bridging fibrosis.

Canal of Hering. The canal of Hering is a thin, linear, intralobular biliary structure formed by cuboidal cells that extend from the portal tracts into zone 1 of the hepatic lobules. The canal of Hering is formed by both biliary-type cells and by hepatocytes and connects the bile canaliculi (formed entirely by hepatocytes) to the bile ducts (formed entirely by ductular cells). The canal of Hering is usually not visible on H&E, but can be seen as a thin line of single cuboidal cells extending from the portal tracts, when using immunohistochemistry for cytokeratin 19 (Figure A.1.15). When looking at a single slide, the canals of Hering typically appear as a discontinuous line of cells, but serial sections show a continuous line of cells extending from the portal tracts into the lobules.

Cholate stasis; *synonyms: feathery degeneration, pseudoxanthomatous change (no longer in common usage).* Cholate stasis is used to describe swollen and pale periportal hepatocytes (located in zone 1) of livers with chronic cholestasis. Cholate stasis is most commonly seen in cirrhotic livers, but can be seen in noncirrhotic livers.

Cholate stasis (Figure A.1.16) results from injury to zone 1 hepatocytes as a result of chronic exposure to bile acids. The hepatocytes appear somewhat similar to ballooned hepatocytes, but often are not quite as swollen as balloon cells in steatohepatitis. In addition, cholate stasis affects the zone 1 hepatocytes, often in a contiguous fashion, in contrast to balloon cells in steatohepatitis, which are often in zone 3 and are usually found as scattered single cells or small clusters of cells.

A copper stain is typically positive in hepatocytes with cholate stasis, but not in balloon cells from fatty liver disease or in ballooning degeneration from lobular hepatitis. Essentially all hepatocytes with cholate stasis

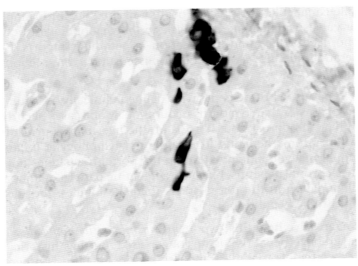

FIGURE A.1.15 **Canal of Hering.** A CK7 immunostain highlights a canal of Hering that extends from the portal tract into the lobules.

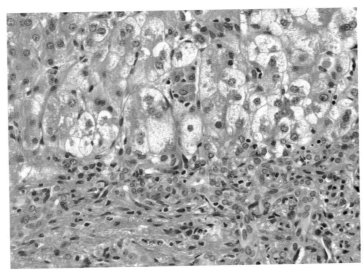

FIGURE A.1.16 **Cholate stasis.** The periportal hepatocytes are swollen, with rarified cytoplasm.

are intermediate hepatocytes (CK7 positive), although not all intermediate hepatocytes show cholate stasis.

Cholestasis; *synonym: bilirubinostasis.* Cholestasis, simply put, is the presence of bile in the liver that is visible on H&E stains. It may be present in hepatocytes, in bile canaliculi, in proliferating ductules, or in the bile duct proper. The most common place to see cholestasis is within hepatocytes and/or bile canaliculi. The precise location of the bile, for example, hepatocellular versus canicular, offers little in the way of diagnostic value, so there is no need to mention the location in pathology reports. Bile plugs in proliferating ductules is rare and discussed under the section for *bile ductular cholestasis*.

Chronic hepatitis. Chronic hepatitis is defined clinically as serum enzyme elevations of greater than 6 months in duration. Many cases of chronic hepatitis will have no fibrosis, but fibrosis on the liver biopsy provides strong evidence for chronic hepatitis. The finding of lymphocytic inflammation, or lymphoplasmacytic inflammation, in the portal tracts does not by itself constitute a chronic hepatitis; likewise, a hepatitic pattern of injury that has more inflammation in the portal tracts then the lobules does not always indicate a chronic hepatitis.

Chronic aggressive hepatitis; *synonym, chronic active hepatitis.* The term chronic aggressive hepatitis[23] is no longer used, but has historical significance. Early attempts to understand risk factors for fibrosis progression in patients with chronic hepatitis divided cases into two histological injury patterns: (1) chronic aggressive hepatitis or (2) chronic persistent hepatitis. This classification was based on piecemeal necrosis, which we now call interface activity, and what was then called periportal fibrosis, both of which are present in chronic aggressive hepatitis, but absent in chronic persistent hepatitis, which instead shows absent or "slight" piecemeal necrosis and either no fibrosis or portal fibrosis. In this model, chronic aggressive hepatitis had a worse prognosis.

This basic approach, one that focused on interface activity and the distinction of portal fibrosis versus periportal fibrosis as key components of prognostication, was not easily applied in many cases and eventually was abandoned in favor of current approaches, where disease is classified primarily by etiology and inflammatory grade is fully separated from fibrosis stage.

Nonetheless, the notion of interface activity is still relevant today, although we now understand that it has no special significance over that of portal inflammation or lobular inflammation, and all three are routinely assessed in scoring systems. In addition, the distinction of portal fibrosis versus periportal fibrosis has persisted in some staging systems, an interesting intellectual fossil representing important, early steps in understanding chronic hepatitis (see separate entry on portal fibrosis for more details).[24]

Chronic persistent hepatitis. This term is no longer used, but was defined as a chronic hepatitis with absent or "slight" piecemeal necrosis and no fibrosis. Please see the entry for "chronic aggressive hepatitis" for more information.

Cirrhosis. Cirrhosis is defined as diffuse scarring of the liver, leading to regenerative nodules of hepatocytes surrounded by bands of fibrosis. The history of the term includes major figures in the history of medicine, notably Rene Laennec (1781-1826), a distinguished French physician who invented the stethoscope. Laennec is often credited with the first description of a cirrhotic liver, which he named "kirrhos," after the Greek word for "tawny," which in turn became the English word *cirrhosis*.

Laennec, it turns out, only thought he was the first to describe cirrhosis. Instead, cirrhosis was described earlier and more accurately by two British pathologists, John Browne (1642-1700) and Matthew Baillie (1761-1823). History, however, is rarely fair and subsequently Sir William Osler (1849-1919), a dominant North American physician, one of the four founders of the Johns Hopkins Hospital, gave the credit to Laennec in his very influential medical text books, and this credit has stuck to this day.[25]

For over 100 years, cirrhosis was thought to be permanent, but studies over the past 20 years have convincingly shown that cirrhosis can regress, given enough time and cessation of the chronic injury.[24,26] This remarkable advance in understanding cirrhosis, made possible by the development of highly effective treatments for chronic liver disease, has even led some authors to suggest abandoning the term cirrhosis itself.[27]

Councilman body; *synonyms: Councilman hyaline body, acidophil, apoptotic body, spotty necrosis.* Councilman bodies are essentially synonymous with acidophil bodies. They are named after the American pathologist William Councilman (1854-1933), who described hepatocyte necrosis in the pathology of yellow fever. In current literature, however, the term apoptotic body or acidophil body is most commonly used. Some authors prefer to use Councilman bodies only in reference to the histology of yellow fever.

Confluent necrosis. Confluent necrosis refers to apoptosis or necrosis that affects a grouping of hepatocytes that is larger than a single cell or a small cluster of a few cells (which would be called spotty necrosis). Confluent necrosis may be limited to clusters of hepatocytes around the central veins or, in more severe cases, can lead to bridging necrosis that extends from central veins to portal tracts, or from central veins to central veins.

There is no data-driven cut-off for the minimum size of the necrotic foci needed to separate spotty necrosis from confluent necrosis. Some pathologists like the cut-off of three cells or more as defining confluent necrosis, but it is often very hard to be sure how many hepatocytes actually died in any given small focus of necrosis.

In any case, the temptation to count dead cells is probably missing the point, and at least for clinical care, the distinction between single cell necrosis and confluent necrosis should be based on common sense, with the goal of accurately conveying what you see in the biopsy. For example, if a biopsy specimen shows a hepatitic pattern of injury, with predominately mild lobular spotty necrosis, but after carefully searching you find a single focus with three adjacent dead hepatocytes, the best descriptor is still spotty necrosis for the overall pattern of injury.

Ductal plate malformation; *synonyms: von Meyenburg complex, bile duct hamartoma.* A ductal plate malformation is an abnormally shaped structure composed of bile ducts. The term is used in two distinct situations. First, a ductal plate malformation can refer to irregular, anastomosing biliary structures, often with focally open lumens, that encircle the portal tracts in cases of congenital hepatic fibrosis. Secondly, *ductal plate malformation* can be used to as a synonym for von Meyenburg complexes/bile duct hamartomas (Figure A.1.17).

Ductopenia; *synonym: bile duct loss.* Ductopenia is defined as the morphological loss of bile ducts. The most common cause is chronic biliary tract disease, but bile duct loss can also be seen in other conditions such as drug-induced liver injury and paraneoplastic syndromes.

When evaluating a specimen for bile duct loss, the size of the portal tract matters, as about 10% of normal but smaller sized portal tracts will not have bile ducts apparent on H&E, while medium-sized and larger portal tracts should essentially always have a bile duct visible on H&E. Portal inflammation may at times obscure bile ducts and immunostains can be very helpful to confirm bile duct loss. In some cases, looking for unpaired hepatic arteries can also help identify a portal tract with bile duct loss.[28] Be aware, however, that scarred central veins in fatty liver disease can recruit hepatic arteries[29] and, by so doing, can mimic a portal tract with an unpaired hepatic artery.

A commonly used guideline for the formal diagnosis of ductopenia is that 50% or more of smaller sized portal tracts are without bile ducts, assuming a reasonable sized biopsy of at least 10 portal tracts. The use of a 50% cut-off increases the specificity of the histological diagnosis, but

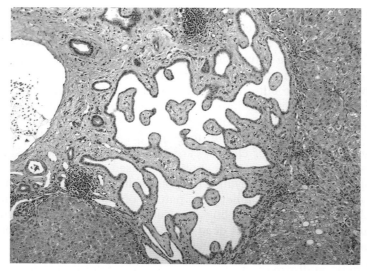

FIGURE A.1.17 **Ductal plate malformation.** These lesions are also called bile duct hamartomas or von Meyenburg complexes.

does lead to some loss of sensitivity. In those cases where bile duct loss falls between 50% and 20%, the possibility of early ductopenia can still be raised in the pathology report. Also, make sure to correlate the histological findings with the serum alkaline phosphatase levels, as a normal alkaline phosphatase level would be very unlikely with true ductopenia. CK7 typically shows intermediate hepatocytes in ductopenia, and a copper stain is commonly positive.

Elastosis. In the liver, elastosis is typically a mixture of elastic fibers as well as other material, principally reticulin. It has a distinctive, gray, paucicellular, homogeneous appearance, one that can mimic amyloid. Elastosis in the liver typically results from focal injury but can also be seen as part of the desmoplastic response in some cases of adenocarcinoma involving the liver. In the nonneoplastic setting, elastosis can be a very focal finding around an isolated central vein, a focal change in the liver capsule, or form a mass lesion in response to a subacute vascular injury.

Emperipolesis. Emperipolesis is a terrific word of Greek origin that literally means the presence of one intact cell inside the cytoplasm of another intact cell. In terms of liver pathology, emperipolesis became relevant when studies suggested the finding of lymphocytes within hepatocyte cytoplasm (emperipolesis) was a helpful microscopic criterion in making the diagnosis of autoimmune hepatitis.[30] In fact, for a while, it was heralded as one of the most important criterion to diagnose autoimmune hepatitis. This finding, however, appears to be more of an indicator of the severity of the lobular hepatitis[31] and not a specific finding for any etiology *per se*, including autoimmune hepatitis. In addition, the very presence of emperipolesis is somewhat elusive, as some pathologists report seeing it a lot, and others hardly ever—I'm in the latter group. In fact, after years of looking through all kinds of cases, lurking, waiting, I finally found a few cases that I thought had very nice emperipolesis, which I thus photographed from numerous different angles, in numerous different fields, to use in book chapters and talks for the rest of my life, since there is no guarantee that I will ever see it again (Figure A.1.18).

Fatty change. Fat and steatosis are synonyms and can be used interchangeably (the term "fat" retains its Middle English roots, while "steatosis" is derived from New Latin with Greek roots). The terms "fat," "fatty change," and "fatty degeneration" are used interchangeably, although the usage of the latter term is no longer common. Please see the steatosis entry for more information.

Feathery degeneration; *synonyms: cholate stasis, pseudoxanthomatous change.* This term refers to pale swollen hepatocytes in periportal or periseptal locations (or the edge of cirrhotic nodule) in livers with chronic cholestasis. Feathery degeneration is occasionally used to describe any swollen hepatocyte or groups of hepatocytes regardless of context.

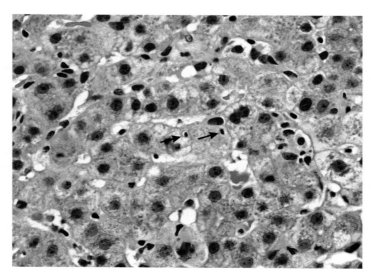

FIGURE A.1.18 **Emperipolesis.** A few lymphocytes appear to be located in the cytoplasm of hepatocytes (arrows), from a cause of autoimmune hepatitis.

Fibrous cap. Biopsies from livers with known cirrhosis are sometimes badly fragmented, and when this happens, small fragments of hepatocyte nodules can show a thin or thick rim of blue collagen on the trichrome stain, which has been called a *fibrous cap*. This observation is sometimes carried over to biopsies of livers where the fibrosis stage is not known beforehand. It is true that thick fibrous caps that surround much/most of the nodule most likely represents advanced fibrosis/cirrhosis, but caps that are thin and incomplete are insufficient for diagnosing cirrhosis, representing a potential diagnostic pitfall.

Fibrous septa. This term is most often used as a synonym for bridging fibrosis. In other situations, however, authors use *fibrous septa* to refer to irregular fibrous extensions from the portal tract, regardless of whether there is full bridging fibrosis. Thus, its meaning can only be understood by its context. As a pathology term, bridging fibrosis has the advantage of greater clarity and thus is preferable in diagnostic reports.

Fibro-obliterative duct lesion. This lesion is defined as a round or oval fibrous scar located in a portal tract, a scar that has replaced a bile duct (Figure A.1.19; eFigs. A.1.2 and A.1.3). Fibro-obliterative duct lesions are seen in a small of cases with chronic obstructive biliary tract disease. In most cases, the obstruction is due to chronic strictures that can either represent primary diseases, such as primary sclerosing cholangitis, or secondary strictures, for example, from an ischemic stricture.

Fibrin ring granuloma; *synonyms (not widely used, not recommended): doughnut hole granuloma, doughnut granuloma.* Fibrin ring granulomas

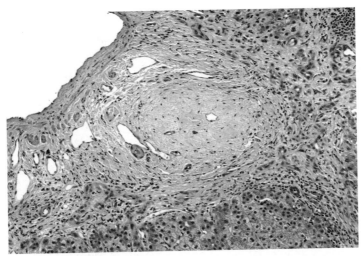

FIGURE A.1.19 **Fibro-obliterative duct lesion.** A fibro-obliterative duct lesion is seen in this case of long-standing primary sclerosing cholangitis. A fibrous plug has completely replaced the normal bile duct.

are small to medium sized and are always noncaseating, but have architecture that is a bit more complicated than ordinary granulomas. They have (1) a central plump droplet of lipid that is (2) surrounded by a thin, eosinophilic "fibrin" ring, followed by (3) an outer rim of epithelioid histiocytes. Sometimes, another layer is seen between the central lipid droplet and the fibrin: a thin ring of histiocytes, evident by a subtle, attenuated rim of nuclei.

In most specimens, not all fibrin ring granulomas have this picture-perfect morphology, and there will some granulomas with very small lipid droplets and others that have less evident or incomplete fibrin rings. Furthermore, in most biopsies with fibrin ring granulomas, there also will be other, often more numerous granulomas with a typical epithelioid appearance. Thus, the composite picture in most biopsy specimens is one of a continuum, extending from the complete, perfectly shaped fibrin ring granuloma to more ordinary epithelioid granuloma.

In most cases, the background liver shows fatty change and the fibrin ring morphology appears to reflect acute granuloma-inducing injury to a liver with steatosis, as opposed to indicating a specific etiology. Nevertheless, they are famously associated with Q-fever. They have also been reported in many other injuries superimposed on fatty liver disease, including drug reactions, EBV and other viral infections, and Hodgkin disease.

Florid duct lesion. A florid duct lesion is defined by lymphohistiocytic inflammation that is centered on a septal sized bile duct and is associated with bile duct epithelial damage and reactive epithelial changes (Figure A.1.20).

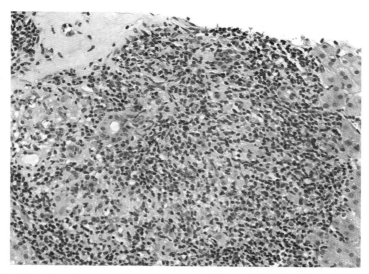

FIGURE A.1.20 **Florid duct lesion in primary biliary cholangitis (PBC).** This medium-sized bile duct (also called septal-sized) shows intense chronic inflammation with bile duct lymphocytosis and injury.

Occasionally, true epithelioid granulomas may be present, but the histiocytic component of the inflammation in most florid duct lesions is more loosely organized. Florid duct lesions can be seen in PBC and rarely in drug-induced liver injury.

Foam cell arteriopathy; *synonym: foam cell arteritis, foam cell endoarteritis, transplant arteriopathy.* Foam cell arteriopathy is defined as a hepatic artery with walls that are thickened and contain clusters of foamy macrophages. The lumen is typically narrowed. This distinctive pattern of injury is seen in medium and larger arteries in cases of chronic liver rejection and is only rarely sampled by peripheral liver biopsies.[32] In addition, portal veins can rarely show the same pattern of injury, with vessel walls that are thickened and filled with foamy macrophages, a finding called foam cell venopathy.[33]

Foamy degeneration. This term describes hepatocytes with a microvesicular steatosis pattern of injury and is used most commonly in the context of *acute foamy degeneration of the liver,* a rare form of alcohol-related liver disease.[9]

Focal biliary cirrhosis. This term is used almost exclusively in the cystic fibrosis literature. The basic notion is that the liver shows focal areas of histological cirrhosis in some parts of the biopsy, but not others. These focally cirrhotic areas also show portal tract inflammation and bile ductular proliferation. Of note, however, the term *focal biliary cirrhosis* is used inconsistently, and in some papers, the term has been used to describe patchy fibrosis of any degree, as long as it is associated with portal inflammation and bile ductular proliferation, regardless of whether the fibrosis reaches the level of cirrhosis. The concept of focal biliary cirrhosis is further complicated by the occurrence of nodular regenerative hyperplasia in some livers affected by cystic fibrosis.

Giant cell change/giant cell transformation. Giant cell change (Figure A.1.21) or giant cell transformation is defined as cells with three or more nuclei. In hepatocytes, this nonspecific reactive change can be seen in a variety of conditions. Rarely, similar findings are seen in biliary epithelium (Figure A.1.22).

Glycogen-storing foci. Glycogen-storing foci are well-circumscribed aggregates of hepatocytes with clear cytoplasm; they are best seen at low power, where they stand out from the background liver (Figure A.1.23). The clear cell change results from glycogen accumulation. These are incidental findings and do not need to be mentioned in surgical pathology reports.

Glycogenated nuclei. Glycogenated nuclei have clear or white vacuoles that typically fill up most of the nuclei, leaving only a thin rim of chromatin at the nuclear edges (Figure A.1.24). Sometimes the inclusions may be more eosinophilic, depending on the stain. Glycogenated nuclei can be found anywhere in the lobules but are somewhat more common

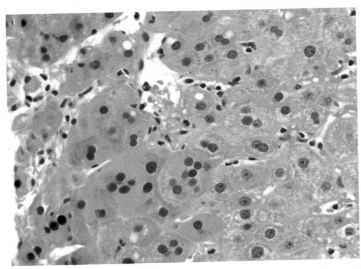

FIGURE A.1.21 **Hepatocyte giant cell transformation.** There is focal giant cell transformation in this liver biopsy.

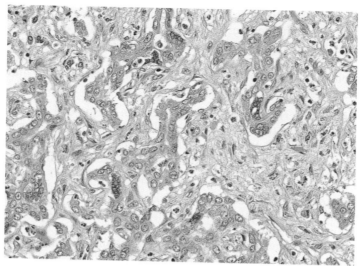

FIGURE A.1.22 **Bile duct multinucleation.** The proliferating bile ducts show focal multi-nucleation, an uncommon finding of uncertain significance.

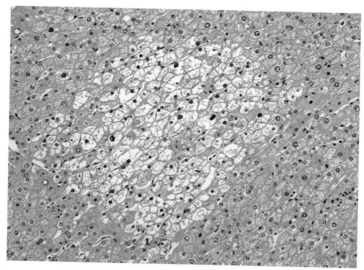

FIGURE A.1.23 **Glycogen-storing foci.** A well-delineated cluster of hepatocytes with clear cell change is seen. They are otherwise normal in their morphology.

in zone 1. They often cluster into small discrete patches. Glycogenated nuclei are a common finding, one that is not useful diagnostically and does not need to be mentioned in pathology reports. They are most commonly seen in fatty liver disease, where they are associated with diabetes mellitus.[34]

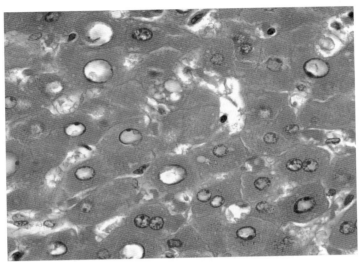

FIGURE A.1.24 **Glycogenated nuclei.** The hepatocyte nuclei in this field have a distinctive homogenous, clear appearance, called glycogenated nuclei.

Granuloma. A granuloma is a discrete collection of epithelioid histiocytes. Granulomas often have varying degrees of admixed lymphocytes. Depending on their appearance, granulomas can be further described as epithelioid, necrotizing, fibrin ring, lipid, or fibrotic. Granulomas can be found in the portal tracts or lobules and are commonly seen in both areas. When they are associated with bile duct inflammation and injury, they can be part of a florid duct lesion. Related terms are defined in the associated box.

Granuloma Terminology

- Granuloma: Cluster of epithelioid histiocytes.
- Granulomatous disease: A disease that has granulomas as a common or characteristic finding; examples include sarcoidosis, PBC.
- Granulomatous hepatitis: Lobular granulomas in the setting of a definite lobular hepatitis, usually a hepatitis that is moderate or severe.
- Granulomatous inflammation: A focal lesion composed of inflammation and a poorly formed granuloma. An example is a florid duct lesion.
- Microgranuloma: Small cluster of histiocytes marking the site of focal hepatocyte injury; this is an old term that is best left unused; instead use *Kupffer cell aggregate* if needed.

Ground glass change/ground glass inclusions. Hepatocytes infected with hepatitis B virus (HBV) can accumulate viral particles in their smooth endoplasmic reticulum, giving rise to a large, amphophilic, circumscribed inclusion in the cytoplasm (Figure A.1.25). These inclusions will be strongly

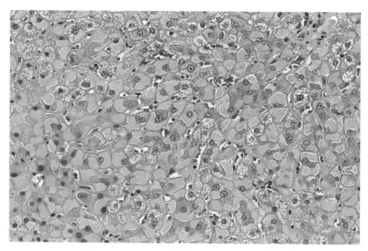

FIGURE A.1.25 **Hepatitis B ground glass**. The hepatocytes show numerous large round amphophilic cytoplasmic inclusions that represent accumulation of hepatitis B surface antigen in the smooth endoplasmic reticulin.

HBsAg positive. There are many conditions that can closely mimic HBV ground glass inclusions on the H&E morphology, so do not make a diagnosis of chronic HBV-associated ground glass changes without a confirmed clinical history or a positive immunostain.

Halo sign. The "halo sign" is a pattern best seen at low power, one that is most commonly found in cirrhotic livers with underlying chronic cholestatic liver diseases, such as PBC or primary sclerosing cholangitis. The cirrhotic nodules are surrounded by a thin rim of edema and cholate stasis that give the impression, on low-power examination, of a halo surrounding the cirrhotic nodule (Figure A.1.26).

Hepatic plate thickening. Hepatocytes in the normal liver are organized into plates or cords that are typically two cells in thickness in the quiescent liver. In an actively regenerating liver, however, the hepatic plates can be focally three to four cells in thickness. The reticulin stain is used to examine plate thickness. In the setting of a mass lesions, plates that are too thick suggest the possibility of hepatocellular carcinoma. Please see the entry for reticulin loss for additional discussion.

Hepatoportal sclerosis. This term technically refers to sclerosis (eg, fibrosis) of the intrahepatic portal veins, but in common usage refers to the atrophy or loss of portal veins, even if they are not specifically fibrotic on H&E.

Hyaline body. Hyaline bodies are seen in hepatocellular carcinomas as dense, eosinophilic inclusions located with the cytoplasm of tumor cells (Figure A.1.27). They are composed of various proteins, but presumably represent some sort of autophagy defect, as they stain for p62 and ubiquitin.

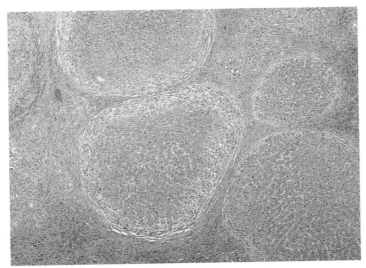

FIGURE A.1.26 **Halo sign.** In this case of cirrhosis from primary sclerosing cholangitis, the cirrhotic nodules have a light-colored "halo" due to cholate stasis.

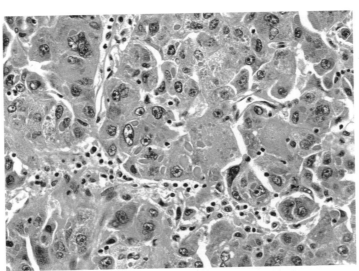

FIGURE A.1.27 **Hyaline body.** The tumor cells in this hepatocellular carcinoma have numerous eosinophilic globules in their cytoplasm.

Incomplete septal cirrhosis. This term is defined by the presence of delicate thin fibrous bands, which are often incomplete, in a liver with nodularity. The nodularity can be subtle and typically shows a macronodular pattern. Incomplete septal cirrhosis appears to represent cirrhosis undergoing regression.[26,35]

The clinical and histological features of incomplete septal cirrhosis can overlap with nodular regenerative hyperplasia, and partial nodular

transformation and the overlapping histological findings complicate interpretation of the published data. A useful approach is to classify a case
as incomplete septal cirrhosis if it clearly has thin delicate fibrous bands
accompanying the nodularity. If the nodularity is not accompanied by
fibrosis, then the best diagnosis is nodular regenerative hyperplasia. In partial nodular transformation, there is nodularity that is accentuated in the
hilum but largely absent in the periphery.

Induced hepatocyte. This term refers to a hepatocyte that has a smooth
amphophilic change affecting part of its cytoplasm (Figure A.1.28). It is
caused by smooth endoplasmic reticulum proliferation, usually in response
to a medication. In some cases, the hepatocytes can have a distinctive "two-
tone" or "tram-track" appearance to their cytoplasm.

Interface activity/interface hepatitis. When the row of hepatocytes that
immediately surrounds a portal tract (ie, the limiting plate) is inflamed and
damaged, the finding is called *interface activity* (Figure A.1.29). Interface
activity can be seen in acute and chronic hepatitis from many different
causes. Interface activity is commonly given a separate score when using a
formal grading system for chronic hepatitis. Older (now obsolete) terms for
this finding include *piecemeal necrosis* and *periportal hepatitis*.

Historically, some pathologists believed they could reliably distinguish
interface activity from lymphocytes that had harmlessly "spilled over" from
the portal tract into the zone 1 region, based on whether the inflammation
at the interface was accompanied by "hepatocyte damage." This approach
seems quite reasonable on paper and was historically important as part of

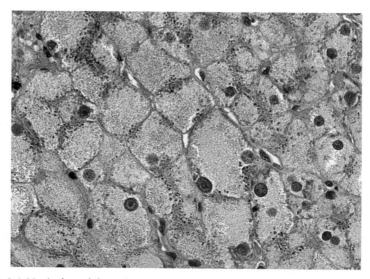

FIGURE A.1.28 **Induced hepatocytes.** These hepatocytes show changes of smooth
endoplasmic reticulum proliferation as a response to chronic medication. The hepatocytes
also show some lipofuscin.

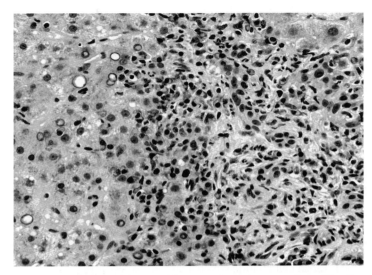

FIGURE A.1.29 **Interface activity.** In this case of autoimmune hepatitis, there is brisk inflammation at the interface between the portal tract and the lobules, obscuring the normally crisp interface.

efforts to classify hepatitis into chronic aggressive versus chronic persistent hepatitis, but in practice, this concept did not stand the test of time, in no small part because the notion of what constituted "hepatocyte damage" was rather subjective. Thus, there currently is no need to expend effort in deciding whether there is innocuous "spill-over" versus true interface activity; it is all considered interface activity. If some pathologists still believe that they can reliably distinguish between the two, there is no harm, as long as it does not influence diagnostic interpretation.

Iron-free foci. In cirrhotic livers that have severe iron deposition, the iron tends to be uniformly distributed throughout the many nodules. Some nodules, however, can stand out grossly because they have less iron accumulation; these should be well sampled because they are enriched for macroregenerative nodules, dysplastic nodules, small hepatocellular carcinoma, and small cholangiocarcinomas.

Lamellar fibrosis. Lamellar fibrosis is found most prominently in scirrhous hepatocellular carcinomas and in fibrolamellar carcinomas, where intratumoral bands of fibrosis tends to align in parallel arrays. The reason(s) for this distinctive pattern of fibrosis is not known. Interestingly, metastatic deposits of fibrolamellar carcinoma to lymph nodes or other organs can show the same distinctive pattern of fibrosis, indicating the lamellar fibrosis is not a reflection of underlying liver architecture.

Large cell change. Large cell change is defined as hepatocytes that have both increased amounts of cytoplasm and increased nuclear size, but with relative preservation of the normal nuclear:cytoplasmic ratio. The nuclei are typically enlarged and hyperchromatic and maybe be binucleated (Figure A.1.30).

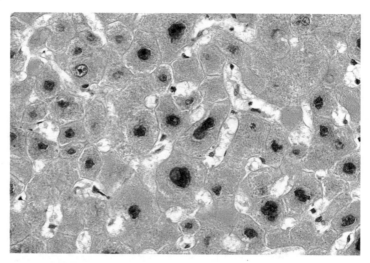

FIGURE A.1.30 Large cell change. The hepatocytes show large cell change in a patient with chronic HBV; the nuclei are enlarged and hyperchromatic, but there also is abundant cytoplasm, with a near-normal N:C ratio.

Large cell change is commonly encountered in cirrhotic livers from chronic hepatitis B, but can be seen with many different liver diseases. Overall, large cell changes are considerably more common in cirrhotic than noncirrhotic livers. Large cell change can be associated with DNA damage and potentially could be a marker of increased hepatocellular carcinoma risk, while in other cases, large cell change is thought to be degenerative. This distinction is based on molecular findings, one that cannot reliably be made on H&E alone. Large cell change does not need to be specifically mentioned in pathology reports.

Large cell change can be seen in macroregenerative nodules, dysplastic nodules, and hepatocellular carcinoma. Of note, large cell change can also be seen in other settings, such as inflammatory hepatic adenomas and androgen-related hepatic adenomas. Large cell change is more common than small cell change (see separate entry).

Limiting plate. The limiting plate is the single layer of hepatocytes immediately surrounding the portal tract.

Lipofuscin. Lipofuscin is a granular, yellow-brown pigment seen in the hepatocyte cytoplasm, typically with a strong zone 3 distribution (Figure A.1.31). It is composed of highly oxidized fatty acids and proteins that are cross linked, rendering them insoluble and no longer degradable by either lysosomal enzymes or by the proteasome.[36] Lipofuscin can be mistaken for iron or bile on H&E stains, but the true nature of the pigment can be readily sorted out by doing an iron stain to rule out iron, checking the serum bilirubin levels to rule out cholestasis, or doing a Fontana-Masson stain, which will stain the lipofuscin in a granular black pattern (Figure A.1.32).

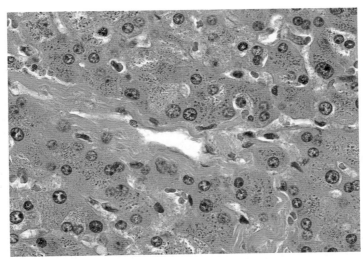

FIGURE A.1.31 **Lipofuscin.** The zone 3 hepatocytes show marked lipofuscin accumulation in their cytoplasm.

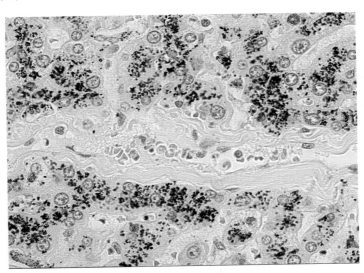

FIGURE A.1.32 **Lipofuscin, Fontana-Masson stain.** The lipofuscin has a black granular staining pattern.

Lipofuscin is often referred to as a "wear and tear pigment" and is more abundant in liver biopsies of the elderly.[37] In general, the more lipofuscin that is present in a postmitotic cell, the shorter the cell's life span.[36] Thus, lipofuscin accumulation may reflect the age of the cell better than the age of individual.[38] In this regard, there is a wide variation between lipofuscin density and a person's age, and its true significance in the liver remains unclear, although the significance is generally thought to be minimal or none in terms of sporadic cases (those not associated with Dubin-Johnson or Gilbert syndrome). Ceroid pigment is essentially a synonym, though some would argue that there are subtle differences.

Lobule. In common usage, the term *lobule* refers to "where the hepatocytes are located" and is not meant to indicate anything more than that. In formal usage, at least when discussing microanatomy, the lobule is defined as the smallest unit of the liver that has portal tracts, hepatocytes, and central veins.

The anatomic lobule, using the formal definition, is conceptualized in three main ways. First, the "classic" lobule is shown as a hexagonal structure with one portal tract at each of the six corners and the central vein in the middle. This hexagonal lobule works well in cartoons, but is hardly ever seen in its ideal form in human livers. Second, the lobule can be conceptualized as a "hepatic acinus," which is shaped like a short, fat diamond, with top and bottom corners located at portal tracts, and the side corners located in central veins (see entry for *hepatic acinus*). The hepatic acinus attempts to capture the microanatomy according to blood flow and gives rise to the notion of hepatic zones, with zone 1 hepatocytes (periportal hepatocytes) receiving blood that is the most nutrient and oxygen rich. Third, the lobule can be drawn as a "portal lobule," a triangle-shaped structure with a central vein at each edge and a single portal tract in the middle. Three-dimensional reconstruction of the liver acinus adds additional layers of complexity that are interesting,[39] but the basic notions of zones 1, 2, and 3 are the most important for practical pathology.

Lobular collapse. Severe liver injury can lead to parenchymal collapse. Early lesions show the loss of hepatocytes replaced by a robust ductular proliferation and mixed inflammation. Later lesions show less ductular proliferation, variable amounts of chronic inflammation, hepatocyte regeneration, and sometimes early fibrosis. In both early and later cases, the portal tracts can be closer together than in normal livers.

Macrovesicular steatosis. This term is used both for single cells and for an important pattern of injury. A single hepatocyte with macrovesicular steatosis shows a large droplet of fat that distends the cytoplasm and pushes the nucleus to the side.

In pathology reports, the term *macrovesicular steatosis* typically refers to the pattern of injury, not an individual cell. When used in this context, macrovesicular steatosis indicates the predominant pattern of fatty change in the lobules, and some degree of small and intermediate fat is invariably present.

Mallory hyaline. Mallory hyaline is also referred to as Mallory-Denk bodies.[40] Mallory hyaline is seen as eosinophilic clumps and irregular aggregates of cytoplasmic proteins, usually in ballooned hepatocytes (Figure A.1.33; eFig. A.1.4). Mallory hyaline is most often found in the setting of steatohepatitis, but can be seen in a wide variety of chronic liver diseases outside of fatty liver disease, in particular with chronic cholestasis. Mallory hyaline represents damaged and ubiquitinated cytoskeleton proteins and can be immunostained, if you so desire, with ubiquitin (Figure A.1.34), p62, or cytokeratins 8 and 18.[41-43]

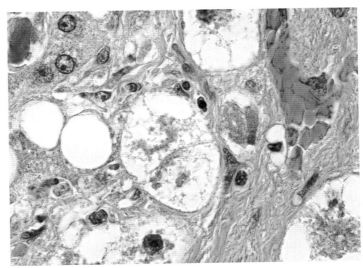

FIGURE A.1.33 **Mallory hyaline.** Mallory hyaline forms pink ropy aggregates in the cytoplasm of these ballooned hepatocytes.

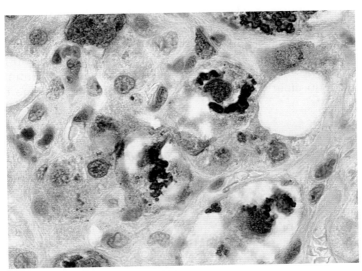

FIGURE A.1.34 **Mallory hyaline, ubiquitin.** The Mallory hyaline is strongly ubiquitin positive.

    Classic Mallory hyaline is easily identified. There can be a lot of subtle cytoplasmic changes on H&E stains that may or may not be Mallory hyaline, depending on the eye of the beholder. This has led to considerable variation in the frequency of Mallory hyaline reported in various studies. Not surprisingly, Mallory hyaline that is readily seen and is typically located in ballooned hepatocytes is the most reproducibly identified. Subtle cytoplasmic changes on H&E stain that may or may not represent Mallory hyaline do not need to be further evaluated by special stains. In fact, for practical purposes, there is little diagnostic importance for even classic Mallory hyaline, as its diagnostic value is fully captured in most cases by the balloon cell itself. Thus, immunostains for Mallory hyaline are best used for fun and interest.

Microabscess. Also called a mini-microabscess, this lobular finding is composed of a small distinct cluster of neutrophils in the sinusoids (Figure A.1.35). This finding is nonspecific, but typically prompts a CMV immunostain in the transplanted population.

Microgranuloma. A microgranuloma was historically defined as a small collection of lobular Kupffer cells (typically 3-7), located in a site of recent hepatocyte death and drop out. The macrophages may be pigmented (Figure A.1.36) and are typically PASD positive. This finding is common and does not have the same biological or clinical meaning as true granulomas. Since the term "microgranuloma" can be confused by clinical teams to mean true granulomas, the term is probably best avoided in surgical pathology reports. If you need a good term, *Kupffer cell aggregate* is a better option.

Micronodular cirrhosis/macronodular cirrhosis. Before the major etiologies for cirrhosis were known, cirrhotic livers were classified by their morphological findings into *micronodular cirrhosis* and *macronodular cirrhosis*, an early approach that attempted to better understand potential risk factors for cirrhosis.

In this classification system, cases were categorized by the average size of the individual cirrhotic nodules, typically using a cut off of 3 mm or less to define micronodular cirrhosis, but sometimes 5 mm or less. If there was no clear pattern for the predominant size of the cirrhotic

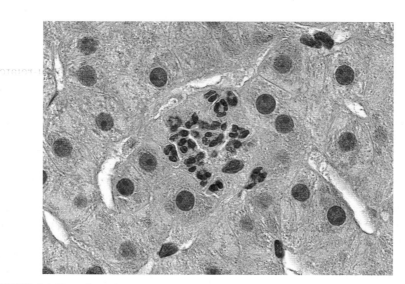

FIGURE A.1.35 **Microabscess**. The lobules contain a small cluster of neutrophils in the sinusoids.

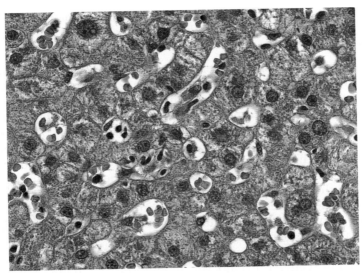

FIGURE A.1.36 **Micrograntulomas.** These small Kupffer cell aggregates are sometimes called *microgranulomas,* but a better term is *Kupffer cell aggregates.*

nodules, if the numbers of micro- and macro-sized nodules were approximately equal, then the term *mixed micro- and macronodular cirrhosis* was used. As research studies were undertaken, it became clear that this classification system was not entirely stable, as micronodular patterns of cirrhosis could evolve into macronodular patterns, especially if the injury abated.[44]

Over the years, other terms were used as synonyms for *micronodular cirrhosis* and *macronodular cirrhosis.* Synonyms for micronodular cirrhosis included *portal cirrhosis, regular cirrhosis, monolobular cirrhosis,* and *nutritional cirrhosis* (the latter because it was not clear if the alcohol-related cirrhosis, which typically causes a micronodular pattern, resulted from the alcohol itself or from nutritional deficiencies). The term *Laennec cirrhosis* was also commonly used for alcohol-related cirrhosis, alcohol being one of the first etiologies for cirrhosis demonstrated by medicine. For macronodular cirrhosis, synonyms included *postnecrotic cirrhosis, posthepatitic cirrhosis, irregular cirrhosis,* and *multilobular cirrhosis.*

As specific etiologies were discovered for cirrhosis, the etiologies naturally became the basis for classifying liver disease, and this older nomenclature, which is based on the size of the cirrhotic nodules and not etiology, is obsolete. Early studies did, however, go back and map these old patterns to specific etiologies. In general, they found these correlates for the micronodular pattern of cirrhosis: alcoholic cirrhosis, alpha-1 antitrypsin deficiency, Indian childhood cirrhosis, vascular outflow disease, cirrhosis from biliary obstruction, PBC, and hemochromatosis. In contrast, macronodular cirrhosis generally correlated with these etiologies: chronic viral hepatitis B, chronic viral hepatitis C, autoimmune hepatitis, and Wilson disease, but also some cases of alcoholic liver disease and alpha-1 antitrypsin deficiency.

Microvesicular steatosis. This term is used in two ways, one as a descriptor of an individual cell and one as a pattern of injury. Individual hepatocytes show microvesicular steatosis when they have very small droplets of fat that diffusely fill their cytoplasm. But this is not enough to make a *diagnosis* of a microvesicular steatosis pattern of injury, which requires that microvesicular steatosis be the dominant pattern of injury, diffusely present throughout the liver. Not all hepatocytes need to be affected to qualify for a diagnosis of microvesicular steatosis, as zone 1 hepatocytes are often spared, and there can be scattered large droplet fat, but the microvesicular changes should be seen in essentially all zone 3/2 areas of the liver. The diagnosis of microvesicular steatosis has its own distinct differential, usually indicating mitochondrial injury.

In contrast, microvesicular steatosis at the individual cell level is commonly seen in scattered hepatocytes in all forms of fatty liver disease and many different acute injuries; this usage in pathology reports leads to a lot of confusion. The good news is that there is no need to use the term *microvesicular steatosis* in a pathology report unless you mean the microvesicular steatosis pattern of injury.

For diagnostic purposes, microvesicular steatosis should be diagnosed on H&E and not solely on Oil red O stains. Of note, Oil red O stains show extensive small droplet staining in many different liver diseases that are not microvesicular steatosis.[45] Diagnostic misadventures are quite possible in cases where a pathologist overrelies on Oil red O stains.

Megamitochondria. Megamitochondria are round to oval eosinophilic structures located in the hepatocyte cytoplasm (Figure A.1.37). Megamitochondria represent damaged mitochondria and are most commonly seen in fatty liver disease, both alcoholic and nonalcoholic, but can be found in a wide range of liver conditions. Hepatocytes with megamitochondria can be located anywhere within the hepatic lobules. In some cases, megamitochondria can mimic alpha-1-antitrysin globules on H&E stain; when necessary, the two can be distinguished by special stains, including a PASD for alpha-1-antitrysin globules and a phosphotungstic acid-hematoxylin stain (PTAH) for megamitochondria (Figure A.1.38).

Multilocular. The term *multilocular* is used to describe a single large cystic structure that has internal septations. A cut grape fruit is often used as an illustration, with the grape fruit rind forming the walls of the cyst and the pulp divided into multilocular segments by thin membranous septations.

Multicystic. Multicystic refers to cystic structures that are individually unilocular but cluster together. A cluster of grapes is often used to illustrate the concept, with each grape representing a single cyst.

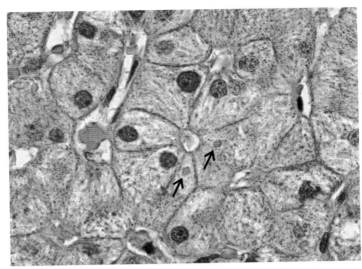

FIGURE A.1.37 **Megamitochondria in hepatocytes.** The megamitochondria are seen as small pink cytoplasmic inclusions that are round to oval in shape (arrows).

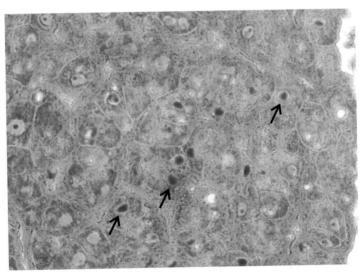

FIGURE A.1.38 **Megamitochondria, phosphotungstic acid-hematoxylin stain (PTAH) stain.** The megamitochondria stain dark blue and often have a thin surrounding halo (arrows).

Nodular regenerative hyperplasia. Nodular regenerative hyperplasia is a reactive parenchymal change due to irregular blood flow within the liver. On low-power histological examination, the liver has a nodular appearance, but the nodularity is not due to fibrosis. Instead, the nodularity results from areas of zone 3 hepatocyte atrophy, alternating with areas of normal-sized or even somewhat enlarged hepatocytes centered on zone 1. These changes can be enhanced by using a reticulin stain.

Onion-skin fibrosis. Onion-skin fibrosis has a concentric, laminated appearance (Figure A.1.39) and most commonly affects medium-sized bile ducts. This finding typically indicates chronic biliary tract obstruction. As onion-skin fibrosis progresses, it can lead to fibro-obliterative duct lesions. Of note, the bile ducts in medium and larger sized portal tracts often have a normal collar of dense collagen, and this should not be overinterpreted as onion-skin fibrosis.

Pancreatic acinar cell metaplasia. In about 4% of explants and autopsy livers, small clusters of cells with acinar cell differentiation are located in the soft tissue surrounding the large bile ducts of the hilum (Figure A.1.40).[46,47] Pancreatic acinar cell metaplasia can be identified in both cirrhotic and noncirrhotic livers. These changes are assumed to represent metaplasia, although they are sometimes referred to as heterotopias in the literature, and rare examples may be true heterotopias. In most cases, however, pancreatic acinar cell metaplasia arises in benign, reactive peribiliary glands.

Pale body. Pale bodies are single large cytoplasmic inclusions found in malignant hepatocytes, most commonly in fibrolamellar carcinomas but also in a small number of conventional hepatocellular carcinomas. The pale body is round, fills much of the cytoplasm, and is gray in color (Figure A.1.41). Electron microscopy studies suggest they originate from dilated bile canaliculi that are mislocated within the tumor cell cytoplasm, and then get filled with various proteins.[48,49] Pale bodies stain variably for fibrinogen, p62, and a number of other proteins.

Panacinar necrosis; *synonym: panlobular necrosis.* Panacinar necrosis is a severe form of confluent necrosis where entire lobular fields of hepatocytes are absent. In their place, there may be a brisk ductular reaction,

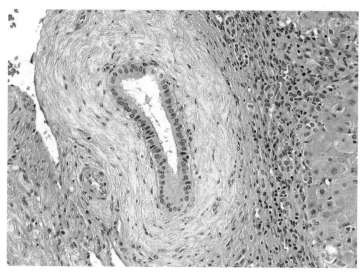

FIGURE A.1.39 **Onion-skin fibrosis.** The bile duct has a thick rim of layered fibrosis, also called as "onion-skin" fibrosis.

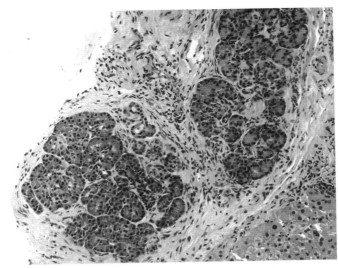

FIGURE A.1.40 **Pancreatic acinar cell metaplasia.** This finding is most commonly seen in explants or biopsies that include hilar tissue. It is not specific for any pattern of disease injury.

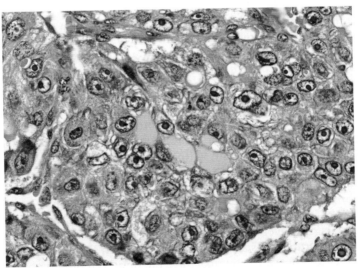

FIGURE A.1.41 **Pale body in conventional hepatocellular carcinoma.** Several tumor cells have large amphophilic cytoplasmic inclusions. Pale bodies are common in fibrolamellar carcinoma, but can also be seen in conventional hepatocellular carcinoma.

inflammatory cells, and pigment-laden macrophages. The portal tracts will often be more closely approximated than in the normal liver.

Partial nodular transformation. This term refers to distinct nodularity in the hilar area of the liver. The nodularity is not due to fibrosis but instead is essentially an exuberant form of nodular regenerative hyperplasia, but one that is localized to the hilum/center of the liver. Partial nodular transformation is typically associated with portal vein thrombosis or other vascular flow abnormalities, but can also be seen in a subset of livers with primary sclerosing cholangitis. The parenchyma in the periphery of the liver can be normal or atrophic.

Pericholangitis. Pericholangitis is an older term, for the most part obsolete, that describes a bile ductular reaction that is accompanied by neutrophilic inflammation.

Historically, before primary sclerosing cholangitis (PSC) was recognized as a distinct entity, *pericholangitis* was used to described the histological findings in patients with ulcerative colitis who also had what was then an undefined chronic biliary tract disease, one that we now know as PSC. Since the pathology community now recognizes the histological changes of PSC, there is little use for this older term.

Its use, however, has persisted, with some pathologists using the term as originally defined, essentially as synonym for the histology findings in PSC patients, while others use the term for a ductular reaction from any etiology, and still others as a synonym for the small duct variant of PSC. Because of the fuzzy use of the term, and because other, better terms are available, abandoning its use in liver pathology was suggested 30 years ago,[50] a good suggestion both then and now.

Periportal hepatitis/piecemeal necrosis. Both of these terms are historically interesting but largely obsolete and have been replaced by *interface activity*. While there was nothing terribly wrong with either of the older terms, it is best to use *interface activity* for clarity of communication; at this point, only very old people know the meaning of, or have ever used, the terms *periportal hepatitis* or *piecemeal necrosis*.

Periportal fibrosis. The term *periportal fibrosis* is used inconsistently in the literature and in pathology reports. Preferences for *periportal* fibrosis versus *portal* fibrosis tend to correlate with where pathologists did their training. In many ways, the terms are synonymous, both capturing a mild form of fibrosis affecting the portal tracts. *Portal fibrosis* emphasizes the structure that is fibrotic (portal tract), while *periportal fibrosis* emphasizes where the new collagen is being laid down (next to the original portal region).

There is, however, significant variation in what is precisely meant by the term *periportal fibrosis*. The different uses can be grouped into at least five major categories, and you may have encountered others not listed here: (1) as a synonym for portal fibrosis (most common usage); (2) to indicate that there is "spiky" portal fibrosis, with irregular edges that show thin or thick, but short, fibrous extensions that extend into zone 1; (3) as a specific fibrosis stage that includes both portal fibrosis and early bridging fibrosis, for example, in the Batts-Ludwig staging system[51]; (4) as an indicator of "newly laid fibrosis," where the user believes the original portal tract is still visible on trichrome by a dark blue color, with an outer rim of newly-laid, lighter-blue fibrosis; and, finally, (5) a finding that can suggest fibrosis regression.[52] In many cases, an author's precise meaning for the term *periportal fibrosis* is difficult to discern with confidence. For all of these reasons, *periportal fibrosis* as pathology term lacks the clarity of communication possessed by *portal fibrosis*.

Pericellular fibrosis; *synonyms: sinusoidal fibrosis, perisinusoidal fibrosis.* Pericellular fibrosis is defined as irregular strands of fibrosis within the hepatic parenchyma, with collagen deposited between hepatocytes and the sinusoids (Figure A.1.42; eFig. A.1.5). Another more colorful term is "chicken wire fibrosis." Pericellular fibrosis is most commonly encountered in fatty liver disease but can also be seen with vascular outflow disease, drug induced liver injury, and many other conditions (see Chapter 2, Table 6). It can also be observed as an idiosyncratic finding in long-standing liver allografts. In most cases, the pericellular fibrosis is located in zone 3, but in some diseases, it can be located in zone 1, for example, fibrosing cholestatic hepatitis C.

Portal vein herniation. Portal veins are normally located in the center of portal tracts, but in some cases of noncirrhotic portal hypertension, they can be located at the periphery of the portal tract, focally bulging or extending out into the lobules (Figure A.1.43). When well-developed and present in multiple portal tracts, this finding supports a diagnosis of hepatoportal sclerosis. Subtler changes are common in diseased livers and are not as specific.

Phospholipidosis. This is a rare finding where Kupffer cells show distinctive, abundant foamy cytoplasm. The background liver often shows fatty change. Phospholipidosis is a response to drugs; over 50 drugs have been linked to this pattern, most commonly antidepressants, antimalarials, antianginals, and cholesterol-lowering agents.[53]

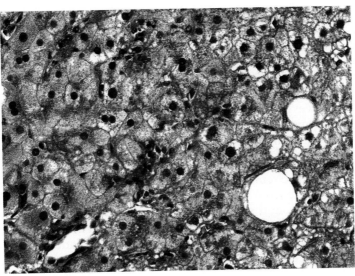

FIGURE A.1.42 **Pericellular fibrosis.** Pericellular fibrosis is seen on trichrome stain in a case of steatohepatitis.

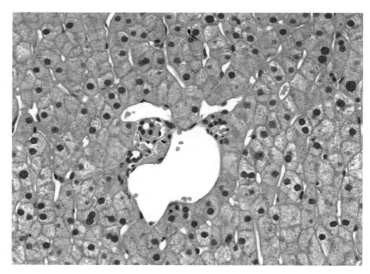

FIGURE A.1.43 **Portal vein herniation.** The portal vein is dilated and appears to herniate out of the portal tract into the hepatic lobules.

Pipestem fibrosis; *synonym, Symmers fibrosis.* This term describes bulky fibrosis that involves the portal vein, a pattern most commonly seen with schistosomiasis, where the organisms can elicit a granulomatous response that causes fibrosis of the portal veins. In addition, the overall portal tracts tend to be fibrotic and round.

Portal hepatitis; *synonyms: chronic portal inflammation, triaditis.* This term refers to inflammation within the portal tracts, typically lymphocytic. The term *chronic portal inflammation* is more widely used.

Poulsen lesion *synonym: Poulsen-Cristoffersen lesions.* Bile duct lymphocytosis and reactive epithelial changes define this lesion. This lesion is seen in both chronic hepatitis C and B and in some medication effects. In a classic Poulsen lesion, the affected bile duct will be associated with a lymphoid aggregate. However, many times, the term is used more loosely to indicate any bile duct lymphocytosis and injury, mostly in the setting of chronic hepatitis C or B. The finding has no particular diagnostic or clinical significance.

Pseudoglands; *synonym: pseudoacinar.* Pseudoglands are found in hepatocellular tumors as circular structures with a centrally dilated lumen, which can varying in size from small to huge (Figure A.1.44). The cells lining the pseudoglands look and stain like ordinary hepatocytes. Pseudoglands are seen in a subset of hepatocellular carcinomas, which tend to be enriched for *CTNNB1* mutations, as well as in atypical hepatic adenomas.

Pseudoground glass. This term refers to large, amphophilic, cytoplasmic inclusions in hepatocytes. In most cases, they represent smooth endoplasmic reticulum proliferation in response to drugs. The histological findings

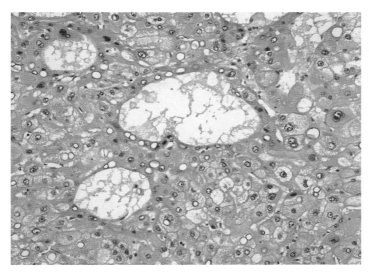

FIGURE A.1.44 **Pseudoglands in a hepatocellular carcinoma.** Some hepatocellular carcinomas have focal dilated space lined by tumor cells. They are not true glands.

closely mimic the ground glass inclusions that can be seen in chronic hepatitis B infection.

Pseudorosettes; *synonym: hepatic rosettes.* Pseudorosettes are seen as small circular structures in the lobules, formed by a group of hepatocytes (Figure A.1.45). They occur in two primary settings. First, livers with marked inflammation from any cause can have active regeneration and show scattered pseudorosettes; one good example is acute autoimmune hepatitis. The second common setting is when there is significant lobular cholestasis, leading to cholestatic rosettes. Cholestatic rosettes tend to be more common in zones 2 and 3, while regenerative rosettes tend to be more common in zones 1 and 2.

Pseudoxanthomatous change; *synonyms: feathery degeneration, cholate stasis.* This term is used to describe cluster of hepatocytes with pale foamy cytoplasm in the setting of chronic cholestasis. The cytoplasm has some resemblance to lipid-laden (xanthomatous) macrophages, thus the term, "pseudoxanthomatous." Affected hepatocytes are usually located in zone 1, or at the edges of cirrhotic nodules.

Reticulin loss; *synonym: reticulin reduction.* Reticulin loss in a neoplastic process supports a diagnosis of hepatocellular carcinoma, separating it from benign liver proliferations, which retain a normal reticulin pattern.

In nonmalignant hepatocellular lesions, the hepatic cords or plates are two or three cells thick and essentially every hepatocyte touches reticulin on at least one of its borders. In hepatocellular carcinoma, this reticulin framework is disrupted and there are foci, or even larger groups, of

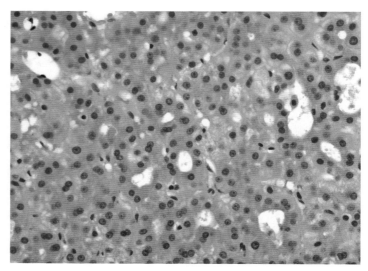

FIGURE A.1.45 **Pseudorosettes cholestatic.** Pseudorosettes are seen in this biopsy that showed bland lobular cholestasis.

hepatocytes that have no associated reticulin. As with all special stains, reticulin needs to be interpreted in the context of the morphology, as there can be focally thickening of the hepatic plates, beyond the two to three cells seen normally, in rapidly proliferating livers following acute injury. In addition, there can be physiological loss of reticulin in the setting of fatty liver disease.[54]

Riedel lobe. Riedel lobes are a fairly common anatomic variant and are not an abnormality *per se*, although they are often classified as an accessory lobe. They were first described in 1888 in a case series of 10 women who all underwent surgery for a palpable abdominal mass.[55] The prevalence is about 9%, and they are more common in women.[8] Riedel lobes project from the anterior right lobe of the liver, usually along its lateral side, extending inferiorly into the right flank and/or iliac fossa. Riedel lobes can be fairly uniform in width or can be more like an upside down pyramid.

Sanded glass nuclei. This term refers to hepatocyte nuclei with eosinophilic inclusions that largely fill the entire nuclei and have a finely granular appearance (Figure A.1.46). They are most commonly seen with hepatitis B infection and represent accumulation of HBV core antigen, but are not specific, occasionally being present in other diseases. Even in HBV they are uncommon.

Small cell change; *synonym, small cell dysplasia.* Small cell change is seen as small aggregates of hepatocytes with relatively little cytoplasm but otherwise normal, or nearly normal, nuclear and cytoplasmic cytology (Figure A.1.47). Hepatocytes with small cell change tend to have increased proliferative rates, but no loss of reticulin has been shown. Molecular studies

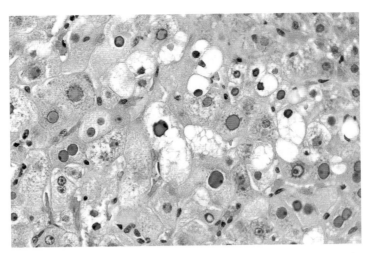

FIGURE A.1.46 **Sanded glass nuclei.** The hepatocytes have reddish appearing smooth nuclear inclusions. This case is from hepatitis B infection, and the nuclear change represents accumulation of hepatitis B core antigen.

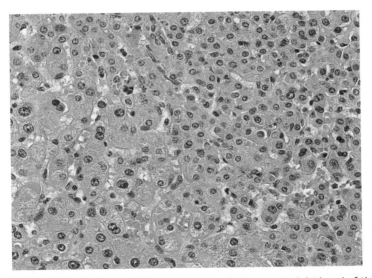

FIGURE A.1.47 **Small cell change.** The hepatocytes in the upper right hand of this image show small cell change.

have identified chromosomal damage and other DNA changes that support a role as a precursor for hepatocellular carcinoma, although the prognostic value for future cancer risk remains poorly defined.

Spotty necrosis. This term is used to indicate the presence of scattered small foci of hepatocyte loss, typically associated with a small cluster of lobular inflammation composed of lymphocytes and Kupffer cells. You may or may not see the actual dead hepatocytes. Sometimes these foci are referred to as "tombstones" because they mark the sites of hepatocyte death.

Steatosis; *synonyms, fat, fatty change.* Fat and steatosis are synonyms and can be used interchangeably, though there tends to be a general usage preference for *steatosis* as a microscopic finding and *fat* as a gross observation. Histological steatosis is further divided into microvesicular and macrovesicular steatosis patterns (Figures A.1.48 and A.1.49), which have distinctly different differentials.

Microvesicular steatosis is defined by numerous small droplets of fat that are often barely visible at the resolution of light microscopy. In contrast, macrovesicular steatosis typically has a single large droplet of fat that fills the entire cell cytoplasm.

In most diseases, however, there will be some admixture of both, and it is the predominant pattern that should be the histological focus. For example, the fatty change associated with the metabolic syndrome is of the macrovesicular pattern, but there invariably is some degree of hepatocytes with microvesicular steatosis mixed in, as well as a fair number of fat droplets whose sizes are intermediate between that of microvesicular and macrovesicular.

Stellate cell; *synonym (historical). Ito cell* Stellate cells were first described in 1898, by Karl Wilhelm Ritter von Kupffer, for whom of course the Kupffer cell is named; he believed, however, that they were phagocytic cells.[56] Subsequently, in 1951, Toshio Ito described them and differentiated them from Kupffer cells.

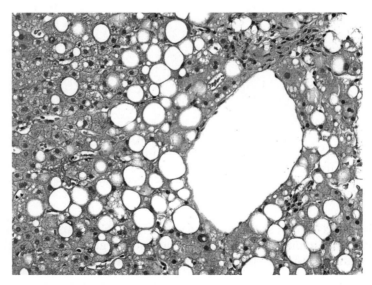

FIGURE A.1.48 **Macrovesicular steatosis.** Macrovesicular steatosis is seen in a case of obesity. Note that the size of fat droplets varies, but this pattern is still called macrovesicular steatosis.

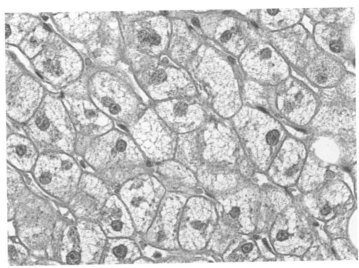

FIGURE A.1.49 **Microvesicular steatosis.** The hepatocytes show tiny droplets of fat that fill the cytoplasm and diffusely affect the hepatocytes.

Stellate cells are inconspicuous cells located in the space of Disse. They are not evident by H&E in normal liver tissue or in most liver diseases. In the normal liver, they store vitamin A and likely having many other functions we are unaware of. Ultrastructural studies have shown stellate cells have dendritic processes that extend around the liver sinusoids. When activated by chronic liver injury, stellate cells lose their vitamin A, become myofibroblastic in morphology, and are major drivers of fibrosis.

Stellate cells can be seen on H&E in the setting of hypervitaminosis A as small sinusoidal cells containing multiple tiny vacuoles that indent the nuclei (Figure A.1.50). Despite a lot of effort, no sensitive or specific immunostain marker for stellate cells in human tissue have been reported to date.

Triaditis. This term refers to inflammation in the portal tract. It does not mean that any of the structures that form the "triad"–the portal tract, hepatic artery, portal vein–are actually inflamed; only that there is some degree of inflammation in the connective tissue within portal tract. This term is largely obsolete, replaced by *portal inflammation.*

Small Hepatocellular carcinoma. Small hepatocellular carcinomas are defined as those that are less than 2 cm in size and arise in a background of cirrhosis. These designations are mostly for research purposes and do not need to be included in the pathology report.

Small hepatocellular carcinomas are further subdivided into tumors that are well circumscribed and stand out from the background cirrhotic nodules (*distinctly nodular*) or those that have less distinct boundaries (*vaguely nodular*).[57] The vaguely nodular pattern of early hepatocellular

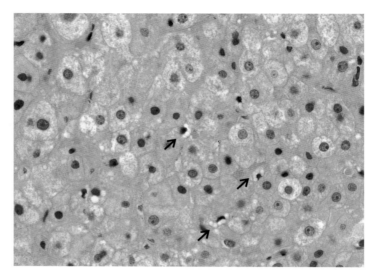

FIGURE A.1.50 **Stellate cell hyperplasia.** The sinusoids contain small cells (arrows) with cytoplasm extended by small droplets of fat—a subtle finding!

carcinoma often develops from dysplastic nodules and so may have residual areas of dysplastic nodules at their edges, including a few portal tracts. They are hypovascular on imaging, lack a well-developed pseudocapsule, are well-differentiated (>90%), and rarely show vascular invasion (5%). In contrast, the distinctly nodular pattern is hypervascular on imaging, often has a pseudocapsule (50%), is more likely to be moderately differentiated (60%), and is more likely to have vascular invasion (40%).[57]

von Meyenburg Complex; *synonym: bile duct plate malformation, bile duct hamartoma.* A von Meyenburg Complex is a small tangle of bile ducts, typically located in or adjacent to a portal tract. They are primarily located in the smaller branches of the biliary tree. This lesion was named after the Swiss pathologist Hanns von Meyenburg (1887-2013;1971), who was chair of pathology at Zurich. When sporadic, these benign lesions are typically single or few in number. They are, however, also routinely present in livers with polycystic kidney/liver disease, in which case they are diffusely distributed throughout much of the liver.

Zones 1, 2, and 3; *synonym: Rappaport zones.* The lobules can be divided into zones, reflecting the blood flow through the sinusoids, from zone 1 near the portal tracts through the sinusoids to zone 3 near the central veins (see Figure A.1.4). Zone 2 is defined more by default, being the portion of the lobules that is in between zones 1 and 3. The widths of the zones are not precisely defined, but the most common approach is to divide the lobules into three approximately equal zones, going from the portal tracts to the central veins.

REFERENCES

1. Kakar S, Torbenson M, Jain D, et al. Immunohistochemical pitfalls in the diagnosis of hepatocellular adenomas and focal nodular hyperplasia: accurate understanding of diverse staining patterns is essential for diagnosis and risk assessment. *Mod Pathol.* 2015;28:159-160.

2. Torbenson M, Yasir S, Anders R, et al. Regenerative hepatic pseudotumor: a new pseudotumor of the liver. *Hum Pathol.* 2020;99:43-52.

3. Krings G, Can B, Ferrell L. Aberrant centrizonal features in chronic hepatic venous outflow obstruction: centrilobular mimicry of portal-based disease. *Am J Surg Pathol.* 2014;38:205-214.

4. Mall F. A study of the structural unit of the liver. *Am J Anat.* 1906;5(3):227-308.

5. Koga C, Murakami M, Shimizu J, et al. A Case of Extrahepatic Hepatocellular Cancer Discovered during Gynecological Laparoscopic Surgery. Article in Japanese. *Gan To Kagaku Ryoho.* 2015;42:1866-1868.

6. Leone N, De Paolis P, Carrera M, et al. Ectopic liver and hepatocarcinogenesis: report of three cases with four years' follow-up. *Eur J Gastroenterol Hepatol.* 2004;16:731-735.

7. Arakawa M, Kimura Y, Sakata K, et al. Propensity of ectopic liver to hepatocarcinogenesis: case reports and a review of the literature. *Hepatology.* 1999;29:57-61.

8. Glenisson M, Salloum C, Lim C, et al. Accessory liver lobes: anatomical description and clinical implications. *J Visc Surg.* 2014;151:451-455.

9. Uchida T, Kao H, Quispe-Sjogren M, et al. Alcoholic foamy degeneration—a pattern of acute alcoholic injury of the liver. *Gastroenterology.* 1983;84:683-692.

10. Lackner C, Gogg-Kamerer M, Zatloukal K, et al. Ballooned hepatocytes in steatohepatitis: the value of keratin immunohistochemistry for diagnosis. *J Hepatol.* 2008;48:821-828.

11. Guy CD, Suzuki A, Burchette JL, et al. Costaining for keratins 8/18 plus ubiquitin improves detection of hepatocyte injury in nonalcoholic fatty liver disease. *Hum Pathol.* 2012;43:790-800.

12. Abraham S, Torbenson M. Von-Meyenburg complexes increase with age and are specifically associated with alcoholic cirrhosis and end-stage hepatitis B infection. *Lab Invest.* 2006;86:266A.

13. Wu TT, Levy M, Correa AM, et al. Biliary intraepithelial neoplasia in patients without chronic biliary disease: analysis of liver explants with alcoholic cirrhosis, hepatitis C infection, and noncirrhotic liver diseases. *Cancer.* 2009;115:4564-4575.

14. Tobe K. Electron microscopy of liver lesions in primary biliary cirrhosis. I. Intrahepatic bile duct oncocytes. *Acta Pathol Jpn.* 1982;32:57-70.

15. Ray MB, Mendenhall CL, French SW, et al. Bile duct changes in alcoholic liver disease. The Veterans Administration Cooperative Study Group. *Liver.* 1993;13:36-45.

16. Roskams TA, Theise ND, Balabaud C, et al. Nomenclature of the finer branches of the biliary tree: canals, ductules, and ductular reactions in human livers. *Hepatology.* 2004;39:1739-1745.

17. Lefkowitch JH. Bile ductular cholestasis: an ominous histopathologic sign related to sepsis and "cholangitis lenta". *Hum Pathol.* 1982;13:19-24.

18. Lin CC, Sundaram SS, Hart J, et al. Subacute nonsuppurative cholangitis (cholangitis lenta) in pediatric liver transplant patients. *J Pediatr Gastroenterol Nutr.* 2007;45:228-233.

19. Torous VF, De La Cruz AL, Naini BV, et al. Cholangitis Lenta: a clinicopathologic study of 28 cases. *Am J Surg Pathol.* 2017;41:1607-1617.

20. Altamirano J, Miquel R, Katoonizadeh A, et al. A histologic scoring system for prognosis of patients with alcoholic hepatitis. *Gastroenterology.* 2014;146:1231-1239.e1-e6.

21. Popper H, Kent G, Stein R. Ductular cell reaction in the liver in hepatic injury. *J Mt Sinai Hosp N Y.* 1957;24:551-556.

22. Popper H. The relation of mesenchymal cell products to hepatic epithelial systems. *Prog Liver Dis.* 1990;9:27-38.

23. De Groote J, Desmet VJ, Gedigk P, et al. A classification of chronic hepatitis. *Lancet.* 1968;2:626-628.

24. Torbenson M, Washington K. Pathology of liver disease: advances in the last 50 years. *Hum Pathol.* 2020;95:78-98.

25. Duffin JM. Why does cirrhosis belong to Laennec? *Can Med Assoc J.* 1987;137:393-396.

26. Wanless IR, Nakashima E, Sherman M. Regression of human cirrhosis. Morphologic features and the genesis of incomplete septal cirrhosis. *Arch Pathol Lab Med.* 2000;124:1599-1607.

27. Hytiroglou P, Snover DC, Alves V, et al. Beyond "cirrhosis": a proposal from the International Liver Pathology Study Group. *Am J Clin Pathol.* 2012;137:5-9.

28. Moreira RK, Chopp W, Washington MK. The concept of hepatic artery-bile duct parallelism in the diagnosis of ductopenia in liver biopsy samples. *Am J Surg Pathol.* 2011;35:392-403.

29. Gill RM, Belt P, Wilson L, et al. Centrizonal arteries and microvessels in nonalcoholic steatohepatitis. *Am J Surg Pathol.* 2011;35:1400-1404.

30. Hennes EM, Zeniya M, Czaja AJ, et al. Simplified criteria for the diagnosis of autoimmune hepatitis. *Hepatology.* 2008;48:169-176.

31. Gurung A, Assis DN, McCarty TR, et al. Histologic features of autoimmune hepatitis: a critical appraisal. *Hum Pathol.* 2018;82:51-60.

32. Neil DA, Hubscher SG. Histologic and biochemical changes during the evolution of chronic rejection of liver allografts. *Hepatology.* 2002;35:639-651.

33. Jain D, Robert ME, Navarro V, et al. Total fibrous obliteration of main portal vein and portal foam cell venopathy in chronic hepatic allograft rejection. *Arch Pathol Lab Med.* 2004;128:64-67.

34. Abraham S, Furth EE. Receiver operating characteristic analysis of glycogenated nuclei in liver biopsy specimens: quantitative evaluation of their relationship with diabetes and obesity. *Hum Pathol.* 1994;25:1063-1068.

35. Schinoni MI, Andrade Z, de Freitas LA, et al. Incomplete septal cirrhosis: an enigmatic disease. *Liver Int.* 2004;24:452-456.

36. Jung T, Bader N, Grune T. Lipofuscin: formation, distribution, and metabolic consequences. *Ann N Y Acad Sci.* 2007;1119:97-111.

37. Schmucker DL. Age-related changes in liver structure and function: Implications for disease ? *Exp Gerontol.* 2005;40:650-659.

38. Tauchi H, Hananouchi M, Sato T. Accumulation of lipofuscin pigment in human hepatic cells from different races and in different environmental conditions. *Mech Ageing Dev.* 1980;12:183-195.

39. Lamers WH, Hilberts A, Furt E, et al. Hepatic enzymic zonation: a reevaluation of the concept of the liver acinus. *Hepatology.* 1989;10:72-76.

40. Zatloukal K, French SW, Stumptner C, et al. From Mallory to Mallory-Denk bodies: what, how and why? *Exp Cell Res.* 2007;313:2033-2049.

41. Schirmacher P, Dienes HP, Moll R. De novo expression of nonhepatocellular cytokeratins in Mallory body formation. *Virchows Arch.* 1998;432:143-152.

42. Stumptner C, Fuchsbichler A, Zatloukal K, et al. In vitro production of Mallory bodies and intracellular hyaline bodies: the central role of sequestosome 1/p62. *Hepatology.* 2007;46:851-860.

43. Lowe J, Blanchard A, Morrell K, et al. Ubiquitin is a common factor in intermediate filament inclusion bodies of diverse type in man, including those of Parkinson's disease, Pick's disease, and Alzheimer's disease, as well as Rosenthal fibres in cerebellar astrocytomas, cytoplasmic bodies in muscle, and mallory bodies in alcoholic liver disease. *J Pathol.* 1988;155:9-15.

44. Fauerholdt L, Schlichting P, Christensen E, et al. Conversion of micronodular cirrhosis into macronodular cirrhosis. *Hepatology.* 1983;3:928-931.

45. Fraser JL, Antonioli DA, Chopra S, et al. Prevalence and nonspecificity of microvesicular fatty change in the liver. *Mod Pathol.* 1995;8:65-70.

46. Kuo FY, Swanson PE, Yeh MM. Pancreatic acinar tissue in liver explants: a morphologic and immunohistochemical study. *Am J Surg Pathol.* 2009;33:66-71.

47. Terada T, Nakanuma Y, Kakita A. Pathologic observations of intrahepatic peribiliary glands in 1000 consecutive autopsy livers. Heterotopic pancreas in the liver. *Gastroenterology.* 1990;98:1333-1337.

48. An T, Ghatak N, Kastner R, et al. Hyaline globules and intracellular lumina in a hepatocellular carcinoma. *Am J Clin Pathol.* 1983;79:392-396.

49. Sato S, Masuda T, Oikawa H, et al. Bile canaliculi-like lumina in fibrolamellar carcinoma of the liver: a light- and electron-microscopic study and three-dimensional examination of serial sections. *Pathol Int.* 1997;47:763-768.

50. Ludwig J. Small-duct primary sclerosing cholangitis. *Semin Liver Dis.* 1991;11:11-17.

51. Batts KP, Ludwig J. Chronic hepatitis. An update on terminology and reporting. *Am J Surg Pathol.* 1995;19:1409-1417.

52. Hytiroglou P, Theise ND. Regression of human cirrhosis: an update, 18 years after the pioneering article by Wanless et al. *Virchows Arch.* 2018;473:15-22.

53. Donato MT, Gomez-Lechon MJ. Drug-induced liver steatosis and phospholipidosis: cell-based assays for early screening of drug candidates. *Curr Drug Metab.* 2012;13:1160-1173.

54. Singhi AD, Jain D, Kakar S, et al. Reticulin loss in benign fatty liver: an important diagnostic pitfall when considering a diagnosis of hepatocellular carcinoma. *Am J Surg Pathol.* 2012;36:710-715.

55. Riedel I. Ueber den zungenfrmigen Fortsatz des rechten Leberlappens und seine pathognostische Bedeutung für die Erkrankung der Gallenblase nebst Bemerkungen über. *Berliner klinische Wochenschrift.* 1888;25:577-602.

56. Suematsu M, Aiso S. Professor Toshio Ito: a clairvoyant in pericyte biology. *Keio J Med.* 2001;50:66-71.

57. Kojiro M. *Pathology of Hepatocellular Carcinoma.* Replika Presss Pvt. Ltd.; 2006:174.

INDEX

Note: Page numbers followed by "f" indicate figures, "t" indicate tables and "b" indicate boxes.